THE LEUCOCYTE ANTIGEN
FactsBook

Second Edition

THE LEUCOCYTE ANTIGEN *FactsBook*

Second Edition

A. Neil Barclay
Marion H. Brown
S.K. Alex Law
Andrew J. McKnight
Michael G. Tomlinson
P. Anton van der Merwe

MRC Cellular Immunology Unit,
MRC Immunochemistry Unit and the
Sir William Dunn School of Pathology
University of Oxford, Oxford, UK

Academic Press
Harcourt Brace & Company, Publishers
SAN DIEGO   LONDON   BOSTON   NEW YORK
SYDNEY   TOKYO   TORONTO

This book is printed on acid-free paper

Academic Press
525B Street, Suite 1900, San Diego, California 92101-4495, USA
http://www.apnet.com

Academic Press Limited
24–28 Oval Road, London NW1 7DX, UK
http://www.hbuk.co.uk/ap/

ISBN 0-12-078185-9

A catalogue record for this book is available from the British Library

Typeset in Great Britain by Alden, Oxford, Didcot and Northampton
Printed in Great Britain by WBC, Bridgend, Mid Glamorgan

97 98 99 00 01 02 EB 9 8 7 6 5 4 3 2 1

Contents

Section I THE INTRODUCTORY CHAPTERS

Section II THE LEUCOCYTE ANTIGENS

V

Preface

Due to the very large increase in data on leucocyte antigens since the first edition was published, all the entries have been completely revised. In addition, about a further 70 new entries have been added. The introductory chapters have been revised and reorganized. The chapter in the first edition on gene locations has been deleted in the second edition as these data will rapidly become outdated as the genome project progresses.

The authors acknowledge all those that helped in the completion of the second edition of this book. In particular we thank our colleagues for their patience and advice during the period in which this book, known colloquially as the CD book, was being written. Many colleagues around the world communicated unpublished information and helped with parts of the manuscript. These included Iain Campbell, Marco Colonna, Paul Crocker, Simon Davis, Anthony Day, Mark Gorrell, Peter Gough, Vicky Heath, David Jackson, William James, Lewis Lanier, Peter Linsley, Don Mason, Steve Rosen, Dave Simmons, Antony Symons and Masahide Tone. We also thank Tessa Picknett of Academic Press for her contributions.

The authors acknowledge their funding by the UK Medical Research Council in the MRC Cellular Immunology Unit (ANB, MHB, MGT, and PAV), the MRC Immunochemistry Unit (AL) and the Sir William Dunn School of Pathology (AJM).

The authors hope that there are a minimum of omissions and inaccuracies and that these can be recitified in later editions. We would appreciate if such points were forwarded to the Editor, Leucocyte Antigen FactsBook, Academic Press, 24–28 Oval Road, London NW1 7DX, UK.

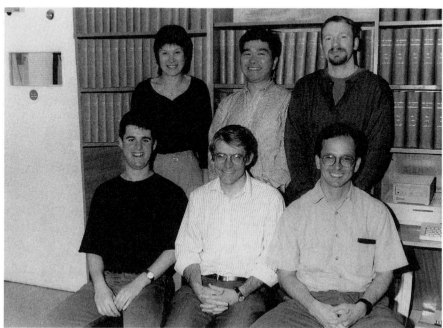

From top left: *Marion Brown, Alex Law, Andrew McKnight;*
bottom left: *Michael Tomlinson, Neil Barclay and Anton van der Merwe.*

Abbreviations

CCP	Complement control protein
CS	Chondroitin sulfate
CSF	Colony-stimulating factor
CTL	Cytotoxic T cell
EGF	Epidermal growth factor
fMET	Formyl MetLeuPhe
Fn	Fibronectin
GAG	Glycosaminoglycan
GAP	p21 *ras* GTPase-activating protein
GCSF	Granulocyte colony-stimulating factor
GMCSF	Granulocyte-macrophage colony-stimulating factor
GPI	Glycosyl-phosphatidylinositol
IFNγ	Interferon γ
Ig	Immunoglobulin
IgSF	Immunoglobulin superfamily
IL-1 etc.	Interleukin 1 etc.
kDa	Kilodalton
LRR	Leucine-rich repeat
LDLR	Low-density lipoprotein receptor
mAb	Monoclonal antibody
MHC	Major histocompatibility complex
M-CSF	Macrophage colony-stimulating factor
mIg	Membrane immunoglobulin
MLR	Mixed lymphocyte reaction
NGFR	Nerve growth factor receptor
N-linked glycosylation	Asparagine-linked glycosylation
NMR	Nuclear magnetic resonance
NK	Natural killer
O-linked glycosylation	Hydroxyl-linked glycosylation
PI 3-kinase	Phosphatidylinositol 3′-kinase
PLC-γ1	Phospholipase C-γ1
PBL	Peripheral blood lymphocytes
PCR	Polymerase chain reaction
PMA	Phorbol 12-myristate 13-acetate
R	Receptor
RTPCR	Reverse transcriptase polymerase chain reaction
SRCR	Scavenger receptor cysteine-rich
SD	Standard deviation
SDS-PAGE	Polyacrylamide gel electrophoresis in sodium dodecyl sulfate
SF	Superfamily
TM4	Membrane protein with four transmembrane regions
TCR	T cell receptor for antigen
TNF	Tumour necrosis factor
WWW	World Wide Web

DEDICATION

This book is dedicated to the memory of

Alan F. Williams

THE INTRODUCTORY CHAPTERS

1 Introduction

AIMS OF THE BOOK

The primary aim of this book is to provide a compendium of the molecules that are found at leucocyte surfaces. The book includes entries for 206 antigens. Prior to the entries there are three chapters that provide a perspective for thinking about cell surface molecules. These chapters deal with the architecture of cell surfaces and with the domain types which can be found in leucocyte surface proteins.

A systematic approach to the naming of leucocyte antigens was made with the "cluster of differentiation" designation (CD) for human leucocyte antigens identified with monoclonal antibodies (mAbs)[1]. MAbs were submitted to workshops and were placed into groups based on fluorescent labelling patterns for different leucocyte populations. In this classification, antigens are given a CD number and we provide in this book, entries on the CD antigens defined in the 5th International Workshop in 1993. We also include entries on antigens from any species which are known to be expressed on the surface of leucocytes, that have been characterized at the level of their primary sequence, including those that were given a CD number at the 6th International Workshop in 1996 and also those that have not been given a CD number. Molecules that have been sequenced but for which there are no additional data are not included.

The CD numbering was extended to endothelial antigens in the 6th International Workshop in 1996 but these are not included. The cytokine receptors often have more than one polypeptide chain and the cytokine receptor designation is given first together with the CD numbers. Thus CD25 appears under IL-2R rather than between CD24 and CD26. The cytokine receptor for a particular CD number can be found from the index. Table 1 lists all the entries in the book and Table 2 contains a brief summary of those CD antigens for which entries are not included, that is the endothelial antigens mentioned above, those CD numbers between CD1 and CD166 which have not yet been allocated and CDs in the range CD131–CD166 which had not been included on the above criteria at the time of completion of the book.

ORGANIZATION OF THE DATA

Name

The CD nomenclature is used for both the human antigens and their homologues in rat and mouse. This nomenclature is now being used for other species homologues as illustrated in the recent swine workshop on leucocyte markers[2]. In some cases the antigens are known by several other names and the most common of these are also given. The term homologue is reserved for equivalent molecules between species and is not used to indicate related molecules in a superfamily. In cases where the CD nomenclature is not widely used (e.g. cytokine receptors and integrins) the commonly used names are used in the introductory chapters.

Molecular diagram

This gives a visual representation of the molecule and includes details such as the mode of membrane attachment, the protein domains that are present, and the degree of glycosylation. Figure 1 shows the symbols that are used to represent the

Table 1 *Distribution of domains in leucocyte surface molecules. The names of the antigens are those given in the entries in Section II and the abbreviations of the domain types are those defined in Fig. 1. The data are for single polypeptides although some will form homo- or heterodimers. Some of the cytokine receptors have polypeptide chains in common and these are indicated in each case.*

Antigen name	CCP	Cytokine R	EGF	Fn2	Fn3	Galectin	IgSF	Integrin	Lectin C-type	Link	LRR	LDLR	Ly-6	MHC	TNFSF	TNFRSF	ScavengerCR	Somatomedin	Number	GPI	Type	Tyr kinase	PTPase	Page number
CD1							1							2					1		I			132
CD2							2												1		I			134
CD3 δ, γ, ε							1												1		I			137
ζ or η																			1		I			137
TCRα, β, γ, δ							2												1		I			137
pre-TCRα							1												1		I			137
CD4							4												1		I			141
CD5																	3		1		I			143
CD6																	3		1		I			145
CD7							1												1		I			147
CD8α							1												1		I			149
β							1												1		I			149
CD9																			4		III			152
CD10																			1		II			154
CD11a								α											1		I			156
CD11b								α											1		I			158
CD11c								α											1		I			161
Integrin αD								α											1		I			161
CDw12 (NS)																								165
CD13																			1		II			166
CD14																				1				169
CD15 (CHO)																								171
CD15s (CHO)																								172
CD16							2												1 or 1		I			173
CDw17 (CHO)																								176
CD18								β											1		I			177
CD19							2												1		I			179
CD20																			4		III			181
CD21	15 or 16																		1		I			183
CD22							5 or 7												1		I			186
CD23									1										1		II			189
CD24																				1				192
CD26																			1		II			194
CD27																2			1		I			197
CD28							1												1		I			199
CD29								β											1		I			201
CD30																5			1		I			204
CD31							6												1		I			206
CD32							2												1		I			209
CD33							2												1		I			213

Antigen name	CCP	Cytokine R	EGF	Fn2	Fn3	Galectin	IgSF	Integrin	Lectin C-type	Link	LRR	LDLR	Ly-6	MHC	TNFSF	TNFRSF	ScavengerCR	Somatomedin	Number	GPI	Type	Tyr kinase	PTPase	Page number
CD34																			1		I			215
CD35	30																		1		I			217
CD36																			2		VI			221
CD37																			4		III			224
CD38																			1		II			226
CD39																			3		III			228
CD40																4			1		I			230
CD41								α											1		I			232
CD42a											1								1		I			235
CD42bα											7								1		I			235
CD42bβ											1								1		I			235
CD43																			1		I			238
CD44										1									1		I			240
CD45																			1		I		2	244
CD46	4																		1		I			248
CD47							1												5		III			251
CD48							2													1				253
CD49a								α											1		I			255
CD49b								α											1		I			257
CD49c								α											1		I			260
CD49d								α											1		I			262
CD49e								α											1		I			265
CD49f								α											1		I			267
CD50							5												1		I			269
CD51								α											1		I			271
CD52																				1				274
CD53																			4		III			276
CD54							5												1		I			278
CD55	4																			1				281
CD56				2			5												1 or 1		I			284
CD57 (CHO)																								287
CD58							2												1 or 1		I			288
CD59													1							1				290
CD60 (CHO)																								292
CD61								β											1		I			293
CD62ᴇ	6	1							1										1		I			295
CD62ʟ	2	1							1										1		I			298
CD62ᴘ	9	1							1										1		I			301
CD63																			4		III			304
CD64							3												1		I			306
CD65 (CHO)																								309
CD66a							4												1		I			310
CD66b							3													1				310
CD66c							3													1				310
CD66d							1												1		I			310
CD68																			1		I			314

Antigen name	Extracellular regions																		TM regions			Cytoplasm		Page number
	CCP	Cytokine R	EGF	Fn2	Fn3	Galectin	IgSF	Integrin	Lectin C-type	Link	LRR	LDLR	Ly-6	MHC	TNFSF	TNFRSF	ScavengerCR	Somatomedin	Number	GPI	Type	Tyr kinase	PTPase	
CD69									1										1		II			316
CD70															1				1		II			318
CD71																			1		II			320
CD72									1										1		II			323
CD73																				1				325
CD74																			1		II			327
CDw75 (CHO)																								329
CDw76 (CHO)																								330
CD77(CHO)																								331
CD79α and β							1												1		I			332
BCR e.g. IgM (H chain)							5												1		I			332
CD80							2												1		I			335
CD81																			4		III			337
CD82																			4		III			339
CD83							1												1		I			341
CDw84 (NS)																								343
CD85 (NS)																								344
CD86							2												1		I			345
CD87													3							1				347
CD88																			7		III			349
CD89							2												1		I			351
CD90							1													1				353
CD91			22									31							1		I			355
CDw92 (NS)																								359
CD93 (NS)																								360
CD94									1										1		II			361
CD95																3			1		I			363
CD96							3												1		I			365
CD97			3																7		III			367
CD98																			1		II			369
CD99																			1		I			371
CD100							1												1		I			373
CD101							7												1		I			375
CD102							2												1		I			377
CD103								α											1		I			379
CD104								β											1		I			381
CD105																			1		I			384
CD106							7												1		I			386
CD107a/b																			1		I			389
CDw108 (NS)																								392
CD109 (NS)																								393
CD117							5												1		I	1		394
CD120a/b																4			1		I			397
CD134																3			1		I			400
CD135							5												1		I	1		402
CDw137																2			1		I			404

Antigen name	Extracellular regions																		TM regions			Cytoplasm		Page number
	CCP	Cytokine R	EGF	Fn2	Fn3	Galectin	IgSF	Integrin	Lectin C-type	Link	LRR	LDLR	Ly-6	MHC	TNFSF	TNFRSF	ScavengerCR	Somatomedin	Number	GPI	Type	Tyr kinase	PTPase	
CD138																			1		I			406
CD147							2												1		I			408
CD148					10														1		I		1	410
CDw150							2												1		I			412
CD151																			4		III			414
CD152							1												1		I			415
CD153															1				1		II			417
CD154															1				1		II			419
CD161									1										1		II			421
CD162																			1		I			424
CD163																	9		1		1			427
CD166							5												1		I			429
114/A10		3																	1		I			431
2B4							2												1		I			433
4-1BBL															1				1		II			435
Aminopeptidase A																			1		II			437
B-G							1												1		I			439
Chemokine Rs																			7		III			441
c-kitL																			1		I			443
CMRF35							1												1		I			445
DEC-205			1						10										1		I			447
DNAM-1							2												1		I			450
ESL-1																			1		I			452
F4/80			7																7		III			454
FasL															1				1		II			456
FcεRIα							2												1		I			458
β																			4		III			458
γ																			1		I			458
FLT3 ligand																			1		I			461
FPR (fMLPR)																			7		III			463
Galectin-3						1													0					465
G-CSFR/CD114		1			4		1												1		I			467
GM-CSFR/CD116		1			1														1		I			470
CDw131		2			2														1		I			470
GlyCAM-1																			0					473
gp42							2													1				475
gp49							2												1		I			476
HTm4																			4		III			478
IFNγR					2														1		I			479
AF-1					2														1		I			479
IL-1R/CD121a							3												1		I			482
CD121b							3												1		I			482
IL-1RAcP							3												1		I			482
IL-2R/CD25	2																		1		I			486
CD122		1			1														1		I			486
CD132		1			1														1		I			486

Antigen name	CCP	Cytokine R	EGF	Fn2	Fn3	Galectin	IgSF	Integrin	Lectin C-type	Link	LRR	LDLR	Ly-6	MHC	TNFSF	TNFRSF	ScavengerCR	Somatomedin	Number	GPI	Type	Tyr kinase	PTPase	Page number
IL-3R/CDw123		1			1														1		I			490
CDw131		2			2														1		I			490
IL-4R/CD124		1			1														1		I			493
CD132		1			1														1		I			493
IL-13R α		1			1														1		I			493
IL-5R/CDw125		1			1														1		I			496
CDw131		2			2														1		I			496
IL-6R/CD126		1			1		1												1		I			498
CD130		1			4		1												1		I			498
IL-7R/CD127		1																	1		I			501
CD132		1			1														1		I			501
IL-8Ra/CDw128																			7		III			503
IL-8RB																			7		III			503
IL-9Rα (CD129)		1			1														1		I			506
CD132		1			1														1		I			506
IL-10R					2														1		I			508
IL-11R α		1			1		1												1		I			510
CD130		1			4		1												1		I			510
IL-12R β					5														1		I			512
IL-13R α		1			1														1		I			514
CD124		1			1														1		I			514
IL-14R (NS)																								516
IL-15R α	1																		1		I			517
CD122		1			1														1		I			517
CD132		1			1														1		I			517
IL-17R																			1		I			520
Integrin β7								β											1		I			522
KIR family (e.g. CD158a and b)							2												1		I			524
(e.g. NKAT3)							3												1		I			524
L1					3		6												1		I			528
LAG-3							4												1		I			531
LDLR			3									7							1		I			533
LPAP																			1		I			536
ltk																			1		I	1		538
Ly-6													1							1				540
Ly-9							4												1		I			543
Ly-49									1										1		II			545
Mac-2 binding protein																	1		?					548
Macrophage lectin									1										1		II			550
MAdCAM-1							2												1		I			552
Mannose R				1					8										1		I			554
MARCO																	1		1		II			557
M-CSFR/CD115							5												1		I	1		559
MDR1																			12		III			562
MHC Class I α							1							2					1		I			564
β 2M							1												0					564

Antigen name	CCP	Cytokine R	EGF	Fn2	Fn3	Galectin	IgSF	Integrin	Lectin C-type	Link	LRR	LDLR	Ly-6	MHC	TNFSF	TNFRSF	ScavengerCR	Somatomedin	Number	GPI	Type	Tyr kinase	PTPase	Page number
						Extracellular regions													TM regions			Cyto-plasm		
MHC Class II α							1							1					1		I			567
β							1							1					1		I			567
MS2																			1		I			569
NKG2									1										1		II			571
OX2							2												1		I			573
OX40L															1				1		II			575
PC-1																		2	1		II			577
PD-1							1												1		I			579
RT6																				1				581
Sca-2													1							1				583
Scavenger RI																	1		1		II			585
Sialoadhesin							17												1		I			588
Thrombopoietin R		2			2														1		I			591
WC1																	11		1		I			593

TM, Transmembrane regions; Number, the number of predicted passes through the membrane; GPI, whether or not the molecule has a GPI anchor; Type, whether it is a type I, II, III or VI transmembrane protein (see Chapter 4); Cytoplasm, number and type of domains in the cytoplasm; Integrin, α or β chain. In the antigen section the terms NS indicate that the sequence has not been determined and CHO that the determinant is dependent on carbohydrate.

various domains and their N- and O-linked oligosaccharide structures. A summary of the domains present in the leucocyte molecules is given in Table 1 which also includes the page numbers of the individual entries.

For molecules attached to the cell surface by glycosyl-phosphatidylinositol (GPI) anchors, the anchors are shown in the diagrams by an arrow. The orientation of molecules with protein transmembrane sequences is evident from the labelling of the N- and/or the C-termini. This scheme for the diagrams is chosen in preference to that being standardized by SWISSPROT in order to illustrate features such as glycosylation which may be important in leucocyte function. The SWISSPROT system is aimed more at describing the modular content of proteins [3,4].

The criteria used for assigning sequences to domain types or superfamilies are discussed in Chapter 3. In those cases where no assignment can be made, the extracellular region or domain is shown as a circle containing a question mark with the diameter of the circle being proportional to the size of the extracellular region or domain. If the protein sequence contains a high proportion of Ser, Thr and Pro residues and is probably heavily O-glycosylated (see below), it is shown as an extended structure to distinguish it from regions likely to have a folded conformation. It is not possible to show the positions of all the disulfide bonds in the diagrams and these bonds are shown only for the inter-sheet disulfides of Ig superfamily (IgSF) domains since this has been traditionally done in illustrating this domain type. The majority of the cytoplasmic domains do not have recognizable domains and are represented by squiggly lines whose length is proportional to the sequence length.

The number and approximate positions of potential N-linked glycosylation sites are deduced from the presence of the sequences Asn-Xaa-Thr or Asn-Xaa-Ser where Xaa is

Table 2 *CD antigens for which there are no individual entries in this book*

	Name	Distribution	M_r (kDa)
CD67	Reassigned to CD66b		
CDw78	MHC Class II		
CD110	Not assigned		
CD111	Not assigned		
CD112	Not assigned		
CD113	Not assigned		
CD118	Interferon α/β receptor	Broad	
CD133	Not assigned		
CDw136	Macrophage-stimulating protein receptor		180
CD139	Germinal centre B cells		209, 228
CD140a,b	PDGF receptor	Broad	180
CD141	Trombomodulin		100
CD142	Tissue factor	Activated monocytes and endothelium	45
CD143	Angiotensin-converting enzyme	Endothelial subsets	170
CD144	VE-cadherin		135
CDw145		Endothelium, stromal	25, 90, 110
CD146	MUC-18	Endothelium, activated T cells	115
CDw149		Broad	
CD155	Poliovirus receptor	Monocytes, macrophages, thymocytes	80–90
CD156	ADAM-8	Monocytes, macrophages, granulocytes	80
CD157	BST-1	Monocytes, neutrophils, endothelium	42–45
CD159	Not assigned		
CD160	Not assigned		
CD164	MGC-24	Haematopoietic cells	80
CD165	AD2/gp37	Thymocytes, thymic epithelial cells	37

Note: CDw78 has been found to be an MHC Class II antigen (Slack, J.L. et al. (1995) Int. Immunol. 7, 1087–1092).

any amino acid except for Pro. The nature of the Xaa may affect the degree of glycosylation. Thus Pro prevents glycosylation and *in vitro* studies indicate that Trp, Asp, Glu and Leu give relatively inefficient glycosylation[5]. Asn-Xaa-Ser-Pro and Asn-Xaa-Thr-Pro are variably glycosylated and in the entries they are assumed to be glycosylated unless there are contrary biochemical data[6-8]. O-linked glycosylation occurs at Ser or Thr amino acids but there is no sequence motif that invariably indicates this type of glycosylation. However O-linked glycosylation is usually found in stretches of sequence with a preponderance of Ser, Thr and Pro[9,10]. In many cases there are biochemical data to support the assignment of O-glycosylation to the Ser, Thr, Pro rich regions.

Glycosaminoglycans (GAG) have been identified in three leucocyte membrane glycoproteins CD44, CD138 (syndecan) and F4/80. The number of these sites has not been confirmed biochemically and the symbols indicate only their approximate number and positions. Where the GAG has been characterized, for example, the chondroitin sulfate in CD44, this is shown in the diagram.

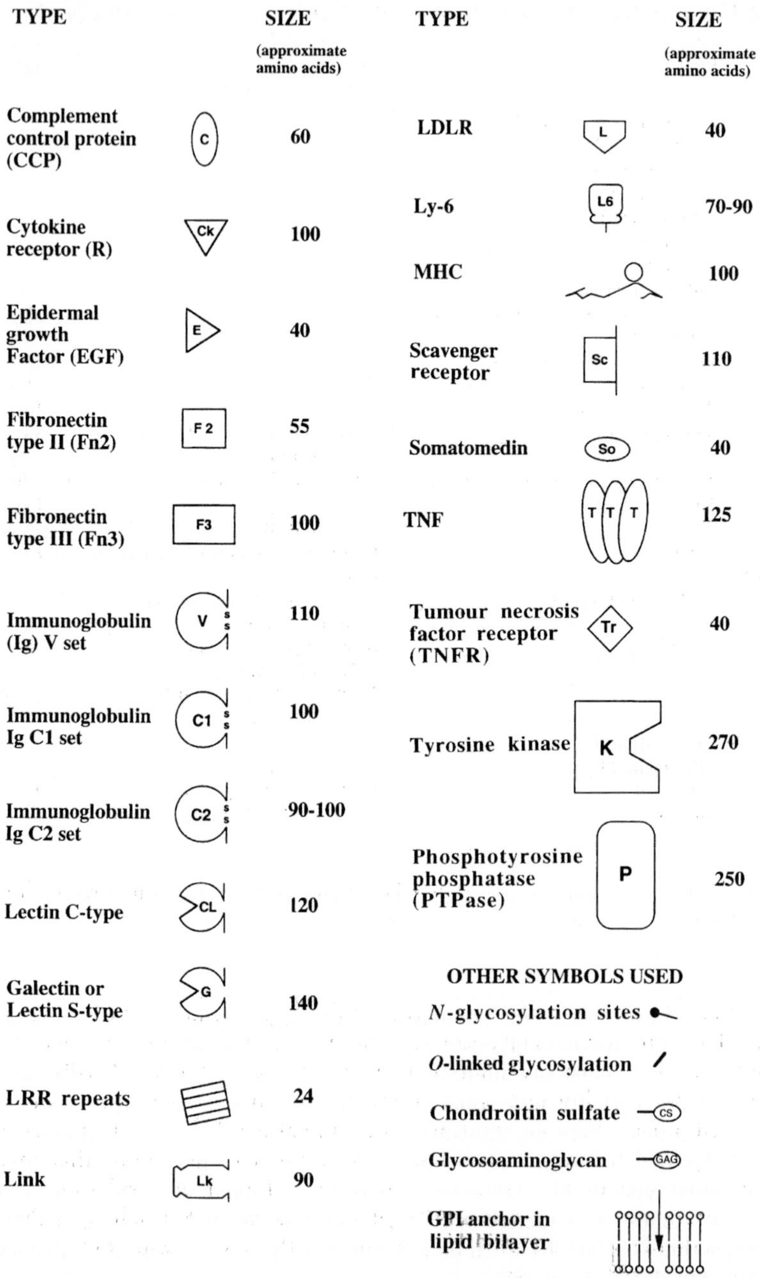

TYPE		SIZE (approximate amino acids)	TYPE		SIZE (approximate amino acids)
Complement control protein (CCP)	C	60	LDLR	L	40
Cytokine receptor (R)	Ck	100	Ly-6	L6	70-90
			MHC		100
Epidermal growth Factor (EGF)	E	40	Scavenger receptor	Sc	110
Fibronectin type II (Fn2)	F 2	55	Somatomedin	So	40
Fibronectin type III (Fn3)	F3	100	TNF	T T T	125
Immunoglobulin (Ig) V set	V	110	Tumour necrosis factor receptor (TNFR)	Tr	40
Immunoglobulin Ig C1 set	C1	100	Tyrosine kinase	K	270
Immunoglobulin Ig C2 set	C2	90-100			
Lectin C-type	CL	120	Phosphotyrosine phosphatase (PTPase)	P	250
Galectin or Lectin S-type	G	140			

OTHER SYMBOLS USED

N-glycosylation sites

O-linked glycosylation

Chondroitin sulfate — CS

LRR repeats		24
Link	Lk	90

Glycosoaminoglycan — GAG

GPI anchor in lipid bilayer

Figure 1 *Icons used for the protein domains and repeats which are present in leucocyte membrane proteins. These icons are used to depict all the molecules described in Section II. Additional abbreviations used in the domain diagrams are: S, signal sequence; TM, transmembrane sequence; CY, cytoplasmic sequence; G, GPI anchor signal sequence.*

Size of the processed form of the molecule

The calculated relative molecular weight (M_r) of the mature fully processed polypeptide backbone is given together with the M_r values obtained from polyacrylamide gel electrophoresis in sodium dodecyl sulfate (SDS-PAGE) under reducing and/or unreducing conditions. There can be considerable variation according to the conditions used for the SDS-PAGE and the values are typical of those in the literature.

The degree of glycosylation

The number of potential N-linked glycosylation sites in the extracellular portions of membrane glycoproteins is shown as determined by the presence of the consensus sequence Asn-Xaa-Thr/Ser (see above). To obtain a rough idea of the weight of the glycoprotein likely to be accounted for by N-linked oligosaccharides an average value of 3000 M_r can be used per N-linked structure. It should however be noted that some oligosaccharides can be considerably larger, due, for example, to the presence of repeating lactosamine units or complex blood group antigens and not all potential N-linked sites are necessarily occupied.

The number of O-linked sites cannot be directly predicted from the sequence and thus the following terms are used to describe the extent of O-glycosylation:

1 Unknown: There are no data from sequence or immunochemical studies to indicate the level of O-glycosylation.
2 Nil: No O-linked oligosaccharides indicated by biochemical analysis or the M_r determined by SDS-PAGE analysis is fully accounted for by the polypeptide M_r and any N-linked oligosaccharides.
3 Probable +:   Sequence data suggest the likelihood of O-glycosylation.
4 + abundant: There are biochemical data to indicate a high level of O-glycosylation.

Gene location and size

The chromosome location of the human gene from the Genome Data Base [11,12] is given together with the approximate size of the region encompassing the exons.

Domain and exon organization

A diagrammatic representation of the positions of domains and exons is given for those proteins containing clear domains. These diagrams are not drawn to scale. Domain positions are defined by indicating the positions of two key conserved residues within the domain. The first residue is shown with two flanking residues on the C-terminal side and the second with two flanking residues on the N-terminal side. The sequences which are shown in the upper part of the domain diagram can be used to identify the domain within the full sequence given at the end of the entry. The key conserved residues for each domain type are marked with asterisks in the superfamily sequence alignments given in Chapter 3. Internal positions are identified rather than domain boundaries since in some cases the end of one domain overlaps with the beginning of another (e.g. between CD4 domains 1 and 2 [13]). The identification of conserved internal residues allows a domain to be analysed by comparison with the alignment of other superfamily members shown in Chapter 3. Also the ends of the domains seldom have conserved residues.

Exon junctions are identified by three or four residues of protein sequence in the lower part of the diagram. The amino acid(s) encoded at the splice junction is aligned with the intron/exon boundary marker. The type of intron/exon boundary is indicated as type 1 (splicing after the first nucleotide of the triplet), type 2 (splicing after the second nucleotide) and type 0 (splicing between the codons) [14]. Thus if the junction was type 1 and a Trp residue was shown at the boundary of an exon/intron splice site, the point of junction would be after the T of the TGG codon. By comparing the intron/exon boundaries and the domain designations it can be seen whether a given domain is encoded within one exon. Where exons are known to be alternatively spliced a space is inserted between the rectangles that represent the exons; otherwise exons are drawn contiguously.

Tissue distribution

A brief description is given of the cells and tissues that have been clearly shown to express the antigen. In many cases a full analysis of the tissue distribution has not been done. A failure to mention a cell type cannot be taken as meaning that it is known that the cell type does not express the antigen. The distribution of the CD antigens in humans is reviewed in reports from the Leucocyte Typing Workshops [15] and a computerized database of tissue distributions based on the 5th Workshop, called LDAD is available for downloading by anonymous FTP from the NIH site, e.g. using the URL ftp://anonymous@balrog.nci.nih.gov/. The Leucocyte Typing Workshop reference is used for each of the entries on the CD antigens but is not explicitly cited. There are often considerable differences in the tissue distribution between species and this is indicated where data are available. A pullout diagram of the distribution of the human CD antigens on leucocyte populations is enclosed inside the back cover.

Structure

Biochemical and structural data are summarized in this section.

Ligands and associated molecules

Many of the cell surface proteins interact through their extracellular domains with soluble proteins (e.g. cytokines) or other cell surface proteins (adhesion molecules). Those that have been identified are listed together with proteins that interact through the membrane or cytosolic regions of the antigens.

Function

Functional data are summarized in this section.

Database entries

Accession numbers are given for the amino acid sequences in the PIR (Protein Identification Resource) and SWISSPROT databases and the nucleic acid sequences in the GENBANK and EMBL databases. Every new sequence submitted to the databases is given an accession number. These are then incorporated into entries which are given a specific identifier. One problem is that identifiers can change if, for instance, two entries are merged or when sequences become fully annotated. Therefore the only definitive way to identify a sequence is through the accession numbers and these are given in the entries. Where there are multiple accession numbers for a sequence the primary number is given. In some cases genomic but not cDNA sequence is available and is spread over several database entries. In these cases more than one accession number is given. Apart from some early entries EMBL and GENBANK use the same accession number for each entry. If available, the accession numbers are given for human, rat and mouse homologues but not generally for other species.

Retrieval of sequences from databases
Most sequence analysis software will identify and retrieve sequences from local computers using the accession number. Sequences can also be obtained directly through the Internet from computer servers at the database centres, again using the accession number. These procedures are changing rapidly as more servers become available. The simplest and most powerful methods use the World Wide Web (WWW) browsers such as Netscape™. A selection of currently available WWW sites of relevance to protein and DNA sequences and protein structures is given below. It should be stressed that new resources are becoming available all the time. New WWW sites can often be identified by checking the links available from well-established sites [16-18] (see below). A guide to the Internet has been published on the WWW by Elsevier Trends Journals [19] and there are regular articles in the "Computing Corner" of *TIBS*, in *Current Biology* and various books (e.g. ref. 20). Several of the major databases are available from more than one site, i.e. "mirrored" copies exist. It is usually quicker to use a local site. For instance EMBL is available from many sites with one official EMBnet node in each European country [21] and the SWISSPROT database is based in Geneva [22] but a mirror version exists in Cambridge, UK [16]. The Protein Database (PDB) is based in the US but there are mirror sites in China, Israel and the UK (see ref. 23).

In addition to retrieving data directly from the databases many sites offer services for searching databases using programmes such as BLAST or BLITZ, together with other modelling and alignment programmes.

WWW sites for DNA and protein databases
Entrez (http://www3.ncbi.nlm.nih.gov/Entrez/)
An interlinked database of DNA sequences, protein sequences, protein structures and a subsection of MEDLINE containing references including abstracts, for those references with sequence-related information.

European Bioinformatics Institute (EBI) (http://www.ebi.ac.uk/)
A wide range of databases including the Protein Data Bank (PDB), SWISSPROT, EMBL and many more specialized databases.

GenBank (http://www.ncbi.nlm.nih.gov)
The complete nucleotide database along with many other databases and searching tools such as BLAST (see below for Email).

Genome Database (GDB) (http://gdbwww.gdb.org/)
The central repository for genomic mapping data resulting from the Human Genome Initiative.

OMIM©, On-line Mendelian Inheritance in Man (http://www3.ncbi.nlm.nih.gov/Omim/)
This database is a catalogue of human genes and genetic disorders with many links to the Entrez database (see above).

Protein Data Bank (PDB) (http://pdb.pdb.bnl.gov/)
An archive of experimentally determined three-dimensional structures of biological macromolecules compiled at the Brookhaven National Laboratory.

SwissProt (http://expasy.hcuge.ch/)
This contains all the SWISSPROT entries. The database has links to entries in the protein structure database (PDB) and references in ENTREZ (see above).

Email servers for biological databases
A comprehensive list of useful servers is given by SWISSPROT on WWW
http://expasy.hcuge.ch/info/serv_ema.txt
A good starting point is to send Email containing the single word HELP to the Email address (e.g. see below).

A. Obtaining DNA and protein sequences from the EMBL and SWISSPROT databases
The Email address is: NetServ@ebi.ac.uk
The commands used are: GET to specify the request and NUC or PROT to specify the EMBL or SWISSPROT databases, respectively.
A typical file might look like:

GET PROT:P01830
GET NUC:X03152

This file would request the sending of two entries, one from SWISSPROT (protein) and one from EMBL (DNA).

B. Obtaining protein sequences from the PIR databases
The Email address is: fileserv@nbrf.georgetown.edu
The file should contain the command GET followed by the accession number.
A typical file would look like:

GET A02107

C. Obtaining DNA sequence from the GENBANK database
The Email address is: retrieve@ncbi.nlm.nih.gov
List the DATABASE required, the command <Begin> and then the identifiers or accession numbers in a single column.
A typical file would look like:

DATALIB GenBank
Begin
J02852
J02855

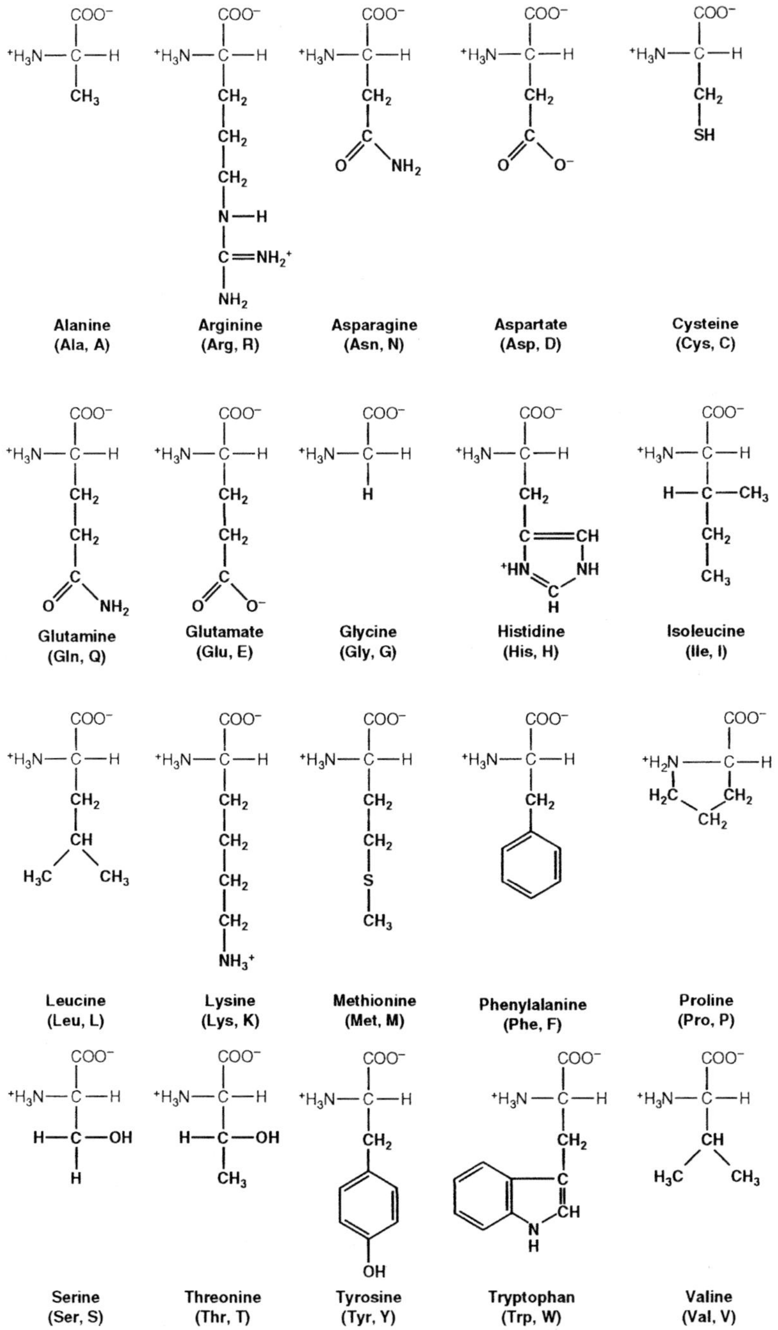

Alanine
(Ala, A)

Arginine
(Arg, R)

Asparagine
(Asn, N)

Aspartate
(Asp, D)

Cysteine
(Cys, C)

Glutamine
(Gln, Q)

Glutamate
(Glu, E)

Glycine
(Gly, G)

Histidine
(His, H)

Isoleucine
(Ile, I)

Leucine
(Leu, L)

Lysine
(Lys, K)

Methionine
(Met, M)

Phenylalanine
(Phe, F)

Proline
(Pro, P)

Serine
(Ser, S)

Threonine
(Thr, T)

Tyrosine
(Tyr, Y)

Tryptophan
(Trp, W)

Valine
(Val, V)

Figure 2 *Chemical formulae for the amino acids found in proteins. The single letter amino acid code is used in the entries and the three letter code when discussing particular amino acids in the text. The side-chains are shown in bold.*

D. Database searching
Several sites allow database searching by BLAST, BLITZ and FASTA. For example for details send "help" message to
blast@ncbi.nlm.nih.gov
blitz@ebi.ac.uk
fasta@ebi.ac.uk

Sequence

The human amino acid sequence is given if it is known. If a sequence has only been obtained in a different species, then this is given. The single letter code for amino acids is used and this is defined in Fig. 2 together with their chemical formulae. In most cases where structural and functional data are discussed it is with respect to sequence numbering of the fully processed form of the molecule. If the N-terminus has not been defined by sequence analysis the signal sequence for secretion is predicted from comparisons with sequences where the position of signal cleavage has been determined. The consensus rules for defining cleavage sites are reviewed in ref. 24. The signal sequence is shown on a separate line. For molecules likely to have transmembrane sequences the proposed hydrophobic regions are underlined. For GPI anchors, signal sequences are predicted using criteria discussed in Chapter 4 and the GPI signal sequence is shown on a separate line below the proposed processed sequence. Thus the amino acid length of the predicted mature protein is given (and used in the M_r value given at the beginning of the entry) as well as the length of the GPI signal sequence if present. Variants produced by alternative splicing are shown only where they are known to be expressed.

References

It is not feasible to give a comprehensive list of references. The references that are given are recent ones that should allow access to the rest of the literature and key references are highlighted in bold. In some cases these are recent reviews but in others it is the most recent paper containing relevant references.

References
[1] Bernard, A. et al. (1984) Leukocyte Typing. Springer-Verlag, Berlin, pp. 1–814.
[2] Saalmuller, A. (1996) Characterization of swine leucocyte differentiation antigens. Immunol. Today 17, 352–354.
[3] Bork, P. and Bairoch, A. (1995) Extracellular protein modules: A proposed nomenclature. Trends Biochem. Sci. 20, Suppl. March, CO3
[4] http://swan.embl-heidelberg.de:8080/Modules/. Modules in extracellular proteins.
[5] Shakin-Eshleman, S. et al. (1996) The amino acid at the X position of an Asn-X-Ser sequon is an important determinant of N-linked core-glycosylation efficiency. J. Biol. Chem. 271, 6363–6366.
[6] Bause, E. and Hettkamp, H. (1979) Primary structure requirements for N-glycosylation of peptides in rat liver. FEBS Lett. 108, 341–344.
[7] Kornfeld, R. and Kornfeld, S. (1985) Assembly of asparagine-linked oligosaccharides. Annu. Rev. Biochem. 54, 631–664.

[8] Gavel, Y. and von Heijne, G. (1990) Sequence differences between glycosylated and non-glycosylated Asn-X-Thr/Ser acceptor sites: implications for protein engineering. Protein Eng. 3, 433–442.

[9] Wilson, I.B.H. et al. (1991) Amino acid distributions around O-linked glycosylation sites. Biochem. J. 275, 529–534.

[10] Gooley, A.A. et al. (1991) Glycosylation sites identified by detection of glycosylated amino acids released from Edman degradation: the identification of Xaa-Pro-Xaa-Xaa as a motif for Thr-O-glycosylation. Biochem. Biophys. Res. Commun. 178, 1194–1201.

[11] http://gdbwww.gdb.org/gdb/gdbtop.html. The Genome Database.

[12] http://www.hgmp.mrc.ac.uk/gdb/gdbtop.html. The Genome Database.

[13] Ryu, S.E. et al. (1990) Crystal structure of an HIV-binding recombinant fragment of human CD4. Nature 348, 419–426.

[14] Sharp, P.A. (1981) Speculations on RNA splicing. Cell 23, 643–646.

[15] Schlossman, S. et al. (1995) Leucocyte Typing V. Oxford University Press, Oxford, UK, pp. 1–2044.

[16] http://www.ebi.ac.uk/. European Bioinformatics Institute (EBI).

[17] http://www.fmi.ch/biology/research_tools.html. Pedro's BioMolecular Research Tools.

[18] http://www.ncbi.nlm.nih.gov/. National Center for Biotechnology Information (NCBI).

[19] http://www.elsevier.com/locate/trendsguide. The Trends Guide to the Internet.

[20] Swindell, S. et al. (1996) Internet for the Molecular Biologist. Horizon Scientific Press, Wymondham.

[21] Harper, R. (1996) EMBnet: an institute without walls. Trends Biochem. Sci. 21, 150–152.

[22] http://expasy.hcuge.ch/. SWISSPROT.

[23] http://pdb.pdb.bnl.gov/mirror_sites.html. Protein database.

[24] von Heijne, G. (1983) Patterns of amino acids near signal-sequence cleavage sites. Eur. J. Biochem. 133, 17–21.

2 The discovery and biochemical analysis of leucocyte surface antigens

EARLY STUDIES ON CELL MEMBRANES

In the 1960s and early 1970s there were few useful techniques for the analysis of the cell surface molecules of eukaryotic cells and important early data were obtained from studies on cells that had relatively simple plasma membranes such as human erythrocytes. Studies with the electron microscope established the concept of a lipid bilayer encompassing eukaryotic cells and it was demonstrated by radiolabelling inner and outer membranes of erythrocytes, that the membrane proteins glycophorin and Band 3 spanned this bilayer[1]. This was later confirmed by the sequencing of glycophorin which established the presence of a stretch of hydrophobic amino acids sufficient to traverse the bilayer[2]. The concept of a fluid membrane with proteins surrounded by lipids and free to move in the bilayer was proposed[3], along with the concept that signal transduction would occur by an event outside the cell somehow being transmitted to the interior via a surface molecule with a transmembrane sequence and a cytoplasmic domain. These ideas were given credence by the observation that molecules could mix between membranes when cells were fused together[4], and by the finding that reactions with antibodies could lead to a cell surface molecule capping at one pole of a cell with cytoskeletal proteins accumulating underneath the cap[5]. The interpretation of the capping phenomenon has not become simple with further study, for example capping can occur via glycolipids or GPI-anchored molecules that do not traverse the bilayer. Despite these complications the phenomenon was of considerable conceptual influence in the early 1970s.

The early studies on the erythrocyte and other model systems did not give a general method for analysing complex cell membranes. However considerable progress was possible with the introduction of techniques for solubilizing membrane molecules using detergents[6] and affinity chromatography[7] (reviewed in ref. 8). It was established that ionic detergents like sodium dodecyl sulfate (SDS) would bind to both hydrophilic and hydrophobic parts of protein sequences and this led to the technique of SDS polyacrylamide gel electrophoresis, which allowed resolution of proteins roughly in proportion to their molecular weight[9]. SDS was of minimal use in the purification of membrane molecules since it often destroyed biological activities and led to the loss of antigenic determinants. Weakly ionic detergents like deoxycholate were more useful since they bound predominantly to the hydrophobic parts of cell surface molecules. They did interfere with some ionic interactions, notably the binding of histones to DNA and thus deoxycholate could not be used on whole cells but instead membranes had to be prepared prior to extraction. The advantages of deoxycholate were that it gave very good solubilization of molecules and that it had a small micelle size such that its binding did not interfere with the behaviour of solubilized molecules in fractionation techniques such as gel filtration. Also it could be removed from proteins by dialysis against deoxycholate-free buffer. Non-ionic detergents bound only to hydrophobic domains forming a micelle of lipid-like molecules around the hydrophobic region. These detergents have the disadvantage that they interfere with molecular properties due to their large micelle size and are difficult to remove from proteins. In addition they sometimes yield membrane molecules in complexes, rather than as a single molecule plus detergent.

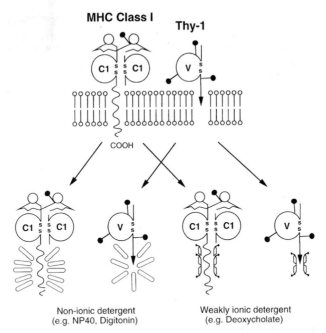

Figure 1 *Detergent binding to cell membrane proteins. The binding of detergent to the solubilized monomeric forms of two cell surface antigens, one GPI-anchored and one with a conventional transmembrane is illustrated. The non-ionic detergents can form large micelles and complexes with more than one protein. The size of deoxycholate micelles is generally much smaller but depends on the pH and salt concentrations. The symbols for each molecule of non-ionic detergent are (⌒) and for the weakly ionic detergent, deoxycholate (⌂).*

For purification studies this was a disadvantage [10], but what was formerly a problem is now exploited as a way of studying multimolecular complexes in the membrane that may be of biological relevance. The differences between deoxycholate and non-ionic detergents in solubilizing cell surface molecules are illustrated in Fig. 1.

The technique of affinity chromatography was developed in the late 1960s with the highly effective cyanogen bromide coupling method being first reported in 1967 [7]. However, whilst antibodies against known antigens could be purified, the converse of purifying a cell surface antigen with antibody affinity chromatography was not considered to be useful. Poor results with the method were probably due to the inability to raise high titre, specific sera against molecules that were not available in pure form (reviewed in ref. 8). In contrast, affinity chromatography with lectins was developed as a most useful technique for purifying cell surface glycoproteins [11] and was a key element of the first studies in which leucocyte antigens were purified.

MOUSE IMMUNOGENETICS AND THE SEROLOGICAL APPROACH TO CELL SURFACE ANTIGENS

Mouse H2 antigens were discovered by Gorer using haemagglutination assays on red

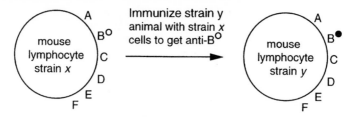

Figure 2 *Mouse immunogenetic approach to the identification of cell surface antigens. Production of alloantisera by the immunization of strain "y" mice with cells from strain "x" that differ only in a polymorphic determinant of the antigen "B".*

cells, with the first antiserum that reliably identified a polymorphism being an absorbed rabbit anti-mouse erythrocyte serum (reviewed in ref. 12). Then sera were raised between mouse strains and the concept was introduced of backcrossing a strain to isolate one polymorphic antigenic determinant against a background of molecules identical and thus non-immunogenic between the strains (Fig. 2)[13]. In this way one molecule could be confidently recognized from a complex mixture of other molecules. Agglutination assays could not be used to study nucleated cells but an effective cytotoxicity assay was developed[14]. With this assay, alloantigens of mouse thymocytes and lymphocytes were sought, leading to the discovery of the Tla (MHC-like molecules)[15] and Thy-1 antigens[16] and later to the Ly-1 (CD5), Ly-2 (CD8α) and Ly-3 (CD8β) antigens[15]. Other antigens to be discovered at an early stage were the rat ART-1 (or Ly-1 antigen)[17,18] and the mouse Ly-5 antigen that were later both established as polymorphic determinants of the CD45 antigen. Studies on Thy-1 antigen were of major importance in delineating B from T lymphocytes[19] and work on the Ly-1 and Ly-2,3 antigens led to the discovery of subsets amongst T cells[20].

Studies on mouse alloantigens presented a major step forward in the analysis of lymphocyte surfaces but this approach had considerable problems. It was applicable only to rodents, where inbred strains could be produced, and sera were often weak and dependent on the use of the cytotoxicity assay for analysis. Many sera contained heterophilic and anti-viral antibodies and specificity was probably often achieved by the antibody to an alloantigen giving the final increment of binding necessary to achieve cell death in the cytotoxicity assay which is of an all-or-none nature. In quantitative binding assays alloantisera often gave poor specificity. The dependence on cytotoxicity assays was a major problem for biochemical studies involving the detergents necessary for solubilization (see below) because these detergents in trace amounts also caused cell lysis.

QUANTITATIVE SEROLOGY AND XENOGENEIC ANTIBODIES

The first quantitative binding studies were done for Thy-1 and H2 antigens using ^{3}H-labelled antibodies[21] and in the analysis of the amount of surface Ig on B cells using ^{125}I-labelled antibodies[22]. Anti-Ig antibodies could be purified by affinity chromatography but saturating binding was not obtained with such antibodies due to aggregation involving the uncharacterized interactions of the Fc regions of acid-eluted antibodies. However ^{125}I-labelled purified antibody in the form of F(ab')$_2$ fragments did give saturating binding[23] and also avoided any problems due to

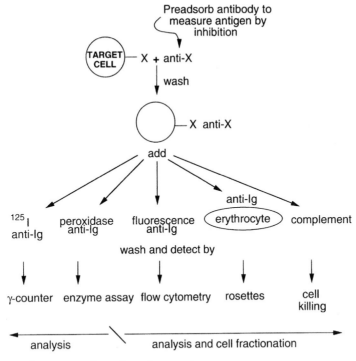

Figure 3 *Binding assays for cell surface antigens.*

binding by Fc receptors. Thus purified F(ab')$_2$ antibodies became the preferred reagent for the serological detection of antigen by an indirect binding assay using a variety of markers to reveal the reactions (Fig. 3). Protein A was also used as an alternative to F(ab')$_2$ anti-immunoglobulin as a second reagent[24]. Binding in the presence of detergents was possible if glutaraldehyde-fixed cells were used and antigen in extracts could then be measured by inhibition assays[25]. The development of flow cytometry revolutionized studies on cell subsets[26] and analysis of the apparent molecular weight of an antigen was often made simple by the finding that indirect binding assays could be performed on antigens after SDS-PAGE (Western blotting or immunoblotting[27]). Thus binding serology replaced the cytotoxicity assay and a quantitative and biochemical approach to the cell surface became possible[28].

The major problem in using antibodies to study cell surface molecules was to produce a specific antibody against a cell surface molecule. If an immunization was made across a species barrier then potentially all cell surface molecules might be antigenic due to divergence in evolution and thus antibodies to previously unknown cell surface molecules could be produced, but the problem was that unless a pure antigen was used, a mixture of antibodies would result. Various attempts to overcome this problem were made with one approach being to try to identify antigens via inhibition assays with absorbed xenoantisera and use this assay to follow the purification of the antigens. Then strong specific antisera could be produced against the purified antigen. This scheme was successful for obtaining anti-Thy-1 xenoantisera[29] and in initial studies on the CD45 antigen (T200 or the leucocyte common antigen), but there was no general solution to resolving the complexity of xenoantisera (reviewed in ref. 28).

MONOCLONAL ANTIBODIES

In 1975 the hybridoma method to produce monoclonal antibodies was described and initially was discussed in terms of producing antibodies "of predetermined specificity"[30]. A more interesting possibility from the viewpoint of analysis of the cell surface was to use the method in a "shot gun" technique to resolve the complexity of a xenogeneic immunization and to discover new cell surface molecules[31]. The principles are shown in Fig. 4. The method was investigated in a mouse anti-rat thymocyte fusion and five new antigens that all marked subsets of lymphoid cells were discovered including the CD4 (W3/25) and CD43 (W3/13) antigens[31]. Binding serology as in Fig. 3 was essential for the effective use of the mAb approach since a single antibody against one epitope is not usually effective in a cytotoxicity assay. The xenogeneic approach was applicable to human cells and mAbs to human antigens were soon produced including antibodies to MHC Class I antigen[32], CD1[33], CD3, CD4 and CD8[34] in the earliest studies.

The use of mAbs was particularly effective in combination with flow cytometry since background binding was almost non-existent and flow cytometry became increasingly used to characterize new mAbs. In studies on human antigens the use of flow cytometry labelling became the basis for grouping antigens in "Clusters of Differentiation" or CD antigens[35]. Those mAbs that gave the same patterns of labelling on different cell types were considered to label the same antigen and the naming of antigens was formalized in these workshops on human leucocytes[36]. This systematic approach has been of great benefit in the field since the CD names have allowed a common nomenclature not only for human antigens but also for the homologous antigens of other species. The CD groupings have mostly identified

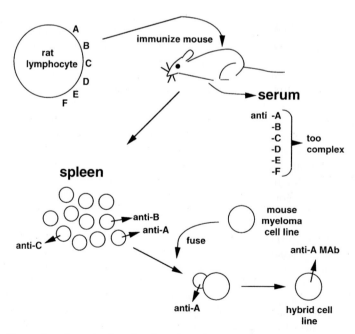

Figure 4 *Monoclonal antibodies for the identification of cell surface proteins.*

unique antigens and a CD antigen is validated when it is cloned and sequenced at the cDNA level and expressed in soluble or cell-bound form to provide a reagent to check that relevant mAbs all react with the same gene product.

As well as identifying antigens, mAbs have been of great use in analysing cellular and molecular functions. It was found that the W3/25 (CD4) mAb could be used to separate functional subpopulations of T cells[37] and would block the mixed lymphocyte response[38] and an autoimmune disease *in vivo*[39]. MAbs that could activate responses were seen in the activation of T cells with CD3 mAbs[40]. Inhibition or stimulation of cell responses have subsequently been seen in many other cases and while the meaning of such results can sometimes be difficult to interpret, the use of mAbs in functional studies has been of major importance.

MOLECULAR ANALYSIS – AMINO ACID SEQUENCING

Molecular analysis of leucocyte antigens began with the purification of the papain fragment of mouse MHC Class I antigen[41] and the demonstration that radiolabelled antigens could be immunoprecipitated from detergent extracts[42]. Biochemical purification of leucocyte membrane molecules was difficult but was achieved for Thy-1 antigen by use of lentil lectin affinity chromatography and gel filtration. Antibody affinity chromatography using polyclonal antisera was used and elution at high pH in deoxycholate was introduced[43]. The only leucocyte antigens to be entirely sequenced at the protein level were Ig[44,45], β_2 microglobulin[46], MHC Class I[47] and II[48] and Thy-1[49].

MOLECULAR ANALYSIS – NUCLEIC ACID SEQUENCING OF LEUCOCYTE GENES

Apart from the antigens described in the paragraph above, all other leucocyte antigens have been sequenced first at the DNA level and this has been achieved in a variety of ways.

1 MAb affinity columns were found to be very effective for antigen purification[50,51] and from the pure protein, peptide sequence could be obtained to allow the prediction of a mixture of oligonucleotides that would encode the sequence in question. The oligonucleotide mixture could be synthesized and then used to screen a cDNA library and isolate the relevant clone[52–55]. In some recent cases the mixture of oligonucleotides has been used in the polymerase chain reaction to amplify cDNA. As far as we are aware, the primary cloning of the following antigens was achieved in this way: CD2, CD3δ, CD3ζ, CD5, CD8β, CD9, CD10, CD11a, CD11b, CD11c, CD18, CD21, CD23, CD25, CD32, CD35, CD43, CD45, CD46, CD47, CD49a, CD49f, CD50, CD52, CD54, CD55, CD58, CD61, CD62L, CD62P, CD69, CD87, CD103, CD107a, CD120a, CD132, CD151, CD158, aminopeptidase A, BP1/6C3, DEC-205, DNAM-1, E-selectin ligand, FcεRIα, FcεRIβ, FcεRIγ, FLT3 ligand, GlyCAM-1, L1, LPAP, Ly-6, Ly-49, M130, Mac-2 binding protein, mannose receptor, OX2, PC-1, scavenger receptor, sialoadhesin, TCRα.

2 DNA was transfected into recipient cells and expression of antigen at the cell surface assayed. This was followed by re-isolation of the transfected DNA which

was used for screening cDNA or genomic libraries [56,57]. With this procedure the following antigens were cloned: CD4, CD8α, CD33, CD63, CD98.

3 Bacterial expression systems were used in which cDNA was cloned into λ phage and screened with antibodies [58]. This gave rise to cloning of: CD2, CD3ε, CD3γ, CD9, CD13, CD26, CD29, CD30, CD31, CD41, CD42a, CD42bα, CD42bβ, CD44, CD48, CD49b, CD49c, CD49d, CD49e, CD51, CD96, CD99, CD105, CD119, CD130, CD147, CD166, B-G, gp42, F4/80, RT6.

4 Differential subtraction of cDNA was used to isolate clones specific for a certain cell type [59]. This gave rise to the cloning of: CD20, CD22, CD45, CD62L, CD79a, CD79b, CD82, CD83, CD124, CDw137, CD152, HTm4, LAG-3, MS2, NKG2, PD1, TCRβ, TCRγ.

5 Crosshybridization using probes for related proteins was used [60]. This gave rise to cloning of: CD24, CD66, CD88, CD91, CD117, CD128b, CD135, CD158, ltk, mannose R, MARCO, macrophage lectin, MDR1, M-CSFR (CD115), thrombopoietin receptor.

6 Methods were used such as "hybrid arrest translation", involving the purification of mRNA by antibody selection of mRNA on membrane-associated polysomes or testing of cDNA clones for their ability to bind to specific mRNA. The mRNA was assayed by translation *in vitro* or in *Xenopus* oocytes [61,62]. This gave rise to cloning of: CD1, CD56, CD71, CD74.

7 A major impetus to cloning of leucocyte antigens was provided by the expression cloning system devised by Seed in which cDNA is cloned into a bacterial vector that will also replicate and give expression in eukaryotic cells. The cDNA library is transfected into COS cells and those cells expressing the required antigens are selected using antibody in a panning or similar technique. The plasmids are recovered from the positive COS cells, amplified in bacteria and the cycle is repeated until a single clone giving expression of the antigen is isolated [63-65]. In some cases ligands such as cytokines were used instead of antibodies (e.g. ref. 66). This method has been highly effective and has resulted in the primary cloning of the following antigens: CD2, CD6, CD7, CD14, CD16, CD19, CD22, CD24, CD27, CD28, CD31, CD33, CD34, CD36, CD37, CD38, CD40, CD44, CD50, CD52, CD53, CD54, CD58, CD59, CD62L, CD64, CD66, CD68, CD69, CD70, CD72, CD80, CD81, CD85, CD86, CD94, CD95, CD100, CD101, CD120b, CD121a, CD121b, CD122, CDw123, CDw125, CD126, CD127, CDw128, CD129, CDw131, CD134 (OX40), CDw150, CD161, CD162, CD40 ligand, 114/A10, 2B4, 4-1BB ligand, CMRF35 antigen, Fas ligand, FcαR, G-CSFR (CD114), GM-CSFRα (CD116), IL-1R AcP, IL-10R, IL-12Rβ, IL-13Rα, IL-15Rα, IL-17R, Ly-9, Ly-49, OX40 ligand, Sca-2, WC-1.

8 The isolation of related proteins by polymerase chain reaction has been successful for many antigens in general although only a few leucocyte surface proteins [67]. In some cases the method was combined with oligonucleotides based on peptide data or expression cloning in phage [68]. This method gave rise to cloning of: β7 integrin, β4 integrin (CD104), CD11d, CD50, CD91, CD148, IL-11Rα.

9 A strategy based on direct cloning of human transcripts from hybrid cell lines using a PCR strategy together with Alu repeats was successful in cloning the EMR1 antigen which is probably the human homologue of the F4/80 antigen [69]. A comparable strategy using cosmids for chromosome 21 to screen a cDNA library was successful for IFNγR AF-1.

10 Many new sequences are being determined by random sequencing of cDNA clones or by genomic sequencing. Many of the former are available in the "expressed

sequence tag or EST" databases. This has revealed a number of new genes often related to those already identified. They are not included in the entries in this book where additional data are required such as evidence of expression, tissue distribution and availability of antibodies recognizing the antigens.

One exception to the above methods is the TCRδ which was isolated first at the genomic level by sequencing clones encoding the TCRα V-genes [70]. In some cases the same cDNA was cloned independently by more than one group at about the same time and hence appears more than once in the above list.

A plot of the progress of sequence determination of cell surface molecules versus time is shown in Fig. 5. Currently the Seed method is the cloning method of choice with the proviso that it has drawbacks for very large molecules and for molecules that cannot be expressed as single chains. The method via protein purification is reliable but it can be tedious to isolate enough pure antigen for sequence determination, particularly if an antigen is present at very low numbers or on a minor cell type. However, techniques of microsequencing have been improving rapidly, including the development of sensitive mass spectrographic methods [71].

AMINO ACID SEQUENCES AND THE SUPERFAMILY CONCEPT

The amino acid sequences of most leucocyte surface proteins contain regions of sequence that have similarities to regions present in other proteins. These are termed superfamilies [72] and it was predicted that these sequences were derived by divergent evolution from common precursors and would have similar structures and types of functions. The first superfamily of leucocyte surface proteins to be defined was the immunoglobulin superfamily (IgSF) [73] and this is now one of the largest

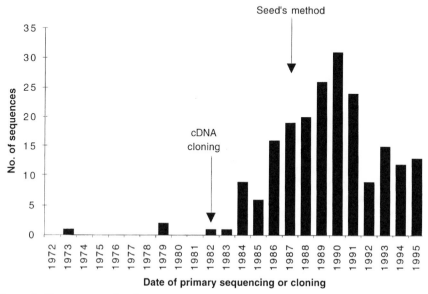

Figure 5. *Time course for the primary cloning of leucocyte antigens. The number of new leucocyte antigens cloned each year is indicated.*

with more than 100 different polypeptides expressed by a variety of cell types [74]. In protein superfamilies there is often only 15–25% sequence identity and these initial assignments were controversial [74]. However the determination of structures of several of these proteins such as CD2 and CD4 (see below) confirmed the predictions. One important aspect of the superfamilies is that they often correspond to domains. The conserved residues tend to relate to important structural features that are characteristic of the superfamily in question, as shown for IgSF domains where these residues are clustered mainly in regions corresponding to the in-pointing residues of β strands of the Ig-fold with a subset of these forming the core of the fold [75]. In contrast, the regions corresponding to the loops at the ends of the strands mostly show greater sequence diversity.

Several different superfamilies have been identified among leucocyte surface molecules and these are described in Chapter 3 together with their relationship to protein domains.

MOLECULAR ANALYSIS – PROTEIN STRUCTURE

The presence of a transmembrane or GPI anchor in membrane proteins hinders the preparation of soluble protein at the high concentrations necessary for techniques of structure determination such as NMR and X-ray crystallography. NMR is not suitable for large proteins but the structures of several single domains have been determined. The first structural information came from the X-ray crystallography of membrane proteins that also occurred naturally as soluble forms, namely immunoglobulin light chain dimers (Bence Jones proteins) [76] and β_2-microglobulin from urine [77]; later fragments of immunoglobulins were prepared by limited proteolysis and their structure determined [76]. Subsequently the structures of the intra- and extracellular parts of membrane proteins have been determined separately. The first structure determined was the extracellular region of MHC Class I antigen which could be cleaved by papain to give a soluble fragment [78]. A key to this success was the ability to select cell lines that expressed the antigen at high levels and the good efficiency of the papain cleavage. This approach in combination with recombinant expression in insect cells was successful for MHC Class II [79]. The structure of the Ly-6SF domain of CD59 was determined by NMR from native soluble fragments found in urine [80].

With the introduction of recombinant DNA techniques and a variety of different expression systems many structures of domains of leucocyte surface antigens have been determined. NMR structures were obtained by expressing single domains in *E. coli*, e.g. rat CD2d1 [81], in transfected cell lines such as Chinese hamster ovary (CHO) cell lines, e.g. human CD2d1 [82] and CD59 [83] and in yeast expression systems such as *Pichia*, e.g. NCAM (CD56) domain 1 [84]. All these systems have been used for X-ray crystallography studies, e.g. CHO cells for CD4d1+2 [85,86], CD4d3+4 [87], rat CD2 [88], human CD2 [89], CD8α [90], CD62Ed1+2 [91], *E. coli* for integrin I-domain [92], T cell receptor α chain [93], TNFR [94], VCAM-1d1 [95], a myeloma expression system for T cell receptor β chain [96] and yeast (*Pichia pastoris*) for CD40L [97]. In addition, crystal structures for the T cell receptor and complexes of TCR with MHC Class I antigens have recently been determined using expression in insect cells [98] and in *E. coli* [99].

Structures for nearly all the domain types found on the extracellular side of leucocytes have now been determined [100]. Many antigens contain large numbers of domains in a single polypeptide and the complete polypeptides are less amenable to structural analysis than single domains, probably because of flexibility between some of the domains. In most of the cases above the structures are for only one or two domains unless the polypeptides form a larger complex, e.g. the TNFR contains four domains but the structure determined was of a complex of the trimeric TNF and three TNFR chains[94]. However, recently the structure of a stretch of four Fn3 domains from fibronectin has been determined[101]. Electron microscopy has been valuable in examining the overall topology of domains of larger proteins and this is discussed further in Chapter 4.

References

[1] Bretscher, M.S. (1971) Major human erythrocyte glycoprotein spans the cell membrane. Nature New Biol. 231, 229–232.

[2] Tomita, M. and Marchesi, V.T. (1975) Amino-acid sequence and oligosaccharide attachment sites of human erythrocyte glycophorin. Proc. Natl Acad. Sci. USA 72, 2964–2968.

[3] Singer, S.J. and Nicolson, G.L. (1972) The fluid mosaic model of the structure of cell membranes. Science 175, 720–731.

[4] Frye, L.D. and Edidin, M. (1970) The rapid intermixing of cell surface antigens after formation of mouse-human heterokaryons. J. Cell. Sci. 7, 319–335.

[5] Taylor, R.B. et al. (1971) Redistribution and pinocytosis of lymphocyte surface immunoglobulin induced by anti-immunoglobulin antibodies. Nature New Biol. 233, 225–229.

[6] Helenius, A. and Simons, K. (1975) Solubilization of membranes by detergents. Biochim. Biophys. Acta 415, 29–79.

[7] Axen, R. et al. (1967) Chemical coupling of peptides and proteins to polysaccharides by means of cyanogen halides. Nature 214, 1302–1304.

[8] Arvieux, J. and Williams, A.F. (1988) Antibodies, a Practical Approach, Catty, D., ed. IRL Press, Oxford, pp. 113–136.

[9] Weber, K. and Osborn, M. (1969) The reliability of molecular weight determinations by dodecyl sulfate-polyacrylamide gel electrophoresis. J. Biol. Chem. 244, 4406–4412.

[10] Muirhead, M.L. et al. (1974) Preliminary characterization of Thy-1.1 and Ag-B antigens from rat tissues solubilized in detergents. Biochem. J. 143, 51–61.

[11] Allan, D. et al. (1972) Glycoprotein receptors for concanavalin A isolated from pig lymphocyte plasma membrane by affinity chromatography in sodium deoxycholate. Nature New Biol. 236, 23–25.

[12] Klein, J. (1975) Biology of the Mouse Histocompatibility-2 Complex. Springer-Verlag, Berlin.

[13] Snell, G.D. (1981) Studies in histocompatibility. Science 213, 172–178.

[14] Gorer, P.A. and O'Gorman, P. (1956) The cytotoxic activity of isoantibodies in mice. Transplant. Bull. 3, 142–143.

[15] Boyse, E.A. and Old, L.J. (1969) Some aspects of normal and abnormal cell surface genetics. Annu. Rev. Genet. 3, 269–290.

[16] Reif, A.E. and Allen, J.M.V. (1964) The AKR thymic antigen and its distribution in leukemias and nervous tissue. J. Exp. Med. 120, 413–433.

[17] Lubaroff, D.M. (1973) An alloantigenic marker on rat thymus and thymus-derived cells. Transplant. Proc. 5, 115–118.

[18] Fabre, J.W. and Morris, P.J. (1974) The definition of a lymphocyte-specific alloantigen system in the rat (Ly-1). Tissue Antigens 4, 238–246.

19 Raff, M.C. (1971) Surface antigenic markers for distinguishing T and B lymphocytes in mice. Transplant. Rev. 6, 52–80.

20 Kisielow, P. et al. (1975) Ly antigens as markers for functionally distinct subpopulations of thymus-derived lymphocytes of the mouse. Nature 253, 219–220.

21 Hammerling, U. and Eggers, H.J. (1970) Quantitative measurement of uptake of alloantibody on mouse lymphocytes. Eur. J. Biochem. 17, 95–99.

22 Nossal, G.J.V. and Lewis, H. (1972) Variation in accessible cell surface immunoglobulin among antibody-forming cells. J. Exp. Med. 135, 1416–1422.

23 Jensenius, J.C. and Williams, A.F. (1974) The binding of anti-immunoglobulin antibodies to rat thymocytes and thoracic duct lymphocytes. Eur. J. Immunol. 4, 91–97.

24 Dorval, G. et al. (1975) A radioimmunoassay of cellular surface antigens on living cells using iodinated soluble protein A from Staphylococcus aureus. J. Immunol. Methods 7, 237–230.

25 Williams, A.F. (1973) Assays for cellular antigens in the presence of detergents. Eur. J. Immunol. 3, 628–632.

26 Bonner, W.A. et al. (1972) Fluorescence activated cell sorting. Rev. Sci. Instrum. 43, 404–409.

27 Towbin, H. et al. (1979) Electrophoretic transfer of proteins from polyacrylamide gels to nitrocellulose sheets: procedure and some applications. Proc. Natl Acad. Sci. USA 76, 4350–4354.

28 Williams, A.F. (1977) Differentiation antigens of the lymphocyte cell surface. Contemp. Top. Mol. Immunol. 6, 83–116.

29 Morris, R.J. and Williams, A.F. (1975) Antigens on mouse and rat lymphocytes recognized by rabbit antiserum against rat brain: the quantitative analysis of a xenogeneic antiserum. Eur. J. Immunol. 5, 274–281.

30 Kohler, G. and Milstein, C. (1975) Continuous cultures of fused cells secreting antibody of predefined specificity. Nature 256, 495–497.

31 Williams, A.F. et al. (1977) Analysis of cell surfaces by xenogeneic myeloma-hybrid antibodies: differentiation antigens of rat lymphocytes. Cell 12, 663–673.

32 Barnstable, C.J. et al. (1978) Production of monoclonal antibodies to group A erythrocytes, HLA and other human cell surface antigens—new tools for genetic analysis. Cell 14, 9–20.

33 McMichael, A.J. et al. (1979) A human thymocyte antigen defined by a hybrid myeloma monoclonal antibody. Eur. J. Immunol. 9, 205–210.

34 Terhorst, C. et al. (1980) Biochemical analysis of human T lymphocyte differentiation antigens T4 and T5. Science 209, 520–521.

35 Bernard, A. et al. (1984) Leucocyte Typing. Springer-Verlag, Berlin, pp. 1–814.

36 Knapp, W. et al. (1989) Leucocyte Typing IV. Oxford University Press, Oxford, pp. 1–1182.

37 White, R.A.H. et al. (1978) T-lymphocyte heterogeneity in the rat: separation of functional subpopulations using a monoclonal antibody. J. Exp. Med. 148, 664–673.

38 Webb, M. et al. (1979) Inhibition of mixed lymphocyte response by monoclonal antibody specific for a rat T lymphocyte subset. Nature 282, 841–843.

39 Brostoff, S.W. and Mason, D.W. (1984) Experimental allergic encephalomyelitis: successful treatment in vivo with a monoclonal antibody that recognises T helper cells. J. Immunol. 133, 1938–1942.

[40] Van Wauwe, J.P. et al. (1980) OKT3: a monoclonal anti-human T lymphocyte antibody with potent mitogenic properties. J. Immunol. 124, 2708–2713.

[41] Shimada, A. and Nathenson, S.G. (1969) Murine histocompatibility-2 (H-2) alloantigens. Purification and some chemical properties of soluble products from H-2b and H-2d genotypes released by papain digestion of membrane fractions. Biochemistry 8, 4048–4062.

[42] Schwartz, B.D. et al. (1973) H-2 histocompatibility alloantigens. Some biochemical properties of the molecules solubilized by NP-40 detergent. Biochemistry 12, 2157–2164.

[43] Letarte-Muirhead, M. et al. (1975) Purification of the Thy-1 molecule, a major cell-surface glycoprotein of rat thymocytes. Biochem. J. 151, 685–697.

[44] Hill, R.L. et al. (1966) The evolutionary origins of the immunoglobulins. Proc. Natl Acad. Sci. USA 56, 1762–1769.

[45] Hilschmann, N. and Craig, L.C. (1965) Amino acid sequence studies with Bence Jones proteins. Proc. Natl Acad. Sci. USA 59, 613–619.

[46] Cunningham, B.A. et al. (1973) The complete amino acid sequence of beta 2-microglobulin. Biochemistry 12, 4811–4822.

[47] Orr, H.T. et al. (1979) The heavy chain of human histocompatibility antigen HLA-B7 contains an immunoglobulin-like region. Nature 282, 266–270.

[48] Gotz, H. et al. (1983) Primary structure of human class II histocompatibility antigens 3rd communication. Amino acid sequence comparison between DR and DC subclass antigens derived from a lymphoblastoid B cell line homozygous at the HLA loci (HLA-A3,3; B7,7; Dw2,2; DR2,2: MT1,1; Dc1,1: MB1,1). Hoppe Seylers Z. Physiol. Chem. 364, 749-755.

[49] Campbell, D.G. et al. (1981) Rat brain Thy-1 glycoprotein. The amino acid sequence, disulfide bonds and an unusual hydrophobic region. Biochem. J. 195, 15–30.

[50] Sunderland, C.A. et al. (1979) Purification with monoclonal antibody of a predominant leukocyte-common antigen and glycoprotein from rat thymocytes. Eur. J. Immunol. 9, 155–159.

[51] Parham, P. (1979) Purification of immunologically active HLA-A and -B antigens by a series of monoclonal antibody columns. J. Biol. Chem. 254, 8709–8712.

[52] Wallace, R.B. et al. (1981) The use of synthetic oligonucleotides as hybridization probes. II. Hybridization of oligonucleotides of mixed sequence to rabbit beta-globin DNA. Nucleic Acids Res. 9, 879–894.

[53] Stetler, D. et al. (1982) Isolation of a cDNA clone for the human HLA-DR antigen alpha chain by using a synthetic oligonucleotide as a hybridization probe. Proc. Natl Acad. Sci. USA 79, 5966–5970.

[54] Moriuchi, T. et al. (1983) Thy-1 cDNA sequence suggests a novel regulatory mechanism. Nature 301, 80–82.

[55] Cosman, D. et al. (1984) Cloning, sequence and expression of human interleukin-2 receptor. Nature 312, 768–771.

[56] Kavathas, P. et al. (1984) Isolation of the gene encoding the human T-lymphocyte differentiation antigen Leu-2 (T8) by gene transfer and cDNA subtraction. Proc. Natl Acad. Sci. USA 81, 7688–7692.

[57] Maddon, P.J. et al. (1985) The isolation and nucleotide sequence of a cDNA encoding the T cell surface protein T4: a new member of the immunoglobulin gene family. Cell 42, 93–104.

[58] Young, R.A. and Davis, R.W. (1983) Efficient isolation of genes by using antibody probes. Proc. Natl Acad. Sci. USA 80, 1194–1198.

59 Hedrick, S.M. et al. (1984) Isolation of cDNA clones encoding T cell-specific membrane-associated proteins. Nature 308, 149–153.

60 Qiu, F.H. et al. (1988) Primary structure of c-kit: relationship with the CSF-1/ PDGF receptor kinase family – oncogenic activation of v-kit involves deletion of extracellular domain and C terminus. EMBO J. 7, 1003–1011.

61 Korman, A.J. et al. (1982) cDNA clones for the heavy chain of HLA-DR antigens obtained after immunopurification of polysomes by monoclonal antibody. Proc. Natl. Acad. Sci. USA 79, 1844–1848.

62 Long, E.O. et al. (1982) Isolation of distinct cDNA clones encoding HLA-DR beta chains by use of an expression assay. Proc. Natl Acad. Sci. USA 79, 7465–7469.

63 Seed, B. and Aruffo, A. (1987) Molecular cloning of the CD2 antigen, the T-cell erythrocyte receptor, by a rapid immunoselection procedure. Proc. Natl Acad. Sci. USA 84, 3365–3369.

64 Seed, B. (1987) An LFA–3 cDNA encodes a phospholipid-linked membrane protein homologous to its receptor CD2. Nature 329, 840–842.

65 Aruffo, A. and Seed, B. (1987) Molecular cloning of two CD7 (T-cell leukemia antigen) cDNAs by a COS cell expression system. EMBO J. 6, 3313–3316.

66 Yamasaki, K. et al. (1988) Cloning and expression of the human interleukin-6 (BSF-2/IFN beta 2) receptor. Science 241, 825–828.

67 Vazeux, R. et al. (1992) Cloning and characterization of a new intercellular adhesion molecule ICAM-R. Nature 360, 485–488.

68 Van der Vieren, M. et al. (1995) A novel leukointegrin, $\alpha d\beta 2$ binds preferentially to ICAM-3. Immunity 3, 683–690.

69 Corbo, L. et al. (1990) Direct cloning of human transcripts with HnRNA from hybrid cell lines. Science 249, 652–655.

70 Chien, Y.H. et al. (1987) A new T-cell receptor gene located within the alpha locus and expressed early in T-cell differentiation. Nature 327, 677–682.

71 Wilm, M. et al. (1996) Femtomole sequencing of proteins from polyacrylamide gels by nano-electrospray mass spectrometry. Nature 379, 466–469.

72 Dayhoff, M.O. et al. (1983) Establishing homologies in protein sequences. Meth. Enzymol. 91, 524–545.

73 Williams, A.F. and Gagnon, J. (1982) Neuronal cell Thy-1 glycoprotein: homology with immunoglobulin. Science 216, 696–703.

74 Williams, A.F. and Barclay, A.N. (1988) The immunoglobulin superfamily – domains for cell surface recognition. Annu. Rev. Immunol. 6, 381–405.

75 Harpaz, Y. and Chothia, C. (1994) Many of the immunoglobulin superfamily domains in cell-adhesion molecules and surface-receptors belong to a new structural set which is close to that containing variable domains. J. Mol. Biol. 238, 528–539.

76 Amzel, L.M. and Poljak, R.J. (1979) Three-dimensional structure of immunoglobulins. Ann. Rev. Biochem. 48, 961–997.

77 Becker, J.W. and Reeke, G.J. (1985) Three-dimensional structure of beta 2-microglobulin. Proc. Natl Acad. Sci. USA 82, 4225–4229.

78 Bjorkman, P.J. et al. (1987) Structure of the human class I histocompatibility antigen, HLA-A2. Nature 329, 506–512.

79 Brown, J.H. et al. (1993) Three-dimensional structure of the human class II histocompatibility antigen HLA-DR1. Nature 364, 33–39.

80 Fletcher, C.M. et al. (1994) Structure of a soluble, glycosylated form of the human-complement regulatory protein CD59. Structure 2, 185–199.

81 Driscoll, P.C. et al. (1991) Structure of domain 1 of rat T lymphocyte CD2 antigen. Nature 353, 762–765.

82 Wyss, D. et al. (1993) 1H resonance assignments and secondary structure of the 13.6 kDa glycosylated adhesion domain of human CD2. Biochemistry 32, 10995–11006.

83 Kieffer, B. et al. (1994) 3-dimensional solution structure of the extracellular region of the complement regulatory protein CD59, a new cell-surface protein domain related to snake-venom neurotoxins. Biochemistry 33, 4471–4482.

84 Thomsen, N. et al. (1996) The three-dimensional structure of the first domain of neural cell adhesion molecule. Nature Struct. Biol. 3, 581–585.

85 Ryu, S.E. et al. (1990) Crystal structure of an HIV-binding recombinant fragment of human CD4. Nature 348, 419–426.

86 Wang, J. et al. (1990) Atomic structure of a fragment of human CD4 containing two immunoglobulin-like domains. Nature 348, 411–418.

87 Brady, R.L. et al. (1993) Crystal structure of domains 3 and 4 of rat CD4: relationship to the N-terminal domains. Science 260, 979–983.

88 Jones, E.Y. et al. (1992) Crystal structure of a soluble form of the cell adhesion molecule CD2 at 2.8 Å. Nature 360, 232–239.

89 Bodian, D.L. et al. (1994) Crystal structure of the extracellular region of the human cell adhesion molecule CD2 at 2.5 Å resolution. Structure 2, 755–766.

90 Leahy, D.J. et al. (1992) Crystal structure of a soluble form of the human T cell coreceptor CD8 at 2.6 Å resolution. Cell 68, 1145–1162.

91 Graves, B.J. et al. (1994) Insight into E-selectin/ligand interaction from the crystal structure and mutagenesis of the lec/EGF domains. Nature 367, 532–538.

92 Qu, A. and Leahy, D.J. (1995) Crystal structure of the I-domain from the CD11a/CD18 (LFA-1, alpha(L)beta2) integrin. Proc. Natl Acad. Sci. USA 92, 10277–10281.

93 Fields, B.A. et al. (1995) Crystal structure of the V(alpha) domain of a T cell antigen receptor. Science 270, 1821–1824.

94 Banner, D.W. et al. (1993) Crystal structure of the soluble human 55kd TNF receptor-human TNFβ complex: implications for TNF receptor activation. Cell 73, 431–445.

95 Jones, E.Y. et al. (1995) Crystal structure of an integrin-binding fragment of vascular cell adhesion molecule-1 at 1.8 Å resolution. Nature 373, 539–544.

96 Bentley, G.A. et al. (1995) Crystal structure of the beta chain of a T cell antigen receptor. Science 267, 1984–1987.

97 Karpusas, M. et al. (1995) 2 Å crystal structure of an extracellular fragment of human CD40 ligand. Structure 3, 1031–1039.

98 Garcia, K. et al. (1996) An $\alpha\beta$ T cell receptor structure at 2.5 Å and its orientation in the TCR-MHC complex. Science 274, 209–219.

99 Garboczi, D. et al. (1996) Structure of the complex between T-cell receptor, viral peptide and HLA-A2. Nature 384, 134–141.

100 Bork, P. et al. (1996) Structure and distribution of modules in extracellular proteins. Q. Rev. Biophys. 29, 119–167.

101 Leahy, D.J. et al. (1996) 2.0 A Crystal structure of a four-domain segment of human fibronectin encompassing the RGD loop and synergy region. Cell 84, 155–164.

3 Protein superfamilies and cell surface molecules

CONCEPTS CONCERNING PROTEIN SUPERFAMILIES

Introduction

The amino acid sequences of most leucocyte surface proteins contain regions of sequence that have similarities to regions present in other proteins and are termed superfamilies](see Chapter 2). It has now been established that these regions often correspond to structural units or domains or modules (see below) and the general sequence term "superfamily" is often dropped in favour of the predicted structural terms "domains" and "modules". This chapter describes the methods for the identification of superfamilies and shows alignments of some sequences to illustrate the key residues that are often conserved in these superfamilies together with examples of their structures.

Nomenclature for superfamilies, protein domains, modules, repeats and motifs

The nomenclature for terms like superfamily, domains, repeats and motifs is not hard and fast, and in this book we have tried to conform to the most commonly used names and in some cases to introduce abbreviations that might be useful. The domains and repeats discussed in this chapter include only those present on leucocyte surface molecules. Additional domains have been described for secreted molecules and for surface molecules of other cell types. These include cadherin, Fn type I, kringle, perforin, serine protease and thrombospondin domains [1-3]. Recently, a single example of a semaphorin domain has been reported in CD100 and a cytokine domain on a transmembrane protein (FLT3 ligand). Details of these domain types have not been included but are reviewed in refs 4 and 5.

Domain

The term "domain" is used where it is likely that a segment of sequence forms a discrete structural unit, i.e. a peptide sequence whose three-dimensional conformation is not determined by other parts of the total protein sequence but is "self-contained" (discussed in ref. 6). Although at one time the term was used exclusively for regions of known structure, it is now used where this seems likely by analogy to other structures. Three criteria are used here. Proof of a domain structure comes from tertiary structure determination and domains established at this level include: IgSF, complement control protein (CCP), cytokineR, EGF, fibronectin type III (Fn3), integrin I domain, lectin C-type, galectin, link, LDLR, LRR and Ly-6. The MHC domain has also been revealed by X-ray crystallography in MHC Class I and II antigens and it might be argued that this should not be referred to as a domain since it is not clear that this domain will be found as an isolated unit rather than appearing always as a structural pair as for the $\alpha 1$ and $\alpha 2$ domains. However we will follow the precedent in the field and refer to these segments as domains. TNF and CD40L are members of an increasingly large superfamily whose structures show that they usually exist as trimers. They have not been found as multiples or in association with other superfamily types but the folds for TNF and all the above domains are illustrated later in this chapter and are discussed further in the commentary on each superfamily.

Secondly, a domain structure can also be argued for any superfamily segments that occur as the sole component of an extracellular sequence, or as sequence (or sequences) within proteins that is contiguous with hinge-like regions of sequence containing a high content of Ala, Gly, Pro, Ser, and Thr residues. Most Ly-6 domains fall into this category and a structure now confirms this [7,8].

A third criterion for defining a sequence as a domain is that the superfamily segments are found in the genome in single exons that can be readily spliced with other exons to form a new gene with an open reading frame. Proteins containing a variety of structural domains could then arise by recombination. The scavenger receptor cysteine-rich domain provides an example based on the last two criteria.

Module
The term module is used for the subset of domains that are often used as building blocks in functionally diverse proteins. In the majority of extracellular proteins the modules correlate with exons with phases suitable for "exon shuffling" (see below and ref. 9). However other methods of shuffling are possible and the term module is no longer restricted to domains with compatible exon boundaries [10].

Repeat
In other cases it is not clear that a superfamily segment is an independent structural unit and for these the term "repeat" is used in cases such as the leucine-rich repeats (LRR) which are usually present only as multiples forming a larger structure [11,12] and the short repeats of segments of sequence found in individual proteins such as CD43 and P-selectin glycoprotein ligand 1 (CD162).

Motif
The term "motif" is used to describe a smaller sequence pattern than might be expected to form a folded structural unit. Thus the patterns of signal sequences for protein secretion and GPI attachment (see Chapter 2) would be considered as motifs, albeit of rather ill-defined character in terms of sequence identities. A good example of a motif is the conserved sequence pattern found in the cytoplasmic domains of the CD3, CD79a, and CD79b antigens and other molecules of signal transduction complexes, now called the ITAM or immunoreceptor tyrosine-based activation motif. Alignments identifying this motif are shown in Fig. 37.

Superfamily
The term "superfamily" was widely used to describe sequence similarities predicted to give rise to similar structures. As discussed in Chapter 2, this concept has been proven in many cases by structure determination and it is more common to assume the prediction and to talk about domains or modules. However the term "superfamily" is useful in discussing sequence similarities in general and also when one wants to distinguish between, for example, an Ig domain meaning a domain in immunoglobulins and an Ig-like domain found in many leucocyte proteins. We use the commonly used name IgSF in the latter. We also use TNFSF and TNFRSF to prevent confusion between TNF and TNFR and related proteins. Finally, the term superfamily is often used to describe a protein, e.g. "Thy-1 is a member of the IgSF". When IgSF domains were first described, there were very few cases in which they were found together

with other superfamily domains (see ref. 13). Since then many examples have been found with two or even more superfamilies (see Table 1 in Chapter 1) and these are often termed "mosaic" proteins. It is confusing to name these mosaic proteins as members of a superfamily and it is more useful to discuss the proteins in terms of their content of domains, i.e. CD62L contains one C-type lectin, one EGF and two CCP domains. In other cases there is no ambiguity, for example phosphotyrosine phosphatase where the name signifies a family rather than a single example.

The term superfamily is also used to describe proteins with clear sequence similarity but no clear domain or module structure. These include the proteins with multiple membrane spanning regions such as the TM4SF. Integrins are also likely to have domains but apart from the I-domain discussed below, integrins tend not to show sequence similarities with other proteins and the full extracellular sequences are discussed as a single superfamily.

Identifying domains and repeats: testing the significance of relationships

The main difficulty in identifying superfamily domains and repeats is in their low level of amino acid sequence identity, but many methods have been developed to analyse the data from the various large-scale sequencing projects and these are reviewed in detail in refs 14–17 and only an outline is given here. A first step is to use a database searching program such as FASTA[17,18] or BLAST[19]. In many cases these programs will pick up some of the members of a superfamily that the new protein sequence matches. However, no search program picks up all superfamily members and it is not uncommon for a relationship to be entirely missed. A second approach is to look by eye, or apply various computer programs[20]. A third method is to make a consensus sequence for a particular domain type, for example the PROSITE database contains a large compilation of patterns and sites found in protein sequences (see ref. 21 and see also SWISSPROT[22] and Chapter 1). These patterns can then be used to search a novel sequence for the presence of domains or to search the databases. With the wealth of sequence data these tools are becoming more reliable. Problems arise in aligning sequences if there is variability in the lengths of sequences and also if there is only a low level of identity. This is the case for IgSF domains although there are small patches of characteristic sequence patterns. For example, in the IgSF one would look for Cys residues with the patterns L/I/VXL/IXC and DXGXYXC for candidate regions that might occur around the conserved disulfide bond. In relation to these there should be other patches, for example V/L/YXW corresponding to β strand C. If the various conserved patterns fall into place then a possible domain has been identified. The candidate domain can be defined in relation to conserved sequence positions and then tested for statistical significance. For example in the IgSF, the positions of the conserved Cys residues, or equivalent residues if the domain lacks the typical disulfide bond, are nominated and the domain is defined as beginning and ending 20 residues before and after these positions. This proposed domain is then tested for the statistical significance of sequence similarities against a set of domains that are accepted to be in the IgSF. For other superfamilies, other conserved residues would be chosen and the domain defined in relation to these. Possible key conserved residues are shown on the diagrams in this chapter and the designated residues are used to identify the domains in the entries for the molecules.

In testing for statistical significance of a superfamily relationship it could be argued that the conserved pattern for a domain should be defined and the extent to which this occurs in the new sequence should be tested. This works well for many superfamilies (see PROSITE discussed above). However, it can be difficult to define precisely a pattern for use in a statistical analysis since at many positions in the conserved pattern, one of a group of alternative amino acids can occur. Moreover it is difficult to know how to treat sequence gaps in defining a pattern. For example in the IgSF there can be very large differences in the length of the middle of the domain and this creates problems in defining a pattern that is characteristic of the IgSF to use in statistical analysis.

An alternative method to testing a sequence against a single superfamily sequence pattern is to test it against a set of sequences (e.g. 20 sequences) that are accepted as being members of the superfamily in question. In such an analysis a simple statistical program that compares sequences pairwise for similarity can be used and the ALIGN program[23] has proved satisfactory for this purpose[13]. In these comparisons no account is taken of superfamily patterns. However if a set of good scores is obtained against a family of sequences, then the superfamily pattern must be present since this is the only pattern in common amongst the family of sequences against which the new domain is being tested. This method is discussed in detail in ref. 13.

One feature of both the comparison of sequences using methods like ALIGN and database searches is the requirement for a matrix to assess the scores for the likelihood of amino acid exchange within a protein during evolution. One of the widest used matrices was the 250 PAMS mutation matrix of Dayhoff[24]. However the availability of very many more sequences now makes it possible to construct more accurate matrices such as the BLOSUM62 which is shown in comparison with the Dayhoff 250 PAMS in Table 1. The amino acids are grouped according to structure and the full formulae are given in Chapter 1 (Fig. 2), together with the single and three letter amino acid codes. The derivation and applications of these matrices are discussed in refs 16, 17, 24 and 25.

The importance of inspection of sequences is illustrated by the example of LAG-3. This protein contains four IgSF domains with similarities to the four domains of CD4. It seems likely that both these proteins arose by gene duplication from the same precursor. However domain 1 of LAG-3 is atypical in that it contains about 30 residues of extra sequence that is predicted to form an extended loop. The patterns of sequence are also compatible with an unusual disulfide bridge between strands B and G rather than B and F[26].

Domain sequence and structure: divergent and convergent evolution

In the above section, criteria for defining a superfamily have been based on identifying a sequence pattern that is shared in a non-trivial way between sequences of different molecules. It is then argued that the presence of the sequence pattern indicates a relationship in evolution such that the domains that share the sequence pattern derive from one primordial domain. However it could be argued that a certain structure dictates a sequence pattern and the sharing of the pattern is due to convergent evolution from different ancestral molecules rather than divergent evolution from a primordial domain. Conversely it may be found that sequences with no detectable common pattern form similar tertiary structures and thus that these are in the same superfamily even though there is no detectable sequence relationship.

Table 1 The 250 PAMS Mutation Matrix and BLOSUM62 matrix of scores for amino acid substitutions used in database searching and sequence comparisons

	C	S	T	P	A	G	N	D	E	Q	H	R	K	M	I	L	V	F	Y	W	Group
Cysteine (C)	12/9	-1	-1	-3	0	-3	-3	-3	-4	-3	-3	-3	-3	-1	-1	-1	-1	-2	-2	-2	Sulfhydryl
Serine (S)	0	2/4	1	-1	1	0	1	0	0	0	-1	-1	0	-1	-2	-2	-2	-2	-2	-3	Small hydrophilic
Threonine (T)	-2	1	3/5	-1	0	-2	0	-1	-1	-1	-2	-1	-1	-1	-1	-1	0	-2	-2	-2	
Proline (P)	-3	1	0	6/7	-1	-2	-2	-1	-1	-1	-2	-2	-1	-2	-3	-3	-2	-4	-3	-4	
Alanine (A)	-2	1	1	1	2/4	0	-2	-2	-1	-1	-2	-1	-1	-1	-1	-1	0	-2	-2	-3	
Glycine (G)	-3	1	0	-1	1	5/6	0	-1	-2	-2	-2	-2	-2	-3	-4	-4	-3	-3	-3	-2	
Asparagine (N)	-4	1	0	-1	0	0	2/6	1	0	0	1	0	0	-2	-3	-3	-3	-3	-2	-4	Acid, acid amide hydrophilic
Aspartic (D)	-5	0	0	-1	0	1	2	4/6	2	0	-1	-2	-1	-3	-3	-4	-3	-3	-3	-4	
Glutamic (E)	-5	0	0	-1	0	0	1	3	4/5	2	0	0	1	-2	-3	-3	-2	-3	-2	-3	
Glutamine (Q)	-5	-1	-1	0	0	-1	1	2	2	4/5	0	1	1	0	-3	-2	-2	-3	-1	-2	
Histidine (H)	-3	-1	-1	0	-1	-2	2	1	1	3	6/8	0	-1	-2	-3	-3	-3	-1	2	-2	Basic
Arginine (R)	-4	0	-1	0	-2	-3	0	-1	-1	1	2	6/5	2	-1	-3	-2	-3	-3	-2	-3	
Lysine (K)	-5	0	0	-1	-1	-2	1	0	0	1	0	3	5/5	-1	-3	-2	-2	-3	-2	-3	
Methionine (M)	-5	-2	-1	-2	-1	-3	-2	-3	-2	-1	-2	0	0	6/5	1	2	1	0	-1	-1	Small hydrophobic
Isoleucine (I)	-2	-1	0	-2	-1	-3	-2	-2	-2	-2	-2	-2	-2	2	5/4	2	3	0	-1	-3	
Leucine (L)	-6	-3	-2	-3	-2	-4	-3	-4	-3	-2	-2	-3	-3	4	2	6/4	1	0	-1	-2	
Valine (V)	-2	-1	0	-1	0	-1	-2	-2	-2	-2	-2	-2	-2	2	4	2	4/4	-1	-1	-3	
Phenylalanine (F)	-4	-3	-3	-5	-4	-5	-4	-6	-5	-5	-2	-4	-5	0	1	2	-1	9/6	3	1	Aromatic
Tyrosine (Y)	0	-3	-3	-5	-3	-5	-2	-4	-4	-4	0	-4	-4	-2	-1	-1	-1	7	10/7	2	
Tryptophan (W)	-8	-2	-5	-6	-6	-7	-4	-7	-7	-5	-3	2	-3	-4	-5	-2	-6	0	0	17/11	

The amino acids are arranged in groups according to their physicochemical properties. The single-letter and three-letter codes are given in addition to the full names. The upper panel shows the 250 PAMS Mutation Matrix and the lower panel the BLOSUM62 matrix. Data are from refs 24 and 25. The Mutation Matrix is based on the frequency of evolutionary replacements of one amino acid for another at homologous positions between present-day sequences and inferred ancestral sequences. One PAM unit is the unit of evolution represented by the matrix corresponding to one accepted amino acid substitution per 100 residues. This is discussed in detail in ref. 24. The BLOSUM series of matrices are calculated differently in that substitution probabilities are calculated from amino acid pairs of multiple alignments of related sequences. Thus the BLOSUM62 (blocks substitution matrix at 62%) is the log-odds matrix derived from pair counts between sequence segments that are less than 62% identical [16,25].

It now seems unlikely that a general structure will dictate a unique sequence pattern. This can be seen from a consideration of sequences that can give rise to domains with the Ig fold. There are now four different sets of sequence found at the surface of cells with no convincing sequence similarity between them but which all give rise to an Ig-like fold. These are the sequences of IgSF, Fn3, cytokineR and cadherin domains [2,3,27–31]. There is also enormous diversity of sequences within the IgSF that leads to the argument that there is no unique sequence required to determine any part of the IgSF fold. Thus it seems rather unlikely that convergent evolution yielding the same structure would give rise to any common sequence pattern.

The converse argument is that all the sequences that give the same folding structure have derived by divergent evolution and that all sequences with this structure should be included in the same superfamily. For example, the four sets of sequences referred to above might all be considered as IgSF sequences. It does not seem useful to take this point of view since there may be a relatively limited number of small stable protein folds that can occur and these may have evolved on numerous occasions in evolution. In this case each of the sets of sequences with the Ig fold would have an independent primordial ancestor. Alternatively, there may have been one primordial structure which acquired mutations such that a new solution to the structure was produced, ultimately giving rise to sequences that were not detectably similar to the ancestor family of sequences. At this stage there is no way to estimate the probability of the divergent versus the convergent case for generation of the same structure without recognizable sequence similarity and it seems best to stick to sequence patterns as the criteria for defining superfamilies. This is sensible from a practical as well as a theoretical standpoint since sequence data are much more readily obtained than tertiary structural data. The superfamilies defined on the basis of sequence would be grouped as subsets within superfamilies based on tertiary structure considerations. Thus it seems better to retain the sequence criterion and to note that certain superfamilies have the same folding patterns in their domains.

Given that the same structure can arise from various sequences, the question arises as to why sequence patterns are conserved in evolution. Molecules on the cell surface present unique determinants for interaction with a soluble molecule or with other cell surface receptors. Such interactions require diversity between molecules and not conservation of epitopes. However the sequence patterns shared within a superfamily conserve the fold of the molecule and usually involve residues pointing inwards in the folded structure rather than out-pointing residues that are available for intermolecular interactions. Thus the question arises as to what evolutionary force can operate to preserve the tertiary structure of the molecule.

For cell surface molecules it can be argued that the key evolutionary pressure is the requirement for molecular stability and in particular resistance to proteolysis. The small, tightly folded domains that make up most of the leucocyte molecules may have evolved as parts of stable coat proteins on single cell eukaryotes [32]. These coat proteins then gave rise to the families of molecules that evolved along with the evolution of multicellular organisms, to mediate cell division and regulation of cell differentiation. Surface molecules are generally resistant to proteolytic enzymes and this resistance is based on the folded structure, since denatured molecules are easily digested. One could argue that mutation to give new recognition epitopes would be constrained by the necessity of preserving the folded structure of the domain. In general this led to preservation of certain sequence patterns that determine one particularly stable solution for the fold. Numerous alternative sequence patterns may exist that could also give a stable fold, but to reach these a number of simultaneous mutations may be required and hence a switch to a new pattern may be a rare event in evolution. If a new pattern did form this may have become the founder of a new set of sequences in which the new pattern is retained, again because of the pressure of proteolysis. From this viewpoint it seems likely that the IgSF, Fn3 and cytokineR domains all arose from a common ancestor via sequence shifts as described above. This view might be favoured because these domains are found in molecules with similar functions and often a molecule may contain combinations of IgSF domains and Fn3 and cytokineR domains. In particular, IgSF and Fn3 domains are often found together in a single polypeptide and examples of these are particularly common in nervous tissue.

Genomic structure and evolution of proteins with mixtures of domain types

The number of domains in a cell surface protein can vary greatly. In the Thy-1 antigen (CD90) there is a single IgSF domain making up the whole of the extracellular segment, whilst for the complement receptor 1 protein (CD35) the extracellular region consists of 30 CCP domains in a linear array. In these molecules only one domain type is present but in other proteins there can be a mixture of domain types. For example the L-selectin (CD62L) antigen contains lectin C-type, EGF and CCP domains.

The efficient build-up of proteins from individual domains during evolution appears to depend on two aspects of genomic structure. First, there should be an approximate concordance of the domain ends with intron/exon boundaries. Secondly the position of the intron with respect to the reading frame of a gene should be such that an open reading frame results from the recombination of an exon into the intron of an existing sequence [34]. The term "module" is often used for these types of domains [1]. Introns that are inserted after the first base of a codon are called phase 1, those after the second base, phase 2, and those between codons, phase 0 [35]. Analysis of the intron/exon boundaries of domains present on leucocyte surface molecules shows that they are usually of phase 1 type as illustrated in Table 2. Duplication and recombination of such exons may lead to a different combination of exons within a gene but because of the continuity of phase of the intron/exon boundaries (Table 2), a new open reading frame is still formed. The domain does not need to be contained within a single exon to allow shuffling as long as the outermost intron/exon boundaries, corresponding to the ends of domains, are compatible. For instance some IgSF domains are coded for by two exons [13] and the cytokineR domain in the CD132 is also coded by two exons. In the latter case the internal splice site is phase 2 whilst the external ones are phase 1; thus it is not possible to get half of the domain integrated into a sequence containing phase 1 splice sites although multiples of the full domain can be duplicated.

One of the consequences of the mechanisms of domain duplication and shuffling discussed above is that the domains are unlikely to be found either with insertions or as partial domains. However the fact that some domains can be found with introns within the coding sequence for a module leads to the possibility that insertions are possible. So far, examples of this are rare with one example in the neural cell adhesion molecule (NCAM or CD56) where a short exon is alternatively spliced leading to a sequence called VASE of 10 amino acids being inserted into the

Table 2 *Exon boundaries for domains present in leucocyte surface molecules*

Domain or repeat type	Do the domain boundaries coincide with introns with same splice sites?	Splice site	Usual number of exons per domain
Complement control protein (CCP)	Yes	type 1	1
CytokineR	Yes	type 1	2
Death domain	No		
EGF	Yes	type 1	1
Fibronectin type II	Yes	type 1	1
Fibronectin type III	Yes	type 1	1
Galectin (lectin S-type)	No		
IgSF	Yes	type 1	1 or 2
ITAM motif	No		
Lectin C-type (e.g. selectins)	Yes	type 1	1
Lectin C-type (e.g. Kupffer cell R)	No		
Leucine-rich repeat	No		
Link	Yes	type 1	1
LDLRSF	Yes	type 1	1
Ly-6	No		
MHC	Yes	type 1	1
Protein tyrosine phosphatase	No		
Protein tyrosine kinase	No		
ScavengerR cysteine-rich	Yes	type 1	1[a]
Somatomedin B	Yes	type 1	1
Tumour necrosis factorSF	No		
Tumour necrosis factorRSF	No		

In both IgSF and CCP domains there are examples where a domain is encoded by two exons and also where two domains are encoded by one exon. Only limited data are available on some of the domains and it is possible that other examples with different numbers of exons per domain or motif may be found.
[a] See recent data on CD6[36].

fourth IgSF domain[37]. A similar mechanism seems likely to be responsible for the large insertion in domain of the LAG-3 protein although there is no evidence that this is alternatively spliced. The possibility that domains originated from smaller subdomains is possible but difficult to prove. The finding that an IgSF domain of CD2 can form a folding intermediate involving half domains from two polypeptides suggests that the domain may have arisen from a homodimer of half domains[38]. Galectin 2 is unusual in that three β strands within one sheet are formed by a contiguous sequence contained within one exon and all residues involved in carbohydrate binding are present in this region. This raises the possibility that this region originated as a functional mini-domain[39]. It is notable that the cytoplasmic parts of membrane proteins, or indeed most cytosolic proteins, do not contain modules as defined above. For instance the CD45 antigen contains two domains with sequence similarity to phosphotyrosine phosphatases and one has clear enzymatic activity but the intron/exon boundaries do not correlate with these structural features[33].

Another feature of the extracellular parts of leucocyte membrane proteins is that they are often poorly conserved between species, e.g. around 40–50% amino acid identity for CD4, CD8 and CD45 between rodents and man which contrasts with around 90% for the cytoplasmic part of CD45 and many cytosolic proteins. One suggestion is that cytosolic proteins need to interact with more than one protein and so mutations in one protein would need to be compensated by complementary mutations in two or more proteins to maintain the desired interactions. Alternatively, a higher rate of mutations will increase the risk of new, "non-specific interactions" occurring. Although these may be of very low affinity, they may cause unwanted interactions at the high concentrations of proteins found in the cytosol. Weak, non-specific interactions may be less of a problem at the cell surface because the surface proteins are continuously recycling and are usually glycosylated. It is possible that a major function of glycosylation, which is a feature of most cell surface proteins, is to provide a shield to prevent unwanted interactions. Receptor aggregation is often a key step in signalling events across the cell membrane and fortuitous aggregation due to non-specific interactions could affect the balance of signalling with potentially undesirable effects. Although this rapid divergence of extracellular domains is particularly common in leucocyte membrane proteins, it may not be general to all tissues. Thus there are several examples in the nervous system of high levels of conservation between membrane proteins, e.g. IgSF proteins such as myelin protein P_0 and NCAM.

THE DOMAINS AND SUPERFAMILIES THAT ARE FOUND IN LEUCOCYTE CELL SURFACE MOLECULES

The frequency of the different types of domains and motifs found in leucocyte membrane proteins are summarized in Table 3 and itemized in Table 1 of Chapter 1. It is clear that IgSF domains are the most common domain type, present in about 34% of leucocyte antigens and these are often involved in protein interactions. Fn3 and cytokineR domains have a similar Ig-like fold to the IgSF domains. Thus about 54% of leucocyte membrane proteins contain at least one domain with an Ig fold. TNFSF domains are often present as trimeric proteins and exist in membrane-associated and soluble forms and the latter have cytokine activities. Integrins are involved in adhesion events with membrane proteins and extracellular matrix. IgSF and Fn3 domains are common in cytokine receptors and these are usually complexes of two or three different polypeptides. Thus by analysis of the sequence some idea of the function of a protein may be obtained.

The superfamilies that are present in leucocyte surface molecules are discussed below, together with alignments of their amino acid sequences. The alignments were made using a variety of computer programs, ALIGN[23], AMPS[40], PILEUP[41], and then modified after visual examination. The ends of the domains can be difficult to define from the sequence and this problem is illustrated by consideration of the structure for CD4. In CD4 the last β strand of domain 1 continues directly into domain 2 and the last β strand of domain 3 also continues to form the first β strand of domain 4[42-44]. Thus in the alignments shown, the domains are defined with respect to key internal residues that are marked with an asterisk and the beginnings and ends can be taken for statistical comparisons as being a constant number of residues before and after the conserved positions. For example, in the case of the IgSF this is taken as 20 residues before and after the conserved Cys positions. If the goal was to express a single domain in an expression system then sequence alignments and structure should be taken into account and a structural prediction would be attempted on the basis of all the data to decide on the

Table 3 *Analysis of structural features of leucocyte surface molecules*

Domain type	% of leucocyte antigens where domain is present
A Distribution of superfamily domains or motifs in extracellular parts of leucocyte antigens	
CCP	5
CytokineR	8
EGF	4
Fibronectin type II	1
Fibronectin type III	12
Galectin (lectin S-type)	<1
IgSF	34
Integrin	8
Lectin C-type	6
LRR	2
Link	<1
LDLR	1
Ly-6	2
MHC	2
TNFSF	3
TNFRSF	3
ScavengerRCR	3
Somatomedin B	<1
B Percentage of domains in the intracellular parts of leucocyte antigens	
Phosphotyrosine phosphatase (PTPase)	1
Tyrosine kinase	2

Note that leucocyte polypeptides often contain more than type of domain or motif.

sequence that should be expressed. In order to obtain stable proteins it may be advantageous to have a few extra amino acids at the N-terminus of a domain as discussed in ref. 45.

Complement control protein (CCP) domains (Figs 1 and 2)

This domain is named CCP because it is commonly found in proteins that control the complement cascade [46]. For instance Factor H consists solely of 20 CCP domains whilst other complement components contain CCP domains mixed with other domains, e.g. Factor B and C2 each contain three CCP domains together with a serine protease domain. The CCP domain is also commonly called the short consensus repeat (SCR) or Sushi [46]. It is present in widely different numbers in cell surface molecules, ranging from 30 domains in complement receptor 1 (CD35) to two in L-selectin (CD62L). These domains are clearly involved in protein binding and the CR1 (CD35) and CR2 (CD21) complement binding regions have been mapped to the first four CCP domains of each of the first three groups of seven domains in CD35 and to the first two domains of CD21.

The structure of a pair of CCP domains from complement control protein Factor H (domains 15+16), has been solved using NMR [47]. Each domain consists of two segments of antiparallel β sheet and a short triple-stranded β sheet with no α-helical structure [47,48]. The folding pattern for this domain is shown in Fig. 2 and the β strand positions are marked above the sequence alignments shown in Fig. 1.

```
Factor H    L P C K S - P P E I S H G V V A H M - - - - - S D S Y Q Y G E E V T Y K C F E G
CD35 d12    R V C Q P - P P D V L H A E R T Q R D K - - - - D N F S P G Q E V F Y S C E P G
Factor B    G S C S L - - - E G V E I K G G S F R L - - - - - - L Q E G Q A L E Y V C P S G
CD62L       I Q C E - - P L E A P E L G T M D C T H P - - L G N F N F N S Q C A F S C S E G
C4BPA       N S C I N - L P D I P H A S W E T Y P R P T K E D V Y V V G T V L R Y R C H P G
IL-2R1      E L C D D D P P E I P H A T F K A M - - - - - - A Y K E G T M L N C E C K R G
FXIII       E P C T V - N V D Y M R N N I E M K W - K Y E G K V L H G D L I D F V C K Q G
              *

Factor H    F G I D G P A - - - - - I A K C L G - E K W S H P - - - - - - - - - P S C I
CD35 d12    Y D L R G A A - - - - - S M R C T P Q G D W S P A A - - - - - - - - - P T C E
Factor B    F Y P Y P V Q - - - - - T R T C R S T G S W S T L K T Q D Q K T V R K A E C R
CD62L       T N L T G I E - - - - - E T T C E P F G N W S S P E - - - - - - - - P T C Q
C4BPA       Y K P T T D E P T - - - T V I C Q K N L R W T P Y Q - - - - - - - - - G C E
IL-2R1      F R R I K S G S L - - - Y M L C T G N S S H S S W D N Q C - - - - - Q C T
FXIII       Y D L S P L T P L S E L S V Q C N R - G E V K Y - - - - - - - - - - P L C T
                                                                                   *
```

Figure 1 *CCP domains. Residues identical in four or more sequences are boxed. The lines above the sequences correspond to the positions of the β strands determined from the structure of Factor H domain 16, residues 927–985 (see Fig. 2)[48]. The asterisks mark the positions of the conserved residues used to identify domains for the corresponding entries in Section II. The sequences of the following proteins are from the SWISSPROT database unless otherwise indicated and the database accession number and residue numbers are given in brackets. Factor H, human complement Factor H precursor domain 16 (P08603, 929–985); CD35 d12, complement receptor 1 precursor domain 12 (P17927, 745–799); Factor B, human complement Factor B precursor (P00751, 35–99); CD62L, human CD62L or L-selectin precursor (P14151, 195–252); C4BPA, human complement C4 binding protein (P04003, 249–313); IL-2R1, human interleukin 2 receptor α chain (CD25) precursor (P01589, 22–83); FXIII, human coagulation Factor XIII B chain precursor (P05160, 452–516).*

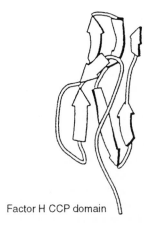

Factor H CCP domain

Figure 2 *The folding pattern of a CCP domain. Ribbon diagram showing the folding pattern of CCP domain 16 from Factor H determined by NMR[48]. The β strands are shown as broad arrows pointing from the N- to C-terminal direction and the connecting loops as thinner lines.*

Cytokine receptor (cytokineR) domains (Figs 3 and 4)

The cytokine receptor domain is often found in association with Ig and Fn3 domains in receptors for cytokines. A common arrangement is to have a single N-terminal cytokineR domain followed by a Fn3 domain, but there are variations on this theme. Initially these two domain types were not distinguished [20] and the term haematopoietin receptor superfamily was widely used for molecules containing this pair of domain types [49,50]. We use the term cytokine receptor domain for the region of about 100 amino acids usually found N-terminal to the Fn3 domain and alignments of domains from this superfamily are shown in Fig. 3. The IL-7 receptor contains a clear Fn3 domain but the sequence at the N-terminal region shows only a marginal similarity to the cytokineR domains. The possible cytokineR domain in the IL-7 receptor [50,51] is shown below the other sequences in Fig. 3 but the correctness or otherwise of this assignment will require validation by tertiary structure determination.

The structures of the extracellular region of the growth hormone receptor and the related prolactin receptor have been solved by X-ray crystallography [29,52]. This has revealed the fold for the cytokineR and the Fn3 domains that constitute the extracellular portion of this receptor. (The structure of Fn3 domains from fibronectin and neuroglian have been solved by NMR and X-ray crystallography – see below.) Both the cytokineR and the Fn3 domains have similar folds which are also similar to the folds of IgSF C2-set domains, e.g. in CD4 [42–44], CD2 [53,54] and telokin (Fig. 4) [55]. Bazan [56] had previously argued that there may be structural similarities between cytokineR domains, Fn3 domains and IgSF domains on the basis of predicting patterns of β strands in the sequences. Despite the success of these predictions the degree of sequence similarity between these domain types is low. The cytokineR domains have a characteristic Cys-X-Trp sequence together with three other conserved Cys residues, whilst the Fn3 domains lack a conserved pattern of Cys residues. The possible origin of the cytokineR, Fn3 and IgSF domains by divergent evolution is discussed above (see **Domain sequence and structure**).

Epidermal growth factor (EGF) domains (Figs 5 and 6)

EGF domains are found in EGF itself and in transforming growth factor α (TGFα). This domain type is also found in a variety of secreted proteins such as blood coagulation factor IX and cell surface molecules such as in three selectins, L-selectin, E-selectin and P-selectin (CD62). The structures of several EGF domains have been determined and all show similarity in folding pattern, e.g. EGF [57], TGFα [58], Factor IX EGF domain [59,60] and the EGF domain found in CD62$_E$ [61]. The structures of EGF and Factor IX EGF domains are shown in Fig. 6. The latter is slightly smaller than EGF itself but is probably representative of the repeating EGF domains found in many proteins (see Fig. 5). The single EGF domain from Factor IX has functional activities distinct from the EGF itself, for example it has Ca^{2+} binding activity [59,62]. The structure of a pair of calcium binding EGF domains in human fibrillin 1 have been determined by NMR and it is likely that the orientation of tandem EGF domains can vary [63]. In addition to mediating interactions directly, EGF domains may be important in giving the correct spacing and orientation of other domains.

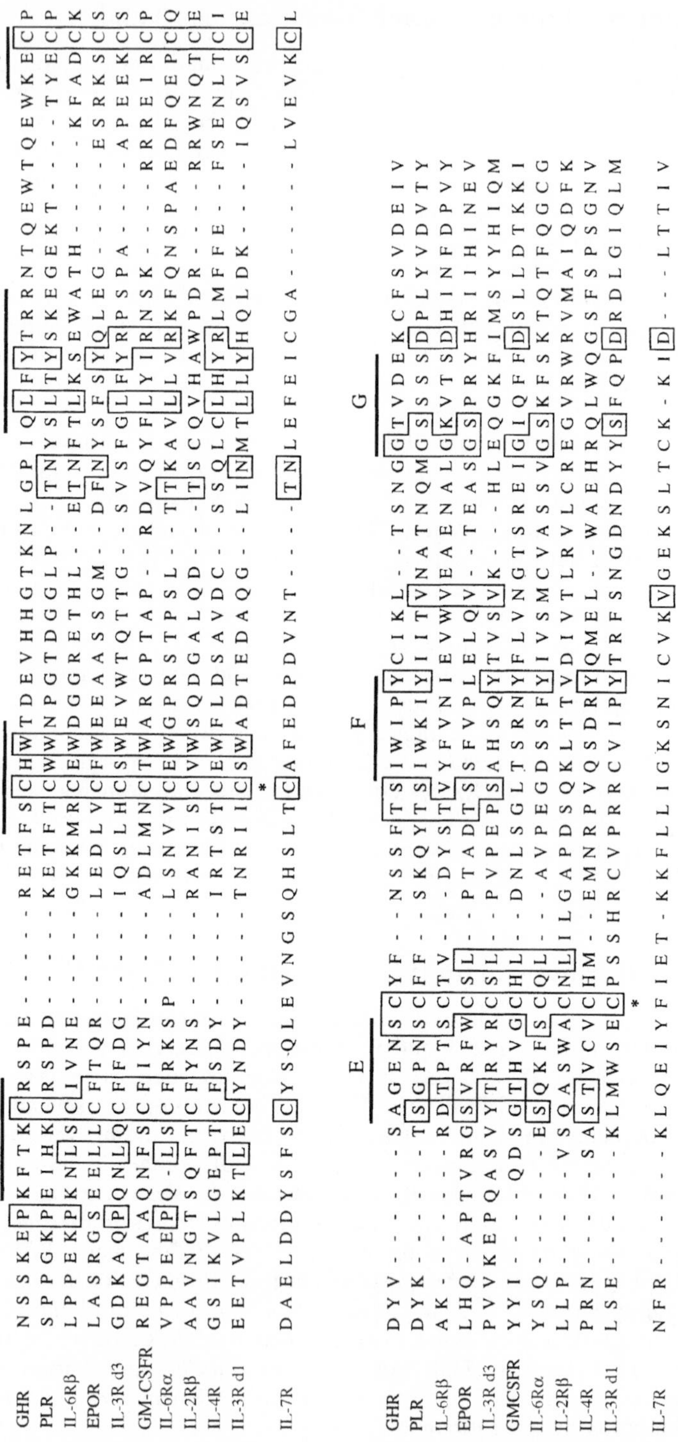

Figure 3 *Cytokine receptor (cytokineR) domains*

Figure 3 (opposite) *CytokineR domains. Residues identical in four or more sequences are boxed. The asterisks mark the positions of the conserved residues used to identify domains for the corresponding entries in Section II. The sequences of the following proteins are from the SWISSPROT database unless otherwise indicated and the database accession number and residue numbers are given in brackets. GHR, human growth hormone receptor precursor (P10912, 46–147); PLR, rat prolactin receptor precursor (P05710, 21–116); IL-6Rβ, human IL-6 receptor β (CD130, gp130) precursor (P40189 124–218); EPOR, mouse erythropoietin receptor precursor (P14753, 42–140); IL-3R, mouse IL-3 receptor precursor (CDw123) domains 1 and 3 (PIR: A35782, d1 29–127; d3 243–347); GM-CSFR, human GM-CSFR precursor (CD116) (P15509, 116–214); IL-6Rα, human IL-6 receptor α chain precursor (CD126) (P08887, 112–214); IL-2Rβ; human IL-2 receptor β chain precursor (CD122) (P14784, 26–125); IL-4R, mouse IL-4 α chain receptor precursor (CD124) (P16382, 24–122); IL-7R, human IL-7 receptor α chain precursor (CD127) (P16871, 32–127). The sequence alignments are from 20 amino acids N-terminal from the conserved CXW. The sequence start corresponds to residue 2 in the prolactin receptor. The C-terminus is more difficult to define due to the lack of conserved residues and that shown is close to the predicted boundary between the cytokineR domains and the Fn3 domains in GHR, PLR, IL-6R (CD126) . The evidence for a cytokineR domain in IL-7R (CD127) is controversial and this sequence is given below the main alignments.*

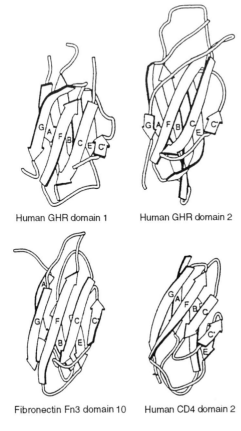

Human GHR domain 1

Human GHR domain 2

Fibronectin Fn3 domain 10

Human CD4 domain 2

Figure 4 *The folding patterns of the cytokineR and fibronectin type III (Fn3) domains. Ribbon diagrams for the cytokineR (domain 1) and Fn3 (domain 2) from human growth hormone receptor*[29]*, and Fn3 domain 10 from human fibronectin*[30]*. The IgSF C2-set domain from human CD4 domain 2 is included for comparison*[42,43]*. The β strands are shown as broad arrows pointing from the N- to C-terminal direction and the connecting loops as thinner lines. Some gaps are present in the loops of the growth hormone receptor where the structure has not been fully resolved*[29]*. Each β strand is labelled using the same nomenclature as in the IgSF. This lettering corresponds to that in the sequence alignments (Figs 3, 8 and 15).*

```
FA9-1    V D G D Q C - - E S N P C L N G G S C K D - - D I N S Y E C W C P F G F E G K - - N C E L
FA9-2    - D V T C C N I - K N G R C - - E Q F C K N S - A D N K V V C S C T E G Y R L A E N Q K S C E P
EGF      N S D S E C P L S H D G Y C L H D G V C M Y I E A L D K Y A C N C V V G Y I G E - - - R C Q Y
CD62L    - - T A S C - - Q P W S C S G H E C V E - - I I N N Y T C N C D V G Y Y G P - - - Q C Q F
CD62P    - - T A S C - - Q D M S C S K Q G E C L E - - T I G N Y T C S C Y P G F Y G P - - - E C E Y
CD62E    - - T A A C - - T N T S C G H G E C V E - - T I N N Y T C K C D P G F S G L - - - K C E Q
PRTC     P L E H P C - - A S L C C G H G T C I D - - G I G S F S C D C R S G W E G R - - F C Q R
114/A10  G P S D L C - - N P N P C K G T A S C V K - - L H S K H F C L C L E G Y Y N S S L S S C V K
NOTCH    T N D E D C - - T E S S C L N G G S C I D - - G I N G Y N C L C L A G Y S G A - - - N C Q Y
              *                                                           *
```

Figure 5 *EGF domains. Residues identical in five or more sequences are boxed. The asterisks mark the positions of the conserved residues used to identify domains for the corresponding entries in Section II. The sequences of the following proteins are from the SWISSPROT database and the database accession number and residue numbers are given in brackets. FA9-1 and FA9-2, human coagulation Factor IX precursor (P00740, 92–130 and 131–172); EGF, human epidermal growth factor precursor (P01133, 971–1014), CD62L, human CD62L or L-selectin precursor (P14151, 157–193); CD62P, human CD62P or P-selectin precursor (P16109, 160–196); CD62E, human CD62E or E-selectin precursor (P16581, 138–176); PRTC, human protein C precursor (P04070, 96–133), NOTCH; Drosophila notch protein (P19467, 232–274), 114/A10; mouse haematopoietic cell surface protein 114/A10 precursor (P07207, 1021–1059). The ends of the alignment correspond to those of the coagulation Factor IX EGF domain whose structure has been determined*[59]*. The structure of EGF itself has been determined for a sequence that extends a further four residues beyond that shown (see Fig. 6)*[57]*.

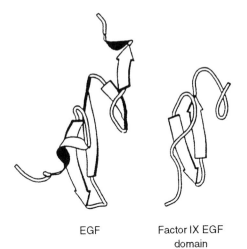

Figure 6 *The folding pattern of EGF domains. Ribbon diagrams of EGF[57] and a coagulation Factor IX EGF domain[59]. The β strands are shown as broad arrows pointing from the N- to C-terminal direction and the connecting loops as thinner lines. The N-terminal core of the structure is similar in both domains but the EGF structure extends further with two more short β strands.*

EGF

Factor IX EGF
domain

Fibronectin type II (Fn2) domains (Fig. 7)

The Fn2 domains were first identified as one of three different repeating sequence patterns within the fibronectin molecule. The Fn2 domain has been found in few other proteins and the only leucocyte molecules with this domain are the mannose receptor and DEC-205 which each contain one Fn2 domain. The structure of a sequence from bovine seminal fluid protein PDC-109 that shows sequence

```
                                                    *
Fibr d1      T A V T Q T Y G G N S N G E P C V L P F T Y N G R T F Y S
Fibr d2      T V L V Q T Q G G N S N G A L C H F P F L Y N N H N Y T D
Mannose R    Y E A M Y T L L G N A N G A T C A F P F K F E N K W Y A D
Factor XII   K A E E H T V V L T V T G E P C H F P F Q Y H R Q L Y H K
Collag       R A D S T V M G G N S A G E L C V F P F T F L G K E Y S T

                                                    *
C T T E G R Q D G H L W C S T T S N Y E Q D Q K Y S F C T D H T
C T S E G R R D N M K W C G T T Q N Y D A D Q K F G F C P M A A
C T S A G R S D G W L W C G T T T D Y D T D K L F G Y C P L K F
C T H K G R P G P Q P W C A T T P N F D Q D Q R W G Y C L E P K
C T S E G R G D G R L W C A T T S N F D S D K K W G F C P D Q G
```

Figure 7 *Fibronectin type II (Fn2) domains. Residues identical in three or more sequences are boxed. The asterisks mark the positions of the conserved residues used to identify domains for the corresponding entries in Section II. The sequences of the following proteins are from the SWISSPROT database and the database accession number and residue numbers are given in brackets. Fibr, human fibronectin precursor (P02751; d1, 345–405; d2, 405–465); Mannose R, human mannose receptor precursor (P22897, 153–212); Factor XII, human coagulation factor XII precursor (P00748, 32–91); Collag, human type V collagenase precursor (EC 3.4.24.7) (P14780, 332–391). The ends of the alignments are based on the exon boundaries of the fibronectin type II domains.*

similarity over part of the Fn2 domain alignment shown in Fig. 7 has been determined by NMR [64].

Fibronectin type III (Fn3) domains (Figs 4 and 8)

The largest group of Fn3 domains in leucocytes is found in many of the receptors for cytokines. These polypeptides also contain cytokineR domains (see above) and often have a characteristic WSXWS sequence between β strands F and G. The Fn3 domain is also particularly common in membrane molecules found in the nervous system, which in addition often have IgSF domains [13,65]. Fn3 domains are also found within cells including large numbers in the group of muscle proteins that bind myosin such as twitchin in *Caenorhabditis elegans* [66] and also in titin in vertebrates [67,68]. Fn3 domains, together with IgSF domains, are one of the few examples of domains present both intracellularly and extracellularly in leucocytes. Another example of cytoplasmic localization of Fn3 domains is in the cytoplasmic segment of the integrin $\beta4$ chain [69] (note the external regions of integrins do not contain any Fn3 domains). This is currently the only example of a domain found at the surface of leucocytes which is also present on the cytoplasmic side of a trans-membrane protein (the muscle proteins discussed above are not membrane associated).

Several structures for Fn3 domains have been solved by NMR [30] and X-ray crystallography [29,52,70]. This domain consists of two β sheets with a similar folding pattern to the IgSF fold, the cytokineR domain and the domains of the PapD chaperone protein [28]. However, there is no significant sequence similarity amongst these proteins as analysed by the methods discussed above. Recently, the structures of a pair of Fn3 domains from neuroglian and four domains of fibronectin have been determined by X-ray crystallography [70,71]. These structures have shown that the orientations between domains can vary considerably within and between proteins.

Figure 8 (opposite) *Fibronectin type III (Fn3) domains. Residues identical in five or more sequences are boxed. The positions of the β strands determined for domain 10 of human fibronectin are indicated above the sequences [30]. See Fig. 4 for folding patterns of Fn3 domains from fibronectin and growth hormone receptor. The asterisks mark the positions of the conserved residues used to identify domains for the corresponding entries in Section II. The sequences of the following proteins are from the SWISSPROT database unless otherwise indicated and the database accession number and residue numbers are given in brackets. GHR, human growth hormone receptor precursor (P10912, 148–251); Fibr, human fibronectin precursor (P02751: d1 605–700, d2 719–809, d5 996–1085, d10 1447–1541); LAR, human LAR precursor (P10586, 596–694); TWIT, twitchin cytoplasmic protein from* Caenorhabditis elegans *(PIR: S07571 1761–1854); L1, mouse neural adhesion molecule L1 precursor (P11627, 916–1012); IL-7R, human IL-7 receptor precursor (CD127) (P16871, 128–231); IL-6Rβ, human IL-6 receptor β chain precursor (gp130) (PIR: A36337, 221–324); PLR, rat prolactin receptor precursor (P05710, 121–224); IL-3LR, mouse IL-3 receptor-like protein precursor (AIC2B) (PIR: A35782, d2 135–243, d4 342–441).*

Figure 8 *Fibronectin type III (Fn3) domains*

A

Fibr-10	V S D V P R D L E V V A A T P T - - - - -
GHR	Q P D P P I A L N W T L L N V S L T G I H A D I Q K
Fibr-1	Y P I S S S G P V F I T E T P S - - - - -
Fibr-2	S P L V A T S E S V T E I T A - - - - -
Fibr-5	K L D A P T N L Q F V N E T - - - - -
LAR	P S A P P Q K V M C V S M G S - - - - -
TWIT	R P D R P G R P E P T D W D S - - - - -
L1	V P G H P E A L H L E C Q S D - - - - -
IL-7R	K P E A P F D L S V I Y R E G A - - - - -
IL-6Rβ	K P N P P H N L S V I N S E E L S - - - - -
PLR	I V E P P R N L T L E V K Q L K D - - - - -
IL-3LR d2	Q P P L P K N V S I S S S E D - - - - -
IL-3LR d4	I Q M E P P T L N L T K N R D - - - - -

B

Fibr-10	S L L I S W D A P A V T - - - - -
GHR	R W E A P R N A D I Q K - - - - -
Fibr-1	Q V R W E A P R N A D I Q K - -
Fibr-2	H P I Q W N A P Q P S H - - - - -
Fibr-5	S I S F V R W T P P R A Q - - - - -
LAR	T T V R V S W V P P A D S R N G - -
TWIT	D H V D L K W D P P L S D G G A - -
L1	T S L L L H W Q P P L S H N G - - - -
IL-7R	N D F V T F N T S H L Q K K Y V - -
IL-6Rβ	S I L K L T W T N P S I K S V - - - -
PLR	R F L L E W S V S L G D A Q V S W L S S K D I E F E V A Y K R L Q
IL-3LR d2	S I Y S L H W E T Q K M A Y - - - -
IL-3LR d4	*

C

Fibr-10	V R Y Y R I T Y G E T G
GHR	G W M V L E Y E L Q Y K E V N
Fibr-1	I S K Y I L R W R P K N
Fibr-2	V S G F R V E Y E L S -
Fibr-5	I T G Y R L T V G L T R
LAR	V I T Q Y S V A H E A V D
TWIT	P I E E Y Q I E K R T K Y
L1	V L T G L L S Y H P V E
IL-7R	K V L M H D V A Y R Q E K
IL-6Rβ	I L K Y N I Q Y R T K D
PLR	G W F T M E Y E I R L K P E E
IL-3LR d2	S F I E H T F Q V Q Y K K K S

C'

Fibr-10	G N S P V Q E F T V P G S - -
GHR	- E T K W K M M D P I L - -
Fibr-1	S V G R W K E A T I P G -
Fibr-2	E E G D E P Q Y L D L P S -
Fibr-5	- R G Q P R Q Y N V G P S -
LAR	G E D R G R H V V D G I S -
TWIT	- G R W E P I T V P G -
L1	G E S K E Q L F F N L S D P -
IL-7R	D E N K W T H V N L S S T -
IL-6Rβ	- A S T W S Q I P P E D T A S T R S S
PLR	- A E E W E I H F T G - -
IL-3LR d2	- D S W E D A Y S L H T S K F
IL-3LR d4	- D S W E D S K T E N L - D R A H S

E

Fibr-10	K S T A T I S G L K
GHR	T T S V P V Y S L K
Fibr-1	H L N S Y T I K G L K
Fibr-2	T A T S V N I P D L L P
Fibr-5	V S K Y P L R N L Q
LAR	R E H S S W D L V G L E
TWIT	G Q T T A T V P D L T
L1	E L R T H N L T N L N P
IL-7R	K L T L L Q R K L Q
IL-6Rβ	S F T V Q D L K P F
PLR	H Q T Q F K V F D L
IL-3LR d2	Q V N F E P K L F
IL-3LR d4	M D L S Q L E P D T S

F

Fibr-10	P G V D Y T I T V Y A V T G R G D S P - -
GHR	V D K E Y E V R V R S K Q R N S G - -
Fibr-1	P G V V Y E G Q L I S I Q Q Y G H - -
Fibr-2	R K Y I V N V Y Q I S E D G E - - - -
Fibr-5	A S E Y T V S L V A I K G N Q E - - -
LAR	K W T E Y R V W V R A H T D V G P G - -
TWIT	P N E E Y E F R V V A V N K G G P - - -
L1	O Y R F Q L Q A T T Q Q G G - - -
IL-7R	A A M Y E I K V R S I P D H Y F -
IL-6Rβ	T E Y V F R I R C M K E D G -
PLR	Y P G Q K Y L V Q T R C K P D H G -
IL-3LR d2	L P N S I Y A P R V R T R L Y P G
IL-3LR d4	K F Q V N Y C A R V R V K P I S N Y -

G

Fibr-10	A S S K P I S I N Y R T E
GHR	- N Y G E F S E V L Y V T L
Fibr-1	- Q E V R F D F T T T
Fibr-2	- Q S L I L S T S Q T T
Fibr-5	- S P K A T G V F T T L
LAR	- P E S S P V L V R T D
TWIT	- S I D P S D A S K A V I
L1	- P G E A I V R E G G T M
IL-7R	K G F W S E W S P S Y Y F R T P E I
IL-6Rβ	K G Y W S D W S E E A S G I T Y E D
PLR	- Y W S R W S Q E S S V E M P N D
IL-3LR d2	S S L S G R P S R W S P E A H W D S Q P Q
IL-3LR d4	- D G I W S K W S E E Y T W K T D W V

49

Galectin or the lectin S-type domains (Figs 9 and 10)

Galactoside binding proteins have been sequenced from several species and shown to contain a sequence pattern different from that of the lectin C-type domain. These were termed S-type to distinguish them from lectin C-type because the first examples contained free accessible thiol groups[72]. However, they are now generally referred to as galectins[73]. They are found both intracellularly and extracellularly and a region with strong sequence similarity is found in the Mac-2 leucocyte antigen now called galectin 3 (Fig. 9). However in this case analysis of protein produced by recombinant DNA techniques shows no requirement for a reducing environment for lectin activity and no accessible thiol groups[74]. Thus the thiol requirement is no longer general for this domain type.

The structures of galectins determined by X-ray crystallography show two anti-parallel β sheets, with five and six strands each, which associate to form a β sandwich (Fig. 10). The topology is different from the Ig fold with one sheet made up of strands AJCDEF and the other sheet strands KBGHI (see Fig. 12 for topology of IgSF domains). However the galectin 2 structure does resemble some leguminous plant lectins although they lack significant sequence similarity[39].

G protein-coupled receptor or transmembrane 7 superfamily (Fig. 11)

This large superfamily of several hundred proteins are expressed by a wide range of cell types and are characterized by the presence of seven hydrophobic membrane-spanning sequences (reviewed in ref. 75 and see WWW site at ref. 76). The proteins are oriented with the N-terminus on the extracellular side and the C-terminus on the cytoplasmic side of the plasma membrane. Several names have been used to describe this superfamily such as G protein-coupled receptor, 7TMS (seven-transmembrane) and rhodopsin superfamilies and about six different groups of receptors have been distinguished[76]. We use the term G protein-coupled receptor as this is the most widely used name.

The sequence conservation is highest in the potential transmembrane segments, with most diversity in the N- and C-termini and the cytoplasmic loop between trans-membrane segments 5 and 6. Most members of the G protein-coupled receptor superfamily have been shown to couple to various G proteins and include a large family of receptors for chemokines. Many more examples may be found on leucocytes as the monoclonal antibody approach may not recognize them well because of their low site number per cell and the high degree of amino acid sequence identity between species homologues. Experiments using chimeric proteins have shown that the sequences contributing to G protein attachment are found in transmembrane segments 5 and 6 and the cytoplasmic loop between them. A subset of closely related G protein-coupled R members is found on leucocytes and includes the C5aR (CD88), fMLPR (FPR) and IL-8Rs (CDw128 and IL-8Rb). Two further members, the F4/80 and CD97 antigen are unusual in that they contain several EGF domains in their first extracellular regions[77].

Immunoglobulin (Ig) superfamily domains (Figs 12–15)

Immunoglobulin superfamily (IgSF) domains are the most abundant domain type found in leucocyte membrane proteins, as is evident from the collated data in Table

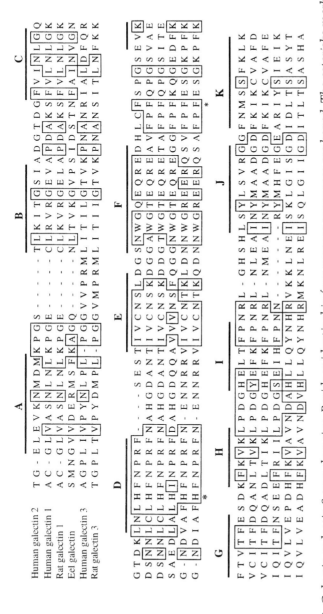

Figure 9 *Galectin or lectin S-type domains. Residues identical in four or more sequences are boxed. The asterisks mark the positions of the conserved residues used to identify domains for the corresponding entries in Section II. The positions of the β strands present in galectin 2[39] are indicated above the sequences and on the fold (Fig. 10). The sequences of the following proteins are from the SWISSPROT database and the database accession number and residue numbers are given in brackets except where the full sequence is given. Human galectin 2, human galectin 2 precursor or HL14 (P05162, 2–131); Human galectin 1, human galectin 1 or β-galactoside binding lectin (P09382); Rat galectin 1, rat galectin 1 or β-galactoside binding lectin (P11762); Eel galectin, electric eel β-galactoside binding lectin (P08520); Human galectin 3, human galectin 3 or Mac-2 antigen precursor (P17931, 111–248); Rat galectin 3, rat galectin 3 or Mac-2 antigen precursor (P08699, 123–260).*

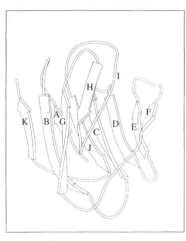

Figure 10 *The folding pattern of a galectin or lectin S-type domain. Ribbon diagram of the one domain of the homodimer of galectin 2 [39]. The β strands are shown as broad arrows pointing from the N- to C-terminal direction. Each strand is labelled and corresponds to the labels in the alignments (Fig. 9).*

3 which shows that approximately 34% of leucocyte membrane polypeptides contain IgSF domains. The structures of several IgSF domains have been determined by X-ray crystallography including Ig V- and C-domains, β_2-microglobulin [27], MHC Class I antigen $\alpha 3$ domain [78], MHC Class II $\alpha 2$ and $\beta 2$ domains [79–81], CD4 domains 1+2 and CD4 domains 3+4 [42–44], CD8α [82], CD2 [53,54,83], VCAM domain 1 [84] and T cell antigen receptor α and β V- and C-domains [85–88]. These structures show that the IgSF domains characterized by sequence similarities over about 100 amino acids correspond to structural units with distinct folding patterns referred to as the Ig fold (reviewed in ref. 27). The Ig fold consists of a sandwich of two β sheets, each consisting of antiparallel β strands of 5–10 amino acids with a conserved disulfide between the two sheets in most but not all domains (Fig. 12). The sequence similarities are mainly found at the positions of in-pointing residues in the β strands with considerable differences in the loops that connect the strands and the out-pointing residues on the faces of the β sheets. The core of the fold is made up of three β strands labelled ABE and GFC and the positioning of these is shown in the various folds illustrated in Fig. 12. The folds vary considerably in length in the middle of the sequence with Ig V-domain folds being the archetype for the longer fold. The extra sequence in comparison with C-domains forms an additional pair of β strands (C' and C" in Fig. 12) and the connection between these forms the second complementarity determining region in antibody and TCR V-domains.

In IgSF domains there are limited sequence patterns in β strands B, C, E and F that are common across the superfamily (Figs 13–15) and other patterns that allow a subdivision of the domains. Ig and TCR V-domains have a characteristic pattern in

Figure 11 (*opposite*) *G protein-coupled receptors. Residues identical in four or more sequences are boxed. The bars over the sequences indicate the transmembrane regions. The sequences of the following proteins are from the SWISSPROT database and the database accession numbers are given in brackets. IL-8R, human high-affinity IL-8 receptor [192]; C5aR, human C5a anaphylatoxin chemotactic receptor (P21730); fMLPR, human fMet-Leu-Phe receptor (P21462); Rhodopsin, human rhodopsin (P08100); NeurokininR, human neurokinin A receptor (P21452); DopaR, human D(1) dopamine receptor (P21728).*

Figure 11 *G protein-coupled receptor or transmembrane 7 superfamily*

```
                                                                    I
IL-8R        MSNITDPQMWDFDDLNFTGMPPADEDYSPCMLETETLNKYVVIIAYALVFLLSLLGNSLVMLVILYSRVGRS-
C5aR         --MNSFNYTTPDYGHYDDKDTLDLNTPVDKTSNTLRVPDILALVIFAVVFLVGVLGNALVVWVTAF-EAKRT-
fMLPR        --------------METNSSLPTNISGGTPAVSAGYLFLDIITYLVFAVTFVLGVLGNGLVIWVAGF-RMTHT-
Rhodopsin    -MNGTEGPNFYVPFSNATGVVRSPFEYPQYYLAEPWQFSMLAAYMFLLI-VLGFPINFLTLYVTVQHKKLRT-
NeurokininR  -----MGTCDIVTEANISSGPESNTTGITAFSMPSWQLALWAPAYLALV-LVAVTGNAIVIWIILAHRRMRT-
DopaR        ------------------MRTLNTSAMDGTGLVVERDFSVRILTACFLSLLILSTLLGNTLVCAAVIRFRHLRSK

            II                                      III
VTDVYLLNLALADLLFALTLPIWAASKVNG--WIFGTFLCKVVSLLKEVNFYSGILLLACISVDRYLAIVHATRTLTQKRH-LV
INAIWFLNLAVADFLSCLALPILFTSIVQHHHWPFGGAACSILPSLILLNMYASILLLATISADRFLLVFKPIWCQNFRGAGLA
VTTISYLNLAVADFCFTSTLPFFMVRKAMGGHWPFGWFLCKFLFTIVDINLFGSVFLIALIALDRCVCVLHPVWTQNHRTVSLA
PLNYILLNLAVADLFMVLGGFTSTLYTSLHGYFVFGPTGCNLEGFFATLGGEIALWSLVVLAIERYVVVCKPMSNFRFGENH-A
VTNYFIVNLALADLCMAAFNAAFNFVYASHNIWYFGRAFCYFQNLFPITAMFVSIYSMTAIAADRYMAIVHPFQP-RLSAPS-T
VTNFFVISLAVSDLLVAVLVMPWKAVAEIAGFWPFGS-FCNIWVAFDIMCSTASILNLCVISVDRYWAISSPFRYERKMTPKAA

      IV                                                          V
KFVCLGCWGLSMNLSLPFFLFRQAYHPNNSSPV-CYEVLGNDTAKWR----------MVLRILPHTFGFIVPLFVMLFCYGFTLRT
WIACAVAWGLALLLTIPSFLYRVVREEYFPPKVLCGVDYSH--DKRRER---------AVAIVRLVLGFLWPLLTLTICYTFILLR
KKVIIGPWVMALLLTLPVII-RVTTVPGKTGTVACTFNFSPWTNDPKERINVAVAMLTVRGIIRFIIGFSAPMSIVAVSYGLIATK
IMGVAFTWVMALACAAPPLAGWSRYIPEGLQCS-CGDYI----------YTLKPEVNNESFVIYMFVVHFTIPMIIIFFCYGQLVFT
KAVIAGIWLVALALASPQCFYSTVTMDQGATK--CVAWV----------PEDSGGKTLLLYHLVVIALIYFLPLAVMFVAYSVIGLT
FILISVAWTLSVLISFIPVQLSWHKAKPTSPSDGNATSLAETID------NCDSSLSRTYAISSSVISFYIPVAIMIVTYTRIYRI

                                                           VI
LFK---------------------------------AHMGQKHRAMRVIFAVVLIFLLCWLPYNLVLLADTLMRTQVIQET
TWS---------------------------------RRATRSTKTLKVVVAVVASFFIFWLPYQVTGIM--MSFLEPSSPT
IHK---------------------------------QGLIKSSRPLRVLSFVAAAFFLCWSPYQVVALIATVRIRELLQGM
V---------------------------KEAAAQQQESATTQ--KAEKEVTRMVIIMVIAFLICWVPYASVAFYIFTHQG------
LWR---------------------------RAVPGHQAHGANLRHLQAKKKFVKTMVLVVLTFAICWLPYHLYFILGSFQEDIYCHK-
AQKQIRRIAALERAAVHAKNCQTTTGNGKPVECSQPESSFKMSFKRETKVLKTLSVIMGVFVCCWLPFFILNCILPFCGSGETQPF

                   VII
CERRNNIGRALDATEILGFLHSCLNPIIYAFIGQNFRHGFLKILA---MHGLVSKEFLARHRVTSYTSSSVNVSSNL ------
F---LLLNKLDSLCVSFAYINCCINPIIYVVAGQGFQGRLRKSLPSLLRNVLTEESVVRESKSFTRSTVDTMAQKTQAV------
Y---KEIGIAVDVTSALAFFNSCLNPMLYVFMGQDFRERLIHALPASLERALTEDS-TQTSDTATNSTLPSAEVALQAK------
SNFGPIF---MTIPAFFAKSAAIYNPVIYIMMNKQFRNCMLTTI-CCGKNPLGDDEASATVSKTETSQVAPA-----------
-FIQQVY----LALFWLAMSSTMYNPIIYCCLNHRFRSGFRLAFRCCPWVTPTKEDKLELTPTTSLSTRVNRCHTKETL  39 amino acids
CIDSNTF----DVFVWFGWANSSLNPIIYAF-NADFRKAFSTLLGCYRLCPATNNAIETVSINNNGAAMFSSHHEPRGS  64 amino acids
```

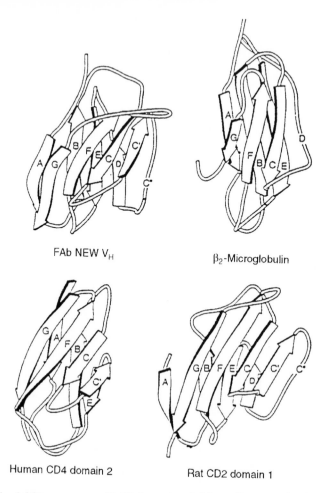

FAb NEW V$_H$

β$_2$-Microglobulin

Human CD4 domain 2

Rat CD2 domain 1

Figure 12 *The folding pattern of IgSF domains. Ribbon diagrams for four IgSF domains: Ig V-set (V$_H$ of human NEW Fab), Ig C1-set (β$_2$-microglobulin), Ig C2-set (CD4 domain 2) and Ig V-set lacking the normally conserved disulfide between β strands B and F (rat CD2 domain 1). These are labelled with the corresponding strand letters used in the alignments for the Ig V-set, C1-set and C2-set sequences (Figs 13–15) and in the Fn3 domains (Figs 4 and 8). The data are from the Brookhaven Protein Structure Database* [83].

the region leading into β strand F of Asp-X-Gly/Ala-X-Tyr-X-Cys. The receptor C-domains have a characteristic pattern between β strands B and C of Gly-Phe-Tyr-Pro and another on the C-terminal side of β strand F of Cys-X-Val-X-His. The Ig, TCR and MHC antigen C-type domains all share the same types of sequence patterns and are referred to as the C1-set within the IgSF. With the sequencing of various cell surface molecules a third category of domains became evident, namely domains of length similar to C-domains but with some of the sequence patterns of V-domains. These domains are referred to as the C2-set [13]. They have V-type patterns in the β

Figure with strand labels A, B, C, C′, C″ (first block) and D, E, F, G (second block).

First block (strands A, B, C, C′, C″):

```
                   A                    B                      C              C'               C''
Ig λ       A V V T Q E S A L T T S P G E T V T L T C R S S T G A V - T T S N Y A N W V Q Q K P - D H L F T G L I G G - - T N N R A P G V - - -
Ig κ       Q M T Q S P S S L S A S V G D R V T I T C Q A S Q D - - I S I F L N W Y Q Q K P G - K A P K L L I Y D A - - S K L E A G V - - -
IgG heavy  Q L E Q S G P G L V R P S Q T - L S L T C T V S G S - - T F S N D Y Y T W V R Q P P G - R G L E W I G Y V F Y H - G T S D D T T P L
TCRβ       G V I Q S P R H E V T E M G Q E V T L R C K P I S G H - - - N S L F W Y R Q T M M - R G L E L L I Y F N - - N V P I D D S G M P
TCRα       N V Q Q S P E S L I V P E G A R T S L N C T F S D S - - A S Q Y F W W Y R Q H S G - K A P K A L M S I F S - - N G E K E - - -
CD8 β      A L L Q T P S S L L V Q T N Q T A K M S C E A K T F P K - - G T T I Y W L R E L Q D S N K N K N K H F E F L A S R T S T K G I K Y - -
CD8 α      Q L Q L S P K K V D A E I G Q E V K L T C E V L R D T S - - - Q G C S W L F R N S S S E L L Q P T F I I Y V S S S R S K L N D I L D
CD4 d1     A A T Q G K K V V L G K K G D T V E L T C T A S Q K K - - - S I Q F H W K N S N - - - Q I K I L G N Q G - - S F L T K G P S K L
Thy-1      R G Q R V I S L T A C L V Q N L R L D C R H E N N T N L P I Q H E F S L T R E - - - K K K H V L S G T L - - G V P E H T Y - - -
CD2 d1     A D C R D S G T V W G A L G H G I N L N I P N F Q M T D - D I D E V R W E R G S - - - - T L V A E F K R K M K P F L K S G - - - -
                                        *
```

Second block (strands D, E, F, G):

```
                  D                E                        F                     G
Ig λ       P A R F S G S L I - - - - G N K A A L T I T G A Q T E D E A I Y F C A L W Y S N - - - - H W V F G G G T K L T V L
Ig κ       P S R F S G T G S - - - G T D F T F T I S S L Q P E D I A T Y Y C Q Q F D N L - - - P L T F G G G T K V D F K
IgG heavy  R S R V T M L V D T S - K N Q F S L R L S S V T A A D T A V Y Y C A R N L I A G - - C I D V W G Q G S L V T V S
TCRβ       E D R F S A K M P N A - - S F S T L K T Q P S E P R D S A V Y F C A S S F S T C S A N Y G Y T F G S G T R L T V V
TCRα       E G R F T I H L N K A - - S L H F S L H I R D S Q P S D S A L Y L C A V T L Y G G - S G N K L I F G T G T L L S V K
CD8 β      G E R V K K N M T L S F N S T L P F L K I M D V K P E D S G F Y F C S F T K N Q G G Y F C S D T Y I C E V E
CD8 α      P N L F S A R K E - - N N K Y I L T L S K F S T K N Q G Y F C S I T S N S - - - - - V M Y F S P L V P V F Q K
CD4 d1     N D R A D S R R S L W D - Q G N F P L I I K N L K I E D S D T Y I C E V E - - - - - - D Q K E E V Q L L V F
Thy-1      R S R V N L F S D R - - - F I K V L T L A N F T T K D E G D Y M C E L R V S G Q N P T S S N K T I N V I R D K L V
CD2 d1     - A F E I L A - - - - - N G D L K I K N L T R D D S G T Y N V T V Y S T N G - - - T R I L D K A L D L R I L
                                                      *
```

Figure 13 Immunoglobulin V-set domains. Residues identical in five or more sequences are boxed. The positions of the β strands are indicated above the sequences. The asterisks mark the positions of the conserved residues used to identify domains for the corresponding entries in Section II. The sequences of the following proteins are from the SWISSPROT database and the database accession number and residue numbers are given in brackets. Ig λ; mouse Ig λ chain precursor (MOPC 104E) (P01724, 21–129); Ig κ, human Ig κ chain Roy (P01608, 3–107); IgG heavy, human IgG heavy chain NEWM (P01825, 3–116); TCR β, human TCR β chain precursor (P05541, 21–134); TCR α, mouse TCR α chain precursor (P01733, 22–135); CD8 β, rat CD8 β chain precursor (P01739, 23–132); CD8 α, rat CD8 α chain precursor (P07725, 27–138); CD4 d1, human CD4 precursor domain 1 (P01730, 21–123); Thy-1, rat Thy-1 precursor (P01830, 18–128); CD2 d1, rat CD2 precursor domain 1 (P08921, 20–120).

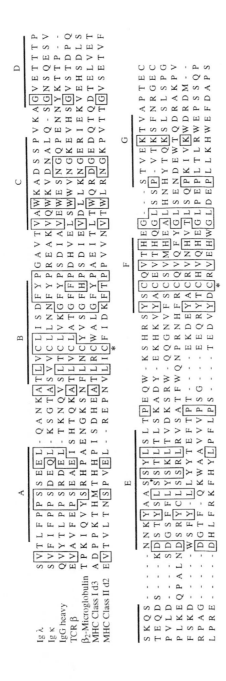

Figure 14 *Immunoglobulin C1-set domains. Residues identical in four or more sequences are boxed. The positions of the β strands are indicated above the sequences. The asterisks mark the positions of the conserved residues used to identify domains for the corresponding entries in Section II. The sequences of the following proteins are from the SWISSPROT database unless otherwise indicated and the database accession number and residue numbers are given in brackets. Ig λ, human Ig λ chain C region (P01842, 7–104); Ig κ, human Ig κ chain C region (P01834, 6–106); IgG heavy, human Ig γ-1 C region (P01857, 230–329); TCRβ, human TCRβ chain (P01850, 10–117); β₂-Microglobulin, human β₂-microglobulin precursor (P01884, 24–119); MHC Class I d3, human MHC Class I HLA α chain precursor domain 3 (PIR: A02189, 203–301); MHC Class II d2, human MHC Class II DR α chain precursor domain 2 (PIR: A02206, 113–209).*

```
                    A                         B                          C                              C'
CD4 d2       F G L T A N S D T H L L Q G Q S L T L T L E S - P P G S S P S V Q C R S P R G - - - - - - - - - K N I Q G - -
L1d3         F P T N S S S R L V A L Q G Q S L I L E C I A - E G F P T P T I K W L H P S D P M P - - - - T D R V I Y Q N
MAG d4       W K P T V N G T V V A V E G E T V S I L C S T - Q S N P D P I L T I F K E K Q I L - - - - - - A T V I Y E S
Amalgam d3   Q I A V Q R P K I A Q M V S H S A E L E C S V - Q G Y P A P T V V W H K N G V P L Q S - S R H H E V A N T A
NCAM         R A R Q S T M N A T A N L S Q S V T L A C D A - D G F P E P T M T W T K D G E P I E Q E D N E E K Y S F N Y
CEA d4       P F I T S N N S N P V E D E D A V A L T C E P - - E I Q N T T Y L W W V N N Q S L P - - - V S P R L Q L S N
IgFcRII      V V K L E P P W I Q V L K E D T V T L T C E G T H N P G N S S T Q W F H N G R - - - - - - - - - S I R S Q V
CD2 d2       Q E R V S K P - K I S W T C I N T T L T C E V M N G - T D P E L N L Y Q D G - - - - - - - - - K H L K L S -
CD3 ε        G G I T Q T P Y K V S I S G T T V I L T C - - - - P Q Y P G S E I L W Q H N D K N I G G D E D D K N I G S - -
                                                 *

                      E                        F                      G
- - - - - - G K T L S V S Q L - E L Q D S G T W T C T V L Q N Q - K K V E F K I D I V V L A F
- - - - - H N K T L Q L L N V - G E E D D G E Y T C L A E N S L - G S A R H A Y Y V T V E A A
- - - - - - Q L Q L E L P A V - T P E D D G E Y W C V A E N Q Y - G Q R A T A F N L S V E F A
S S S G T T T S V L R I D S V - G E E D F G D Y Y C N A T N K L - G H A D A R L H L F Q T V I
- - - - - D G S E L I I K K V - D K S D E A E Y I C I A E N K A - G E Q D A T I H L K V F A K
- - - - - D N R T L T L L S V - T R N D V G P Y E C G I Q N E L S V D H S D P V I L N V L Y G
- - - - - - Q A S Y T F K A - - T V N D S G E Y R C Q M E Q T - - - R L S D P V D L G V I S D
- - - - - - - Q R V I T H K W T T - S L S A K F K C T A G N K - - - - V S K E S S V E P V S C
- - - - - D E D H L S L K E F S E L E Q S G Y Y V C Y P R G S - - K P E D A N F Y L Y L R A R
                                                 *
```

Figure 15 *Immunoglobulin C2-set domains. Residues identical in four or more sequences are boxed. The positions of the β strands are indicated above the sequences. The asterisks mark the positions of the conserved residues used to identify domains for the corresponding entries in Section II. The sequences of the following proteins are from the SWISSPROT database unless otherwise indicated and the database accession number and residue numbers are given in brackets. CD4 d2, human CD4 precursor domain 2 (P01730, 123–204); L1 d3, mouse neural cell adhesion molecule L1 precursor domain 3 (P11627, 243–331); MAG d4, rat myelin-associated glycoprotein precursor domain 4 (P07722, 327–412); Amalgam d3,* Drosophila *amalgam protein precursor domain 3 (P15364, 231–327); NCAM, chicken neural cell adhesion molecule precursor (P13590, 203–295); CEA d4, human carcinoembryonic antigen precursor domain 4 (CD66e) (P06731, 325–414); IgFcRII, mouse IgG FcRII precursor (CD32) domain 1 (P08101, 37–116); CD2 d2, human CD2 precursor domain 2 (P06729, 127–203); CD3 ε, human CD3 ε precursor (P07766, 29–117).*

```
CD49a  FCVSFNVDVKNSMSFSGPVEDMFGYTVQQYENEEG--KWVLIGSPLVGQPKA----RTGDVYKCPVGRERAMPCVKLDLPV
CD49b  CCLAYNVGLPEAKIFSGPSSEQFGYAVQQFINPKG--NWLLVGSPWSGFPEN----RMGDVYKCPVDLSTA-TCEKLNLQT
CD51   LCRAFNLDVDSPAEYSGPEGSYFGFAVDFFVPSASSRMFLLVGAPKAN-TTQPGIVEGGQVLKC--DWSSTRRCQPIEFDA
CD49d  TGRPYNVDTESALLYQGPHNTLFGYSV--VLHSHGANRWLLVGAPTANWLANASVINPGAIYRCRIGKNPGQTCEQLQLGS

NTSIP----NVTEIKENMTFGSTLVTNP--NGGFLACGPLYAYRCGHLHY------TTGICSDVSPTFQVVNSFAP-VQECSTQ-
STSIP----NVTEMKTNMSLGLILTRNMG-TGGFLTCGPLWAQQCGNQYY------TTGVCSDISPDFQLSASFSPATQPCPSL-
TGNRDYAKDDPLEFKSHQWFGASVRSK---QDKILACAPLYHWRTEM----KQEREPVGTCFLQDGTKTVEY------APCRSQD
PNGEPCGK-TCLEERDNQWLGVTLSRQPGENGSIVTCG---HRWKNIFYIKNENKLPTGGCYGVPPDLRTELSKRI--APCYQDY

LDIVIVLDGSN-196 Amino acids --SQTGFSAHYS--QDWVMLGAVGAYDWNGTVVMQKANQMV---------IPHNTTFQTEPAKMNE
IDVVVVCDESN-195 Amino acids --SQVGFSADYSSQNDILMLGAVGAFGWSGTIVQKTSHGHLI---------FPKQAFDQILQDRNH-
IDADGQGF------(I Domain)---CQGGFSIDFT-KADRVLLGGPGSFYWQGQLISDQVAEIVSKYDPNVYSIKYN--NQLATRTAQA
VKKFGENFAS------------CQAGISSFYT--KDLIVMGAPGSSYWTGSLF---------------VYNITTNKYKAFLDKQNQV

PL-ASYLGYTVNSATIPGD--VLYIAGQPRYNHT-GQVVIYKMEDGNINILQTLGGEQIGSYFGSVLTTIDIDKDSYTDLLLVGA
---SSYLGYSVAAISTGES--THFVAGAPRANYTGQIVLYSVNENGNITVIQAHRGDQIGSYFGSVLCSVDVDKDTITDVLLVGA
IFDDSYLGYSVAVGDFNGDGIDDFVSGVPRAARTLGMVYIY--DGKNMSSLYNFTGEQMAAYFGFSVAATDINGDDYAD-VFIGA
KF-GSYLGYSVGAGHFRSQHTTEVVGGAPQHEQ-IGKAYIFSIDEKELNILHEMKGKKLGSYFGASVCAVDLNADGFSD-LLVGA

PMYM----GTEKEEQGKVYVYAVNQTRFEYQMSLEPIRQTCCSSLKDNSCTKENKNEPCGARFGTAIAAVKDLNVDGFNDVVIGA
PMYM-----SDLKKEEGRVYLFTIKKGILGQHQFL-----------------EGPEGIENTRFGSAIAALSDINMDGFNDVIVGS
PLFMDRGSDGKLQEVGQVSVSLQRASGDF-------------------QTTKLNGFEVF-ARFGSAIAPLGDLDQDGFNDIAIAA
PM------QSTIREEGRVFVYINSGSGAV---------------MNAMETNLVGSDKYAARFGESIVNLGDIDNDGFEDVAIGA

PL-EDDHAGAVYIYHGSGKTIREAYAQRIPSGGDG--KTLKFFGQSIHGEMDLNGDGLTDVTIGGLG--GAALFWARDVAVVKVT
PL-ENQNSGAVYIYNGHQGTIRTKYSQKILGSDGAFRSHLQYFGRSLDGYGDLNGDSITDVSIGAFG--QVVQLWSQSIADVAIE
PYGGEDKKGIVYIFNGRSTGLNAVPSQILEGQWAA-RSMPPSFGYSMKGATDIDKNGYPDLIVGAFGVDRAILYRARPVITVNAG
P-QEDDLQGAIYIYNGRADGISSTFSQRIEGLQIS-KSLSM-FGQSISGQIDADNNGYVDVAVGAFRSDSAVLLRTRPVVIVDAS

MNFEPNKVNIQKKNCRVEGK--ETVCINATMCFHVKLKSKEDSIYEADLQYRVTLD----SLRQISRSFFSGTQERKIQRNITVR
ASFTPEKITLVNKNAQIILK-----------LCFSAKFRPTKQN-NQVAIVYNITLDADGFSSRVTSRGLFKENNERCLQKNMVVN
LEVYPSILNQDNKTCSLPGTALKVSCFNVRFCLKADGKGV--LPRKLNFQVELLLDKLKQKGAIRRALFLYSRSPSHSKNMTI--
LS-HPESVNRTKFDC--VENGWPSVCIDLTLCFSYKGKEV---PGYIVLFYNMSLD-VNRKAESPPRFYFSSNGTSDVITGSIQV
```

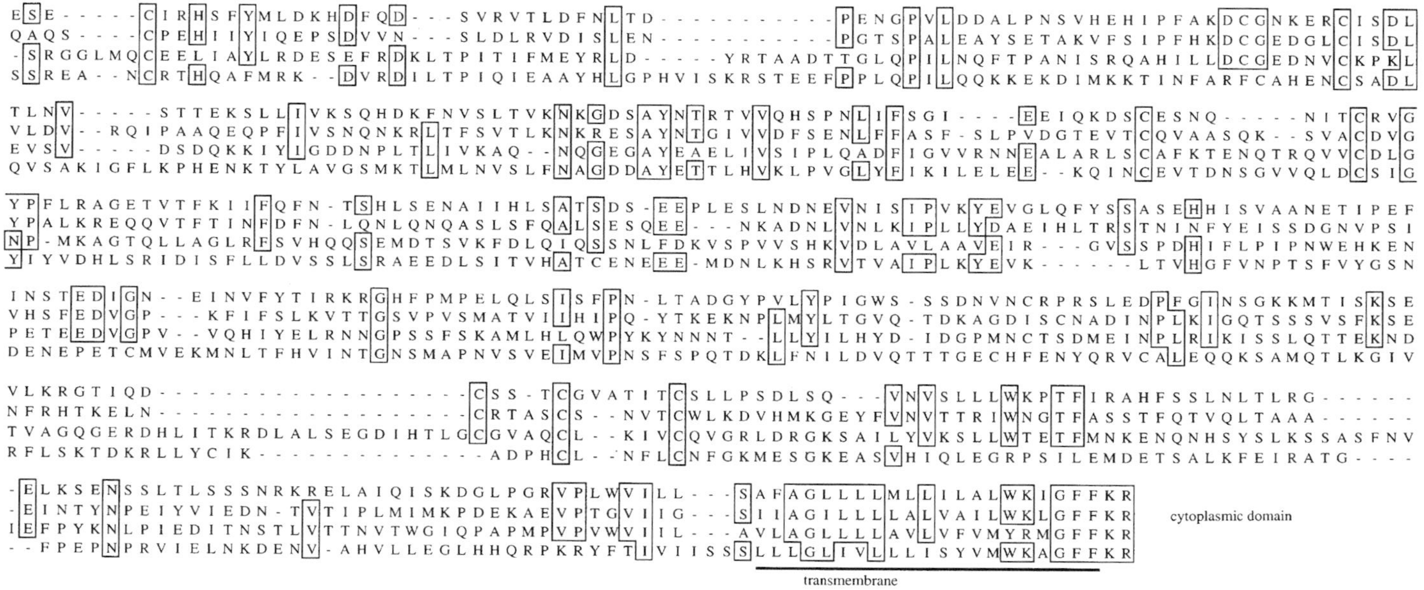

transmembrane

cytoplasmic domain

Figure 16 *Integrin α chains. Residues identical in three or more sequences are boxed. The sequences of the following proteins are from the SWISSPROT database and the database accession number and residue numbers are given in brackets. CD49a, rat integrin α1 precursor (P18614, 25–1172); CD49b, human integrin α2 precursor (P17301, 26–1161); CD51, vitronectin receptor integrin αV precursor (P06756, 27–1023); CD49d, integrin α4 precursor (P13612, 36–1013). The extracellular and transmembrane regions are shown. The position of the I-domain in those sequences where it is present is indicated. Alignments of the I-domain are shown in Fig. 18.*

strand E–F region, a pattern of Pro-X-Pro is relatively common between β strands B and C and the pattern Cys-X-Ala-X-Asn is common after β strand F. This distinction between C2- and C1-sets has been confirmed by structural studies, e.g. CD4 domain 2 is a C2-set sequence and its structure is classified in terms of sheet assignments labelled as ABE/GFCC'. This is in comparison to ABED/GFC for C1-set sequences and ABED/GFCC'C'' for V-set sequences. That is, for C2-set sequences the middle β strand may be generally in line with the GFC β sheet rather than the ABE sheet as is the case with antibody C-domains. So far, none of the structures of C2-set domains has a C1-set structure, i.e. like TCR, MHC antigens and Ig C-domains themselves. In all IgSF domains the structure of the core of the domain is maintained. The C2-set domains are mostly included in an I-set that has been defined on structural grounds (reviewed in refs 89 and 90) but in this review where in most cases only sequence data are available, we use the widely accepted C2-set nomenclature. The points about conserved patterns and the positioning in β sheets are made evident by comparing the sequence alignments in Figs 13–15 with the folding patterns for the domains in Fig. 12. The sequence alignments are discussed in more detail in ref. 13.

Integrins (Figs 16–19)

The integrins have a heterodimeric structure with α and β chains that both traverse the lipid bilayer. There are at least 16 α and 8 β chains which can be found in various but not all possible combinations. Sequence similarities are seen within the α and β chains across all the integrin types (Figs 16 and 17 and discussed in detail in refs 91–93). The integrins are known to be involved in cell interactions and include receptors for the extracellular matrix proteins fibronectin and vitronectin and for cell surface molecules CD54 (ICAM-1) and CD102 (ICAM-2). The integrins are reviewed elsewhere[94] including a companion volume in this FactsBook series[95]. They are expressed on many different cell types; the CD11/CD18 family and the CD49 very late activation antigen family (VLA) are expressed mainly on leucocytes. This family of related proteins does not generally contain other domain types. One exception is the β4 integrin that contains two Fn3 domains in the cytoplasmic region (ref. 69 and see also section on Fn3 domains).

Some integrin α chains contain an inserted sequence or I-domain which shows sequence similarity to sequences in von Willebrand factor (where the domain is usually termed the A-domain!), some matrix proteins and complement factor B (Fig. 18)[96]. The structures of two I-domains from CD11a and CD11b have recently been determined by X-ray crystallography (Fig. 19)[96,97]. The fold consists of alternating amphipathic α helices and hydrophobic β strands that form a classic dinucleotide binding fold that is a common topology of many intracellular enzymes.

Figure 17 (opposite) *Integrin β chains. Residues identical in three out of three of the sequences are boxed. The sequences of the following proteins are from the SWISSPROT database and the database accession number and residue numbers are given in brackets. β1, human fibronectin receptor – integrin β1 precursor (CD29) (P05556, 26–752); β2, human integrin β2 (CD18) precursor (P05107, 24–724); β3, human integrin β3 (CD61) precursor (P05106, 30–742). The extracellular and transmembrane regions are shown.*

Figure 17 *Integrins*

INTEGRIN BETA CHAINS

```
β1  RCLKANAKSCGECIQAGPNCGWCTNSTFLQEGMPTSARCDDLEALKKKGCPPDDIENPRGSKDIKKNKNVT
β2  ECTKFKVSSCRECIESGPGCTWCQKLNFTGPGDPDSIRCDTRPQLLMRGCAADDIMDPTSLAETQEDHNGG
β3  ICTTRGVSSCQQCLAVSPMCAWCSDEAL----PLGSPRCDLKENLLKDNCAPESIEFPVSEARVLEDRPLS

NRSKGTAEKLKPEDIHQIQPQQLVLRLRSGEPQTFTLKFKRAEDYPIDLYYLMDLSYSMKDDLENVKSLGTDLMNE
QK--------------QLSPQKVTLYLRPGQAAAFNVTFRRAKGYPIDLYYLMDLSYSMLDDLRNVKKLGGDLLRA
DKGSGDSS-----QVTQVSPQRIALRLRPDDSKNFSIQVRQVEDYPVDIYYLMDLSYSMKDDLWSIQNLGTKLATQ

MRRITSDFRIGFGSFVEKTVMPYISTTP-AKLRNPCTS-EQNCTTPFSYKNVLSLTNKGEVFNELVGKQRISGNLD
LNEITESGRIGFGSFVDKTVLPFVNTHP-DKLRNPCPNKEKECQPPFAFRHVLKLTNNSNQFQTEVGKQLISGNLD
MRKLTSNLRIGFGAFVDKPVSPYMYISPPEALENPCYDMKTTCLPMFGYKHVLTLTDQVTRFNEEVKKQSVSRNRD

SPEGGFDAIMQVAVCGSLIGWRNVT-RLLVFSTDAGFHFAGDGKLGGIVLPNDGQCHLE-NNMYTMSHYYDYPSIA
APEGGLDAMMQVAACPEEIGWRNVT-RLLVFATDDGFHFAGDGKLGAILTPNDGRCHLE-DNLYKRSNEFDYPSVG
APEGGFDAIMQATVCDEKIGWRNDASHLLVFTTDAKTHIALDGRLAGIVQPNDGQCHVGSDNHYSASTTMDYPSLG

HLVQKLSENNIQTIFAVTEEFQPVYKELKNLIPKSAVGTLSANSSNVIQLIIDAYNSLSSEVILENGKLSEGVTIS
QLAHKLAENNIQPIFAVTSRMVKTYEKLTEIIPKSAVGELSEDSSNVVHLIKNAYNKLSSRVFLDHNALPDTLKVT
LMTEKLSQKNINLIFAVTENVVNLYQNYSELIPGTTVGVLSMDSSNVLQLIVDAYGKIRSKVELEVRDLPEELSLS

YKSYCKNGVNGTGENGRKCSNISIGDEVQFEISITSNKCPKKDSDSFKIRPLGFTEEVEVILQYICECECQSEGIP
YDSFCSNGVTHRNQPRGDCDGVQINVPITFQVKVTATECIQEQ--SFVIRALGFTDIVTV--QVLPQCECRCRDQS
FNATCLNNEVIPGL--KSCMGLKIGDTVSFSIEAKVRGCPQEKEKSFTIKPVGFKDSLIVQVTFDCDCACQAQAEP

ES-PKCHEGNGTFECGACRCNEGRVGRHCECSTDEVNSEDMDAYCRKENSSEICSNNGECVCGQCVCRKRDNTNEI
RDRSLCH-GKGFLECGICRCDTGYIGKNCECQTQGRSSQELEGSCRKDNNSIICSGLGDCVCGQCLCHTSDVPGKL
NS-HRCNNGNGTFECGVCRCGPGWLGSQCECSEEDYRPSQQDE-CSPREGQPVCSQRGECLCGQCVCHSSDFGK--

YSGKFCECDNFNCDRSNGLICG--GNGVCKCRVCECNPNYTGSACDCSLDTSTCEASNGQICNGRGICECGVCKCT
IYGQYCECDTINCERYNGQVCGGPGRGLCFCGKCRCHPGFEGSACQCERTTEGCLNPRRVECSGRGRCRCNVCEC-
ITGKYCECDDFSCVRYKGEMCS--GHGQCSCGDCLCDSDWTGYYCNCTTRTDTCMSSNGLLCSGRGKCECGSCVCI

DPKFQGQTCEMCQTCLGVCAEHKECVQCRAFNKGEK--KDTCTQECSYFNITKVESRDKLPQPVQPDPVSHCKEKD
HSGYQLPLCQECPGCPSPCGKYISCAECLKFEKGPF--GKNCSAACPGLQLSN-----------NPVKGRTCKERD
QPGSYGDTCEKCPTCPDACTFKKECVECKKFDREPYMTENTCNRYCRDE-IESVKELKD-----TGKDAVNCTYKN

VDDCWFYFTYS-VNGNNEVMVHVVENPECPTGPDIIPIVAGVVAGIVLIGLALLLIWK
SEGCWVAYTLEQQDGMDRYLIYVDESRECVAGPNIAAIVGGTVAGIVLIGILLLVIWK     cytoplasmic domain
EDDCVVRFQYYEDSS-GKSILYVVEEPECPKGPDILVVLLSVMGAILLIGLAALLIWK
```

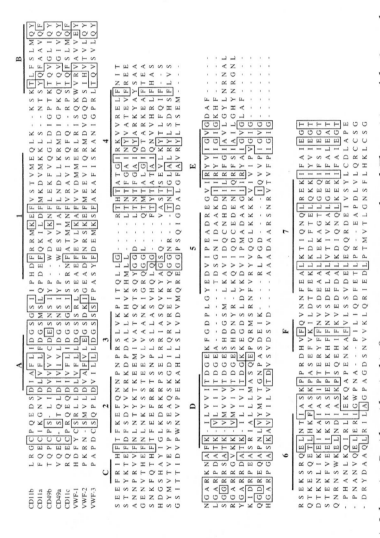

Figure 18 Integrin I-domains. Residues identical in five or more sequences are boxed. The positions of the β strands and α helices are indicated by letters and numbers respectively shown above the sequences as determined for the structure of the I-domain from CD11b[96]. The sequences of the following proteins are from the SWISSPROT database and the database accession number and residue numbers are given in brackets. CD11b, human CD11b precursor (P11215, 141–338); CD11a, human CD11a precursor (P20701, 147–337); CD49b, rat CD49b precursor (P17301, 166–367); CD49a, human CD49a precursor (P18614, 165–365); CD11c, human CD11c precursor (P20702, 142–338); VWF, human von Willebrand factor precursor (P04275; 1268–1463, 1490–1672, 1681–1874).

Lectin C-type domains (Figs 20 and 21)

This family of lectin domains are termed C-type because some members have been shown to require Ca^{2+} to bind carbohydrate[98]. This domain has been found in a number of lectins such as the Kupffer cell fucose/galactose receptor, hepatocyte galactose receptor, mannose binding protein from plasma, and galactose binding proteins in two invertebrate species, the flesh fly and sea urchin[99–101]. Lectin C-type domains are found in leucocyte cell surface antigens such as CD62L (L-selectin) and the low-affinity Fc receptor for IgE (CD23) and in a number of proteins not originally known to bind carbohydrate such as the proteoglycan core protein[102]. In some cases carbohydrate binding for the lectin C-type domain has been established, e.g. CD62E[61].

Two groups of lectin C-type domains can be distinguished on genetic organization and sequence patterns. The L-selectin has the lectin C-type domain plus about 10 residues of the signal sequence contained completely within one exon with phase 1 intron boundaries[103]. In cases other than the selectins[103,104], the lectin domain is usually found spread over three exons which also include the C-terminus of the protein and the 3' untranslated sequence[101]. The majority of lectin C-type domains are found as single domains although the macrophage mannose receptor contains eight domains in tandem[105]. In this case there is no simple correlation between the 26 exons that encode the eight lectin C-type domains which are encoded by 2–4 exons with a variety of phases of intron/exon boundaries[106,107]. As well as the differences in intron/exon organization there are sequence patterns that distinguish the lectin C-type domain present in selectins from the other lectins as shown in the sequence alignments in Fig. 20. There is a characteristic Trp residue at the N-terminus of the selectins E-selectin (CD62E), P-selectin (CD62P) and L-selectin (CD62L), whilst in the other group there is a longer patch of sequence at the N-terminus that shows a conserved sequence pattern of Cys-X-X-X-Trp.

At the N-terminus of the mannose receptor there is a region similar to the carbohydrate binding domain of the B chain of the plant lectin ricin and related lectins[107]. This is part of the galactose binding domain of ricin and is the only example of this domain type at the surface of leucocytes to date.

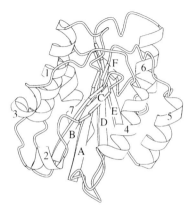

Figure 19 *The folding pattern of the integrin I-domain from CD11b. The β strands are shown as broad arrows pointing from the N- to C-terminal direction and the α helices as coils[96]. The β strands are labelled A–F and the α helices as numbers 1–6 as in the alignments (Fig. 18).*

```
          β1                              α1                                    α2                β2

ManBP  AFSMGKKSGKKFFVTNHERM-PFSKVKALCSELRGTVAIPRNAEENKAIQEVAK---TSAFLGLT
ManR   CPSQWWPYAGHCYKIHRDEKKIQRDALTTCRKEGGDLTSLHTIEELDFLISQLGYEPNDELWIGLN
KUCR   IMQDWKYFNGKFYFSRDKK-SWHEAENFCVSQGAHLASVTSQEEQAFLVQITN--AVDHWIGLT
RHL-1  CPINWVEYEGSCYWFSSSVK-PWTEADKYCQLENAHLVVVTSWEEQRFVQQHMG--PLNTWIGLT
CD23   CPEKWINFQRKCYYFGKGTK-QWVHARYACDDMEGQLVSIIHSPEEQDFLTKHA--SHTGSWIGLR
PGCA   CEEGWTKFQGHCYRHFPDRE-TWVDAERRCREQQSHLSSIVTPEEQEFVNKNA--QDYQWIGLN
CD62E               WSYNTSTEAM-TYDEASAYCQQRYTHLVAIQNKEEIEYLNSILSY-SPSYYWIGIR
CD62P               WTYHYSTKAY-SWNISRKYCQNRYTDLVAIQNKNEIDYLNKVLPY-YSSYYWIGIR
CD62L               WTYHYSEKPM-NWQRARRFCRDNYTDLVAIQNKAEIEYLEKTLPF-SRSYYWIGIR


          L1      L2       L3              L4          β3        β4          β5

ManBP  DEVTEGQFMYVTGRLT----YSNWKKDEPNDHGS-------GEDCVTIVDN-----GLWNDISCQA-SHTAVCEFPA
ManR   DIKIQMYFEWSDGTPVTFTKWLRGEPSHENNRQ------EDCVVMKG----KDGYWADRGCEW-PLGYICKMKS
KUCR   DQGTEGNWRWVDGTPFDYVQSRRFWRKIGQPDNW-RHGNEREDCVHL-----QRMWNDMACGT-AYNWVCKSTD
RHL-1  DQ--NGPWKWVDGTDY--ETGFKNWRPGQPDDWYGHGLGGGEDCAHF------TTDGHWNDDVCRR-PYRWVCETEL
CD23   NLDLKGEFIWVDGSHV---DYSNWAPGEPTSR-------SQGEDCVMM----RGSGRWNDAFCDRKLGAWVCDRLA
PGCA   DRTIEGDFRWSDGHSL---QFEKWRPNQPDNFF--ATGEDCVM--IWHEREWNDVPCNY-QLPFTCKKGT
CD62E  K--VNNVWVWV-GTQKPLTEEAENWADNEPNNK-----QKDEDCVEIYIKREKDVGMWNDERCSK-KKLALCYTAA
CD62P  K--NNKTWTWV-GTKKALTNEAENWADNEPNNK-----RNNEDCVEIYIKSPSAPGKWNDEHCLK-KKHALCYTAS
CD62L  K--IGGIWTWV-GINKSLTEEAENWGDGEPNNK-----KNKEDCVEIYIKRNKDAGKWNDDACHK-LKAALCYTAS
```

Figure 20 Lectin C-type domains. Residues identical in five or more sequences are boxed. The positions of the β strands, α helices and loops (L) determined for the structure of the rat mannose binding protein [108] are shown above the sequences. The asterisks mark the positions of the conserved residues used to identify domains for the corresponding entries in Section II. The sequences of the following proteins are from the SWISSPROT database and the database accession number and residue numbers are given in brackets. ManBP, rat mannose binding protein A precursor (P19999, 117–238); ManR, human mannose receptor precursor (P22897, 362–490); KUCR, Kupffer cell carbohydrate binding receptor (P10716; 412–540); RHL-1, rat hepatic lectin 1 or asialoglycoprotein receptor 1 (P02706; 152–279); CD23, low-affinity IgE receptor (P06734; 163–286); PGCA, cartilage-specific proteoglycan core (P07897; 1914–2038); CD62E, CD62E or E-selectin precursor (P16581; 22–142); CD62P, CD62P or P-selectin precursor (P16109; 42–162); CD62L, human leucocyte CD62L or L-selectin precursor (P14151; 39–159).

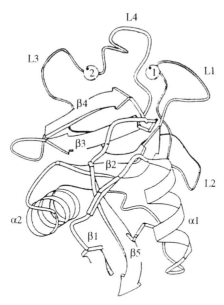

Figure 21 *The folding pattern of a lectin C-type domain. Ribbon diagram of the lectin C-type domain from the rat mannose binding protein [108]. The β strands are shown as broad arrows pointing from the N- to C-terminal direction, α helices as coiled ribbons and the connecting loops as thinner lines. The labelling of the β strands (β1–5), α helices (α1–2) and loops (L1–4) corresponds to that in the sequence alignments in Fig. 20. The numbers 1 and 2 refer to the position of the two holmium ions that are known to stabilize this region that contains a high proportion of non-regular secondary structure [108].*

The structure of a lectin C-type domain from a rat mannose binding protein has been determined by X-ray crystallography [108] and the fold is shown in Fig. 21. The structure contains an unusual region of non-regular secondary structure stabilized by two holmium ions in the crystal structure. The main part of the domain contains both β sheet and α helix and this is unusual as most of the domains for the other cell surface molecules consist solely of β structure (except the link which has a similar fold to the lectin C-type domain, the MHC superfamily and the integrin I-domain). The lectin C-type domain of the human mannose binding protein has also been crystallized with some additional C-terminal sequence. This extra sequence formed a triple α-helical coiled coil structure leading to the display of three lectin C-type domains [109]. This provides a method of increasing the avidity of the interaction as the monomeric affinities of the lectin domains are very low. The structure of the lectin C-type domain of CD62E has also been determined [61]. In both the mannose binding protein [110,111] and CD62E [112] key contact residues in determining the carbohydrate specificity have been determined such that the specificity can be readily modified by mutagenesis. The topology of the fold is similar to that of the link domains (see below).

Leucine-rich repeats (LRR) or leucine-rich glycoprotein (LRG) repeats (Figs 22 and 23)

The leucine-rich repeat (LRR) is characterized by a pattern of conserved residues including about 5 or 6 leucines and some other residues in a tightly defined repeat of about 24–29 residues (Fig. 22). It is found both intracellularly and extracellularly in a variety of species including *Drosophila* and yeast and has also been found in the platelet glycoproteins CD42a and CD42b. It often occurs in an array of tandem repeats[11]. For instance there are nine repeats in the leucine-rich glycoprotein where the repeat was first noted, 26 repeats in the yeast adenyl cyclase, 10 in the proteoglycan protein[113] and three in the trkB protein[114]. In some cases sequence similarities are observed beyond the alignments shown and it has not been clear exactly where the repeat starts. The determination of the structure of porcine ribonuclease inhibitor which contains 15 repeats, shows that each repeat formed a short β strand and an α helix approximately parallel to each other. The β strands and α helices are parallel to a common axis resulting in a horseshoe-shaped molecule with the helices flanking the circumference (Fig. 23)[11]. An unusual property of the repeats is their exposed parallel β sheets which may be useful for protein–protein interactions[12]. Two types of repeat alternate in the ribonuclease inhibitor and in general there is considerable heterogeneity within the LRR (Fig. 22). Thus the dimensions of the α helices and β strands may vary and indeed the sequence alignments for LRR in CD42 should be regarded as tentative (reviewed in ref. 12). The α chain of CD42b contains seven LRRs and these, together with all the remaining coding sequence, are encoded by a single exon[115]. Thus this repeat is not generally coded by single exons.

Link domains (Figs 24 and 25)

Two link domains were originally noted in the link protein that binds hyaluronic acid[116]. This protein also has one IgSF domain. Subsequently a further four link domains were observed in the proteoglycan core protein that has a chondroitin sulfate binding site. This protein also contains one IgSF domain, a CCP domain and a lectin C-type domain[102]. The only link domain found on leucocytes to date is a single domain in CD44 and this domain is known to bind to hyaluronate[117,118].

The structure of a link domain from TSG6, a hyaluronic acid binding protein that can be induced by TNF, has recently been determined by NMR[119]. The fold has a similar topology to that of a lectin C-type domain although there is no significant sequence similarity (Fig. 25). However the large loops that make up the Ca^{2+} binding region in the mannose binding protein are much shorter in TSG6. A small β strand number 2 is indicated in Fig. 25 which is not shown in the lectin C-type domain (Fig. 21). Thus the strand numbering differs with β strands 3–6 in the link corresponding to strands 2–5 in the lectin C-type domain. The link domain also has a similar topology to a domain found in subunits of a toxin from *Bordetella pertussis*[119,120]. The predicted hyaluron binding site is in the same position as the carbohydrate binding site of E-selectin[119].

```
                              β                              α
RNAase inhib A4    Q L E T L R L E N C G L T P A N C K D L C G I V A S Q A
RNAase inhib B4    S L R E L D L G S N G L G D A G I A E L C P G L L S P A
RNAase inhib A5    R L K T L W L W E C D I T A S G C R D L C R V Q A K E -
RNAase inhib B5    T L K E L S L A G N K L G D E G A R L L C E S L L Q P G
CD42a              A F D H L P Q L Q T L D V T Q N P W H C D C S L T Y R L
CD42b              L L D A L P A L R T A H L G A N P W R C D C R L V P L R
A2g-6              L L A N F T L L R T L D L G E N Q L E T L P P D - - - -
A2g-7              L L R G P L Q L E R L H L E G N K L Q V L G K D - - - -
A2g-8              L L L P Q P D L R Y L F L N G N K L A R V A A G A - - -
PG-2               D F K N L K N L H A L I L V N N K I S K V S P G - - - -
PG-3               A F T P L V K L L E R L Y L S K N Q L K E L P E K - - - -
```

Figure 22 *Leucine-rich repeats. Residues identical in four or more sequences are boxed. The positions of the β strand and α helix determined from the structure of the ribonuclease inhibitor[12] are indicated above the sequence. The sequences of the following proteins are from the SWISSPROT database and the database accession number and residue numbers are given in brackets. RNAase inhib, pig ribonuclease inhibitor (P10775; A4 195–222, B4 223–250, A5 252–279, B5 280–307); CD42a, human platelet glycoprotein IX precursor (P14770, 70–98); CD42b, human platelet glycoprotein IB β chain precursor or CD42c (P13224, 74–101); A2g-6, A2g-7, A2g-8, human leucine-rich α2-glycoprotein (LRG) (P02750, 148–171, 172–195, 196–219 respectively); PG-2, PG-3, human bone proteoglycan II precursor (P07585, 100–123 and 124–147 respectively). Note the domain borders have been modified from earlier assignments[193] to account for the recent structural information for LRR from ribonuclease[12].*

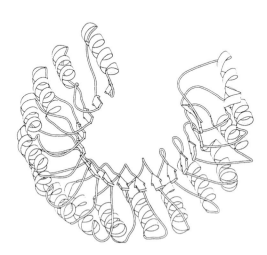

Figure 23 *The folding pattern of the leucine-rich repeats present in the ribonuclease inhibitor. Each repeat consists of a short β strand and a longer α helix[12]. The repeats assemble into an ordered horseshoe-like structure with the curved β sheets lining the interior and the helices flanking the outer circumference.*

β 1   α 1   β 2   α 2   β 3

```
        β1                        α1                              β2                  α2                      β3
TSG6   G - V Y H R E A R S G K Y K L T Y A E A K A V C E F E G G H L A T Y K Q L E A A R K I - G F H V C A A G W
CD44   G - V F H V E - K N G R Y S I S R T E A A D L C K A F N S T L P T M A Q M E K A L S I - G F E T C R Y G F
CORE1  G I V F H Y R A I S T R Y T L D F R A Q R A C L Q N S A I I A T P E Q L Q A A Y E D - G F H Q C D A G W
CORE2  G E V F - Y A T S P E K F T - - F Q E A A N E C R T V G A R L A T T G Q L Y L A W Q G - G M D M C S A G W
CORE3  G V V F H Y R P G S T R Y S L T F E E A Q Q A C I R T G A A I A S P E Q L Q A A W S Q - G Y E Q C D A G W
CORE4  G E V F F A T - Q M E Q F T - - F Q E A Q A F C A A Q N A T L A S T G Q L Y A A W S Q - G L D K C Y A G W
LINK1  G V V F P Y F P R L G R Y N L N F H E A R Q A C L D Q D A V I A S F D Q L Y D A W R G - G L D W C N A G W
LINK2  G - R F Y Y L I H P T K - - L T Y D E A V Q A C L N D G A Q I A K V G Q I F A A W K L L G Y D R C D A G W
                                            *
```

β 4   β 5   β 6

```
        β4                    β5                           β6
TSG6   M A K G R V G Y P I V K P G P N C G F G K - - T G L I D Y G I R - - - L N R S E R W D A Y C Y N P H A
CD44   I E G H V V - I P R I H P N S I C A A N N - - T G V I L T S - - - N T S Q Y D T Y C F N A S A
CORE1  L A D Q T V R Y P I H T P R E G C Y G D K D E F P G V R T V Y L H A N Q T G Y P D P S S R - Y D V Y C F A E E M
CORE2  L A D R S V R Y P I S K A R P N C G G N L L G V R T V Y L H A N Q T G Y P D P S S R - Y D A I C Y T G E D
CORE3  L Q D Q T V R Y P I V S P R T P C V G D K D S S P G V R T V Y L Y P N Q T G L P D D P L S K - H H A F C F R G V S
CORE4  L A D G T L R Y P I V N P R P A C G G D K P G V R T V Y L Y P N Q T G L P D D P L S K - D K D K S R - Y D V F C F T S N F
LINK1  L S D G S V Q Y P I T K P R E P C G G Q N - T V P G V R N Y G F W - - D K D K S R - Y D V F C F T S N F
LINK2  L A D G S V R Y P I S R P W R R C S P T - - E A A V R F V G F - - - P D K K H K L Y G V Y C F R A Y N
                                                                                       *
```

Figure 24 Link domains. Residues identical in four or more sequences are boxed. The positions of the β strands, and α helices determined for the structure of TSG6, a tumour necrosis factor-inducible protein [119], are shown above the sequences. The asterisks mark the positions of the conserved residues used to identify domains for the corresponding entries in Section II. The sequences of the following proteins are from the SWISSPROT database and the database accession number and residue numbers are given in brackets. TSG6, human tumour necrosis factor-inducible protein TSG6 precursor (P98066, 36–132); CD44, human CD44 antigen precursor (P16070, 32–123); CORE1, CORE2, CORE3, CORE4, rat cartilage-specific proteoglycan core protein precursor (P07897, 152–251, 253–353, 486–585 and 587–687 respectively); LINK1, LINK2, rat proteoglycan link protein (P03994, 158–257 and 259–354 respectively).

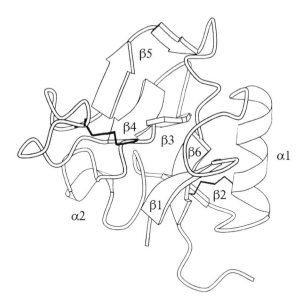

Figure 25 *The folding pattern of a link domain. Ribbon diagram of the link from TSG6, a tumour necrosis factor-inducible protein* [119]. *The β strands are shown as broad arrows pointing from the N- to C-terminal direction, α helices as coiled ribbons and the connecting loops as thinner lines. The short lines in bold indicate the positions of disulfide bridges. The labelling of the β strands (β1–6), and α helices (α1–2) corresponds to that in the sequence alignments in Fig. 24.*

Low-density lipoprotein receptor (LDLR) domains (Figs 26 and 27)

The LDL receptor contains seven domains of about 40 amino acids with six conserved cysteine residues that have been called LDLR domains [121]. The LDLR also contains three EGF domains. LDLR domains have also been found in other proteins, notably some complement components such as C6, C9 and Factor I. In the LDLR, four of the LDLR domains are encoded by individual exons whilst the other three are encoded by a single exon [122]. Mutational analysis has indicated that the LDLR domains are important in the binding of some lipoproteins but otherwise the function of this domain type is not known [123].

The structure of the N-terminal LDLR domain of the LDL receptor has been determined by NMR [124]. It consists of a β hairpin structure followed by a series of β turns (Fig. 27). It lacks extensive α helix and/or β sheet found in many domain types and in this respect it is more like the TNFR [125] although these structures are not particularly similar. However both the LDLR and TNFR contain repeats of about 40 amino acids with a high content of Cys bridges and an unusually low percentage of hydrophobic residues. The LDLR domain shows no resemblance in topology to any other domain type to date.

Ly-6 domains (Figs 28 and 29)

The Ly-6 antigens are a group of leucocyte antigens first identified in the mouse that consist of 70–80 amino acids containing 10 Cys residues [126,127]. Southern blot

```
                           *                                    *
LDLR d1       G T A V G - - D R C E R N E F Q C Q D G - - K C I S Y K W V C D G S A E C Q D G S D E S
LDLR d2       E T C L S - - V T C K S G D F S C G G R V N R C I P Q F W R C D G Q V D C D N G S D E Q
LDLR d3       - G C P P - - K T C S Q D E F R C H D G - - K C I S R Q F V C D S D R D C L D G S D E A
Comp 9        E Q A L P - - S E C S S I E F T C E S G - - A C I K L R L S C N G D Y D C E D G S D E D
Hemo. Linker  D E L E G - - N G C E P R H F Q C G G S A M E C I S D L L T C D G S P D C A N G A D E D
Factor I      E L C C - - - K A C Q G K G F H C K S G - - V C I P S Q Y Q C N G E V D C I T G E D E V
Comp 7        R G C P T E - E G C - G E R F R C F S G - - Q C I S K S L V C N G D S D C E D S A D E
Comp 6        L L C K I E E A D C - K N K F R C D S G - - R C I A R K L E C N G E N D C G D N S D E R
```

Figure 26 *Low-density lipoprotein receptor (LDLR) domains. Residues identical in four or more sequences are boxed. The asterisks mark the positions of the conserved residues used to identify domains for the corresponding entries in Section II. The sequences of the following proteins are from the SWISSPROT database and the database accession number and residue numbers are given in brackets. LDLR, human low-density lipoprotein receptor precursor (P01130, d1 20–59, d2 61–102, d3 103–141); Comp 9, rainbow trout complement C9 (P06682, 72–112); Hemo.Linker, marine worm giant extracellular haemoglobin linker 2 chain (P18208, 61–102); Factor I, human complement factor I precursor (P05156, 253–291); Comp 7, human complement C7 precursor (P10643, 77–116); Comp 6, human complement C6 precursor (P13671, 131–171).*

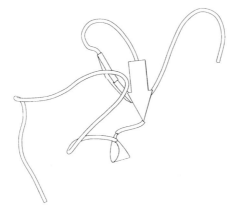

Figure 27 *The folding pattern of a low-density lipoprotein receptor (LDLR) domain from the LDL receptor (domain 1) determined by NMR* [124]. *The domain consists of a β hairpin structure followed by a series of β turns.*

analysis indicates that many Ly-6-related genes are present in the mouse and of these, 10 distinct genes have been identified [128]. The Ly-6 antigens are expressed in non-lymphoid tissues, for example kidney, as well as on leucocytes. Homologues of the Ly-6 antigens have been found in the rat but not yet in other species. In humans the CD59 antigen contains a single Ly-6 domain which causes inhibition of the activity of complement to lyse cells expressing CD59. An invertebrate member of the Ly-6 superfamily has been isolated from squid optic and central nervous tissue [127,129]. All the above molecules consist of a single Ly-6 domain attached to the cell surface by a GPI anchor. The urokinase plasminogen activator receptor (CD87) contains three Ly-6 domains separated by hinge-like sequences and is also attached to the cell surface by a GPI anchor. The alignments for these domains are shown in Fig. 28. No Ly-6 domain has been found in combination with domains of any other superfamily and this may be because the exon structures known for this superfamily are not suited to exon shuffling (Table 3).

The structure of the Ly-6 domain of human CD59 has been determined by NMR [7,8]. It forms a relatively flat disk-like shape consisting of a two stranded β sheet fingers packed against a protein core formed by a three-stranded β sheet and a short α helix (Fig. 29) [7,8]. The topology of the fold is similar to that of snake venom neurotoxins consistent with earlier predictions based on sequence analysis [7,8].

MHC domains (Figs 30–32)

The MHC antigens and related molecules contain membrane-proximal IgSF C1-set domains. However their N-terminal segments, including the α1 and α2 domains of MHC Class I heavy chain and the α1 and β1 domains of the Class II α and β chains, show no sequence similarity to IgSF sequences [130] and the Class I and II domains are known to form an independent structural unit as shown in Fig. 30 [78,79]. Thus in the sequence alignments in Figs 31 and 32 the sequences are shown as an MHC Iα1-set and MHC Iα2-set. There are numerous sequences related to the classical MHC antigens and these show a Class I-type structural organization, including the binding of β_2-microglobulin, with no examples so far of a Class II-like organization.

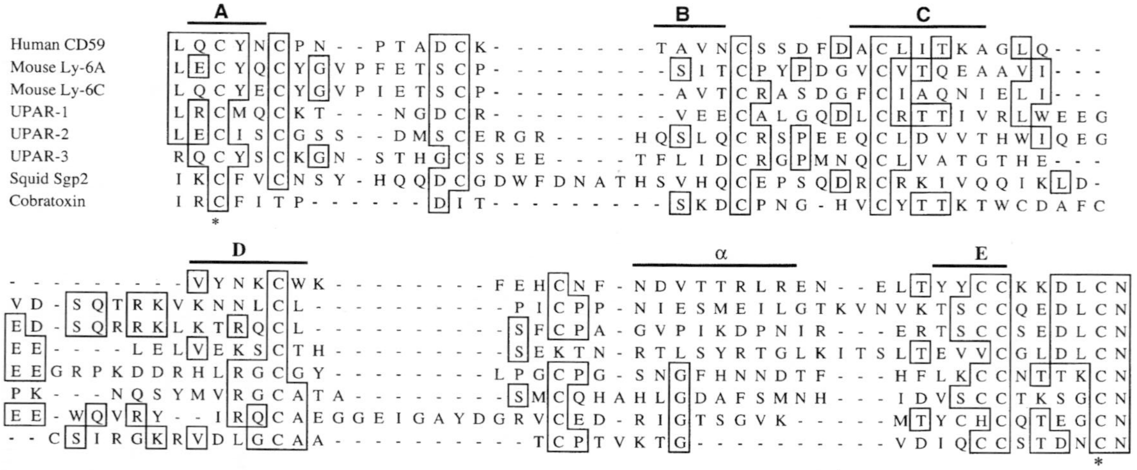

Figure 28 *Ly-6 domains. Residues identical in three or more sequences are boxed. The asterisks mark the positions of the conserved residues used to identify domains for the corresponding entries in Section II. The positions of the β strands (A–E) and single α helix are indicated by the bars above the sequence[8]. The structure of the cobratoxin has also been determined and the strands are in similar positions although the penultimate strand is smaller[8]. The sequences of the following proteins are from the SWISSPROT database unless otherwise indicated and the database accession number and residue numbers are given in brackets. Human CD59, human CD59 antigen (P13987, 26–95); Mouse Ly-6A antigen (P05533, 27–105); Mouse Ly-6C (P09568, 27–102); UPAR-1, UPAR-2, UPAR-3, human urokinase plasminogen activator receptor (CD87) (PIR: S12376, 23–99, 115–199 and 214–294 respectively); Squid Sgp2, squid glycoprotein 2 residues 1–92 [129]; Cobratoxin, Naja siamaensis long neurotoxin (α-cobratoxin, P01391, 1–63).*

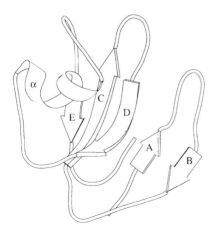

Figure 29 *The folding pattern of a Ly-6 domain. Ribbon diagram showing the β strands of human CD59[8] as broad arrows pointing from the N- to C-terminal direction, the single α helix as a coil and the connecting loops as thinner lines. The labelling of the β strands (A–E) and single α helix (α) corresponds to that in the sequence alignments in Fig. 28.*

The Qa and Tla antigens of mice are very similar in sequence to MHC Class I antigens. Human CD1 antigens, an Fc receptor of rodent neonatal gut [131] and a Class I-related molecule expressed by cytomegalovirus [132] all show sequence identity at the level of about 30%. A more detailed discussion of MHC-related sequences can be found in refs 78, 80 and 133–135.

The MHC Class I α1 and α2 domains show weak sequence similarity to each other and form a similar fold containing a platform of β strands and a single α helix [78]. The two domains together form the peptide binding groove of the MHC molecule. In the MHC Class II molecules the α1 domain shows strong sequence similarity to Class I α1 and the Class II β1 domain is most similar to Class I α2 [133]. The MHC Class II fold is similar to that of MHC Class I with a typical peptide binding groove [79–81]. The rodent neonatal Fc receptor has sequence similarity to MHC Class I and X-ray crystallography showed that it has a typical MHC Class I like structure although the peptide binding groove is closed and unable to bind peptides [136].

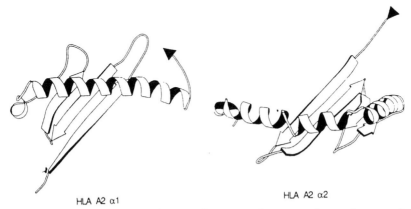

HLA A2 α1

HLA A2 α2

Figure 30 *The folding pattern of MHC domains. The β strands are shown as broad arrows pointing from the N- to C-terminal direction, α helices as coiled ribbons and the connecting loops as thinner lines. The arrowheads indicate where the MHC Class I α1 joins the α2 domain to form the peptide binding groove flanked by the two α helices. The data are from the Brookhaven Protein Database.*

β

		β		β
MHC Class I	G S H S M R Y F F T S - V S R P G R G E P R F I A V G Y V D - D T Q F V R F D S D A A S Q R
CD1 a	S F H V T W I A S F Y - N H S W K Q N L V S G W L S D L Q T H T W D S N S S T I V - - - - -
FcR rat	P R L P L M Y H L A A - V S D L S T G L P S F W A T G W L - G A Q Q Y L T Y N L - - R Q E
HCMV	G M H V L R Y G Y T G I F D - - D T S H M T L T V V G I F D G I Q H F F T Y H V - - - - -
Class II A-B α	A D H V G T Y G I S V Y Q S P G D - - - I G Q Y T F E F D G D E L F Y V D L - - - - -
Class II DQ(3) α	A D H V A S Y G V N L Y Q S Y G P - - - S G Q Y T H E F D G D E Q F Y V D L - - - - -

α

β

	α	
MHC Class I	M E P R A P W I E Q E - G P E Y W D G E T R K V K A H S Q T H R V D L G T L R G Y Y N Q S E A G S
CD1 a	- - F L C P W S R G N F S N E E W K E L E T L F R I R T I R S F E G I R R Y A H E L Q F E Y P F E
FcR rat	A D P C G A W I W E N Q V S W Y W E K E T T D L K S K E Q L F L E A I R T L E N Q I N G T F T L Q
HCMV	N S S D K A S S R A N G T I - S W M A N V S A A Y P T Y L D G E R A K G - - D L I F N Q T E Q N L
Class II A-B α	D K K E T V W M L P E F G Q L - A S F D P Q G G L Q N I A V V K H N L G V L T K R S N S T P A T N
Class II DQ(3) α	G R K E T V W C L P V L R Q - - F R F D P Q F A L T N I A V L K H N L N S L I K R S N S T A A T N

Figure 31 MHC Class I α1-set domains. Residues identical in three or more of the sequences are boxed. The positions of the β strands, α helices determined for the structure of the human HLA Class I are shown above the sequences. The sequences of the following proteins are from the SWISSPROT database and the database accession number and residue numbers are given in brackets. MHC Class I, human HLA Class I A-2 α precursor (P01892, 25–116); CD1a, human CD1a antigen precursor (P06126, 26–112); FcR rat, rat gut Fc receptor precursor (P13599, 25–115); HCMV, human cytomegalovirus glycoprotein H301 precursor (P08560, 19–101); Class II A-B α, mouse MHC Class II A-B α chain precursor (P14434, 21–103); Class II DQ(3) α, human MHC Class II DQ(3) α chain precursor (P01909, 28–109).

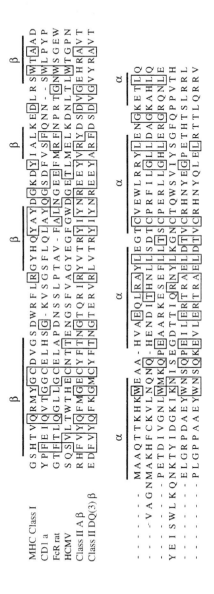

Figure 32 *MHC class I α2-set domains. Residues identical in three or more of the sequences are boxed. The positions of the β strands, α helices determined for the structure of the human HLA Class I are shown above the sequences. The sequences of the following proteins are from the SWISSPROT database and the database accession number and residue numbers are given in brackets. MHC Class I, human HLA Class I A-2α precursor (P01892, 115–203); CD1a, human CD1a antigen precursor (P06126, 109–199); FcR rat, rat gut Fc receptor precursor (P13599, 110–199); HCMV, human cytomegalovirus glycoprotein H301 precursor (P08560, 112–210); Class II A β, mouse H2 Class II A β chain precursor (P14483, 32–122); Class DQ(3) β, human MHC Class II DQ(3) β chain precursor (P06126, 109–199).*

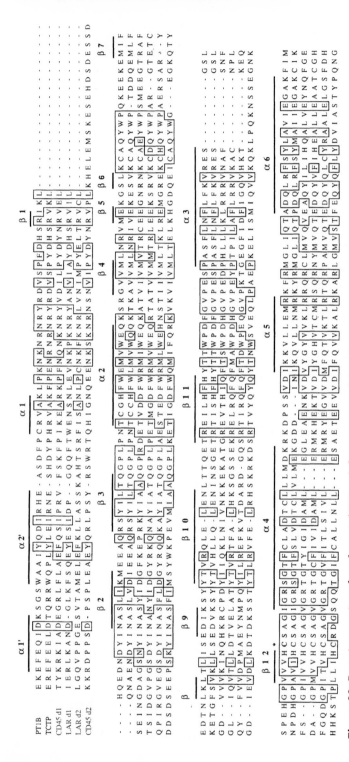

Figure 33 *Protein tyrosine phosphatase (PTPase) domains. Residues identical in four or more sequences are boxed. The positions of the β strands and α helices shown above the sequences are those from the structure of protein tyrosine phosphatase 1B determined by X-ray crystallography[144]. The Cys residue of the active site of this structure is indicated in bold together with the asterisk. The sequences of the following proteins are from the SWISSPROT database and the database accession number and residue numbers are given in brackets. PT1B, human protein tyrosine phosphatase phosphatase PT1B (P18031 4–282); TCTP, human T cell protein tyrosine phosphatase phosphatase (P17706, 25–280); CD45, human CD45 antigen (P08575, d1 639–915, d2 931–1232); LAR, human LAR protein (P10586, d1 1331–1602, d2 1617–1894).*

Protein tyrosine phosphatase (PTPase) (Figs 33 and 34)

The PTPase family of integral membrane proteins was discovered when two cytoplasmic repeats of the CD45 antigen[137] were matched with the sequence of a placental cytoplasmic phosphotyrosine phosphatase[138,139]. Subsequently PTPase activity has been shown for the membrane-proximal cytoplasmic domain of CD45 but as yet not for the C-terminal domain[140]. Subsequently many other sequences have been identified with similarities to these sequences by cross-hybridization with cDNA probes and these include cytosolic proteins and membrane phosphatases. The LAR cell surface protein contains a tandem pair of PTPase domains together with an extracellular portion with three IgSF domains and eight Fn3 domains, although this protein is not expressed widely on leucocytes[141]. Sequences with many similarities to the PTPase domains have also been identified in *Drosophila*[142]. Some examples of the sequences are shown in Fig. 33. The second domain in CD45 is unusual in comparison with other PTPases in that it contains an insertion of 19 amino acids with a very high content of acidic and Ser residues. The Ser residues may be phosphorylated by Ser kinases to produce an extremely negatively charged region of sequence.

The complete genomic structure for mouse CD45[143] shows that the region illustrated in Fig. 33 is encoded by 6 or 8 exons for each domain. However the ends of the domains as defined from the sequence similarities do not correspond to the ends of exons with the same phase of intron/exon boundaries[33]. The genetic origin of these domains is unclear.

The structure of the human protein tyrosine phosphatase 1B domain has been determined (Fig. 34)[144]. This 37 kD domain is organized into eight α helices and 12 β strands with the active Cys in a loop between the final β strand and the fourth α helix (Fig. 34)[144].

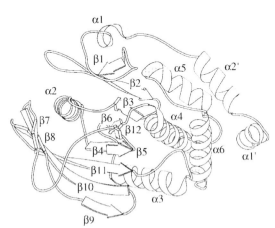

Figure 34 *The folding pattern of protein tyrosine phosphatase domains. Ribbon diagram to show the folding pattern of human protein tyrosine phosphatase 1B determined by X-ray crystallography*[144]. *The structure contains a 10 strand β sheet flanked by regions of α helix. Two α helices at the N-terminus correspond to regions with lower levels of sequence conservation and wrap around the N-terminus of α-6.*

```
                                                                                              *
SREC d4   P K H T R V R I V - G M G Q G Q G R V E V S L G N G W G R - - - - - - - - - - - S D H E A K T V C Y H A G Y K W G A
CD5 d1    D P D F Q A R L T R S N S K C Q G Q L E V Y L K D G W H M - V C S Q S W G R S S K Q W E D P S Q A S K V C Q R L N C G - -
CFAI      E G K F S V S L K H G N T D S E G I V E V K L V D Q D K T M F I C K S S W - - - - - - - - - - S M R E A N V A C L D L G F Q Q G A
CD5 d2    Q P K V Q S R L V G G S S I C E G T V E V R Q G A Q W A A - - - - - - - - - - - K T Q D L E N F L C N N L Q C G S F L
CD5 d3    A V E G N I R L I H G R T E N E G S V E I Y H A T R W G S - - - - - - - - - - - S L R W E E V C R E Q Q C G - -
SREC d1   E P Q G S L R M I L G D V P N E G T L E T F W D G A W G S - - - - - - - - - - - H M E N A N V C Q L G F P - G A
SREC d2   N V E G D I R L M D G S G P H E G R V E I W H D D A W G T - - - - - - - - - - - G T P D G N V A C R Q M G Y S - R G
SREC d3   T P F T K V R L V G G S G P H E G R V E I L H S G Q W G T - - - - - - - - - - - D W A D A N V V C R Q A G Y R - G A
SCAV                                                                                  E V R V G Q V V V C R S L G Y P - G V


                                                                                              *
SRAAGSA - E V S A P F D L E A P F I - - D G I T C S G V E N E T L S Q C Q M K V S A - D M T C A T G - - - - D V G V V C E G
PLSL - - - - G P F L V T Y T P Q S - - S I I C Y G - Q L G S V S - S N C S H - - S R N D M C H - - - - - S L G L T C L E
DTQRRFKLS - - D L S I N S T E C - - L H V H C R G L E T - S L A E C - - T F T K R R T M G Y - - Q D F A D V V C Y T
KHLPETEAGRAQDPG E P R E H Q P L P I Q W K I Q N S S C T S L E H C F R K I K P Q K S G R - - - V L A L L C S G
VNSYR - - - - - - V L D A G D P T S - - R G L F C - - P H Q K L S Q C H - E L W E R N S Y C K - - - K V F V T C Q D
RQFYRR - - - - - A Y F G A H V T T F W V Y - K M N C L G N E T - R L E D C Y H R P Y G R P W L C - N A Q W A A G V E C L P
VKSIKT - - - D G H F G F S T G P I - - I L D A V D C E G T E A - H I T E C N M P V T P Y Q H A C P Y T H N W D V G V V C K P
VKASGFK - - - G E D F G F T W A P I - H T S F V M C T G V E D - R L I D C I L R D - G W T H S C - - Y H V E D A S V V C A T
QAVHKA - - - A H F G Q G T G P I - W L N E V F C F G R E S - S I E E C K I R Q W G - T R A C - - S H S E D A G V T C T L
```

Figure 35 *Scavenger receptor cysteine-rich (SCRC) domains. Residues identical in four or more sequences are boxed. The asterisks mark the positions of the conserved residues used to identify domains for the corresponding entries in Section II. The sequences of the following proteins are from the SWISSPROT database unless otherwise indicated and the database accession number and residue numbers are given in brackets. SREC, sea urchin egg peptide speract receptor precursor (P16264, d1 38–145, d2 148–258, d3 259–367, d4 377–486); CD5, human CD5 antigen (P06127, d1 30–134, d2 156–269, d3 271–369); CFAI, human complement factor I precursor (P05156, 109–216); SCAV, human scavenger receptor type I (P21757, 345–451). Alignments are from 20 residues before the conserved glycine to the C-terminus of the scavenger receptor.*

Scavenger receptor cysteine-rich (SRCR) (Fig. 35)

Three domains with sequence similarities were identified in the extracellular region of the CD5 antigen and later single domains were detected in macrophage scavenger receptors, the complement control protein Factor I, three each in the CD6 antigen and the speract receptor protein present in sea urchins[145], 11 in the bovine WC1 antigen[146] and nine in CD163 (M130) a macrophage cell surface protein[147]. This domain type was first reported in the scavenger receptor and thus is named scavenger receptor cysteine-rich (SRCR) domain[145] and alignments for this superfamily are shown in Fig. 35. However the role of this domain type in the function of the scavenger receptor to bind various ligands is unclear, as some ligands will bind to both scavenger receptors I and II but the latter lacks this type of domain[148]. Initially it was argued that the CD5 antigen domains were related to IgSF domains,[149] and then the PapD bacterial protein[28]. It is now clear that the CD5 domains are related to the SRCR domains. A ligand for CD6 called ALCAM (CD166) has been identified on thymic epithelial cells. It contains five IgSF domains[150] and interacts via its N-terminal IgSF domain with the membrane-proximal domain of the three SRCR domains of CD6[151]. No tertiary structure data are available yet for this domain type.

Signal transduction sequence motifs: ITAM, ITIM and the death domain; motifs in cytoplasmic parts of membrane proteins (Figs 36 and 37)

The cytoplasmic parts of leucocyte membrane proteins tend not to have domains like those found on the extracellular parts. However a number of different motifs have been identified and clearly play an important part in transmitting the effects of signals from the outside of the cell to the nucleus and vice versa. There is a wide range of proteins recognizing these motifs and in turn being recognized by other proteins. The binding may also be dependent on phosphorylation and in addition these regions may interact with components of the cytoskeleton. This is a large field and beyond the scope of this review. However four important motifs will be summarized.

Programmed cell death has been shown to involve signals through cell surface receptors. In the immune system two well-characterized examples involve TNFRI (CD120a) and Fas (CD95)[152,153]. Both these proteins contain a motif in the cytoplasmic region termed the death domain that is necessary for self-association of the receptors leading to signals that lead to cell death[153]. Related sequences have been identified in other proteins including some isolated by the yeast two-hybrid system, e.g. RIP, TRADD (reviewed in refs 152 and 153) and are illustrated in Fig. 36. Thus TNFRI interacts with TRADD which in turn can interact with RIP which has serine threonine kinase activity and can associated with Fas[154]. Some proteins with no apparent involvement in "death", such as the cytoskeletal protein ankyrin, also contain a "death" domain. Unlike the cytoplasmic domains of TNFRI and Fas, these death domains show no significant sequence similarity to "reaper", a protein that is expressed in *Drosophila* cells that are destined to die[155].

One motif that used to be called the signal transduction sequence motif is present in the cytoplasmic regions of several membrane proteins of the antigen receptor

```
Fas      DL SKYITTIAGVMTLSQVKGFVRKNGVNEAKIDEIKND----
TNFR     DDPATLYAVVENVPPLRWKEFVRRLGLSDHEIDRLELQNG----
Ankyrin  EQAEMKMAVISEHLGLSWAELARELQFSVEDLNRIRVENP----
TRADD    PLSLKDQQTFARSVGLKWRKVGRSLQRGCRALRDPALDSLAYEY
RIP      SLTDKHLDPIRENLGKHWKNCARKLGFTQSQIDEIDHDYE----
NFKB     KLQLYKLLEIPDP-DKNWATLAQKLGLGI-LNNAFRLSPA----
NGFR     REEVEKLLNGSA--GDTWRHLAGELGYQPEHIDSFTHEAC----

Fas      NVQDTAEQKVQLLRNWHQLHGKKEA-YDTLIKDLKKANLCTLAEKIQ
TNFR     --RCLREAQYSMLATWRRRTPRREATLELLGRVLRDMDLLGCLEDIE
Ankyrin  --NSLLEQSVALLNLWVIREG-QNANMENLYTALQSIDRGEIVNMLE
TRADD    EREGLYEQAFQLLRRFVQAEG-RRATLQRNLEENELTSLAEDLL
RIP      -RDGLKEKVYQMLQKWVMREGIKGATVGKLAQALHQCSRIDLLSSLI
NFKB     -----PSKTLMDNYEVSG--GTVRELVEALRQMGYTEAIEVIQ
NGFR     -----PVRALLASWA---TQDSATLDALLAALRRIQRADLVESLC
```

Figure 36 *Death domain. Residues identical in four or more sequences are boxed. The sequences of the following proteins are from the SWISSPROT database unless otherwise indicated and the database accession number and residue numbers are given in brackets. Fas, human Fas precursor (P25445, 228–311); TNFR, human TNFR I precursor (P19438, 354–438); Ankyrin, human ankyrin 1 (P16157, 1400–1483); TRADD, human TRADD protein (PIR: A56911, 213–302); RIP, human RIP protein (PIR: I38992, 282–367); NFKB, human NF-κB p105 (P19838, 817–890); NGFR, human low-affinity NGFR precursor (P08138, 344–418).*

Human CD3γ	D K Q T L L P N D Q L Y Q P L K D R E D D Q - Y S H L
Human CD3δ	D T Q A L L R N D Q V Y Q P L R D R D D A Q - Y S H L
Mouse CD3ε	K E R P P P V P N P D Y E P I R K G Q R D L - Y S G L
Human CD3ζ (1)	P P A Y Q Q G Q N Q L Y N E L N L G R R E E - Y D V L
Human CD3ζ (2)	K P R R K N P Q E G L Y N E L Q K D K M A E A Y S E I
Human CD3ζ (3)	E R R R G K G H D G L Y Q G L S T A T K D T - Y D A L
Mouse CD79a	D M P D D Y E D E N L Y E G L N L D D C S M - Y E D I
Mouse CD79b	D G K A G M E E D H T Y E G L N I D Q T A T - Y E D I
Rat FcεR β	F E R S K V P D D R L Y E E L H V Y S P I - - Y S A L
Rat FcεR γ	D I A S R E K S D A V Y T G L N T R N Q E T - Y E T L
Human CD5	E N P T A S H V D N E Y S Q P P R N S R L S A Y P A L

Figure 37 *ITAM (immunoreceptor tyrosine-based activation motif) or signal transduction motifs. Residues identical in five or more sequences are boxed. The sequences of the following proteins are from the SWISSPROT database and the database accession number and residue numbers are given in brackets. Human CD3γ, human CD3γ chain precursor (P09693, 149–181); Human CD3δ, human CD3δ chain precursor (P04234, 138–171); CD3ε, mouse CD3ε chain precursor (P22646, 159–184); CD3ζ, human CD3ζ chain precursor (P20963, 61–94, 99–130, 131–163); CD79a, mouse CD79a (MB1) precursor (P11911, 171–204); CD79b, mouse CD79b (B29) precursor (P15530, 184–217); FcεRβ, rat Igε receptor β subunit (P13386, 207–239); FcεRγ, rat Igε receptor γ subunit precursor (P20411, 54–86); Human CD5, human CD5 antigen precursor (P06127, 442–475).*

complexes on B cells, T cells, and the IgE receptor on mast cells [156]. This is now called ITAM [157,158] or "immunoreceptor tyrosine-based activation motif" and alignments are shown in Fig. 37. One common feature of these molecules is that they are components of membrane complexes which when crosslinked give signals that lead to cell activation. This can result in cell proliferation in the case of the antigen receptors and to degranulation of mast cells. The role of the ITAM motif in this signalling response has been extensively studied. Receptor clustering results in the rapid activation of Src family protein tyrosine kinases which phosphorylate the ITAM on each tyrosine. This results in the association of the Syk and/or Zap tyrosine kinases via their tandem SH2 domains with the phosphorylated ITAM. This leads to the activation of Syk and/or Zap which is a critical step for the generation of a signal transduction cascade (reviewed in refs 159 and 160).

A second motif involved in giving an inhibitory signal is called "immunoreceptor tyrosine-based inhibition motif" or ITIM. In B cells the ITIM motif of the FcγRIIB is thought to be the target for the SH2-containing phosphatase SHP which is critical in determining the threshold by which B cells respond to antigens [157]. Similar motifs are found in CD22, IL-2Rβ (CD122) and IL-3Rβ (CDw131). However the motif is short and not that clearly defined. Thus an alignment is not given but is reviewed in refs 157 and 161.

Both SH2 and SH3 domains are common in cytosolic proteins and recognize phosphotyrosine residues and proline-rich motifs respectively. These motifs are common in other cytosolic proteins, particularly those involved in signal transduction. A proline-rich motif consensus sequence for SH3 domain binding is XpΦPPXP, where X is any amino acid, p is usually a Pro and Φ is a hydrophobic

```
                    *                                                                        *
PC1 d1        K S C - K G R C F E - - R T F S N C R C D A A C V S L G N C C L D F Q E T C V E P T H
PP11          T S C - Q G R C Y E A F D K H H Q C H C N A R C Q E F G N C C K D F E S L C S D H E V
Vitronectin   E S C - K G R C T E G F N V D K K C Q C D E L C S Y Y Q S C C T D Y T A E C K P Q V T
PC1 d2        W T C N K F R C G E K R L S R F V C S C A D D C K T H N D C C I N Y S S V C Q D K K S
```

Figure 38 *Somatomedin B domains. Residues identical in three or more sequences are boxed. The asterisks mark the positions of the conserved residues used to identify domains for the corresponding entries in Section II. The sequences of the following proteins are from the SWISSPROT database and the database accession number and residue numbers are given in brackets. PC1, mouse plasma cell antigen PC1 (P06802; d1 54–93; d2 95–137); PP11, human placental protein precursor (P21128, 47–88); Vitronectin, human vitronectin precursor (P04004; 22–63).*

residue[162]. A putative proline-rich motif has been described in the cytoplasmic domain of CD2 [163].

Somatomedin B domains (Fig. 38)

Somatomedin B is a serum peptide derived from vitronectin (also called serum-spreading factor) by proteolysis. The plasma cell surface antigen PC1 was noted to contain two somatomedin B repeats[99]. This glycoprotein has nucleotide pyrophos-phatase/alkaline phosphodiesterase activity[164] but this is associated with a different region of the molecule than that containing the somatomedin B repeat. The domain has not been found on other cell surface molecules although it is present in placental protein 11 (PP11)[165].

Transmembrane 4 pass (TM4) superfamily and FcεRIβ/CD20 superfamily (Figs 39 and 40)

The TM4 superfamily (also called the tetraspan superfamily) is a large group of proteins that are thought to traverse the lipid bilayer four times with both the N- and C-terminii on the cytoplasmic face of the membrane. This superfamily includes several leucocyte antigens such as CD9, CD37, CD53, CD63, CD81 and CD82[166]. Alignments for the TM4SF are shown in Fig. 39. The genomic organization of the leucocyte TM4SF proteins are similar, pointing to a single primordial gene. The non-leucocyte antigens form a separate group that seems to have branched off in

---

Figure 39 (opposite) *Transmembrane 4 pass (TM4) superfamily. Residues identical in four or more sequences are boxed. The putative positions of the four transmembrane sequences are indicated with a solid bar above the sequences. The dashed line indicates the extracellular loops. The sequences of the following proteins are from the SWISSPROT database and the database accession number is given in brackets (the complete sequences are shown). Sm23, Schistosoma mansoni protein Sm23 (P19331); CD63, human melanoma-associated antigen ME491 (P08962); CD9, human CD9 antigen (P21926); CD81, human CD81 (TAPA-1) antigen (P18582); Co02, human tumour associated antigen Co-029 (P19075); CD82, human CD82 (R2) antigen (P27701); CD37, human CD37 antigen (P11049); CD53, human CD53 antigen (P19397).*

Figure 39 *Transmembrane 4 pass (TM4) superfamily and FcεRIβ/CD20 superfamily*

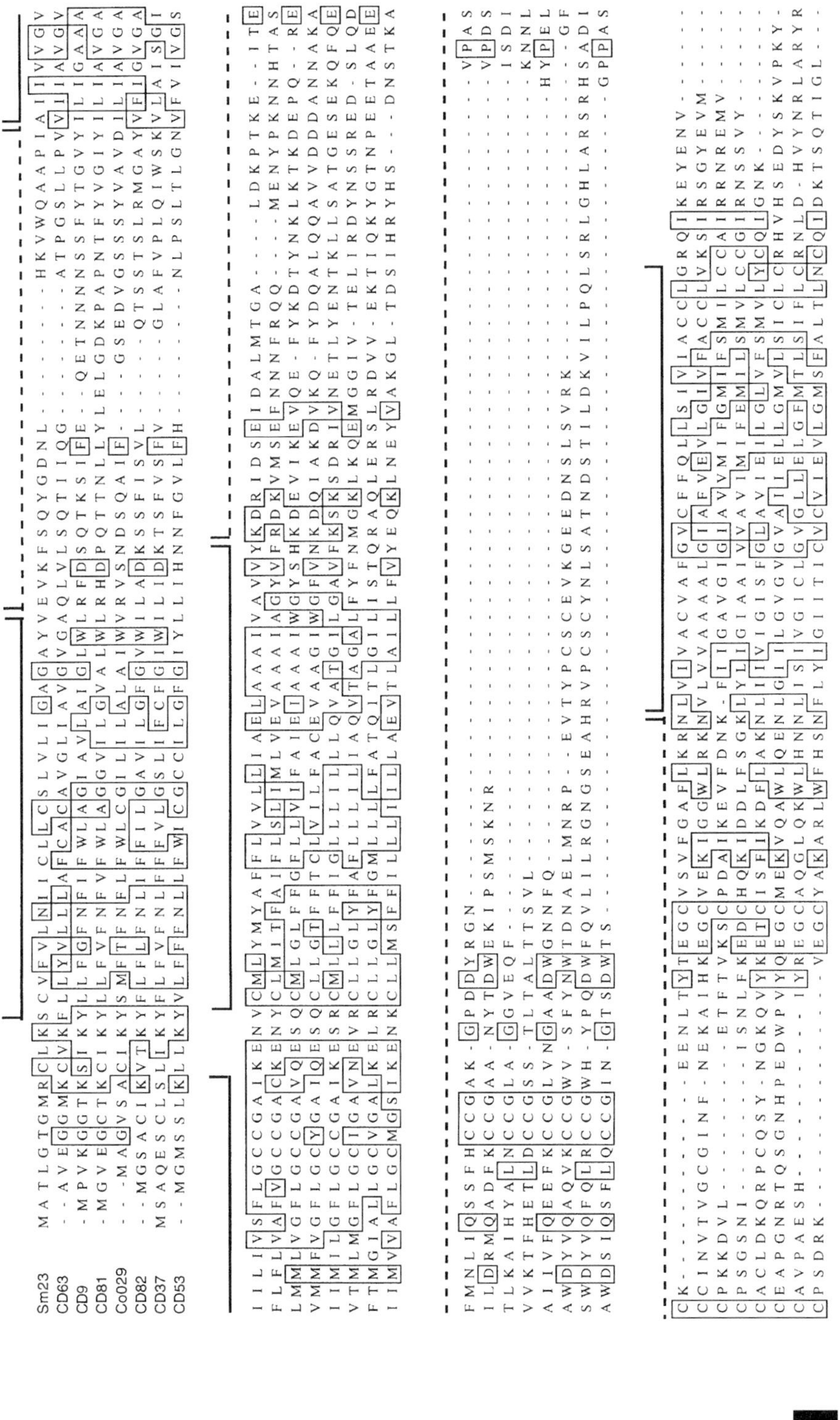

```
CD20    M T T - - - P R N S V N G T F P A E P M K G P - -  I A M Q S G P - - K P L F R R M S
FcεRIβ  M D T E N K S R A D L A L P N P Q E S P S A P D I E L L E A S P P A K A L P E K P A
HTm4    M A S H E V D N A E L G S A S A H G T P G - - - - - S E T G P - - E E L N T S V Y

S L V G P T - - Q S F F M R E S K T L G A V Q I M N G L F H I A L G G L L M I P - - A G I Y
S P P P Q Q T W Q S F L K K E L E F L G V T Q V L V G L I C L C F G T V V C S T L Q T S D F
H P I N G S - - P D Y Q K A K L Q V L G A I Q I L N A A M I L A L G V F L G S L Q Y P Y H F

A P I C V T - - V W Y P L W G G I M Y I I S G S L L A A T E K N S R K C L V K G K M I M N
- D D E V L L L Y R A G Y P F W G A V L F V L S G F L S I M S E R K N T L Y L V R G S L G A N
Q K H F F F F T F Y T G Y P I W G A V F F C S S G T L S V V A G I K P T R T W I Q N S F G M N

S L S L F A A I S G M I L S I M D I L N I K I S H F L K M E S L N F I R A H T P Y I N I Y N
I V S S I A A - - G L G I A I L - I L N L S - - - - - - - - - - - - - N N S A Y M N - Y -
I A S A T I A L V G T A F L S L N I A V N I Q S L - - - - - - - R S C H S S S E S P - - -

C E P A N P S E K N S P S T Q Y C Y S I Q S L F L G I L S V M L I F A F F Q E L V I A G I V
C - - - - - - K D I T E D D G C F V - T S - F I T E L V L M L L F L T I L A F C S A F V L
- - - - - - - - D L C N Y M G S - I S N G M V S L L L I L T L L E L C V T I S T

E N E W K R T C S R P K S N C I V L L S A E E K K E Q T I E I K E E V V G L T E T S S Q P K
L I I Y - - - - - - - - - - - - - - - - R I G Q E F E - R S K V - - - - - - P D D R
I A M W C - - - - - N A N C - - - - - - - - C N S R E E I - - - - - - - - -

N E E D I E I I - P I Q E E E E E E T E T N F P E P P Q D C Q E S S P I E N D S S P
L Y E E L H V Y S P I Y S A L E D T R E A F - - - - - - - - S A P V V S - - - -
- - - - - - - - - - - - - - - - S S P P N S V - - - -
```

Figure 40 *FcεRIβ/CD20 superfamily. Residues identical in two or more sequences are boxed. The putative positions of the four transmembrane sequences are indicated with a bar above the sequences. The sequences of the following proteins are from the SWISSPROT database or the reference given and the database accession number is given in brackets (the complete sequences are shown). Human CD20 (P22836); mouse FcεRI β chain (P20490) and the HTm4 (translated from EMBL accession number L35848).*

evolution from the leucocyte members [167]. The majority of the differences in sequence between TM4SF molecules reside in the extracellular loop between TM sequences 3 and 4 where there are considerable differences in sequence length. This loop of sequence is known to be extracellular because it includes the *N*-linked glycosylation sites and the MRC OX44 epitope, which can be labelled at the cell surface, maps to an Ile/Thr interchange in this region [168]. One feature of this superfamily is the high degree of sequence identity between species homologues, e.g. mouse CD81 is 92% identical to human CD81.

This superfamily appears to have a role outside the immune system because TM4SF members have been identified in schistosomes [169], the nematode *Caenorhabditis elegans* [170] and *Drosophila* [171]. There is no known function for any member of this superfamily although recent data have suggested roles in tumour cell metastasis [172], T cell development [173] and neural synapse formation [171]. TM4SF proteins probably mediate these functions as components of multimolecular complexes since they are known to associate with molecules such as the B and T cell antigen receptor complex, integrins and other TM4SF members (reviewed in ref. 166).

There is one example of a protein predicted to pass through the membrane five times, the CD47 or integrin-associated protein. A related protein has been found in vaccinia but so far a superfamily of TM5 molecules has not been defined.

```
TNFα    K P V A H V V A N - - - P Q A E G Q L Q W L N R R - A N A L L A N G V E L R - - D N Q L V V P S E G L Y L I Y S Q V L
LTα     K P A A H L I G D - - P S K Q N S L L W R A N T - D R A F L Q D G F S L S - - N N S L L V P T S G I Y F V Y S Q V V
LTβ     L P A A H L I G A - - P L K G G Q L G W E T T K - E Q A F L T S G T Q F S - D A E G L A L P Q D G L Y L I Y S Q V L V G
CD40L   Q I A A H V I S E - A S S K T T S V L Q W A E K G - Y Y T M S N N L V T L E - N G K Q L T V K R Q G L Y Y I Y A Q V T
CD30L   K S W A Y L Q V - A K H L N K T K L S W N K D - - Y G I L H - G V K R Y Q - D G N L V I Q F P G L Y F I - C Q L Q
FasL    R K V A H L T G K - S N S R S M P L E W E D T - - Y G I V L L S - G V K Y K - K G G L V I N E T G L Y F V Y S K V Y
OX40L   I Q S I K V Q F - T E Y K K E K G F I L T S - - Q K E D E I M K V Q - N N S V I I N C D G F Y L I S L K G Y
CD27L   W D V A E L Q L N H T G P Q Q D P R L Y W Q G G P A L G R S F L H - G P E L D - K G Q L R I H R D G I Y M V H I Q V T
4-1BBL  G M F A Q L V A Q - N V L L I D G P L S W Y S D P G L A G V S L T G G L S Y K E D T K E L V V A K A G V Y Y V F F Q L E

TNFα    F K G Q G C P - - - - S T H V L L T H T I S R I A V S Y Q T K V N L L S A I K S P C Q R - - - E T P E G A E A K
LTα     F S G K A Y S P K A T - - S S P L Y L A H E V Q L F S S Q Y P F H V P L L S S Q K M V Y - - - - - P G L Q E
LTβ     Y R G R A P P G G G D P Q G R S V T L R S S L Y R A G G A Y G P G T P E L L L E G A E T V T P V L D P A R R Q G Y G P
CD40L   F - - - C S N R E - - A S S Q A P F I A S L C L K S P G R - F E R I L L R A A N T H S - S A K P - - -
CD30L   F - L V Q C P N N - - - S V D Y L S H K V Y M H I K - K Q A L V T V C E S G - - -
FasL    F R G Q S C N - - - - - L P L S L H Y Q K D E - - E P L F Q L K K V - R S V - - -
OX40L   F S Q E - - - - - - V N I S L H Y P T T L A V G I C S P A S R - - S I S L L R L S F H Q G C - - -
CD27L   L - - A I C S S T T A S R H H P T T L A L H L Q P L R S A - - A G A A A L A L T V D L P P A S S E A R
4-1BBL  L R R V V A G E - - - G S G S V S L A L H L Q P L R S A - - A G A A A L A L T V D L P P A S S E A R

TNFα    P W Y E P I Y L G G V F Q L E K G D R L S A E I N R P D Y L D F A - - - E S G Q V Y F G I I A L
LTα     P W L H S M Y H G A A F Q L T Q G D Q L S T H T D G I P H L V L S - - - P S T V F F G A F A L
LTβ     L W Y T S I V G F G G L V Q L R R G E R V I S H P D M V D F A - - - R G K T F F G A V M V
CD40L   C G G Q S I H L G G V F E L Q P G A S V F V N V T D P S Q V S H - - - G T G F T S F G L L K L
CD30L   M Q T K V Y Y Q N L S Q F L L - - D Y L Q V N T T I S V N N D T F Q - Y I D T S T F P L E N V L
FasL    M W A R S S Y L G A V F N L T S A D H L Y V N V S E L S L V N F E - - - E S Q T F F G L Y K L
OX40L   - N S L M V A S - - I T Y K D K V Y L N V T T - D N T S L D - - - D F H V N G G E L I L
CD27L   - T I V S Q R L T P - - L A R G D T L C T N L T G T L L P S R - - - N T D E T F F G V Q W V
4-1BBL  - N S A F G F Q G R L L H L H T E A R A R H A W Q L T Q G A T V L G L F R V
```

Figure 41 *Tumour necrosis factor (TNF) superfamily repeats. Residues identical in five or more sequences are boxed. The positions of the β sheets determined for TNFα[181,182] are indicated by bars above the sequence. The asterisks mark the positions of the conserved residues used to identify domains for the corresponding entries in Section II. The sequences of the following proteins are from the SWISSPROT database and the accession number and residue numbers are given in brackets. TNFα, human tumour necrosis factor α (P01375, 87–233); LTα, human lymphotoxin α (P01374, 62–205); LTβ, lymphotoxin β (Q06643, 87–243); CD40L, human CD40 ligand (P29965, 121–261); CD30L, human CD30 ligand (P32971, 97–225); FasL, human Fas ligand (P48023, 144–281); OX40L, human OX40 ligand (P23510, 58–172); CD27L, human CD27 ligand or CD70 (P32970, 55–191); 4-1BBL, human 4-1BB ligand (P41273, 90–240).*

There are other leucocyte proteins that are predicted to traverse the plasma membrane four times, including CD20 and the FcεRI β chain but these do not show sequence similarity to the TM4SF given above. However, CD20 and the FcεRI β chain show clear sequence similarities to each other [174] in three of the four transmembrane regions of these molecules and a lower similarity to another gene called HTm4 [175], as shown in Fig. 40. All three genes are closely linked in humans to chromosome 11q12–13.1, and CD20 and the FcεRI β chain genes are very closely linked on mouse chromosome 19 [174]. Thus these three sequences form a small distinct superfamily termed FcεRIβ/CD20 superfamily. There are data to suggest that CD20 is a Ca^{2+} channel [176]. It seems likely that CD20 and HTm4 are associated with other membrane proteins since the FcεRIβ is one chain of the complex which forms the high affinity receptor for IgE on mast cells and functions as an amplifier of signals transduced by the FcεRI [177].

Tumour necrosis factor superfamily (TNFSF) (Figs 41 and 42)

This domain type is found in the extracellular domain of type II membrane proteins. It is not associated with any other extracellular domain type. The extracellular regions of

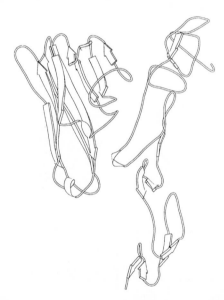

Figure 42 *The folding pattern of tumour necrosis factor (TNF) and TNFR superfamily. The structure shown is of one receptor (TNFR) molecule binding one monomer of TNF and is based on the structure of the complex of TNFR I and TNFβ [125]. The TNF is itself trimeric but the receptor is thought to be monomeric and only made trimeric by binding of ligand. The TNF is on the left of the figure and the receptor on the right. The N-terminus of the receptor is at the top of the figure and the membrane attachment would be at the base of the figure. TNF consist of a group of β sheets arranged into a "jelly-roll" whilst the receptor contains four TNFR repeats characterized by their lack of α helix or β sheet and held together by disulfide bridges.*

Figure 43 *Tumour necrosis factor receptor (TNFR) superfamily repeats. Residues identical in five or more sequences are boxed. The asterisks mark the positions of the conserved residues used to identify domains for the corresponding entries in Section II. The sequences of the following proteins are from the SWISSPROT database unless otherwise indicated and the database accession number and residue numbers are given in brackets. The sequences are contiguous over the four repeats except for OX40 which contains a short sequence in place of the third repeat. OX40, rat OX40 (CD134) antigen precursor (P15725, 25–102, 124–164); TNFRI, human tumour necrosis factor receptor precursor I (CD120a) (P19438, 43–196); TNFRII, human tumour necrosis factor receptor precursor II (CD120b) (P20333, 39–201); NGFR, rat nerve growth factor receptor precursor (P07174, 32–190); CD40, human CD40 antigen precursor (PIR: S04460, 25–187).*

Figure 44 *Tyrosine kinase domains*

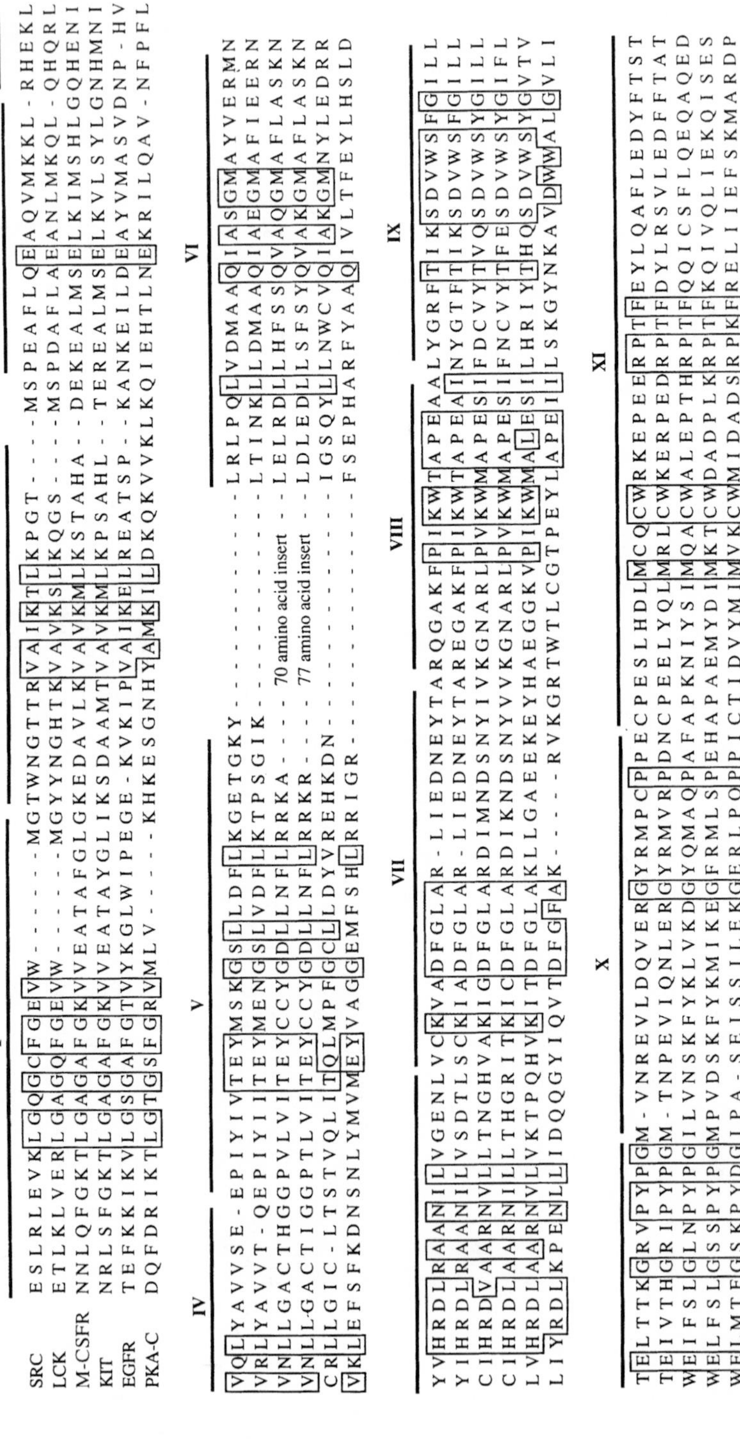

```
                      I                                    II                          III                                IV
SRC     E S L R L E V K L G Q C F G E V W - - - - - M G T W N G T T R V A I K T L K P G T - - - - M S P E A F L Q E A Q V M K K L - R H E K L
LCK     E T L K L V E R L G A G Q F G E V W - - - - - M G Y Y N G H T K V A V K S L K Q G S - - - M S P D A F L A E A N L M K Q L - Q H Q R L
M-CSFR  N N L Q F G K T L G A G A F G K V V E A T A F G L G K E D A V L K V A V K M L K S T A H A - D E K E A L M S E L K I M S H L G Q H E N I
KIT     N R L S F G K T L G A G A F G K V V E A T A Y G L I K S D A A M T V A V K M L K P S A H L - T E R E A L M S E L K V L S Y L G N H M N I
EGFR    T E F K K I K V L G S G A F G T V Y K G L W I P E G E - K V K I P V A I K E L R E A T S P - K A N K E I L D E A Y V M A S V D N P - H V
PKA-C   D Q F D R I K T L G T G S F G R V M L V - - - - K H K E S G N H Y A M K I L D K Q K V V K L K Q I E H T L N E K R I L Q A V - N F P F L

        IV                                      V                                                  VI
SRC     V Q L Y A V V S E - E P I Y I V T E Y M S K G S L L D F L K G E T G K Y - - - - - - - - - L R L P Q L V D M A A Q I A S G M A Y V E R M N
LCK     V R L Y A V V T - Q E P I Y I I T E Y M E N G S L V D F L K T P S G I K - - - - - - - - - L T I N K L L D M A A Q I A E G M A F I E E R N
M-CSFR  V N L L G A C T H G G P V L V I T E Y C C Y G D L L N F L R R K A - - - - 70 amino acid insert - L E L R D L L H F S S Q V A Q G M A F L A S K N
KIT     V N L L G A C T I G G P T L V I T E Y C C Y G D L L N F L R R K R - - - - 77 amino acid insert - L D L E D L L S F S Y Q V A K G M A F L A S K N
EGFR    C R L L G I C - L T S T V Q L I T Q L M P F G C L L D Y V R E H K D N - - - - - - - - - I G S Q Y L L N W C V Q I A K G M N Y L E D R R
PKA-C   V K L E F S F K D N S N L Y M V M E Y V A G G E M F S H L R R I G R - - - - - - - - - - F S E P H A R F Y A A Q I V L T F E Y L H S L D

                        VII                              VIII                          IX
SRC     Y V H R D L R A A N I L V G E N L V C K V A D F G L A R - L I E D N E Y T A R Q G A K F P I K W T A P E A A L Y G R F T I K S D V W S F G I L L
LCK     Y I H R D L R A A N I L V S D T L S C K I A D F G L A R - L I E D N E Y T A R E G A K F P I K W T A P E A I N Y G T F T I K S D V W S F G I L L
M-CSFR  C I H R D V A A R N V L L T N G H V A K I G D F G L A R D I M N D S N Y I V K G N A R L P V K W M A P E S I F D C V Y T V Q S D V W S Y G I L L
KIT     C I H R D L A A R N I L L T H G R I T K I C D F G L A R D I K N D S N Y V V K G N A R L P V K W M A P E S I F N C V Y T F E S D V W S Y G I F L
EGFR    L V H R D L A A R N V L V K T P Q H V K I T D F G L A K L L G A E E K E Y H A E G G K V P I K W M A L E S I L H R I Y T H Q S D V W S Y G V T V
PKA-C   L I Y R D L K P E N L L I D Q Q G Y I Q V T D F G F A K - - - - R V K G R T W T L C G T P E Y L A P E I I L S K G Y N K A V D W W A L G V L I

                        X                                              XI
SRC     T E L T T K G R V P Y P G M - V N R E V L D Q V E R G Y R M P C P P E C P E S L H D L M C Q C W R K E P E E R P T F E Y L Q A F L E D Y F T S T
LCK     T E I V T H G R I P Y P G M - T N P E V I Q N L E R G Y R M V R P D N C P E E L Y Q L M R L C W K E R P E D R P T F D Y L R S V L E D F F T A T
M-CSFR  W E I F S L G L N P Y P G I L V N S K F Y K L V K D G Y Q M A Q P A F A P K N I Y S I M Q A C W A L E P T H R P T F Q Q I C S F L Q E Q A Q E D
KIT     W E L F S L G S S P Y P G M P V D S K F Y K M I K E G F R M L S P E H A P A E M Y D I M K T C W D A D P L K R P T F K Q I V Q L I E K Q I S E S
EGFR    W E L M T F G S K P Y D G I P A - S E I S S I L E K G E R L P Q P P I C T I D V Y M I M V K C W M I D A D S R P K F R E L I I E F S K M A R D P
PKA-C   Y E M A A - G Y P P F F A D - Q P I Q I Y E K I V S G K V R F - P S H F S S D L K D L L R N L L Q V D L T K R F G N L K N G V N D I K N H K W F
```

Figure 44 (opposite) *Tyrosine kinase domains. Residues identical in five or more sequences are boxed. The bars above the sequences represent the subdomains defined in this superfamily and the numbering is as in ref. 191. These correspond to structural features as determined from the structure of the mouse cAMP-dependent protein kinase α subunit illustrated in Fig. 45 and discussed in ref. 194. The sequences of the following proteins are from the SWISSPROT database and the database accession number and residue numbers are given in brackets. SRC, human src proto-oncogene tyrosine kinase (P12931, 268–526); LCK, human T cell-specific tyrosine kinase (P06239, 243–501); M-CSFR, human macrophage colony-stimulating factor receptor precursor (P07333, 580–917); KIT, human kit proto-oncogene precursor (CD117) (P10721, 587–931); EGFR, human EGF receptor precursor (P00533, 710–975); PKA-C, mouse cAMP-dependent protein kinase (P05132, 41–297).*

members are often released by proteolysis to give soluble factors with biological activity such as TNF, lymphotoxin, FasL (reviewed in refs 178–180). Several members have been defined recently and are often called ligands of the respective receptor, e.g. CD40L, CD27L (also called CD70), 4-1BBL, OX40L, FasL (CD95L). The receptors themselves form a superfamily termed the TNFRSF (see below).

Structural studies by X-ray crystallography on TNFα[181,182], TNFβ[125] and CD40 ligand[183] show they form homotrimers with a characteristic "jelly roll" β sandwich. The stoichiometry of the interaction between TNFRI and TNFβ trimer is 3:1[125]. This ratio is probably true for most of the other members of the superfamily although the 4-1BB ligand forms a disulfide-linked homodimer[184,185] and unlike most of the receptors CD27 seems to form a homodimer and may interact with its ligand in a different manner.

The structure of TNFRI complexed with TNFβ is illustrated in Fig. 42 and discussed below.

Tumour necrosis factor receptor superfamily (TNFRSF) (Figs 42 and 43)

This superfamily was previously called nerve growth factor receptor (NGFR) superfamily as NGFR was the first member to be defined of this superfamily. Four cysteine-rich repeats were recognized in the extracellular part of the low-affinity NGFR and subsequently related sequence repeats have been identified in a number of leucocyte cell surface antigens including CD40, CD134 (OX40), CD27, TNF receptors (CD120), CD30 and 4-1BB[178,179]. Figure 43 shows an alignment of some of the repeats. All these examples show more similarity amongst themselves, for instance in gene structure and nature of ligands, than with NGFR. Thus this group is now more generally known as the TNFRSF after the well-characterized TNFR. One unusual feature is that most of the TNFRSF molecules contain 3 or 4 repeats. No single TNFRSF repeat sequence has been found and the repeat has not been associated with any other domain types. The gene structures for TNFRSF members show that the boundaries of each repeat do not correspond to exon boundaries. The gene for NGFR shows a different pattern of intron/exon boundaries to those members on leucocytes which form a separate group[186,187]. It seems possible that a primordial gene with four repeats may have evolved by unequal crossing-over during recombination. This gene probably gave rise to all known members of the TNFR superfamily by duplication and divergence, with the NGFR forming a separate branch from that of the leucocyte members [187]. The ligands for the leucocyte members form a group of type II membrane proteins with sequence similarities to TNF (see above).

The structure of the TNFRI complexed with TNFβ has been determined by X-ray crystallography [125]. Three receptor molecules form a sheath around the trimeric TNFβ. Figure 42 shows the structure of one receptor and one monomer unit of the ligand [125]. The four repeats in the receptor are arranged in a linear array. Each receptor molecule contacts two of the ligand molecules through a combination of hydrophobic and hydrophilic interactions. There is an absence of β sheet or α helix structure, with the three disulfide bridges in each repeat forming a ladder-like pattern. The interaction is intriguing as the two related receptors TNFRI and II share about 24% identity in amino sequence in the Cys-rich region yet both can bind the same ligands TNFα and TNFβ, both of which themselves share only 33% identity.

Tyrosine kinase domains (Figs 44 and 45)

Two groups of tyrosine kinases can be distinguished: receptor tyrosine kinases which are transmembrane proteins where the tyrosine kinase domains are found in the cytoplasmic part, and non-receptor tyrosine kinases which are located in the cytoplasm. The non-receptor group of kinases includes members of the Src family, all of which are anchored to the inner leaflet of the plasma membrane with a myristate moiety. On activation they phosphorylate Tyr residues on their own cytoplasmic domains or on other proteins in the cytoplasm and this is believed to be

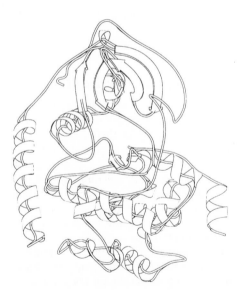

Figure 45 *The folding pattern of a tyrosine kinase domain. The structure shown is that of the mouse cAMP-dependent protein kinase α subunit [194]. The correlation between the secondary structure and the subdomains indicated in Fig. 44 is discussed in ref. 194.*

one of the early events in signal transduction pathways after ligand recognition. The Src kinases are expressed in association with SH2 and SH3 domains which can mediate interactions in the cascade (see details on ITAM earlier under **Signal transduction sequence motifs**). In leucocytes the best studied example is Lck, which associates with the cytoplasmic domains of CD4 and CD8 and regulates signal transduction by these molecules. Other examples are Fyn which associates with the T cell receptor complex [188], and Lyn, Fyn and Blk, which couple to the membrane Ig complex of B cells (reviewed in refs 159 and 189).

Receptor tyrosine kinases are expressed on a wide variety of cells and examples include the PDGF receptor (CD140), EGF receptor and c-kit (CD117). When these receptors bind their natural ligands they oligomerize and the cytoplasmic tyrosine kinase domains become activated and autophosphorylated. This leads to the phosphorylation and activation of various intracellular substrates including phospholipase C-γ, phosphatidylinositol 3-kinase and the c-raf serine kinase. These effector molecules concomitantly associate with the activated receptor kinases.

Tyrosine kinase domains consist of about 260–360 amino acids. The difference in size is due to insertion of a "kinase insert domain" of about 70–100 amino acids in certain receptor kinases, including the PDGFR (CD140), M-CSFR (CD115), and c-kit (CD117) kinases. These insert regions appear to regulate the interaction of the kinase with certain cellular substrates/ effector molecules (reviewed in refs 159 and 190). The tyrosine kinase domain of a particular molecule is particularly well-conserved across species and the identities between molecules within the superfamily are about 40% as illustrated in Fig. 44. This is much higher than for many of the superfamilies with domains that are found at the cell surface.

The amino acid sequences of tyrosine kinase domains are not conserved uniformly, but consist of 11 highly conserved subdomains (I–XI) separated by regions of lower conservation [191]. Subdomain I contains the Gly-X-Gly-X-X-Gly consensus which forms part of the binding site for ATP. Subdomain II contains an invariant lysine, which appears to be directly involved in the phosphotransfer reaction. Subdomain VIII contains a Pro-Ile/Val-Lys/Arg-Trp-Thr/Met-Ala-Pro-Glu consensus which is characteristic of the tyrosine kinases. In the serine/threonine kinases the consensus is Gly-Thr/Ser-X-X-Tyr/Phe-X-Ala-Pro-Glu. These subdomains have now been correlated with structural elements from the X-ray crystallography structure of the cAMP-dependent protein kinase α subunit shown in Fig. 45.

References

[1] Baron, M. et al. (1991) Protein modules. Trends Biochem. Sci. 16, 13–17.

[2] Shapiro, L. et al. (1995) Structural basis of cell-cell adhesion by cadherins. Nature 374, 327–336.

[3] Nagar, B. et al. (1996) Structural basis of calcium-induced E-cadherin rigidification and dimerization. Nature 380, 360–364.

[4] Kolodkin, A.L. (1996) Semaphorins: Mediators of repulsive growth cone guidance. Trends Cell Biol. 6, 15–22.

[5] Mott, H. and Campbell, I. (1995) Four helix bundle growth factors and their receptors: protein-protein interactions. Curr. Opin. Struct. Biol. 5, 114–121.

[6] Doolittle, R. (1995) The multiplicity of domains in proteins. Annu. Rev. Biochem. 64, 287–314.

[7] Fletcher, C.M. et al. (1994) Structure of a soluble, glycosylated form of the human-complement regulatory protein CD59. Structure 2, 185–199.

[8] Kieffer, B. et al. (1994) 3-dimensional solution structure of the extracellular region of the complement regulatory protein CD59, a new cell-surface protein domain related to snake-venom neurotoxins. Biochemistry 33, 4471–4482.

[9] Patthy, L. (1987) Intron-dependent evolution: preferred types of exons and introns. FEBS Lett. 214, 1–7.

[10] Bork, P. et al. (1996) Structure and distribution of modules in extracellular proteins. Q. Rev. Biophys. 29, 119–167.

[11] Kobe, B. and Deisenhofer, J. (1993) Crystal structure of porcine ribonuclease inhibitor, a protein with leucine-rich repeats. Nature 366, 751–756.

[12] Kobe, B. and Deisenhofer, J. (1994) The leucine-rich repeat: a versatile binding motif. Trends Biochem. Sci. 19, 415–421.

[13] Williams, A.F. and Barclay, A.N. (1988) The immunoglobulin superfamily – domains for cell surface recognition. Annu. Rev. Immunol. 6, 381–405.

[14] Brutlag, D. and Sternberg, M. (1996) Sequences and topology, challenges for algorithms and experts. Curr. Opin. Struct. Biol. 6, 343–345.

[15] Bork, P. and Koonin, E. (1996) Protein sequence motifs. Curr. Opin. Struct. Biol. 6, 366–376.

[16] Henikoff, S. (1996) Scores for sequence searches and alignments. Curr. Opin. Struct. Biol. 6, 353–360.

[17] Pearson, W.R. (1995) Comparison of methods for searching protein-sequence databases. Protein Sci. 4, 1145–1160.

[18] Pearson, W.R. and Lipman, D.J. (1988) Improved tools for biological sequence comparison. Proc. Natl Acad. Sci. USA 85, 2444–2448.

[19] Altschul, S.F. et al. (1990) Basic local alignment search tool. J. Mol. Biol. 215, 403–410.

[20] Patthy, L. (1990) Homology of a domain of the growth hormone/prolactin receptor family with type III modules of fibronectin [letter]. Cell 61, 13–14.

[21] Bairoch, A. (1993) The PROSITE dictionary of sites and patterns in proteins, its current status. Nucleic Acids Res. 21, 3097–3103.

[22] WWW. http://expasy.hcuge.ch/

[23] Dayhoff, M.O. et al. (1983) Establishing homologies in protein sequences. Meth. Enzymol. 91, 524–545.

[24] George, D.G. et al. (1990) Mutation data matrix and its uses. Meth. Enzymol. 183, 333–351.

[25] Henikoff, S. and Henikoff, J.G. (1992) Amino acid substitution matrices from protein blocks. Proc. Natl Acad. Sci. USA 89, 10915–10919.

[26] Brady, R.L. and Barclay, A.N. (1995) The structure of CD4. In Current Topics in Microbiology and Immunology, vol. 205: the CD4 Molecule (Littman, D.R., ed.). Springer-Verlag, Berlin, pp. 1–18.

[27] Amzel, L.M. and Poljak, R.J. (1979) Three-dimensional structure of immunoglobulins. Annu. Rev. Biochem. 48, 961–997.

[28] Holmgren, A. and Branden, C.I. (1989) Crystal structure of chaperone protein PapD reveals an immunoglobulin fold. Nature 342, 248–251.

[29] de Vos, A.M. et al. (1992) Human growth hormone and extracellular domain of its receptor: crystal structure of the complex. Science 255, 306–312.

[30] Baron, M. et al. (1992) 1H NMR assignment and secondary structure of the cell adhesion type III module of fibronectin. Biochemistry 31, 2068–2073.

[31] Overduin, M. et al. (1995) Solution structure of the epithelial cadherin domain responsible for selective cell adhesion. Science 386–389.

[32] Williams, A.F. (1987) A year in the life of the immunoglobulin superfamily. Immunol. Today 8, 298–303.

[33] Wong, E. et al. (1993) Leukocyte common antigen-related phosphatase (LRP) gene structure: Conservation of organization of transmembrane protein tyrosine phosphatases. Genomics 17, 33–38.

[34] Patthy, L. (1987) Detecting homology of distantly related proteins with consensus sequences. J. Mol. Biol. 198, 567–577.

[35] Sharp, P.A. (1981) Speculations on RNA splicing. Cell 23, 643–646.

[36] Bowen, M.A. et al. (1997) Structure and chromosomal location of the human CD6 gene. J. Immunol. 158, 1149–1156.

[37] Doherty, P. et al. (1992) The VASE exon downregulates the neurite growth-promoting activity of NCAM 140. Nature 356, 791–793.

[38] Murray, A.J. et al. (1995) One sequence, two folds: a metastable structure of CD2. Proc. Natl Acad. Sci. USA 92, 7337–7341.

[39] Lobsanov, Y.D. et al. (1993) X-ray crystal structure of the human dimeric S-Lac lectin, L-14-II, in complex with lactose at 2.9-A resolution. J. Biol. Chem. 268, 27034–27038.

[40] Barton, G.J. and Sternberg, M.J. (1987) A strategy for the rapid multiple alignment of protein sequences. Confidence levels from tertiary structure comparisons. J. Mol. Biol. 198, 327–337.

[41] Devereux, J. et al. (1984) A comprehensive set of sequence analysis programs for the VAX. Nucleic Acids Res. 12, 387–395.

[42] Ryu, S.E. et al. (1990) Crystal structure of an HIV-binding recombinant fragment of human CD4. Nature 348, 419–426.

[43] Wang, J. et al. (1990) Atomic structure of a fragment of human CD4 containing two immunoglobulin-like domains. Nature 348, 411–418.

[44] Brady, R.L. et al. (1993) Crystal structure of domains 3 and 4 of rat CD4: relationship to the NH_2-terminal domains. Science 260, 979–983.

[45] Politou, A.S. et al. (1994) Immunoglobulin-type domains of titin are stabilized by amino-terminal extension. FEBS Lett. 352, 27–31.

[46] Reid, K.B. and Day, A.J. (1989) Structure-function relationships of the complement components. Immunol. Today 10, 177–180.

[47] Barlow, P.N. et al. (1993) Solution structure of a pair of complement modules by nuclear magnetic resonance. J. Mol. Biol. 237, 268–284.

[48] Barlow, P.N. et al. (1991) Secondary structure of a complement control protein module by two-dimensional 1H NMR. Biochemistry 30, 997–1004.

[49] Idzerda, R.L. et al. (1990) Human interleukin 4 receptor confers biological responsiveness and defines a novel receptor superfamily. J. Exp. Med. 171, 861–873.

[50] Cosman, D. et al. (1990) A new cytokine receptor superfamily. Trends Biochem. Sci. 15, 265–270.

[51] Goodwin, R.G. et al. (1990) Cloning of the human and murine interleukin-7 receptors: demonstration of a soluble form and homology to a new receptor superfamily. Cell 60, 941–951.

[52] Somers, W. et al. (1994) The X-ray structure of growth hormone-prolactin receptor complex. Nature 372, 478–481.

[53] Jones, E.Y. et al. (1992) Crystal structure of a soluble form of the cell adhesion molecule CD2 at 2.8 Å. Nature 360, 232–239.

54 Bodian, D.L. et al. (1994) Crystal structure of the extracellular region of the human cell adhesion molecule CD2 at 2.5 Å resolution. Structure 2, 755–766.

55 Holden, H.M. et al. (1992) X-ray structure determination of telokin, the C-terminal domain of myosin light chain kinase, at 2.8 Å resolution. J. Mol. Biol. 227, 840–851.

56 Bazan, J.F. (1990) Structural design and molecular evolution of a cytokine receptor superfamily. Proc. Natl Acad. Sci. USA 87, 6934–6938.

57 Cooke, R.M. et al. (1987) The solution structure of human epidermal growth factor. Nature 327, 339–341.

58 Tappin, M.J. et al. (1989) A high-resolution 1H-NMR study of human transforming growth factor alpha. Structure and pH-dependent conformational interconversion. Eur. J. Biochem. 179, 629–637.

59 Handford, P.A. et al. (1990) The first EGF-like domain from human factor IX contains a high-affinity calcium binding site. EMBO J. 9, 475–480.

60 Rao, Z. et al. (1995) The structure of a Ca^{2+}-binding epidermal growth factor-like domain: Its role in protein-protein interactions. Cell 82, 131–141.

61 Graves, B.J. et al. (1994) Insight into E-selectin/ligand interaction from the crystal structure and mutagenesis of the lec/EGF domains. Nature 367, 532–538.

62 Handford, P.A. et al. (1991) Key residues involved in calcium-binding motifs in EGF-like domains. Nature 351, 164–167.

63 Downing, A.K. et al. (1996) Solution structure of a pair of calcium-binding epidermal growth factor- like domains: Implications for the Marfan syndrome and other genetic disorders. Cell 85, 597–605.

64 Constantine, K.L. et al. (1991) Sequence-specific 1H NMR assignments and structural characterization of bovine seminal fluid protein PDC-109 domain b. Biochemistry 30, 1663–1672.

65 Brummendorf, T. and Rathjen, F. (1993) Axonal glycoproteins with immunoglobulin and fibronectin type III-related domains in vertebrates: structural features, binding activities, and signal transduction. J. Neurochem. 61, 1207–1219.

66 Benian, G.M. et al. (1989) Sequence of an unusually large protein implicated in regulation of myosin activity in C. elegans. Nature 342, 45–50.

67 Labeit, S. et al. (1990) A regular pattern of two types of 100-residue motif in the sequence of titin. Nature 345, 273–276.

68 Labeit, S. and Kolmerer, B. (1995) Titins: Giant proteins in charge of muscle ultrastructure and elasticity. Science 270, 293–296.

69 Suzuki, S. and Naitoh, Y. (1990) Amino acid sequence of a novel integrin beta 4 subunit and primary expression of the mRNA in epithelial cells. EMBO J. 9, 757–763.

70 Leahy, D.J. et al. (1996) 2.0 Å Crystal structure of a four-domain segment of human fibronectin encompassing the RGD loop and synergy region. Cell 84, 155–164.

71 Huber, A.H. et al. (1994) Crystal structure of tandem type III fibronectin domains from drosophila neuroglian at 2.0 Å. Neuron 12, 717–731.

72 Drickamer, K. (1988) Two distinct classes of carbohydrate-recognition domains in animal lectins. J. Biol. Chem. 263, 9557–9560.

73 Barondes, S. et al. (1994) Galectins: A family of animal β-galactoside-binding lectins. Cell 76, 597–598.

74 Frigeri, L.G. et al. (1990) Expression of biologically active recombinant rat IgE-binding protein in Escherichia coli. J. Biol. Chem. 265, 20763–20769.

[75] Watson, S. and Arkinstall, S. (1994) The G-Protein Linked Receptor FactsBook. Academic Press, London, pp. 1–427.

[76] WWW. http://www.sander.embl-heidelberg.de/7tm/

[77] McKnight, A. and Gordon, S. (1996) EGF-TM7: a novel subfamily of seven-transmembrane-region leukocyte cell surface molecules. Immunol. Today 17, 283–287.

[78] Bjorkman, P.J. et al. (1987) Structure of the human class I histocompatibility antigen, HLA-A2. Nature 329, 506–512.

[79] Brown, J.H. et al. (1993) Three-dimensional structure of the human class II histocompatibility antigen HLA-DR1. Nature 364, 33–39.

[80] Madden, D.R. (1995) The three-dimensional structure of peptide-MHC complexes. Annu. Rev. Immunol. 13, 587–622.

[81] Jardetzky, T.S. et al. (1994) Three-dimensional structure of a human class II histocompatibility molecule complexed with superantigen. Nature 368, 711–718.

[82] Leahy, D.J. et al. (1992) Crystal structure of a soluble form of the human T cell coreceptor CD8 at 2.6 Å resolution. Cell 68, 1145–1162.

[83] Driscoll, P.C. et al. (1991) Structure of domain 1 of rat T lymphocyte CD2 antigen. Nature 353, 762–765.

[84] Jones, E.Y. et al. (1995) Crystal structure of an integrin-binding fragment of vascular cell adhesion molecule-1 at 1.8 Å resolution. Nature 373, 539–544.

[85] Bentley, G.A. et al. (1995) Crystal structure of the beta chain of a T cell antigen receptor. Science 267, 1984–1987.

[86] Fields, B.A. et al. (1995) Crystal structure of the V(alpha) domain of a T cell antigen receptor. Science 270, 1821–1824.

[87] Garboczi, D. et al. (1996) Structure of the complex between T-cell receptor, viral peptide and HLA-A2. Nature 384, 134–141.

[88] Garcia, K. et al. (1996) An $\alpha\beta$ T cell receptor structure at 2.5 Å and its orientation in the TCR-MHC complex. Science 274, 209–219.

[89] Harpaz, Y. and Chothia, C. (1994) Many of the immunoglobulin superfamily domains in cell-adhesion molecules and surface-receptors belong to a new structural set which is close to that containing variable domains. J. Mol. Biol. 238, 528–539.

[90] Thomsen, N. et al. (1996) The three-dimensional structure of the first domain of neural cell adhesion molecule. Nature Struct. Biol. 3, 581–585.

[91] Erle, D.J. et al. (1991) Complete amino acid sequence of an integrin beta subunit (beta 7) identified in leukocytes. J. Biol. Chem. 266, 11009–11016.

[92] Takada, Y. and Hemler, M.E. (1989) The primary structure of the VLA-2/collagen receptor alpha 2 subunit (platelet GPIa): homology to other integrins and the presence of a possible collagen-binding domain. J. Cell Biol. 109, 397–407.

[93] Hemler, M.E. (1990) VLA proteins in the integrin family: structures, functions, and their role on leukocytes. Annu. Rev. Immunol. 8, 365–400.

[94] Stewart, M. et al. (1995) Leukocyte integrins. Current Biol. 7, 690–696.

[95] Piggott, R. and Power, C. (1993) The Adhesion Molecule FactsBook. Academic Press, London.

[96] Lee, J.O. et al. (1995) Crystal structure of the A domain from the alpha subunit of integrin CR3 (CD11b/CD18). Cell 80, 631–638.

[97] Qu, A. and Leahy, D.J. (1995) Crystal structure of the I-domain from the CD11a/CD18 (LFA-1, alpha(L)beta2) integrin. Proc. Natl Acad. Sci. USA 92, 10277–10281.

98 Drickamer, K. (1993) Ca^{2+}-dependent carbohydrate-recognition domains in animal proteins. Curr. Opin. Struct. Biol. 3, 393–400.

99 Patthy, L. (1988) Detecting distant homologies of mosaic proteins. Analysis of the sequences of thrombomodulin, thrombospondin complement components C9, C8 alpha and C8 beta, vitronectin and plasma cell membrane glycoprotein PC-1. J. Mol. Biol. 202, 689–696.

100 Lasky, L.A. et al. (1989) Cloning of a lymphocyte homing receptor reveals a lectin domain. Cell 56, 1045–1055.

101 Hoyle, G.W. and Hill, R.L. (1991) Structure of the gene for a carbohydrate-binding receptor unique to rat kupffer cells. J. Biol. Chem. 266, 1850–1857.

102 Doege, K. et al. (1987) Complete primary structure of the rat cartilage proteoglycan core protein deduced from cDNA clones. J. Biol. Chem. 262, 17757–17767.

103 Collins, T. et al. (1991) Structure and chromosomal location of the gene for endothelial-leukocyte adhesion molecule 1. J. Biol. Chem. 266, 2466–2473.

104 Johnston, G.I. et al. (1990) Structure of the human gene encoding granule membrane protein-140, a member of the selectin family of adhesion receptors for leukocytes. J. Biol. Chem. 265, 21381–21385.

105 Ezekowitz, R.A. et al. (1990) Molecular characterization of the human macrophage mannose receptor: demonstration of multiple carbohydrate recognition-like domains and phagocytosis of yeasts in Cos-1 cells. J. Exp. Med. 172, 1785–1794.

106 Kim, S. et al. (1992) Organisation of the gene encoding the human macrophage mannose receptor (MRC1). Genomics 14, 721–727.

107 Harris, N. et al. (1994) The exon–intron structure and chromosomal localization of the mouse macrophage mannose receptor gene Mrc1: identification of a ricin like domain at the N-terminus of the receptor. Biochem. Biophys. Res. Commun. 198, 682–692.

108 Weis, W.I. et al. (1992) Structure of the calcium-dependent lectin domain from a rat mannose-binding protein determined by MAD phasing. Science 254, 1608–1615.

109 Sheriff, S. et al. (1994) Human mannose-binding protein carbohydrate recognition domain trimerizes through a triple α-helical coiled-coil. Nature Struct. Biol. 1, 789–794.

110 Iobst, S.T. and Drickamer, K. (1994) Binding of sugar ligands to Ca^{2+}-dependent animal lectins. II. Generation of high-affinity galactose binding by site-directed mutagenesis. J. Biol. Chem. 269, 15512–15519.

111 Blanck, O. et al. (1996) Introduction of selectin-like binding specificity into a homologous mannose-binding protein. J. Biol. Chem. 271, 7289–7292.

112 Kogan, T.P. et al. (1995) A single amino acid residue can determine the ligand specificity of E-selectin. J. Biol. Chem. 270, 14047–14055.

113 Hickey, M.J. et al. (1989) Human platelet glycoprotein IX: an adhesive prototype of leucine-rich glycoproteins with flank-center-flank structures. Proc. Natl Acad. Sci. USA 86, 6773–6777.

114 Schneider, R. and Schweiger, M. (1991) A novel modular mosaic of cell adhesion motifs in the extracellular domains of the neurogenic trk and trkB tyrosine kinase receptors. Oncogene 6, 1807–1811.

115 Wenger, R.H. et al. (1988) Structure of the human blood platelet membrane glycoprotein 1b alpha gene. Biochem. Biophys. Res. Commun. 156, 389–395.

[116] Perin, J.P. et al. (1987) Link protein interactions with hyaluronate and proteoglycans. Characterization of two distinct domains in bovine cartilage link proteins. J. Biol. Chem. 262, 13269–13272.

[117] Aruffo, A. et al. (1990) CD44 is the principal cell surface receptor for hyaluronate. Cell 61, 1303–1313.

[118] Miyake, K. et al. (1990) Hyaluronate can function as a cell adhesion molecule and CD44 participates in hyaluronate recognition. J. Exp. Med. 172, 69–75.

[119] Kohda, D. et al. (1996) Solution structure of the link module: a hyaluronan-binding domain involved in extracellular matrix stability and cell migration. Cell 86, 767–775.

[120] Stein, P. et al. (1994) The crystal structure of pertussis toxin. Structure 2, 45–57.

[121] Yamamato, T. et al. (1984) The human LDL receptor: a cysteine-rich protein with multiple Alu sequences in its mRNA. Cell 39, 27–38.

[122] Südhof, T.C. et al. (1985) The LDL receptor gene: a mosaic of exons shared with different proteins. Science 228, 815–822.

[123] Esser, V. et al. (1988) Mutational analysis of the ligand binding domain of the low density lipoprotein receptor. J. Biol. Chem. 263, 13282–13290.

[124] Daly, N. et al. (1995) 3-dimensional structure of a cysteine-rich repeat from the low-density-lipoprotein receptor. Proc. Natl Acad. Sci. USA 92, 6334–6338.

[125] Banner, D.W. et al. (1993) Crystal structure of the soluble human 55 kd TNF receptor-human TNFβ complex: implications for TNF receptor activation. Cell 73, 431–445.

[126] Shevach, E.M. and Korty, P.E. (1989) Ly-6: a multigene family in search of a function. Immunol. Today 10, 195–200.

[127] Williams, A.F. (1991) Emergence of the Ly-6 superfamily of GPI-anchored molecules. Cell Biol. Int. Reports 15, 769–777.

[128] LeClair, K.P. et al. (1986) Isolation of a murine Ly-6 cDNA reveals a new multigene family. EMBO J. 5, 3227–3234.

[129] Williams, A.F. et al. (1988) Squid glycoproteins with structural similarities to Thy-1 and Ly-6 antigens. Immunogenetics 27, 265–272.

[130] Orr, H.T. et al. (1979) Complete amino acid sequence of a papain-solubilized human histocompatibility antigen, HLA-B7.2. Sequence determination and search for homologies. Biochemistry 18, 5711–5720.

[131] Simister, N.E. and Mostov, K.E. (1989) An Fc receptor structurally related to MHC class I antigens. Nature 337, 184–187.

[132] Beck, S. and Barrell, B.G. (1988) Human cytomegalovirus encodes a glycoprotein homologous to MHC class-I antigens. Nature 331, 269–272.

[133] Brown, J.H. et al. (1988) A hypothetical model of the foreign antigen binding site of Class II histocompatibility molecules. Nature 332, 845–850.

[134] Bjorkman, P.J. and Parham, P. (1990) Structure, function, and diversity of class I major histocompatibility complex molecules. Annu. Rev. Biochem. 59, 253–288.

[135] Lawlor, D.A. et al. (1990) Evolution of class-I MHC genes and proteins: from natural selection to thymic selection. Annu. Rev. Immunol. 8, 23–63.

[136] Burmeister, W.P. et al. (1994) Crystal structure at 2.2 Å resolution of the MHC-related neonatal Fc receptor. Nature 372, 336–343.

[137] Thomas, M.L. et al. (1985) Evidence from cDNA clones that the rat leucocyte-common antigen (T200) spans the lipid bilayer and contains a cytoplasmic domain of 80,000 Mr. Cell 41, 83–93.

138 Charbonneau, H. et al. (1988) The leucocyte common antigen (CD45): a putative receptor-linked protein tyrosine phosphatase. Proc. Natl Acad. Sci. USA 85, 7182–7186.

139 Tonks, N.K. et al. (1988) Demonstration that the leucocyte common antigen CD45 is a protein tyrosine phosphatase. Biochemistry 27, 8695–8701.

140 Streuli, M. et al. (1990) Distinct functional roles of the two intracellular phosphatase like domains of the receptor-linked protein tyrosine phosphatases LCA and LAR. EMBO J. 9, 2399–2407.

141 Streuli, M. et al. (1988) A new member of the immunoglobulin superfamily that has a cytoplasmic region homologous to the leukocyte common antigen. J. Exp. Med. 168, 1523–1530.

142 Streuli, M. et al. (1989) A family of receptor-linked protein tyrosine phosphatases in humans and Drosophila. Proc. Natl Acad. Sci. USA 86, 8698–8702.

143 Hall, L.R. et al. (1988) Complete exon-intron organization of the human leukocyte common antigen (CD45) gene. J. Immunol. 141, 2781–2787.

144 Barford, D. et al. (1994) Crystal-structure of human protein-tyrosine-phosphatase 1B. Science 263, 1397–1404.

145 Freeman, M. et al. (1990) An ancient, highly conserved family of cysteine-rich protein domains revealed by cloning type I and type II murine macrophage scavenger receptors. Proc. Natl Acad. Sci. USA 87, 8810–8814.

146 Walker, I.D. et al. (1994) A novel multi-gene family of sheep gammadelta T cells. Immunology 83, 517–523.

147 Law, S.K. et al. (1993) A new macrophage differentiation antigen which is a member of the scavenger receptor superfamily. Eur. J. Immunol. 23, 2320–2325.

148 Freeman, M. et al. (1991) Expression of type I and type II bovine scavenger receptors in Chinese hamster ovary cells: lipid droplet accumulation and nonreciprocal cross competition by acetylated and oxidized low density lipoprotein. Proc. Natl Acad. Sci. USA 88, 4931–4935.

149 Huang, H.J. et al. (1987) Molecular cloning of Ly-1, a membrane glycoprotein of mouse T lymphocytes and a subset of B cells: molecular homology to its human counterpart Leu-1/T1 (CD5). Proc. Natl Acad. Sci. USA 84, 204–208.

150 Bowen, M.A. et al. (1995) Cloning, mapping, and characterization of activated leucocyte-cell adhesion molecule (ALCAM), a CD6 ligand. J. Exp. Med. 181, 2213–2220.

151 Bajorath, J. et al. (1995) Molecular model of the N-terminal receptor-binding domain of the human CD6 ligand ALCAM. Protein Sci. 4, 1644–1647.

152 Feinstein, E. et al. (1995) The death domain – a module shared by proteins with diverse cellular functions. Trends Biochem. Sci. 20, 342–344.

153 Cleveland, J. and Ihle, J. (1995) Contenders in FasL/TNF death signaling. Cell 81, 479–482.

154 Hsu, H.L. et al. (1996) TNF-dependent recruitment of the protein-kinase RIP to the TNF receptor-1 signaling complex. Immunity 4, 387–396.

155 Hofmann, K. and Tschopp, J. (1995) The death domain motif found in Fas (Apo-1) and TNF receptor is present in proteins involved in apoptosis and axonal guidance. FEBS Lett. 371, 321–323.

156 Reth, M. (1989) Antigen receptor tail clue. Nature 338, 383–384.

157 Thomas, M. (1995) Of ITAMs and ITIMs; Turning on and off the B cell antigen receptor. J. Exp. Med. 181, 1953–1956.

[158] Cambier, J. et al. (1994) Signal transduction by the B cell antigen receptor or its coreceptors. Annu. Rev. Immunol. 12, 457–486.

[159] Chan, A.C. and Shaw, A.S. (1996) Regulation of antigen receptor signal transduction by protein tyrosine kinases. Curr. Opin. Immunol. 8, 394–401.

[160] Cambier, J.C. (1995) Antigen and Fc receptor signaling the awesome power of the immunoreceptor tyrosine-based activation motif (ITAM). J. Immunol. 155, 3281–3285.

[161] Daeron, M. et al. (1995) The same tyrosine-based inhibition motif, in the intracytoplasmic domain of FcgammaRIIB, regulates negatively BCR-, TCR-, and FcR-dependent cell activation. Immunity 3, 635–646.

[162] Yu, H. et al. (1994) Structural basis for the binding of proline-rich peptides to SH3 domains. Cell 76, 933–945.

[163] Bell, G.M. et al. (1996) The SH3 domain of p56(lck) binds to proline-rich sequences in the cytoplasmic domain of CD2. J. Exp. Med. 183, 169–178.

[164] Rebbe, N.F. et al. (1991) Identification of nucleotide pyrophosphatase/alkaline phosphodiesterase I activity associated with the mouse plasma cell differentiation antigen PC-1. Proc. Natl Acad. Sci. USA 88, 5192–5196.

[165] Grundmann, U. et al. (1990) Cloning and expression of a cDNA encoding human placental protein 11, a putative serine protease with diagnostic significance as a tumor marker. DNA Cell Biol. 9, 243–250.

[166] Wright, M.D. and Tomlinson, M.G. (1994) The ins and outs of the transmembrane 4 superfamily. Immunol. Today 15, 588–594.

[167] Tomlinson, M.G. and Wright, M.D. (1996) Characterization of mouse CD37: cDNA and genomic cloning. Mol. Immunol. 33, 867–872.

[168] Tomlinson, M.G. et al. (1993) Epitope mapping of anti-rat CD53 monoclonal antibodies. Implications for the membrane orientation of the transmembrane 4 superfamily. Eur. J. Immunol. 23, 136–140.

[169] Wright, M.D. et al. (1990) An immunogenic Mr 23,000 integral membrane protein of *Schistosoma mansoni* worms that closely resembles a human tumor-associated antigen. J. Immunol. 144, 3195–3200.

[170] Tomlinson, M. and Wright, M. (1996) A new transmembrane 4 superfamily molecule in the nematode *C. elegans*. J. Mol. Evol. 43, 312–314.

[171] Kopczynski, C. et al. (1996) A neural tetraspanin, encoded by *late bloomer*, that facilitates synapse formation. Science 271, 1867–1870.

[172] Dong, J.-T. et al. (1995) *KA11*, a metastasis suppressor gene for prostrate cancer on human chromosome 11p11.2. Science 268, 884–886.

[173] Boismenu, R. et al. (1996) A role for CD81 in early T cell development. Science 271, 198–200.

[174] Hupp, K. et al. (1989) Gene mapping of the three subunits of the high affinity FcR for IgE to mouse chromosomes 1 and 19. J. Immunol. 143, 3787–3791.

[175] Adra, C.N. et al. (1994) Cloning of the cDNA for a hemapoietic cell-specific protein related to CD20 and the β subunit of the high-affinity IgE receptor: evidence for a family of proteins with four membrane-spanning regions. Proc. Natl Acad. Sci. USA 91, 10178–10182.

[176] Tedder, T.F. and Engel, P. (1994) CD20: a regulator of cell-cycle progression of B lymphocytes. Immunol. Today 15, 450–454.

[177] Lin, S. et al. (1996) The FcεRIβ subunit functions as an amplifier of FcεRIγ-mediated cell activation signals. Cell 85, 985–995.

[178] Van Kooten, C. and Banchereau, J. (1996) CD40-CD40 ligand: A multifunctional receptor-ligand pair. Adv. Immunol. 1–77.

[179] Armitage, R.J. (1994) Tumor necrosis factor receptor superfamily members and their ligands. Curr. Opin. Immunol. 6, 407–413.

[180] Gruss, H.J. and Dower, S.K. (1995) Tumor necrosis factor ligand superfamily: involvement in the pathology of malignant lymphomas. Blood 85, 3378–3404.

[181] Eck, M.J. and Sprang, S.R. (1989) The structure of tumor necrosis factor-alpha at 2.6 Å resolution. Implications for receptor binding. J. Biol. Chem. 264, 17595–17605.

[182] Jones, E.Y. et al. (1989) Structure of tumour necrosis factor. Nature 338, 225–228.

[183] Karpusas, M. et al. (1995) 2 Å crystal structure of an extracellular fragment of human CD40 ligand. Structure 3, 1031–1039.

[184] Goodwin, R.G. et al. (1993) Molecular cloning of a ligand for the inducible T cell gene 4-1BB: A member of an emerging family of cytokines with homology to tumor necrosis factor. Eur. J. Immunol. 23, 2631–2641.

[185] Camerini, D. et al. (1991) The T cell activation antigen CD27 is a member of the nerve growth factor receptor gene gamily. J. Immunol. 147, 3165–3169.

[186] Sehgal, A. et al. (1988) A constitutive promoter directs expression of the nerve growth factor receptor gene. Mol. Cell. Biol. 8, 3160–3167.

[187] Birkeland, M.L. et al. (1995) Gene structure and chromosomal localization of the mouse homologue of rat OX40 protein. Eur. J. Immunol. 25, 926–930.

[188] Samelson, L.E. et al. (1990) Association of the fyn protein-tyrosine kinase with the T-cell antigen receptor. Proc. Natl Acad. Sci. USA 87, 4358–4362.

[189] Chan, A.C. et al. (1994) The role of protein tyrosine kinases and protein tyrosine phosphatases in T cell antigen receptor signal transduction. Annu. Rev. Immunol. 12, 555–592.

[190] Hardie, G. and Hanks, S. (1995) The Protein Kinase FactsBook. Academic Press, London.

[191] Hanks, S.K. et al. (1988) The protein kinase family: conserved features and deduced phylogeny of the catalytic domains. Science 241, 42–52.

[192] Holmes, W.E. et al. (1991) Structure and functional expression of a human IL-8 receptor. Science 253, 1278–1280.

[193] Barclay, A.N. et al. (1993) The Leucocyte Antigen FactsBook, 1st edn. Academic Press, London.

[194] Hanks, S.K. and Hunter, T. (1995) The eukaryotic protein kinase superfamily: kinase (catalytic) domain structure and classification. FASEB J. 9, 576–596.

4 The architecture and interactions of leucocyte surface molecules

INTRODUCTION

The proteins at the surface of leucocytes play key roles in all aspects of leucocyte functions such as differentiation and maturation, controlling their patterns of migration, response to foreign antigen and the control of the immune response via cytokines and interactions with other cell types. In the previous chapter, the types of domains found in proteins at the surface of leucocytes were described. In this chapter we discuss the organization of these proteins on cells and their interactions under five broad topics: (1) the integration of proteins into the membrane; (2) the carbohydrate structures on leucocyte membrane proteins; (3) the functions of the membrane antigens; (4) the types of interactions they mediate and (5) the architecture of the cell surface including factors such as the distribution of antigens at the cell surface and their abundance.

INTEGRATION OF PROTEINS INTO THE MEMBRANE

Heterogeneity of integration mechanisms

Since the original models for the integration of proteins within a fluid lipid bilayer were established (see Chapter 2), several different methods of protein attachment have been described[1]. Type I and type II proteins have a single transmembrane region whilst type III and IV proteins contain multiple transmembrane regions and type V proteins utilize lipid anchors (Fig. 1). Type IV proteins (not shown) are distinguished from type III proteins by the presence of a water-filled transmembrane channel. They often contain several subunits and are usually transport proteins. Type IV proteins are widely distributed on many cell types, and as we are not aware of any examples restricted to leucocytes, are not discussed further in this review. Two classes of type V proteins, which use lipid to attach to membranes have been described; one involving cell surface proteins linked by glycosyl-phosphatidylinositol (GPI) anchors and the second in which cytoplasmic proteins are linked by lipid moieties such as myristoyl groups. The latter include a large number of signalling proteins such as tyrosine kinases and GTP-binding proteins but these are beyond the scope of this book and are reviewed elsewhere[2,3]. In addition to these common modes of attachment some novel membrane anchors have recently been proposed, although not yet in leucocytes. A type VI membrane anchor has been proposed which contains both an uncleaved leader sequence and a GPI anchor and an example of which is ponticulin in the slime mould *Dictyostelium discoideum*[4]. A comparable orientation is also proposed for CD36 but with two transmembrane regions. X-ray crystallography suggests that the integral membrane glycoprotein prostaglandin H2 synthase-1 integrates into only one leaflet of the lipid bilayer[5]. In this case a patch of hydrophobic side-chains of the amino acids of an α helix integrates with the lipid but is not sufficient to traverse the membrane. This type of protein was termed monotopic[6] but there is now a case for calling it type VII in accordance with the common nomenclature.

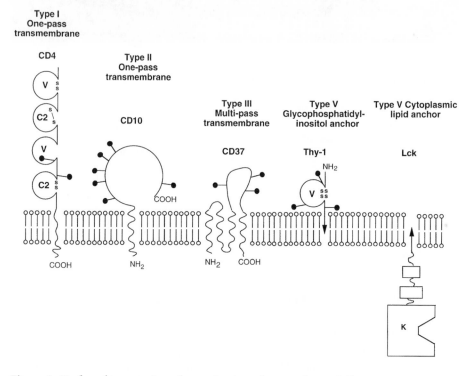

Figure 1 *Modes of integration of proteins into the membrane bilayer.*

A novel method of membrane attachment has been proposed for the peripheral myelin protein P_0 based on the X-ray crystal structure[7]. In addition to a type I transmembrane attachment an additional interaction has been proposed between the lipid bilayer and the single IgSF domain involving the side-chains of two exposed Trp residues. It should be noted that in most cases there is little biochemical evidence for the assignment of the transmembrane sequences of membrane proteins and these are usually predicted from hydrophobicity analysis. It is likely that some of the assignments given will be refined when more structural data become available. The frequency of each type of membrane attachment found in the leucocyte membrane proteins described in this book is summarized in Table 1.

Type I transmembrane attachment

The most common mode of membrane integration is the type I single-pass hydrophobic transmembrane sequence (Table 1). As illustrated for CD4 in Fig. 1, type I molecules have the C-terminus of the molecule in the cytoplasm and the N-terminus outside the cell. In the biosynthesis of a type I molecule an N-terminal signal sequence is cleaved as the molecule passes through the bilayer of the endoplasmic reticulum. This signal sequence has a loose pattern of conserved residues. The features of this pattern plus predictions for signal sequence cleavage points have been reviewed[8]. In the entries for antigens in this volume consensus

Table 1 *Frequency of types of membrane attachment in leucocyte antigens*

Membrane attachment		% of each type
Type I		69
Type II		12
Type III	2 pass	<1
	3 pass	<1
	4 pass	5
	5 pass	<1
	7 pass	3
	12 pass	<1
Type V (GPI)		8

rules are used to predict N-termini in cases where these have not been determined by protein sequencing.

Type I cell surface molecules have a transmembrane sequence of about 25 hydrophobic amino acid residues that is usually followed by a cluster of basic amino acids that are believed to bind to phospholipid head groups inside the membrane bilayer. Amino acids that are usually excluded from transmembrane sequences include Asn, Asp, Glu, Gln, His, Lys and Arg. In the exceptions where the transmembrane sequence contains some charged residues, the transmembrane sequence is usually associated with transmembrane sequences of other cell surface proteins to form a multimeric complex in the membrane. The classical example of this is the TCR complex in which the TCR α and β chains and CD3 δ, ε, γ and ζ chains all have charged residues in their transmembrane sequences. The presence of a charged residue in a type I transmembrane sequence can be reasonably taken as *prima facie* evidence that the molecule in question will be part of a multimeric complex.

Type II transmembrane attachment

Type II single-pass transmembrane molecules have the opposite orientation to type I molecules (Fig. 1). The N-terminus is found in the cytoplasm and the C-terminus is extracellular, e.g. ref. 9. They usually have a small cytoplasmic region and the transmembrane sequence often resembles an uncleaved signal sequence for secretion. A high proportion of extracellular domains with enzymatic activity are type II membrane proteins although overall the type II proteins are much less abundant than type I (Table 1).

Type III multipass transmembrane attachment

The type III category of membrane attachment consists of those molecules that cross the bilayer numerous times (Fig. 1). One very large group of cell surface molecules in this category is composed of G protein-linked receptors that pass through the membrane seven times (see Chapter 3), many of which function as receptors for soluble molecules such as prostaglandins and chemokines [10]. Structural studies have shown that the seven transmembrane regions are all α helices [11]. On leucocytes, members of this group have usually been identified functionally rather than by antigenicity, e.g. the IL-8R (CDw128), C5aR (CD88) and *N*-formyl peptide receptor

(FPR). A new subgroup of seven-pass transmembrane sequences has been recently described which includes the F4/80 and CD97 antigens which contain several extracellular EGF domains [12].

One group of multipass proteins commonly found on leucocytes contains four transmembrane regions and is called the transmembrane 4 (TM4) superfamily [13]. There are seven members in this superfamily present on leucocytes (Table 1) and a model for one (CD37) is illustrated in Fig. 1. All these molecules probably have both their N- and C-termini inside the cell, an orientation indicated by the fact that the loop of sequence between TM sequences 3 and 4 of CD53 is known to be extracellular since it encodes an extracellular antigenic determinant [14]. The CD20 antigen and the FcεR β chain are also four-pass transmembrane proteins but their sequences are not related to the TM4 superfamily (see Chapter 3) [15].

There is one example of a 12-pass transmembrane protein on leucocytes – the multidrug transporter MDR1 [16]. CD47 is the only example thus far of a leucocyte protein predicted to contain five transmembrane sequences. CD47 also contains an IgSF domain which is unusual for a multipass transmembrane protein.

Type V lipid attachment

Glycosyl-phosphatidylinositol (GPI) anchors
This common method of membrane integration utilizes a glycosyl-phosphatidylinositol (GPI) anchor attached to the C-terminal residue of the protein (Fig. 1 and Table 1) [17]. The structures for GPI anchors of the *Trypanosoma brucei* parasite coat protein and the rat Thy-1 antigen [18] are shown in Fig. 2. The backbone components and their linkages have been totally conserved during the evolution of *Trypanosoma* and *Rattus* but side-chain residues can vary between GPI anchors from different species as illustrated in Fig. 2. Within a species there can be cell type-specific differences as shown by differences in attached mannose and galactosamine residues between anchors of Thy-1 from brain and thymus. An additional palmitate

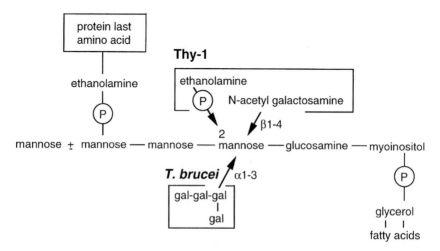

Figure 2 *Glycosyl-phosphatidylinositol anchors (GPI) for* T. brucei *and rat brain Thy-1. The data are from ref. 18.*

residue can also be tissue-specific [18]. GPI anchors can be cleaved by bacterial phosphatidylinositol phospholipase C (PI-PLC) enzymes [18] and the release of an antigen from the cell surface with PI-PLC is diagnostic for GPI anchor attachment. However some GPI-anchored molecules are resistant to PI-PLC cleavage and for instance this occurs when a palmitate residue is attached to the myoinositol ring as is found in bovine, but not human, acetylcholinesterase [19].

The presence of a GPI anchor can be indicated by the predicted protein sequence of a molecule. GPI-anchored molecules have a secretion signal sequence at their N-terminus plus another signal sequence at their C-terminus that is cleaved off and replaced by the GPI-anchor shortly after the biosynthesis of the molecule and entry in the endoplasmic reticulum. Examples of GPI signal sequences in cases where the cleavage site is known, are given in Fig. 3. Thus despite some exceptions, the general rules for a GPI-signal sequence are as follows. (1) The presence of a hydrophobic region at the C-terminus of the molecule that is not followed by a cluster of basic residues. (2) At about 7–12 residues before the hydrophobic region some small amino acids where cleavage of the precursor and attachment site of the GPI anchor occurs. The features of a GPI-signal sequence are quite similar to those of signal sequences for secretion and it has been shown that a secretion signal peptide attached to the C-terminus can function as a GPI-signal sequence [20]. The hydrophobic region can be 10–20 residues long and may seem indistinguishable from a sequence that might form a transmembrane sequence. In fact in the case of the CD58 antigen there are two alternatively spliced forms of the molecule that yield a GPI anchor or a transmembrane form of the molecule [21,22]. The same sequence forms the transmembrane spanning region and the GPI-signal sequence and the outcome is determined by the fact that the transmembrane form has extra sequence following on from the hydrophobic sequence. It is usual for GPI-signal sequences to lack the basic charged residues after the hydrophobic region that are found in the sequences of type I membrane molecules.

The GPI anchor appears to associate specifically with sphingomyelin lipids [23] and follows a different path of transport to the cell surface compared to some protein-anchored molecules following biosynthesis. On polarized cells GPI-anchored molecules are restricted to the apical surface [24]. GPI-anchored molecules are excluded from coated pits but can recycle through the cell via small uncoated vesicles [24]. Complexes enriched in GPI-anchored proteins and Src kinases can be

T. brucei VSG MITat 1.4a	C K D	S S I L V T K K F A L T V V S A A F V A L L F
T. brucei VSG MITat 1.1BC	C C D	G S F L V N K K F A L M V Y D F V S L L A F
T. brucei VSG ILTat 1.1	T G S	N S F V I H K A P L F L A F L L F
T. brucei VSG MITat 1.5b	C R N	G S F L T S K Q F A L M V S A A F V T L L F
Rat Thy-1	V K C	G G I S L L V Q N T S W L L L L L L L S L S F L Q A T D F I S L
DAF	T T S	G T T R L L S G H T C F T L T G L L G T I V T M G L L T
Rat CD48	A R S	S G V H W I A A W L V V T L S I I P S I L L A
Placental ATPase	T T D	A A H P G R S V V P A L L P L L A G T L L L L T A T P
Scrapie prion	R R S	S A V L F S S P P V I L L I S F L I F L M V G
CD59	L E N	G G T S L S E K T V L L L V T P F L A A A W S L H P
CD52	S P S	A S S N I S G G I F L F F V A N A I I H L F C F S
CD73	K F S	T G S H C H G S F S L I F L S L W A V I F V L Y Q

Figure 3 *Signal sequences for glycosyl-phosphatidylinositol (GPI) anchors. The arrow indicates the position of cleavage of the precursor protein. The lipid is attached to the residue immediately preceding the arrow. The data are from refs. 17, 107–111.*

enriched by detergent solubilization. These detergent-insoluble complexes have been equated with calveolae but this seems to be an oversimplification (reviewed in ref. 25).

Fatty acyl or prenyl anchors in cytoplasmic proteins

Many cytoplasmic proteins associate with the lipid bilayer but lack typical hydrophobic transmembrane regions. The commonest examples found in leucocytes and in many other cell types belong to the family of Src-related kinases[26,27]. These often have a myristic acid residue at the N-terminus which is necessary for membrane association[28]. The myristoylation is stable but in addition a cysteine near the N-terminus is often reversibly modified with palmitic acid, e.g. in Lck; palmitoylation enhances interactions with GPI-anchored proteins and subcellular compartments[29]. The myristoyl membrane interactions may be enhanced by interactions of polar headgroups of the phospholipids with groups of charged amino acid side-chains at the N-terminus. This interaction can be modified by phosphorylation, the "myristoyl-electrostatic switch" which may provide a reversible modulator of protein–membrane interactions[30]. It seems likely that the complexity of post-translation modifications with lipid will be revealed when more biochemical data become available[26].

CARBOHYDRATE STRUCTURES ON LEUCOCYTE MEMBRANE PROTEINS

Major glycoproteins and dimensions of carbohydrate structures

A major feature of cell surfaces is the presence of carbohydrate structures on both lipids and proteins. Most of the leucocyte surface antigens are glycoproteins and in this section we will deal exclusively with the carbohydrates of glycoproteins. However it should be noted that glycolipids are an abundant component of the cell surface and the diversity of their carbohydrate structures is as great as that of glycoproteins. N-linked glycosylation occurs on Asn residues within the motif Asn-Xaa-Thr or Asn-Xaa-Ser with the exception of Asn-Pro-Thr/Ser or Asn-Xaa-Thr/Ser-Pro sequences which are not usually glycosylated (see Chapter 1). O-linked glycosylation occurs at Ser or Thr amino acids within stretches of sequence that include a preponderance of the amino acids Ser, Thr and Pro (see Chapter 1).

The levels of glycosylation of membrane proteins vary considerably, with some expressing very high levels of carbohydrate. This can be seen in Fig. 4 which shows the major molecules that display carbohydrate on thymocytes and lymphocytes. These are the main molecules visualized when cells are labelled with [³H]-borohydride in their sialic acid or galactose residues[31,32]. For rat thymocytes three main bands are seen and these correspond to Thy-1, CD43 and CD45; for T cells the main bands are CD43 and CD45; whilst for B cells there is only one strong band and this is accounted for by CD45. On T and B cells the CD45 molecule has a variable amount of extra sequence at the N-terminus due to alternative splicing of exons. This extra sequence has an extended structure which is heavily O-glycosylated[33–35].

Very few membrane proteins lack carbohydrate completely and it seems likely that these unglycosylated polypeptides are associated with glycoproteins, e.g. the CD3 ε chain is part of a multi-polypeptide complex (i.e. the CD3/TCR complex) and CD81 is probably also associated with glycoproteins.

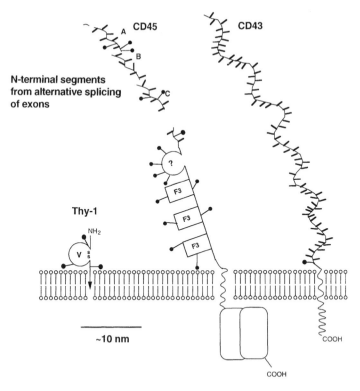

Figure 4 *The three major heavily glycosylated proteins on rat lymphocytes. Thy-1 is present on rat thymocytes and CD43 on thymocytes and T cells. Thymocytes express CD45 without any of the three alternative segments A, B, C whilst various combinations of these are expressed on B and T cells. For further information see entries in Section II and Fig. 9.*

Models such as those in Fig. 4 underestimate the contribution of glycosylation to the glycoprotein structure since the carbohydrates are not drawn to scale. Figures 5 and 6 show typical *N*- and *O*-linked carbohydrates with models for some of the structures drawn to scale. It is evident that for many cell surface molecules much of the protein surface must be obscured by the carbohydrate groups. This is illustrated in Fig. 7, which shows the three *N*-linked carbohydrates of Thy-1 antigen drawn to scale in relation to an immunoglobulin variable domain representing the Thy-1 protein backbone.

Carbohydrate antigenicity

Of the 206 entries in this book only nine antigens are defined by mAbs which recognize carbohydrate epitopes rather than protein epitopes of a glycoprotein or protein molecule. This may be considered surprising given the amount of carbohydrate at the cell surface. Carbohydrate epitopes are not intrinsically non-immunogenic since in other cases where mAbs are raised against cells, the antibodies can be predominantly against carbohydrate epitopes. This is the case for mAbs produced

A

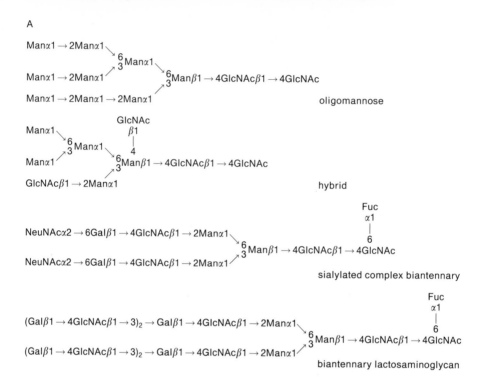

Manα1 → 2Manα1
⁶₃ Manα1
⁶₃ Manβ1 → 4GlcNAcβ1 → 4GlcNAc
Manα1 → 2Manα1
Manα1 → 2Manα1 → 2Manα1

oligomannose

GlcNAc
β1
Manα1
⁶₃ Manα1
4
⁶₃ Manβ1 → 4GlcNAcβ1 → 4GlcNAc
Manα1
GlcNAcβ1 → 2Manα1

hybrid

Fuc
α1
6
NeuNAcα2 → 6Galβ1 → 4GlcNAcβ1 → 2Manα1
⁶₃ Manβ1 → 4GlcNAcβ1 → 4GlcNAc
NeuNAcα2 → 6Galβ1 → 4GlcNAcβ1 → 2Manα1

sialylated complex biantennary

Fuc
α1
6
(Galβ1 → 4GlcNAcβ1 → 3)₂ → Galβ1 → 4GlcNAcβ1 → 2Manα1
⁶₃ Manβ1 → 4GlcNAcβ1 → 4GlcNAc
(Galβ1 → 4GlcNAcβ1 → 3)₂ → Galβ1 → 4GlcNAcβ1 → 2Manα1

biantennary lactosaminoglycan

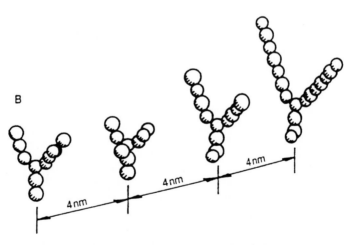

B

Figure 5 *Diagram to show the relative sizes of 4 representative N-linked oligosaccharide side-chains (A) and their structural configurations (B). The terminal GlcNAc is linked to an Asn residue on the glycoprotein. In (B) the structures from left to right are; oligomannose, hybrid, sialylated biantennary, and biantennary lactosaminoglycan. The approximate dimensions of these oligosaccharides are shown. This figure is adapted from ref. 112 with permission from the authors and* Annual Reviews of Biochemistry.

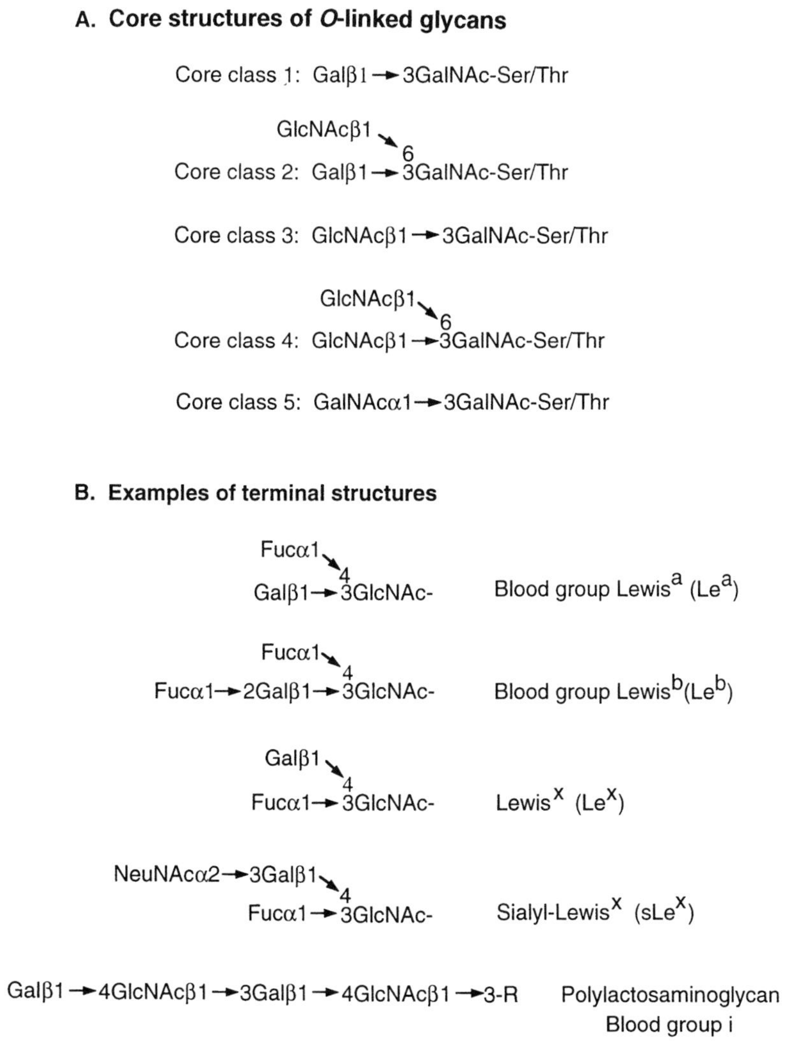

A. Core structures of O-linked glycans

Core class 1: Galβ1 → 3GalNAc-Ser/Thr

GlcNAcβ1 ↘
                    6
Core class 2: Galβ1 → 3GalNAc-Ser/Thr

Core class 3: GlcNAcβ1 → 3GalNAc-Ser/Thr

GlcNAcβ1 ↘
                    6
Core class 4: GlcNAcβ1 → 3GalNAc-Ser/Thr

Core class 5: GalNAcα1 → 3GalNAc-Ser/Thr

B. Examples of terminal structures

Fucα1 ↘
              4
Galβ1 → 3GlcNAc-   Blood group Lewis[a] (Le[a])

Fucα1 ↘
              4
Fucα1 → 2Galβ1 → 3GlcNAc-   Blood group Lewis[b] (Le[b])

Galβ1 ↘
            4
Fucα1 → 3GlcNAc-   Lewis[x] (Le[x])

NeuNAcα2 → 3Galβ1 ↘
                              4
Fucα1 → 3GlcNAc-   Sialyl-Lewis[x] (sLe[x])

Galβ1 → 4GlcNAcβ1 → 3Galβ1 → 4GlcNAcβ1 → 3-R   Polylactosaminoglycan
                                                                                    Blood group i

Figure 6 *The structure of some typical* O-*linked oligosaccharides. (A) Examples of the core residues found commonly in* O-*linked carbohydrate. (B) Examples of terminal residues found on* O-*linked carbohydrates*[113].

against the slime mould *Polysphondylium pallidum*[36]. The main reason that protein epitopes predominate in immunizations between vertebrates is probably because most carbohydrates are shared amongst the higher animals and thus the animal is tolerant to the carbohydrate determinants. It may be that anti-carbohydrate mAbs are raised where this does not hold. For example, a mouse mAb recognizing the human carbohydrate blood group A antigen was one of the first mAbs made against human leucocytes and mice are negative for blood group A[37,38]. In slime moulds the carbohydrate structures seem quite different to vertebrate structures[39,40] and this

A

Manα1
⟍
⁶₃Manα1
⟍
Manα1⟋
⁶₃Manβ1 → 4GlcNAcβ1 → 4GlcNAc
Manα1⟋

Asn 23

Fuc
α1
|
6
Galα1 → 3Galβ1 → 4GlcNAcβ1 → 2Manα1⟍
⁶₃Manβ1 → 4GlcNAcβ1 → 4GlcNAc
(Galβ1 → 4GlcNAcβ1 → 3)₃ → Galβ1 → 4GlcNAcβ1 → 2Manα1⟋

Asn 74

NeuNAcα2 → 6Galβ1 → 4GlcNAcβ1 → 2Manα1⟍
⁶₃Manβ1 → 4GlcNAcβ1 → 4GlcNAc
NeuNAcα2 → 6Galβ1 → 4GlcNAcβ1 → 2Manα1⟋

Asn 98

B

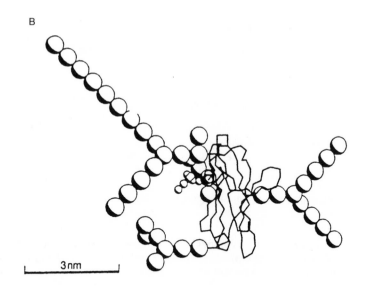

3 nm

Figure 7 *A model for the Thy-1 antigen from rat thymocytes and the major oligosaccharides present at the three N-glycosylation sites (Asn23, Asn74 and Asn98)* [46]. *The structure is a model based on the α-carbon coordinates of the V_L domain of Fab NEW, which Thy-1 resembles in sequence. The three oligosaccharides are shown perpendicular to the protein surface and in an extended conformation. Each sugar residue is represented by a sphere of 0.608 nm in diameter. This figure is adapted from ref. 112 with permission from the authors and* Annual Reviews of Biochemistry.

may explain the strong immunogenicity of carbohydrates in immunizations against these organisms. Terminal α-galactose is not found on human glycoproteins but is common in other species and humans can make a strong response to this carbohydrate; this is an important factor in attempts at organ xenotransplantation[41].

With antibodies against heavily O-glycosylated glycoproteins it is common to find epitopes that are specific to one glycoprotein and yet are apparently dependent on glycosylation[42,43]. A common result is that antigenicity may be lost if sialic acid is removed, or that expression of an epitope may differ between cell types presumably due to differential glycosylation. It might be inferred from this that the epitope consists of both protein and carbohydrate components, but studies on completely unglycosylated forms of the glycoproteins expressed in E. coli make this interpretation unlikely[42,44]. In a number of cases the mAbs whose binding is affected by removal of sialic acid also bind to the unglycosylated forms. This suggests that the epitope specificity is due to the protein sequence but that the availability of the epitope can be influenced by the glycosylation state. In the case of CD45 one antibody has been shown to bind to the native glycosylated protein with an affinity different to that of the unglycosylated backbone[44].

Cell type specificity of glycosylation

One of the key points about glycosylation is that the carbohydrate on a particular protein backbone can vary considerably depending on the cell type in which it is expressed. This was first seen for Thy-1 (CD90) antigen from brain and thymus where it was established that all of the complex N-linked structures differed between the two forms[45,46]. These differences were superimposed upon a site-specific pattern in which Asn23 carried mostly oligomannose structures, Asn74 showed the most extended complex structures, and Asn98 carried smaller complex structures in both forms. It seems as if a site-specific pattern is dictated by the structure of the molecule and that a cell type-specific pattern is superimposed upon this[46].

Major differences in glycosylation are also established between leucocyte populations. A notable example is the differences in O-linked structures on resting T cells, activated T cells and neutrophils. Most of O-linked carbohydrate is present on the CD43 antigen, a major glycoprotein on all three cell types[47,48]. Resting T cells express simple structures (Fig. 8A) whereas more complicated structures are found on activated T cells (Fig. 8B) and neutrophils (Fig. 8C). These differences may be of functional importance since extended mucin-like proteins such as CD43 (and the CD45 N-terminus) are well-suited to display carbohydrates to natural lectins.

Carbohydrates carried by glycoproteins and glycolipids have been shown to be important ligands for the selectin (CD62E, CD62L and CD62P)[49,50] and sialoadhesin (CD22, CD33 and sialoadhesin)[51] families of proteins. The selectin ligands provide a clear example of the importance of cell type-specific glycosylation. Thus GlyCAM-1 is not only expressed in lymph nodes where it is a ligand for L-selectin but is also present in milk[52]. However the GlyCAM-1 present in milk lacks the sulfation of the carbohydrate necessary for CD62L binding[52–54]. The E-selectin ligand (ESL-1) is widely expressed but only that expressed by myeloid cells is a ligand for CD62E[55]. The P-selectin glycoprotein ligand 1 (PSGL-1 or CD162) is also widely distributed but is only an active ligand on a subset of the PSLG-1-expressing leucocytes[56]. Sulfation is also important in the PSLG-1 reaction with P-selectin but in this case it

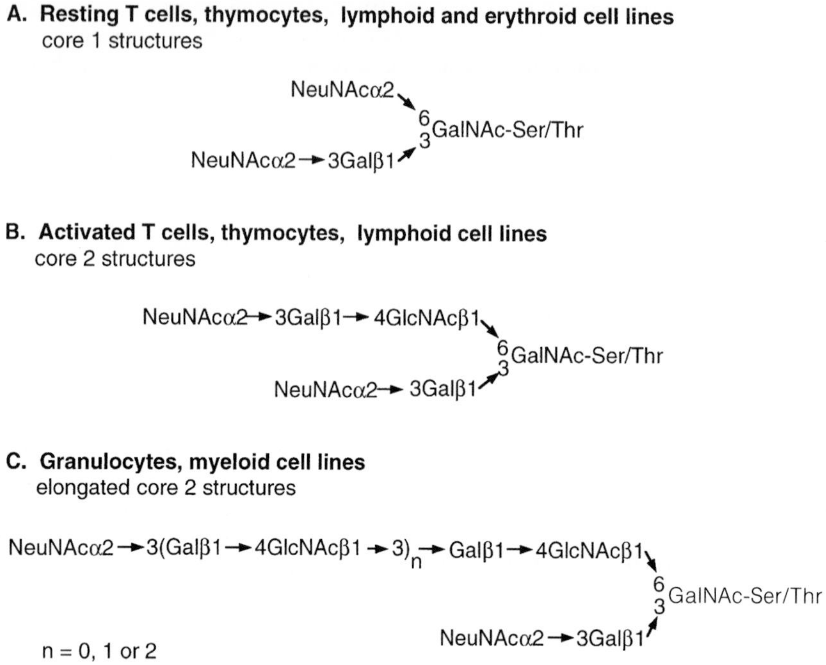

A. Resting T cells, thymocytes, lymphoid and erythroid cell lines
core 1 structures

$$\begin{array}{c}
\text{NeuNAc}\alpha 2 \searrow \\
{}^6_3\text{GalNAc-Ser/Thr} \\
\text{NeuNAc}\alpha 2 \rightarrow 3\text{Gal}\beta 1 \nearrow
\end{array}$$

B. Activated T cells, thymocytes, lymphoid cell lines
core 2 structures

$$\begin{array}{c}
\text{NeuNAc}\alpha 2 \rightarrow 3\text{Gal}\beta 1 \rightarrow 4\text{GlcNAc}\beta 1 \searrow \\
{}^6_3\text{GalNAc-Ser/Thr} \\
\text{NeuNAc}\alpha 2 \rightarrow 3\text{Gal}\beta 1 \nearrow
\end{array}$$

C. Granulocytes, myeloid cell lines
elongated core 2 structures

$$\text{NeuNAc}\alpha 2 \rightarrow 3(\text{Gal}\beta 1 \rightarrow 4\text{GlcNAc}\beta 1 \rightarrow 3)_n \rightarrow \text{Gal}\beta 1 \rightarrow 4\text{GlcNAc}\beta 1 \searrow$$
$${}^6_3\text{GalNAc-Ser/Thr}$$

n = 0, 1 or 2

$$\text{NeuNAc}\alpha 2 \rightarrow 3\text{Gal}\beta 1 \nearrow$$

Figure 8 *Examples of typical heterogeneity of* O-*linked carbohydrate structures found on different leucocytes* [47,48].

is sulfation of tyrosine residues near the N-terminus of the protein rather than carbohydrate that is involved [57,58].

FUNCTIONS OF LEUCOCYTE MEMBRANE ANTIGENS

Leucocytes are characteristically migratory cells which cooperate to recognize and dispose of invasive pathogens or tumour cells. For these functions it is necessary for cell surface antigens to interact with soluble proteins or glycoproteins as well as with the surfaces of other cells and with the extracellular matrix. In addition many of these interactions will lead to signalling events transduced to the cell interior by proteins interacting with the cytoplasmic regions of the cell surface antigens. These signals lead to differentiation and altered migration of the leucocytes. In the entries in Section II there is a section called "Ligands and associated molecules" where the known molecular interactions are listed. Ligands have been identified for about 50% of leucocyte surface proteins and in this chapter we concentrate on the interactions of the extracellular parts of leucocyte antigens. Table 2 summarizes the frequency of different types of functions mediated by membrane proteins of leucocytes. It includes enzymes as a separate small group and these are summarized in Table 3. The leucocyte cell surface must also contain proteins necessary for the metabolism of the cell such as ion channels but these molecules are unlikely to be restricted to leucocytes and hence are not classified as leucocyte antigens. One exception is the CD20 antigen which has ion channel activity [59].

Table 2 *Frequency of the roles of leucocyte surface antigens*

Enzymatic activity in extracellular domains	3%
Receptors for cytokines	13%
Receptors for other soluble proteins (e.g. Fc receptors)	10%
Receptors for cell surface proteins or extracellular matrix	25%
Others (e.g. ion channels and transporters)	1%
Unknown	49%

Enzymatic activity present in leucocyte membrane proteins

The number of enzymes identified at the leucocyte cell surface is low (Table 3). Enzymes may only need to be present at low site numbers per cell, because of their catalytic role, compared to proteins mediating adhesion events where multiple interactions involving large surface areas are likely. Thus it is possible that many more enzymes are present but at low levels not detectable by labelling with mAbs and analysis with flow cytofluorography. It is easy to see how important these might be in providing a method for rapidly decreasing cell surface expression of glycoproteins as shown for CD62L[60]. These proteases often show activities typical of metalloproteases and seem likely to be associated with cell surface molecules rather than secreted proteins[61]. Proteases also provide a powerful way of modifying the activity of cytokines in the vicinity of cell surfaces. Proteolytic activity has been identified in the ectodomains of several antigens (e.g. CD10; Table 3) but its physiological role is not clear. Indeed the role in the immune system of the activities described in Table 3 is poorly understood (reviewed in ref. 62).

Transmembrane proteins containing cytoplasmic regions with kinase and phosphatase activities are common in biology although relatively few are restricted to leucocytes (Table 3). However many of the cytoplasmic regions of transmembrane proteins interact directly with enzymes, for example tyrosine kinases (e.g. CD4 and

Table 3 *Enzymatic activities present in leucocyte membrane proteins*

Extracellular activities
Aminopeptidase A, EC 3.4.11.7

CD10	Neutral endopeptidase, EC 3.4.24.11
CD13	Aminopeptidase N, EC 3.4.11.2
CD26	Dipeptidylpeptidase IV, EC 3.4.14.5
CD38	ADP-ribosyl cyclase
CD39	Ecto (Ca^{2+}, Mg^{2+})-apyrase (ecto-ATPase)
PC1	5'-nucleotidase phosphodiesterase I, EC 3.1.4.1 and nucleotide pyrophosphatase, EC 3.6.1.9
RT6	NAD glycohydrolase

Intracellular activities

CD45	Protein tyrosine phosphatase, EC 3.1.3.48
CD115	Protein tyrosine kinase, EC 2.7.1.112
CD117	Protein tyrosine kinase, EC 2.7.1.112
CD148	Protein tyrosine phosphatase, EC 3.1.3.48
Ltk	Protein tyrosine kinase, EC 2.7.1.112

See refs 62–64 for details of enzymatic activities.

Table 4 *Interactions of leucocyte membrane proteins with soluble proteins*

Cell surface antigen	Domain type involved	Ligand
CD14	Short repeats	LPS binding protein
CD21	CCP	Complement C3d
CD23	Lectin C-type	IgE (not carbohydrate)[a]
CD71	No SF	Transferrin
CD87 (UPAR)	Ly-6	Urokinase plasminogen activator[b]
CD117 (c-kit)	IgSF	Stem cell factor
IL-1R	IgSF	IL-1
IL-4R	CytokineR/Fn3	IL-4
IL-8R	G protein-coupled R	IL-8
LDLR	LDLR	Low-density lipoproteins
Scavenger receptor	No SF	Acetylated lipoproteins[c]
TNFR (CD120)	TNFR	TNF[d]

[a]The lectin C-type domain of CD23 interacts with IgE but not through its carbohydrate and hence is an example of a lectin C-type domain binding an IgSF domain.
[b]The interaction of CD87 has been shown to involve the Ly-6 domain binding to an EGF domain in urokinase plasminogen activator and not the protease domain [66].
[c]The scavenger receptor cysteine-rich domain is not involved in this binding as the form produced by alternative splicing that lacks this domain still binds ligands.
[d]Several members of the TNFSF exist both as soluble and cell surface forms and are also included in Table 6.

CD8) or tyrosine phosphatases (e.g. CD22, FcγRIIB, KIR) and they may also be substrates for enzymes (e.g. CD3 chains). The cytoplasmic regions rarely contain clearly defined domains and may adopt a flexible extended structure. Consistent with this, their interactions usually involve short linear stretches of sequence, such as the ITAM motif (see Chapter 3).

INTERACTIONS OF LEUCOCYTE MEMBRANE PROTEINS

Interactions of leucocyte membrane proteins with soluble protein ligands (Table 4)

This group includes many of the receptors for cytokines. These interactions are generally of high affinity (see below). Apart from TNF and related proteins the cytokines themselves usually contain domain types not found in cell surface proteins and these are reviewed in ref. 65. Table 4 gives examples of interactions of leucocyte membrane proteins with soluble proteins and the different types of domains involved.

Interactions of leucocyte membrane proteins with carbohydrate ligands (Table 5)

The complexity and abundance of carbohydrate indicates that protein–carbohydrate interactions are likely to be important. A number of examples have been identified involving link, IgSF and lectin C-type domains.

Table 5 *Interaction of membrane proteins with carbohydrates. Examples of interactions involving different domain types with carbohydrates*

Cell surface antigen	Domain type involved	Ligand
CD22	IgSF	Sialoglycoconjugates
CD31	IgSF	Glycosaminoglycans
CD44	Link	Hyaluronan
CD62	Lectin C-type	Various carbohydrates including CD15s
Mannose receptor	Lectin C-type	Mannose (in polymeric form)

Interaction of membrane proteins with other membrane-associated ligands (cell adhesion and accessory molecules) (Tables 6 and 7)

A large number of cell surface ligands have been identified for leucocyte surface proteins. Most of these involve heterophilic interactions (Table 6) although there are some homophilic interactions involving IgSF domains (Table 7). IgSF domains are particularly common and interact both with other IgSF domains and a large variety of different domain types. Integrins have various ligands including extracellular matrix proteins and cell surface proteins containing IgSF and cadherin domains.

Table 6 *Heterophilic interactions of leucocyte membrane antigens. Interaction of membrane proteins with other membrane components*

Cell surface antigen	Domain type involved	Ligand	Domain type involved
CD2	IgSF	CD48, CD58	IgSF
CD6	SRCR	CD166 (ALCAM)	IgSF
MHC Class I and II	MHC	Peptide + TCR	IgSF
CD11a/CD18	Integrin	CD50, CD58, CD102	IgSF
CD31	IgSF	$\alpha v \beta 3$ integrin	Integrin
CD40	TNFR	CD40L (CD164)	TNF[a]
CD55	CCP	CD97	EGF or G-protein-coupled receptor TM7 region[b]
$\alpha E\beta 7$	Integrin	E-cadherin	Cadherin

[a]Several members of the TNFSF exist both as soluble and cell-associated forms and are therefore also included in Table 5.
[b]CD97 is a member of the G protein-coupled receptor superfamily but with EGF domains and some other sequence in the extracellular region. The site of interaction with the CCP domains of CD55 has not been determined[67].

Table 7 *Homotypic interactions of membrane proteins*

Cell surface antigen	Domain type involved
CD31	IgSF
CD66a,c	IgSF

There are relatively few examples of homotypic interactions between leucocytes and so far these seem to be confined to proteins containing IgSF domains.

Affinity of interactions of cell surface antigens

The affinities of cell surface receptors for cytokines are generally high with slow dissociation rate constants. This would ensure a high level of occupancy of receptors at relatively low concentrations of cytokine and sufficient time of occupancy to permit signal transduction. In contrast, interactions between cell surface antigens often have very low affinities[68]. For instance the interaction between CD2 and its ligand in rodents, CD48, has been estimated to have a $K_d = {\sim}75\,\mu M$ and a dissociation rate constant of $>6\,s^{-1}$ (see ref. 68). Several other affinities are in the same range (Table 8). A wide range of affinities has been reported for the TCR interaction with MHC peptide complexes but these are much lower than for cytokines and their receptors. Several integrins can exist in one of two states with different binding affinities. It is possible to induce the high-affinity "activated state" by a number of stimuli including signals from within the cell, a phenomenon termed "inside-outside signalling"[69].

The interactions between proteins on opposing cells during cell contact are clearly different from the interactions between proteins in solution. In the latter, diffusion is unlikely to be rate limiting whereas for proteins tethered to the cell surface the movement perpendicular to the cell will be restricted by the attachment to the membrane and the diffusion in the other two dimensions will be dependent on the mobility of the protein in the lipid bilayer. This in turn will depend on whether the proteins are linked by GPI anchors (more mobile) or transmembrane sequences (less mobile) and whether some or all of the protein interacts with other proteins, e.g. through their cytoplasmic regions with the cytoskeleton or other cytoplasmic proteins (discussed in ref. 68). The local distribution of the interacting molecules and their accessibility will also affect their ability to interact (see below, **Architecture of the leucocyte cell surface**).

Table 8 *Monomeric affinities and rate constants for leucocyte membrane protein interactions*

Interaction	Temperature (°C)	K_a (M^{-1})	k_{on} ($M^{-1}.s^{-1}$)	k_{off} (s^{-1})	Refs
Soluble ligands					
IL-1 to IL-1 receptor	8	10^{10}	${\sim}10^6$	${\sim}10^{-4}$	68
Antibody (OX34) to protein (CD2)	37	2×10^9	4×10^5	2×10^{-4}	68
Cell surface ligands					
CD2 to CD58 (human)	37	$4{-}10 \times 10^4$	$\geq 4 \times 10^5$	≥ 4	70
CD2 to CD48 (rat)	37	$1.1{-}1.6 \times 10^4$	$\geq 1 \times 10^5$	≥ 6	68
CD54 to CD11a/CD18 (LFA-1)	37	1.1×10^4	–	–	68
CD80 to CD28	37	2.5×10^5	$\geq 7 \times 10^5$	≥ 1.6	71
CD80 to CTLA-4	37	2.5×10^6	$\geq 9 \times 10^5$	≥ 0.43	71
T cell receptor to peptide/MHC	${\sim}25$	$10^4{-}10^7$	$10^3{-}10^5$	$10^{-3}{-}10^{-1}$	72
CD8$\alpha\beta$ to MHC Class I	${\sim}25$	5×10^4	3×10^3	0.05	73
CD62E to sialyl Le^x	${\sim}25$	10^4	–	–	74
CD62L to GlyCAM-1	37	10^4	$\geq 10^5$	≥ 10	75

Multimeric complexes at the leucocyte surface

Most cell surface antigens are probably present as monomers at the cell surface but there are several examples where the antigens associate to form stable complexes with 2–7 different polypeptides as illustrated in Table 9. Some of the chains are linked by disulfide bonds but others form stable complexes without such bonds, e.g. MHC Class II antigens. The largest complexes are the Fc receptors and the B and T cell antigen receptors. The latter contains a total of six or seven different polypeptide chains, namely, a disulfide-linked heterodimer with antigen binding specificity (TCR$\alpha\beta$), a disulfide-linked homodimer (CD3$\zeta\zeta$) or heterodimer (CD3$\zeta\eta$) important for signalling, and three non-covalently associated chains, CD3δ, CD3γ and CD3ε. All these chains are required in order to get cell surface expression. The exact stoichiometry is not known but there are probably two copies of CD3ε per complex [76].

In addition to the relatively stable multimers mentioned above there are many examples where weak associations have been described. Typically these associations can only be demonstrated when the membrane proteins are solubilized with very weak detergents such as digitonin and often when highly sensitive detection methods are used, e.g. protein kinase assays. For instance most of the TM4SF proteins seem to be associated with other cell surface proteins [77]. The finding that GPI-anchored proteins can give activation signals on crosslinking and can be co-precipitated with cytoplasmic kinases indicated interactions with other components [17]. However these must be indirect as these proteins do not traverse the lipid bilayer and are probably a consequence of the co-localization of these proteins in lipid microdomains which are insoluble in the weak detergents [78].

Stoichiometry of interactions of cell surface antigens

One consequence of the presence of multimers at the cell surface is that they provide variation in the types of interactions with ligands. Table 10 gives examples of cell surface molecules that interact with soluble or membrane molecules with different stoichiometries. This variety of interactions may enable different types of responses to ligand interactions and is very common for the cytokine receptors. A minority of cytokines signal via conformational changes in receptors, e.g. IL-8 binds a G protein-coupled receptor. However the majority of signals transduced by cytokines involve the association of subunits, for example, c-kit ligand forms a dimer and binds a monomeric receptor (CD117) which contains five IgSF domains and a tyrosine kinase domain. This is similar to platelet-derived growth factor receptor (CD140) and c-kit ligand probably also signals by dimerizing the CD117 and activating the

Table 9 *Examples of stable multimeric protein complexes at the cell surface*

Covalently associated	
Homodimers	CD8$\alpha\alpha$, CD28, CD69, CD162, mIg
Homotrimers	Scavenger receptor
Heterodimers	CD8$\alpha\beta$, CD94/NKG2, TCR$\alpha\beta$
Non-covalently associated	
Homodimers	CD10, CD26
Heterodimers	Integrins, MHC Class II
Homotrimers	CD23, CD154
Three or more different chains	CD3δ, γ, ε/TCR complex, IL-2R

Table 10 *Examples of the stoichiometry of interactions of cell surface proteins*

Cell surface antigen	Number of polypeptides	Polypeptides	Ligand
CD2	1	CD2	CD48 (monomer)
CD117 (c-kit)	1	CD117	c-kitL (dimer)
CD120 (TNFR)	1	CD120	TNF (trimer)
IL-2R	3	CD25, CD122, CD132	IL-2 (monomer)
TCR/CD3	8	TCRα, TCRβ, CD3δ, CD3ε(2), CD3γ, CD3ζ(2)	MHC + peptide (monomer)
CD162 (PSLG-1)	2	Dimer	CD62P (monomer)

cytoplasmic tyrosine kinase [79]. TNF and several members of the TNFSF are soluble trimeric proteins and signal by binding and hence associating their monomeric receptors (TNFRSF) [80]. However, TNFSF members may also exist as trimers at the cell surface and further complexity is indicated by their ability to form heterotrimers, e.g. between lymphotoxin β and lymphotoxin α (TNFβ) [81].

The possible relevance of multimeric complexes in providing different sensitivities to ligand availability is illustrated by the IL-2R which consists of three different polypeptides; one chain gives low-affinity binding of IL-2 (a monomeric cytokine), the second chain increases the affinity of binding and a third chain mediates signalling. Thus the sensitivity of a cell to IL-2 can potentially be controlled by the relative expression of each polypeptide. Several other cytokine receptors have similar arrangements and often share the signalling polypeptide, e.g. CD130.

The precise stoichiometry of many of the cell–cell interactions has not been determined and many arrangements are possible due to the presence of dimeric and trimeric proteins (Table 10).

ARCHITECTURE OF THE LEUCOCYTE CELL SURFACE

The binding or enzymatic activities of leucocyte antigens will be affected by factors such as their abundance, accessibility and distribution on the cell surface. On the basis of the accumulated molecular data given in this book it is possible to gain a view of how the cell surface looks with its various molecular forms. In reviewing this subject attention will be focused mainly on the surface proteins of thymocytes and resting T lymphocytes since the membranes of these cells are probably the best characterized of all the leucocytes.

Abundance of leucocyte surface antigens

What proportion of the T cell surface has been accounted for in terms of characterized molecules? It has been estimated that T and B cells differ only in the expression of about 200–300 different genes (see ref. 82). As only about 3% of the mRNA of lymphocytes is in the membrane bound polysome fraction, many of these T cell-specific molecules will not be at the cell surface. If this is the case, most of the surface molecules are probably already known. We believe this is likely, at least in relation to molecules that are susceptible to easy detection by flow cytometry (~5000 molecules per cell), for the following reasons. First, the major bands on T and

B cell surfaces identified by radiolabelling of protein or carbohydrate can be accounted for by known molecules [32]. Secondly, with mAbs made against cells from a variety of species, essentially the same antigens have been discovered. If the known antigens were a minor set of a large total pool that remains to be discovered, one might expect much less overlap between antigens identified in immunizations performed between different species or in different ways. Thirdly, estimates of the surface area of a T lymphocyte covered by known cell surface molecules suggest that much of the surface can be accounted for. Relevant figures for rat thymocytes and T and B lymphocytes are given in Table 11 with areas for molecules derived on the basis of the molecular dimensions discussed below. Obviously there may be errors in these figures but these estimates suggest that known molecules could cover up to 60% of the T lymphocyte surface, if one assumes that the membrane surface is smooth. However scanning electron microscopy shows that it is more likely to be covered

Table 11 *Site numbers for lymphocyte surface antigens and an estimate of the surface area they may cover*

Antigen	Thymocytes		T cells		B cells	
	Numbers	% area	Numbers	% area	Numbers	% area
mIg	–	–	–	–	7×10^4	8.2
MHC Class I	–	–	2×10^5	5.8	2×10^5	5.8
MHC Class II	–	–	–	–	2.4×10^5	7.0
Thy-1	10^6	24	–	–	–	–
CD2	1.4×10^4	0.3	1.4×10^4	0.3	–	–
CD4	1.5×10^4	0.5	3×10^4	1.0	–	–
CD8	4×10^4	1.3	10^5	3.3	–	–
CD43	10^5	19	1.5×10^5	28	–	–
CD44	1.3×10^4	–	*	–	*	–
CD45	7×10^4	13	10^5	23	10^5	27
MRC OX2	1.4×10^4	0.3	–	–	5×10^3	0.08

Values for the site numbers of antigens present on resting rat lymphocytes were determined by binding of [^{125}I]Fab (for CD4 and Thy-1) or by quantitative radioimmunoassay using the numbers obtained with [^{125}I]Fab for CD4 or Thy-1 as standards [86]. The dashes indicate that the antigen is not present on that cell type. Where an antigen is present on a subpopulation of cells the number given is calculated per positive cell. Additional data are from refs 87 and 88 and unpublished. The asterisk denotes that the site number for rat CD44 has not been determined on T cells or B cells but from flow cytometry analysis and comparison with other markers, it is probably in the order of 8×10^4 on thoracic duct lymphocytes.

The percentage of the surface that each antigen may cover was calculated as follows with further information in refs 42, 89 and 90. The surface area of a lymphocyte was assumed to be $120 \, \mu m^2$, with a volume of $125 \, \mu m^3$ (ref. 86). For these calculations Thy-1 was assumed to be a sphere of radius 3 nm, CD43 a rod of 45×5 nm [42]; CD45, thymocyte form 28×8 nm, T cell form 35×8 nm, and B cell form 41×8 nm [90,91]; CD4 13×3 nm [92]; CD2 7×3 nm [93]; MHC Class I 7×5 nm [94]; MHC Class II 7×5 nm [95]. CD8 is assumed to have the same dimensions as CD4, OX2 the same as CD2. The size of IgM is estimated as 3.5 Fab fragments of 8×5 nm [96]. The molecular size of CD44 has not been estimated but it could be quite large due to its post-translational modifications. These calculations are approximate and should be used as an indicator as to the proportion of the surface covered by an antigen. It is notable that a few major molecules make up the majority of the exposed cell surface proteins. The percentages are probably an overestimate as the surface of the lymphocyte could be considerably larger than the smooth sphere assumed due to the presence of microvilli, e.g. possibly 3–4-fold greater [83], and the cell surface molecules may also project away from the surface at least for some of the time.

with microvilli. In the F11 hybrid neuronal line where the surface area was actually measured, it was 3–4-fold greater than that of a smooth sphere[83]. If one assumes a similar figure for lymphocytes and takes into account the fact that many of the molecules are probably not layered over the surface but project outwards from the cell, a figure of about 20% is probably the best estimate of the amount of surface covered by the known, well-characterized proteins. It is notable that the majority of this is due to a few major molecules and it is unlikely that further molecules of this abundance remain to be identified. The proteins will not cover the whole surface, as glycolipids are also readily recognized by antibodies reacting with lymphocytes[84,85].

The levels of expression of cell surface antigens often change rapidly on, for instance, activation of T cells. In addition there are cases where intracellular pools can be directed to the surface giving more rapid increase in cell surface expression as illustrated for CD62P on activation of platelets and endothelial cells. The selectins also provide an example where levels of surface expression are modified by enzyme cleavage and this is discussed above in the section on enzymatic activity of cell surface antigens.

Dimensions of cell surface glycoproteins

The dimensions of many cell surface glycoproteins can now be accurately assessed on the basis of tertiary structure determination of domains, or electron microscopy studies on whole proteins or their extracellular regions. Some of the leucocyte surface molecules with known dimensions are shown in Fig. 9. It is clear that there is a wide variation in size of leucocyte surface antigens and their degree of glycosylation. This, together with the wide range in their abundance (Table 11) will have implications in cell–cell interactions. The TCR and some of the accessory molecules involved in antigen recognition are relatively small. This is illustrated in Fig. 10 which shows the approximate dimensions of some molecules that are involved in B and T cell activation and adhesion between these cells. The dimensions are based on the data in Fig. 9. The recent determination of the structure of the TCR/peptide/MHC ternary complex indicates that the distance between opposing cells at the site of T cell–antigen-presenting cell interaction, is about 14 nm[97,98]. A similar distance (14 nm) has been estimated for the CD2/CD48 complex on the basis of structural and mutagenesis data[93,99] and the CD2/CD58 complex is likely to be similar in size. Structural and mutagenesis data suggest that the CD4/MHC Class II complex will have a similar size[100]. Fewer data are available for CD8/MHC Class I and CD28/CD80 interactions but their predicted structures are consistent with sizes similar to the TCR/MHC complex[101,102]. The CD40/CD154 interaction probably has similar dimensions based on analogy with the structure of the TNFR/TNF complex[80]. This has an overall length of 8.5 nm but there is a short hinge-like sequence in CD154 which may help to span the intercellular difference. Whereas larger adhesion pairs such as LFA-1/CD54 may mediate the initial contacts between cells it is likely that close membrane approximation requires interactions of the smaller molecules such as CD2, CD28 and CD4 or CD8. Furthermore, large, abundant molecules such as CD43 will either need to lie flat on the membrane or move away from the TCR in order to allow close approximation of the membranes. The finding that T cells from a CD43 knockout animal are easier to stimulate and stickier is consistent with the idea that CD43 provides a barrier to the close interactions needed in T cell activation[103].

It is also interesting to consider how this recognition of antigen by T cells might differ from the triggering of B cells by antigens. Figure 10 also shows the dimensions

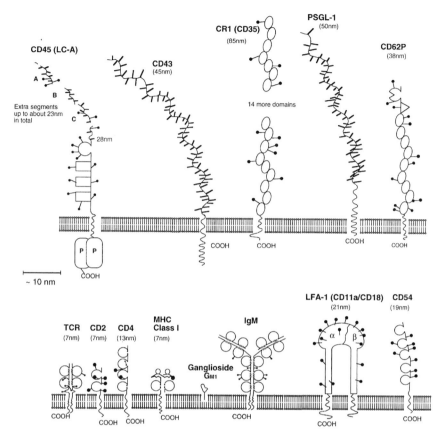

Figure 9 *Schematic view of molecules at the surface of leucocytes for which structural data are available from electron microscopy or X-ray crystallography studies. The molecules shown will not all be expressed simultaneously on the same cell and this figure is solely to illustrate the different sizes of common leucocyte surface antigens. The abundance of the molecules varies considerably and this is illustrated in Table 11. The molecules are drawn roughly to size and shape with the approximate height of the molecule from the cell surface indicated. The N-linked (●—) and O-linked (—) glycosylation sites are indicated. These are not drawn to scale but are shown to indicate the degree of glycosylation. See Figs 5–7 for an idea of the size and types of glycosylation that occur on leucocyte surface proteins. The overall dimensions of the molecules determined by electron microscopy include the contribution for carbohydrate. The model for ganglioside GM_1 is based on the structure and the size of sugar residues (see Fig. 5)[84]. The "P" denotes the phosphotyrosine phosphatase domains in the CD45 cytoplasmic domain. The models are based on the following data: CD4 separate X-ray crystallography studies of the first two[92,114] and second two domains of CD4[115]; X-ray crystallography of CD2[93]; X-ray crystallography of MHC Class I[94]; X-ray crystallography of TCR/MHC Class I complex[97,98]; and electron microscopy of CD35[116], CD43[42], CD45[90,91,117], CD54[118], CD62P[119] and PSGL-1 (CD162)[120]. The CD11a/CD18 model is based on the size determined by electron microscopy for another integrin, the fibronectin receptor[121]. The IgM model is based on the size determined for Fab fragments of IgG[96].*

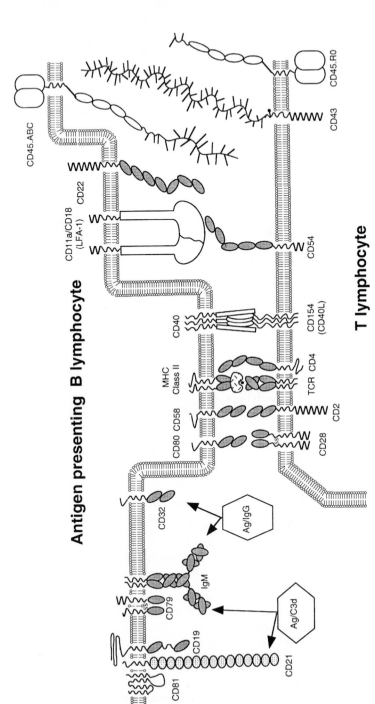

Figure 10 *Models for molecules involved in T and B lymphocyte activation. The dimensions are based on the approximate sizes determined for the molecules in Fig. 9. IgSF domains are indicated by shaded ovals, CCP domains by lightly shaded ovals (CD21) and the fibronectin type III domains in CD45 by clear ovals (the NH$_2$ domain in CD45 shows no sequence similarities and is also indicated by an oval). The CD40/CD154 interaction is based on the structure of TNFR/TNF (see text)[80] and is indiced by the trimeric CD154 binding three copies of the monomeric CD40. See Chapter 3 for more details of the superfamilies and their structures.*

of some molecules involved in B cell antigen recognition. B cell triggering is potentially quite different to that of T cells since presumably surface Ig is crosslinked to give a triggering reaction via antigen complexes. This activation is controlled by interactions of the complement and Fc receptors giving stimulatory and inhibitory signals respectively [104]. In this scheme, B cell triggering via the B cell antigen receptor will occur away from the tight interface between the B cell (acting as an antigen presenting cell) and a T helper cell where T cell activation and lymphokine production occurs.

Distribution of molecules at cell surfaces

Cell surface molecules are not all evenly distributed over the cell surface and there is evidence that the local distribution can play a crucial role in their function. The initial tethering and rolling of leucocytes to endothelial cells under flow conditions can only be mediated by a subset of adhesion molecules on the surfaces of these cells. Interestingly the glycoproteins on leucocytes which participate in adhesion under flow are found on the tips of microvilli (e.g. CD62L, PSGL-1 (CD162) and $\alpha4\beta1$). In contrast, adhesion molecules excluded from the microvilli (e.g. $\alpha M\beta2$) are not able to mediate adhesion under flow although $\alpha M\beta2$ is involved in later adhesion events [105]. Furthermore mutant CD62L (L-selectin) molecules that are excluded from microvilli are much less effective at mediating rolling and tethering of leucocytes under flow [106].

References

[1] Singer, S.J. (1990) The structure and insertion of integral proteins in membranes. Annu. Rev. Cell Biol. 6, 247–296.

[2] Chan, A.C. et al. (1994) The role of protein tyrosine kinases and protein tyrosine phosphatases in T cell antigen receptor signal transduction. Annu. Rev. Immunol. 12, 555–592.

[3] Superti-Furga, G. and Courtneidge, S.A. (1995) Structure–function relationships in Src family and related protein tyrosine kinases. Bioessays 17, 321–330.

[4] Hitt, A.L. et al. (1994) Ponticulin is the major high affinity link between the plasma membrane and the cortical actin network in *Dictyostelium*. J. Cell Biol. 126, 1433–1444.

[5] Picot, D. et al. (1994) The X-ray crystal structure of the membrane protein prostaglandin H2 synthase-1. Nature 367, 243–249.

[6] Blobel, G. (1980) Intracellular protein topogenesis. Proc. Natl Acad. Sci. USA 77, 1496–1500.

[7] Shapiro, L. et al. (1996) Crystal structure of the extracellular domain from P0, the major structural protein of peripheral nerve myelin. Neuron 17, 435–449.

[8] von Heijne, G. (1986) A new method for predicting signal sequence cleavage sites. Nucleic Acids Res. 14, 4683–4690.

[9] Ogata, S. et al. (1989) Primary structure of rat liver dipeptidyl peptidase IV deduced from its cDNA and identification of the NH2-terminal signal sequence as the membrane-anchoring domain. J. Biol. Chem. 264, 3596–3601.

[10] Dohlman, H.G. et al. (1991) Model systems for the study of seven-transmembrane-segment receptors. Annu. Rev. Biochem. 60, 653–688.

[11] Havelka, W.A. et al. (1995) Three-dimensional structure of halorhodopsin at 7 Å resolution. J. Mol. Biol. 247, 726–738.

[12] McKnight, A.J. and Gordon, S. (1996) EGF-TM7: a novel subfamily of seven-transmembrane-region leukocyte cell surface molecules. Immunol. Today 17, 283–287.

[13] Wright, M.D. et al. (1993) Gene structure, chromosomal location and protein sequence of mouse CD53: evidence that the transmembrane 4 superfamily arose by gene duplication. Int. Immunol. 5, 209–216.

[14] Tomlinson, M.G. et al. (1993) Epitope mapping of anti-rat CD53 monoclonal antibodies. Implications for the membrane orientation of the transmembrane 4 superfamily. Eur. J. Immunol. 23, 136–140.

[15] Hupp, K. et al. (1989) Gene mapping of the three subunits of the high affinity FcR for IgE to mouse chromosomes 1 and 19. J. Immunol. 143, 3787–3791.

[16] Gottesman, M.N. and Pastan, I. (1988) The multidrug transporter, a double-edged sword. J. Biol. Chem. 263, 12163–12166.

[17] Ferguson, M.A. and Williams, A.F. (1988) Cell-surface anchoring of proteins via glycosyl-phosphatidylinositol structures. Annu. Rev. Biochem. 57, 285–320.

[18] Homans, S.W. et al. (1988) Complete structure of the glycosyl phosphatidylinositol membrane anchor of rat brain Thy-1 glycoprotein. Nature 333, 269–272.

[19] Roberts, W.L. et al. (1988) Lipid analysis of the glycoinositol phospholipid membrane anchor of human erythrocyte acetylcholinesterase. Palmitoylation of inositol results in resistance to phosphatidylinositol-specific phospholipase C. J. Biol. Chem. 263, 18766–18775.

[20] Caras, I.W. and Weddell, G.N. (1989) Signal peptide for protein secretion directing glycophospholipid membrane anchor attachment. Science 243, 1196–1198.

[21] Wallner, B.P. et al. (1987) Primary structure of lymphocyte function-associated antigen 3 (LFA-3). The ligand of the T lymphocyte CD2 glycoprotein. J. Exp. Med. 166, 923–932.

[22] Seed, B. (1987) An LFA-3 cDNA encodes a phospholipid-linked membrane protein homologous to its receptor CD2. Nature 329, 840–842.

[23] Brown, D.A. and Rose, J.K. (1992) Sorting of GPI-anchored proteins to glycolipid-enriched membrane subdomains during transport to the apical cell surface. Cell 68, 533–544.

[24] Lisanti, M.P. et al. (1989) A glycophospholipid membrane anchor acts as an apical targeting signal in polarized epithelial cells. J. Cell Biol. 109, 2145–2156.

[25] Parton, R. and Simons, K. (1995) Digging into Caveolae. Science 269, 1398–1399.

[26] Resh, M.D. (1994) Myristylation and palmitylation of Src family members: The fats of the matter. Cell 76, 411–413.

[27] Shenoy-Scaria, A.M. et al. (1994) Cysteine3 of Src family protein tyrosine kinases determines palmitoylation and localization in caveolae. J. Cell Biol. 126, 353–363.

[28] Nadler, M. et al. (1993) Treatment of T cells with 2-hydroxymyristic acid inhibits the myristoylation and alters the stability of p56(lck). Biochemistry 32, 9250–9255.

[29] Shenoy-Scaria, A.M. et al. (1993) Palmitylation of an amino-terminal cysteine motif of protein tyrosine kinases p56(lck) and p59(fyn) mediates interaction with glycosyl-phosphatidylinositol-anchored proteins. Mol. Cell. Biol. 13, 6385–6392.

[30] McLaughlin, S. and Aderem, A. (1995) The myristoyl-electrostatic switch: a modulator of reversible protein-membrane interactions. Trends Biochem. Sci. 20, 272–276.

[31] Gahmberg, C.G. et al. (1976) Characterization of surface glycoproteins of mouse lymphoid cells. J. Cell Biol. 68, 642–653.

32 Woollett, G.R. et al. (1985) Molecular and antigenic heterogeneity of the rat leukocyte-common antigen from thymocytes and T and B lymphocytes. Eur. J. Immunol. 15, 168–173.

33 Barclay, A.N. et al. (1987) Lymphocyte specific heterogeneity in the rat leucocyte common antigen (T200) is due to differences in polypeptide sequences near the NH2-terminus. EMBO J. 6, 1259–1264.

34 Jackson, D.I. and Barclay, A.N. (1989) The extra segments of sequence in rat leucocyte common antigen (L-CA) are derived by alternative splicing of only three exons and show extensive O-linked glycosylation. Immunogenetics 29, 281–287.

35 Ralph, S.J. et al. (1987) Structural variants of human T200 glycoprotein (leukocyte-common antigen). EMBO J. 6, 1251–1257.

36 Toda, K. et al. (1984) Monoclonal anti-glycoprotein antibody that blocks cell adhesion in *Polysphondylium pallidum*. Eur. J. Biochem. 140, 73–81.

37 Barnstable, C.J. et al. (1978) Production of monoclonal antibodies to group A erythrocytes, HLA and other human cell surface antigens – new tools for genetic analysis. Cell 14, 9–20.

38 Gooi, H.C. et al. (1985) Differing reactions of monoclonal anti-A antibodies with oligosaccharides related to blood group A. J. Biol. Chem. 260, 13218–13224.

39 Sharkey, D.J. and Kornfeld, R. (1991) Developmental regulation of processing alpha-mannosidases and "intersecting" N-acetylglucosaminyltransferase in *Dictyostelium discoideum*. J. Biol. Chem. 266, 18477–18484.

40 Couso, R. et al. (1987) The high mannose oligosaccharides of *Dictyostelium discoideum* glycoproteins contain a novel intersecting N-acetylglucosamine residue. J. Biol. Chem. 262, 4521–4527.

41 Galili, U. et al. (1993) One percent of human circulating B lymphocytes are capable of producing the natural anti-Gal antibody. Blood 82, 2485–2493.

42 Cyster, J.G. et al. (1991) The dimensions of the T lymphocyte glycoprotein leukosialin and identification of linear protein epitopes that can be modified by glycosylation. EMBO J. 10, 893–902.

43 O'Connell, P.J. et al. (1991) Variable O-glycosylation of CD13 (aminopeptidase N). J. Biol. Chem. 266, 4593–4597.

44 Cyster, J.G. et al. (1994) Antigenic determinants encoded by alternatively spliced exons of CD45 are determined by the polypeptide but influenced by glycosylation. Int. Immunol. 6, 1875–1881.

45 Barclay, A.N. et al. (1976) Chemical characterization of the Thy-1 glycoproteins from the membranes of rat thymocytes and brain. Nature 263, 563–567.

46 Parekh, R.B. et al. (1987) Tissue-specific N-glycosylation, site-specific oligosaccharide patterns and lentil lectin recognition of rat Thy-1. EMBO J. 6, 1233–1244.

47 Fukuda, M. et al. (1986) Structures of O-linked oligosaccharides isolated from normal granulocytes, chronic myelogenous leukemia cells, and acute myelogenous leukemia cells. J. Biol. Chem. 261, 12796–12806.

48 Carlsson, S.R. et al. (1986) Structural variations of O-linked oligosaccharides present in leukosialin isolated from erythroid, myeloid, and T-lymphoid cell lines. J. Biol. Chem. 261, 12787–12795.

49 Varki, A. (1994) Selectin ligands. Proc. Natl Acad. Sci. USA 91, 7390–7397.

50 Lasky, L.A. (1995) Selectin-carbohydrate interactions and the initiation of the inflammatory response. Annu. Rev. Biochem. 64, 113–139.

51 Powell, L. and Varki, A. (1995) I-type lectins. J. Biol. Chem. 270, 14243–14246.

52 Dowbenko, D. et al. (1993) Glycosylation-dependent cell adhesion molecule 1 (GlyCAM-1) mucin is expressed by lactating mammary gland epithelial cells and is present in milk. J. Clin. Invest. 92, 952–960.

53 Hemmerich, S. et al. (1995) Structure of the O-glycans in GlyCAM-1, an endothelial-derived ligand for L-selectin. J. Biol. Chem. 270, 12035–12047.

54 Rosen, S. and Bertozzi, C. (1996) Leukocyte adhesion: Two selectins converge on sulfate. Curr. Biol. 6, 261–264.

55 Steegmaier, M. et al. (1995) The E-selectin-ligand ESL-1 is a variant of a receptor for fibroblast growth factor. Nature 373, 615–620.

56 Vachino, G. et al. (1995) P-selectin glycoprotein ligand-1 is the major counter-receptor for P-selectin on stimulated T cells and is widely distributed in non-functional form on many lymphocytic cells. J. Biol. Chem. 270, 21966–21974.

57 Pouyani, T. and Seed, B. (1995) PSGL-1 recognition of P-selectin is controlled by a tyrosine sulfation concensus at the PSGL-1 amino terminus. Cell 83, 333–343.

58 Sako, D. et al. (1995) A sulfated peptide segment at the amino terminus of PSGL-1 is critical for P-selectin binding. Cell 83, 323–331.

59 Kanzaki, M. et al. (1995) Expression of calcium-permeable cation channel CD20 accelerates progression through the G(1) phase in Balb/c 3T3 cells. J. Biol. Chem. 270, 13099–13104.

60 Chen, A. et al. (1995) Structural requirements regulate endoproteolytic release of the L-selectin receptor from the surface of leukocytes. J. Exp. Med. 182, 519–530.

61 Arribas, J. et al. (1996) Diverse cell surface protein ectodomains are shed by a system sensitive to metallopreotease inhibitors. J. Biol. Chem. 271, 11376–11382.

62 Shipp, M.A. and Look, A.T. (1993) Hematopoietic differentiation antigens that are membrane-associated enzymes: Cutting is the key! Blood 82, 1052–1070.

63 Deterre, P. et al. (1996) Coordinated regulation in human T cells of nucleotide-hydrolyzing ecto-enzymatic activities, including CD38 and PC-1. Possible role in the recycling of nicotinamide adenine dinucleotide metabolites. J. Immunol. 157, 1381–1388.

64 Wang, F. and Guidotti, G. (1996) CD39 is an ecto (Ca^{2+}, Mg^{2+})-apyrase. J. Biol. Chem. 271, 9898–9901.

65 Callard, R. and Gearing, A. (1994) The Cytokine Factsbook. Academic Press, London.

66 Magdolen, V. et al. (1996) Systematic mutational analysis of the receptor-binding region of the human urokinase-type plasminogen activator. Eur. J. Biochem. 237, 743–751.

67 Hamann, J. et al. (1996) The seven-span transmembrane receptor CD97 has a cellular ligand (CD55, DAF). J. Exp. Med. 184, 1–5.

68 van der Merwe, P.A. and Barclay, A.N. (1994) Transient inter-cellular adhesion – the importance of weak protein–protein interactions. Trends Biochem. Sci. 19, 354–358.

69 Schwartz, M. et al. (1995) Integrins: Emerging paradigms of signal transduction. Annu. Rev. Cell Dev. Biol. 11, 549–599.

70 van der Merwe, P.A. et al. (1994) The human cell adhesion molecule CD2 binds CD58 (LFA-3) with a very low affinity and an extremely fast dissociation rate but does not bind CD48 or CD59. Biochemistry 33, 10149–10160.

71 van der Merwe, P. et al. (1997) CD80 (B7-1) binds both CD28 and CTLA-4 with a low affinity and very fast kinetics. J. Exp. Med. 185, 393–403.

[72] Fremont, D. et al. (1996) Biophysical studies of T cell receptors and their ligands. Curr. Opin. Immunol. 8, 93–100.

[73] Garcia, K. et al. (1996) CD8 enhances formation of stable T cell receptor/MHC class I molecule complexes. Nature 384, 577–581.

[74] Jacob, G.S. et al. (1995) Binding of sialyl Lewis X to E-selectin as measured by fluorescence polarization. Biochemistry 34, 1210–1217.

[75] Nicholson, M. et al. unpublished data

[76] Malissen, B. and Malissen, M. (1996) Functions of TCR and pre-TCR subunits: lessons from gene ablation. Curr. Opin. Immunol. 8, 383–393.

[77] Wright, M.D. and Tomlinson, M.G. (1994) The ins and outs of the transmembrane 4 superfamily. Immunol. Today 15, 588–594.

[78] Cerny, J. et al. (1996) Noncovalent associations of T lymphocyte surface proteins. Eur. J. Immunol. 26, 2335–2343.

[79] Arakawa, T. et al. (1991) Glycosylated and unglycosylated recombinant-derived human stem cell factors are dimeric and have extensive regular secondary structure. J. Biol. Chem. 266, 18942–18948.

[80] Banner, D.W. et al. (1993) Crystal structure of the soluble human 55kd TNF receptor-human TNFβ complex: implications for TNF receptor activation. Cell 73, 431–445.

[81] Browning, J. et al. (1993) Lymphotoxin β, a novel member of the TNF family that forms a heteromeric complex with lymphotoxin on the cell surface. Cell 72, 847–856.

[82] Hedrick, S.M. et al. (1984) Isolation of cDNA clones encoding T cell-specific membrane-associated proteins. Nature 308, 149–153.

[83] Yang, P. et al. (1992) Intercellular space is affected by the polysialic acid content of NCAM. J. Cell Biol. 116, 1487–1496.

[84] Stein-Douglas, K.E. et al. (1976) Gangliosides as markers of murine subpopulations. J. Exp. Med. 143, 822–832.

[85] Hershey, P. et al. (1989) Augmentation of lymphocyte responses by monoclonal antibodies to the gangliosides GD3 and GD2: the role of protein kinase C, cyclic nucleotides and intracellular calcium. Cell. Immunol. 119, 263–278.

[86] Williams, A.F. and Barclay, A.N. (1986) Glycoprotein antigens of the lymphocyte surface and their purification by antibody affinity chromatography. In Handbook of Experimental Immunology (Weir, D.M. ed.), Blackwell Scientific Publications, Oxford, pp. 22.1–22.24.

[87] Paterson, D.J. et al. (1987) Antigens of activated rat T lymphocytes including a molecule of 50,000 M_r detected only on CD4 positive T blasts. Mol. Immunol. 24, 1281–1290.

[88] Clark, S.J. et al. (1988) Activation of rat T lymphocytes by anti-CD2 monoclonal antibodies. J. Exp. Med. 167, 1861–1872.

[89] Williams, A.F. et al. (1987) Similarities in sequences and cellular expression between rat CD2 and CD4 antigens. J. Exp. Med. 165, 368–380.

[90] Woollett, G.R. et al. (1985) Visualisation by low-angle shadowing of the leucocyte-common antigen. A major cell surface glycoprotein of lymphocytes. EMBO J. 4, 2827–2830.

[91] McCall, M.N. et al. (1992) Epression of soluble forms of rat CD45. Analysis by electron microscopy and use in epitope mapping of anti-CD45R monoclonal antibodies. Immunology 76, 310–317.

[92] Wang, J. et al. (1990) Atomic structure of a fragment of human CD4 containing two immunoglobulin-like domains. Nature 348, 411–418.

[93] Jones, E.Y. et al. (1992) Crystal structure of a soluble form of the cell adhesion molecule CD2 at 2.8 Å. Nature 360, 232–239.

[94] Bjorkman, P.J. et al. (1987) Structure of the human class I histocompatibility antigen, HLA-A2. Nature 329, 506–512.

[95] Brown, J.H. et al. (1993) Three-dimensional structure of the human class II histocompatibility antigen HLA-DR1. Nature 364, 33–39.

[96] Amzel, L.M. and Poljak, R.J. (1979) Three-dimensional structure of immunoglobulins. Annu. Rev. Biochem. 48, 961–997.

[97] Garcia, K. et al. (1996) An $\alpha\beta$ T cell receptor structure at 2.5 Å and its orientation in the TCR-MHC complex. Science 274, 209–219.

[98] Garboczi, D. et al. (1996) Structure of the complex between T-cell receptor, viral peptide and HLA-A2. Nature 384, 134–141.

[99] van der Merwe, P.A. et al. (1995) Topology of the CD2–CD48 cell-adhesion molecule complex: implications for antigen recognition by T cells. Curr. Biol. 5, 74–84.

[100] Doyle, C. and Strominger, J.L. (1987) Interaction between CD4 and class II MHC molecules mediates cell adhesion. Nature 330, 256–259.

[101] Norment, A.M. et al. (1988) Cell-cell adhesion mediated by CD8 and MHC class I molecules. Nature 336, 79–81.

[102] Linsley, P.S. et al. (1990) T-cell antigen CD28 mediates adhesion with B cells by interacting with activation antigen B7/BB-1. Proc. Natl Acad. Sci. USA 87, 5031–5035.

[103] Manjunath, N. et al. (1995) Negative regulation of T-cell adhesion and activation by CD43. Nature 377, 535–538.

[104] Doody, G. et al. (1996) Activation of B lymphocytes: integrating signals from CD19, CD22 and FcγRIIb1. Curr. Opin. Immunol. 8, 378–382.

[105] Erlandsen, S.L. et al. (1993) Detection and spatial distribution of the beta 2 integrin (Mac-1) and L-selectin (LECAM-1) adherence receptors on human neutrophils by high-resolution field emission SEM. J. Histochem. Cytochem. 41, 327–333.

[106] von-Andrian, U.H. et al. (1995) A central role for microvillous receptor presentation in leukocyte adhesion under flow. Cell 82, 989–999.

[107] Misumi, Y. et al. (1990) Primary structure of human placental 5'-nucleotidase and identification of the glycolipid anchor in the mature form. Eur. J. Biochem. 191, 563–569.

[108] Stahl, N. and Prusiner, S.B. (1991) Prions and prion proteins. FASEB. J. 5, 2799–2807.

[109] Gerber, L.D. et al. (1992) Phosphatidylinositol glycan (PI-G) anchored membrane-amino-acid-requirements adjacent to the site of cleavage and. J. Biol. Chem. 267, 12168–12173.

[110] Sugita, Y. et al. (1993) Determination of carboxyl-terminal residue and disulfide bonds of MACIF (CD59), a glycosyl-phosphatidylinositol-anchored protein. J. Biochem. 114, 473–477.

[111] Xia, M.Q. et al. (1993) Structure of the CAMPATH-1 antigen, a glycosylphosphatidylinositol-anchored glycoprotein which is an exceptionally good target for complement lysis. Biochem. J. 293, 633–640.

[112] Rademacher, T.W. et al. (1988) Glycobiology. Annu. Rev. Biochem. 57, 785–838.

[113] Schachter, H. and Brockhausen, I. (1989) The biosynthesis of branched O-glycans. Symp. Soc. Exp. Biol. 43, 1–26.

[114] Ryu, S.E. et al. (1990) Crystal structure of an HIV-binding recombinant fragment of human CD4. Nature 348, 419–426.

[115] Brady, R.L. et al. (1993) Crystal structure of domains 3 and 4 of rat CD4: relationship to the NH_2-terminal domains. Science 260, 979–983.

[116] Weisman, H.F. et al. (1990) Soluble human complement receptor type 1: in vivo inhibitor of complement suppressing post-ischemic myocardial inflammation and necrosis. Science 249, 146–151.

[117] Barford, D. et al. (1994) Crystal-structure of human protein-tyrosine-phosphatase 1B. Science 263, 1397–1404.

[118] Kirchhausen, T. et al. (1993) Location of the domains of ICAM-1 by immunolabeling and single-molecule electron microscopy. J. Leukocyte Biol. 53, 342–346.

[119] Ushiyama, S. et al. (1993) Structural and functional characterization of monomeric soluble P-selectin and comparison with membrane P-selectin. J. Biol. Chem. 268, 15229–15237.

[120] Li, F. et al. (1996) Visualization of P-selectin glycoprotein ligand-1 as a highly extended molecule and mapping of protein epitopes for monoclonal antibodies. J. Biol. Chem. 271, 6342–6348.

[121] Nermut, M.V. et al. (1988) Electron microscopy and structural model of human fibronectin receptor. EMBO J. 7, 4093–4099.

THE LEUCOCYTE ANTIGENS

Molecular weights
Polypeptide CD1a   35 323

SDS-PAGE
  reduced   43–49 kDa
  unreduced   43–49 kDa

Carbohydrate
N-linked sites   4
O-linked   nil

Human gene location and size
1q22–23; five genes within 190 kb [1]

CD1a

CD1a

Domains

Exon boundaries

CHV LSC

S | | | C1 | TM | CY

DGL   EYP   QVK   WEH

RCF

Tissue distribution

The CD1 antigens are expressed on cortical thymocytes and expression is inversely correlated with that of TCR and MHC Class I [1,2]. CD1 antigens are also expressed on some dendritic cells and cytokine-activated monocytes [1,2]. CD1c is expressed on B cells [1,2]. CD1d but not CD1a, b or c is expressed on intestinal epithelium [1,2]. Different CD1 molecules can be coexpressed on the same cell [1]. Surface expression has been demonstrated for human CD1a, b, c and d [1].

Structure

CD1 has a domain organization similar to that of MHC Class I and is expressed in association with β_2-microglobulin [1,2]. It shows comparable levels of sequence similarity to both MHC Class I and Class II. The CD1 genes form a multigene family with five genes in human, two in mouse, both homologues of human CD1d, and eight in rabbit [1]. However, unlike MHC Class I, CD1 does not show significant polymorphism [1,2]. The N-terminus of human CD1a has been determined [1].

Ligands and associated molecules

Some T cells recognize antigen in a CD1-restricted manner [2]. Mouse NK1+ T lymphocytes which have a restricted TCR repertoire recognize murine CD1, although there are conflicting data [3,4]. Antigens presented by human CD1b were identified as microbial lipids [1,2,5]. A recombinant form of the murine CD1 bound synthetic peptides with micromolar affinities [6]. It showed a preference for longer peptides than seen for Class I and resembles Class II peptide binding.

Function

As suggested by its similarity to MHC antigens and as inferred above there is evidence for roles in presentation of lipid and peptides to T cells[2]. CD1 has a role in positive selection of NK1+ T cells[7]. The pathway for presentation of exogenous antigen by CD1 is different from that for MHC Class I and II[1,2].

Comments

CD1 genes, except CD1b, are transcribed in the same direction and all lack classical promoter elements[1].

Database accession numbers

	PIR	SWISSPROT	EMBL/GENBANK	REFERENCE
Human CD1a	A02242	P06126	X04450	8
Mouse CD1.1	S01297	P11609	X13170	9
Rat CD1			D26439	10

Amino acid sequence of human CD1a

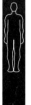

```
MLFLLLPLLA VLPGDGNA                                          -1
DGLKEPLSFH VIWIASFYNH SWKQNLVSGW LSDLQTHTWD SNSSTIVFLW        50
PWSRGNFSNE EWKELETLFR IRTIRSFEGI RRYAHELQFE YPFEIQVTGG       100
CELHSGKVSG SFLQLAYQGS DFVSFQNNSW LPYPVAGNMA KHFCKVLNQN       150
QHENDITHNL LSDTCPRFIL GLLDAGKAHL QRQVKPEAWL SHGPSPGPGH       200
LQLVCHVSGF YPKPVWVMWM RGEQEQQGTQ RGDILPSADG TWYLRATLEV       250
AAGEAADLSC RVKHSSLEGQ DIVLYWEHHS SVGFIILAVI VPLLLLIGLA       300
LWFRKRCFC                                                    309
```

References

1 **Porcelli, S.A. (1995) Adv. Immunol. 59, 1–98.**
2 Melian, A. et al. (1996) Curr. Opin. Immunol. 8, 82–88.
3 Bendelac, A. et al. (1995) Science 268, 863–865.
4 Bendelac, A (1995) Curr. Opin. Immunol. 7, 367–374.
5 Sieling, P.A. et al. (1995) Science 269, 227–230.
6 Castano, A.R. et al. (1995) Science 269, 223–226.
7 Bendelac, A. (1995) J. Exp. Med. 182, 2091–2096.
8 Martin, L.H. et al. (1987) Proc. Natl Acad. Sci. USA 84, 9189–9193.
9 Bradbury, A. et al. (1988) EMBO J. 7, 3081–3086.
10 Ichimiya, S. et al. (1994) J. Immunol. 153, 1112–1123.

Molecular weights
Polypeptide   36 844

SDS PAGE
  reduced   45–58 kDa
  unreduced   45–58 kDa

Carbohydrate
N-linked sites 3
O-linked   nil

Human gene location and size
1p13.1; ~12 kb [1,2]

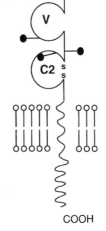

COOH

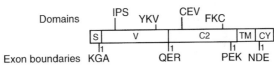

Domains   IPS   YKV   CEV   FKC

| S | V | | C2 | TM | CY |

Exon boundaries KGA   QER   PEK NDE

Tissue distribution

CD2 is expressed on virtually all thymocytes, T lymphocytes and NK cells. CD2 is also expressed on mouse B cells and rat and sheep splenic macrophages [1,3,4].

Structure

CD2 is the best-characterized member of a family of structurally related cell surface IgSF molecules which includes CD48, CD58, 2B4, Ly-9, and CD150 [5]. The gene for CD58 lies 60–250 kb from the CD2 gene. The genes encoding CD48, Ly-9 and 2B4 also lie close together but at a different locus (1q21–23). These two loci encoding CD2-related molecules appear to have arisen by duplication of an entire chromosomal region [6,7]. The structure of the entire extracellular portion of CD2 has been determined by X-ray diffraction [5]. As predicted for other members of this family, it contains a membrane-distal V set domain lacking the canonical inter-β sheet disulfide linked by a somewhat flexible segment to a membrane-proximal C2 set domain with an additional disulfide [5]. The cytoplasmic domain is rich in basic and proline residues and is highly conserved across species [1,3,5]. The V-set domain N-linked glycan has been proposed to be essential for maintaining the structure of CD2, but this is controversial [5]. The N-terminus of the mature polypeptide has been established by protein sequencing [1].

Ligands and associated molecules

The major ligand for the extracellular portion of human CD2 is CD58 [1]. No CD58 homologue has been identified in the rat or mouse and CD48 appears to be the major ligand in these species [5]. Human CD2 has also been reported to bind CD48 and CD59, but this is controversial [5]. CD58 and CD48 both bind to the GFCC'C'' β sheet of the membrane-distal IgSF domain of CD2 [5]. Structural and mutagenesis studies suggest that CD2 interacts with CD48 and CD58 in a head-to-head orientation with the complex predicted to span ~134 Å [5], similar to the dimensions of a T cell receptor/peptide/MHC complex (also ~134 Å) [8]. CD2 binds CD58 in solution with a very low affinity (K_d 9–22 μM) and dissociates rapidly ($k_{off} \geq 4\,s^{-1}$) [5]. Membrane-attached CD58 binds half-maximally to cell surface CD2 at a surface density of ~10–20 molecules/μm^2 and there is rapid exchange of bound and free CD58 at the contact interface [9]. Immunoprecipitation studies indicate an association between CD2 and several transmembrane (T cell receptor/CD3 complex, CD5, CD45 and CD53) and cytoplasmic (Lck, Fyn, phosphatidylinositol 3-kinase, tubulin) proteins [5,10,11]. The interaction with Lck involves two of the proline-rich regions in CD2 which bind the SH3 domain of Lck [12].

Function

The interaction between CD2 and its ligands, CD48 and CD58, enhances T cell Ag recognition [1,3,5]. This is partly a consequence of improved adhesion between T cells and antigen-presenting cells or target cells, but may also be the result of signals transmitted through the CD2 cytoplasmic domain [1,3,4]. No abnormality has been detected in CD2-deficient mice [5,13].

Database accession numbers

	PIR	SWISSPROT	EMBL/GENBANK	REFERENCE
Human	A28967	P06729	M16445	1
Rat	A33071	P08921	X05111	14
Mouse	B28967	P08920	Y00023	15

Amino acid sequence of human CD2

```
MSFPCKFVAS FLLIFNVSSK GAVS                                -1
KEITNALETW GALGQDINLD IPSFQMSDDI DDIKWEKTSD KKKIAQFRKE     50
KETFKEKDTY KLFKNGTLKI KHLKTDDQDI YKVSIYDTKG KNVLEKIFDL    100
KIQERVSKPK ISWTCINTTL TCEVMNGTDP ELNLYQDGKH LKLSQRVITH    150
KWTTSLSAKF KCTAGNKVSK ESSVEPVSCP EKGLDIYLII GICGGGSLLM    200
VFVALLVFYI TKRKKQRSRR NDEELETRAH RVATEERGRK PQQIPASTPQ    250
NPATSQHPPP PPGHRSQAPS HRPPPPGHRV QHQPQKRPPA PSGTQVHQQK    300
GPPLPRPRVQ PKPPHGAAEN SLSPSSN                            327
```

References

1 Moingeon, P. et al. (1989) Immunol. Rev. 111, 111–144.
2 Mitchell, E.L.D. et al. (1995) Cytogenet. Cell Genet. 70, 183–185.
3 Bierer, B.E. and Burakoff, S.J. (1989) Immunol. Rev. 111, 267–94.
4 Beyers, A.D. et al. (1989) Immunol. Rev. 111, 59–77.
5 **Davis, S.J. and van der Merwe, P.A. (1996) Immunol. Today 17, 177–187.**
6 Wong, Y.W. et al. (1990) J. Exp. Med. 171, 2115–2130.
7 Kingsmore, S.F. et al. (1995) Immunogenetics 42, 59–62.
8 Garboczi, D.N. et al. (1996) Nature 384, 134–141.
9 Dustin, M.L. et al. (1996) J. Cell. Biol. 132, 465–474.

[10] Bell, G.M. et al. (1992) J. Exp. Med. 175, 527–36.
[11] Offringa, R. and Bierer, B.E. (1993) J. Biol. Chem. 268, 4979–88.
[12] Bell, G.M. et al. (1996) J. Exp. Med. 183, 169–178.
[13] Killeen, N. et al. (1992) EMBO J. 11, 4329–4336.
[14] Williams, A.F. et al. (1987) J. Exp. Med. 165, 368–380.
[15] Sewell, W.A. et al. (1987) Eur. J. Immunol. 17, 1015–1020.

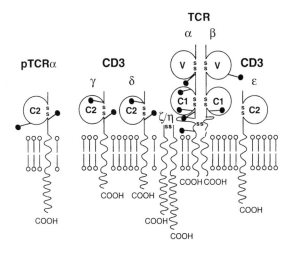

	Molecular weights (reduced)	Carbohydrate (N-linked sites only)	Gene location and size
TCRα	45–60 kDa	5	14q11.2; >800 kb [1]
TCRβ	40–50 kDa	2	7q35; 685 kb [2]
TCRγ	45–60 kDa	4	7p15; 160 kb [3]
TCRδ	40–60 kDa	2	14q11.2; >195 kb [4,5]
pTCRα	33 kDa	2	6p21.2–p12 [6]
CD3γ	25–28 kDa	2	11q23; 9 kb [7]
CD3δ	20 kDa	2	11q23; 3.7 kb [8]
CD3ε	20 kDa	none	11q23; 13 kb [9]
ζ chain	16 kDa	none	1q22–q23
η chain	22 kDa	none	1q22–q23

The CD3/T cell receptor (TCR) gene organization, structure and function have been extensively reviewed (e.g. see ref. 10) and only a brief overview is given here.

Tissue distribution

Expressed during thymopoiesis and on mature T cells in the periphery (reviewed in refs 9 and 10). Less than 10% of human peripheral T cells express the γ/δ TCR complex but in the mouse the great majority of T cells present i]n some epithelial tissues are γ/δ+ and have limited receptor diversity [11]. Pre-TCR α (pTCRα) is expressed in immature but not mature T cells [6].

Structure

CD3/TCR consists of both IgSF and non-IgSF proteins [10,12,13]. The stoichiometry of a CD3/TCR complex is not established but is generally thought to contain a TCR hetrodimer, two CD3ε chains, a CD3γ and a CD3δ chain and a ζ homodimer [13]. The α/β and γ/δ heterodimers are clonotypic and consist of Ig-like variable and constant domains [9,14,15]. The α/β heterodimer has been crystallized and the structure confirms the predicted IgSF domains [14,15]. In immature T cells, pTCRα which is comprised of a single conserved IgSF domain in its extracellular region is expressed instead of TCRα [6,13]. The transmembrane domains of the clonotypic and invariant chains contain oppositely charged amino acids [10]. The ζ chain forms disulfide-linked homodimers or, less frequently, heterodimers with its splicing variant, the η chain [12]. The ζ chain is related to the γ chain of the IgE Fc receptor and can also associate with the Fc receptor CD16 [12]. The cytoplasmic domains of the CD3 and ζ chain contain ITAM motifs [12].

Ligands and associated molecules

The α/β and γ/δ heterodimers recognize peptide antigen bound to MHC antigens [14,15]. The affinity of the interaction between the TCR and the MHC/peptide complex is in the range $10^{-7}-10^{-4}$ M [16]. The cocrystal structure of TCR and peptide-MHC reveals that the TCR VDJC junction, which is equivalent to the third complementarity-determining region (CDR3) of antibodies, interacts directly with the peptide and that the CDR1- and CDR2-like regions of the TCR contact peptide and the MHC antigen [13]. Superantigen binds to non-polymorphic regions of TCRVβ [15]. Intracellularly, Fyn is associated with the CD3/TCR complex [12,17]. Phosphorylated ITAM motifs of the CD3 and ζ chains bind to SH2 domains of intracellular signalling molecules, e.g phosphorylated ζ chains bind to ZAP-70 [12,16-18].

Function

Recognition of antigen leads to signal transduction mediated by the invariant chains and subsequently T cell activation [17]. Consequences of binding by TCR depend on antigen density and affinity of TCR for antigen and may result in unresponsiveness. Signal transduction involves tyrosine kinase and phospholipase C activation followed by phosphoinositide turnover and activation of several second messenger pathways [17,18].

Diversity and ontogeny

Although TCR genes contain fewer variable-region segments [19] than antibody genes, the potential repertoire can be argued to be higher than that of antibodies due to the relative abundance of J-region segments and greater flexibility in the joining of variable (V)-, diversity (D)- and joining (J)-segments [9]. Rearrangement of the TCR genes is similar to that of antibody genes and occurs at the CD4$^-$/CD8$^-$ stage of thymic development, but the TCR genes do not undergo somatic mutation after rearrangement [8]. Selection of the receptor repertoire takes place in the thymic cortex while the thymocytes coexpress CD4 and CD8 and low levels of the TCR. Mature thymocytes expressing CD4 or CD8 and high levels of the TCR complex then leave the medulla for the periphery. Mice deficient in components of the CD3/TCR complex are arrested in development of their T cell repertoire [13].

Database accession numbers

	PIR	SWISSPROT	EMBL/GENBANK	REFERENCE
Human pTCRα chain			U36759	6
Human CD3γ	A25468	P09693	X04145	20
Human CD3δ	A02245	P04234	X03934	21
Human CD3ε	A25769	P07766	X03884	22
Human ζ chain	A31768	P20963	J04132	23
Human η chain			M33158	24

Amino acid sequences of the invariant chains

(The sequences of the clonotypic chains are reviewed in refs 9 and 19.)

pTCRα

```
MAGTWLLLLL ALGCPA                                              -1
LPTGVGGTPF PSLAPPIMLL VDGKQQMVVV CLVLDVAPPG LDSPIWFSAG         50
NGSALDAFTY GPSPATDGTW TNLAHLSLPS EELASWEPLV CHTGPGAEGH        100
SRSTQPMHLS GEASTARTCP QEPLRGTPGG ALWLGVLRLL LFKLLLFDLL        150
LTCSCLCDPA GPLPSPATTT RLRALGSHRL HPATETGGRE ATSSPRPQPR        200
DRRWGDTPPG RKPGSPVWGE GSYLSSYPTC PAQAWCSRSR LRAPSSSLGA        250
FFRGDLPPPL QAGAA                                             265
```

CD3γ

```
MEQGKGLAVL ILAIILLQGT LA                                       -1
QSIKGNHLVK VYDYQEDGSV LLTCDAEAKN ITWFKDGKMI GFLTEDKKKW         50
NLGSNAKDPR GMYQCKGSQN KSKPLQVYYR MCQNCIELNA ATISGFLFAE        100
IVSIFVLAVG VYFIAGQDGV RQSRASDKQT LLPNDQLYQP LKDREDDQYS        150
HLQGNQLRRN                                                   160
```

CD3δ

```
MEHSTFLSGL VLATLLSQVS P                                        -1
FKIPIEELED RVFVNCNTSI TWVEGTVGTL LSDITRLDLG KRILDPRGIY         50
RCNGTDIYKD KESTVQVHYR MCQSCVELDP ATVAGIIVTD VIATLLLALG        100
VFCFAGHETG RLSGAADTQA LLRNDQVYQP LRDRDDAQYS HLGGNWARNK        150
```

CD3ε

```
MQSGTHWRVL GLCLLSVGVW GQ                                       -1
DGNEEMGGIT QTPYKVSISG TTVILTCPQY PGSEILWQHN DKNIGGDEDD         50
KNIGSDEDHL SLKEFSELEQ SGYYVCYPRG SKPEDANFYL YLRARVCENC        100
MEMDVMSVAT IVIVDICITG GLLLLVYYWS KNRKAKAKPV TRGAGAGGRQ        150
RGQNKERPPP VPNPDYEPIR KGQRDLYSGL NQRRI                        185
```

ζ chain

```
MKWKALFTAA ILQAQLPITE A                                        -1
QSFGLLDPKL CYLLDGILFI YGVILTALFL RVKFSRSAEP PAYQQGQNQL         50
YNELNLGRRE EYDVLDKRRG RDPEMGGKPR RKNPQEGLYN ELQKDKMAEA        100
YSEIGMKGER RRGKGHDGLY QGLSTATKDT YDALHMQALP PR                142
```

η chain

```
MKWKALFTAA ILQAQLPITE A                                        -1
QSFGLLDPKL CYLLDGILFI YGVILTALFL RVKFSRSAEP PAYQQGQNQL         50
YNELNLGRRE EYDVLDKRRG RDPEMGGKPR RKNPQEGLYN ELQKDKMAEA        100
YSEIGMKGER RRGKGHDGLY QDSHFQAVQF GNRREREGSE LTRTLGLRAR        150
PKGESTQQSS QSCASVFSIP TLWSPWPPSS SSQL                         184
```

References

1. Wilson, R.K. et al. (1988) Immunol. Rev. 101, 149–172.
2. Rowen, L. et al. (1996) Science 272, 1755–1762.
3. Lefranc, M.-P. et al. (1989) Eur. J. Immunol. 19, 989–994.
4. Satyanarayana, K. et al. (1988) Proc. Natl Acad. Sci. USA 85, 8166–8170.
5. Iwashima, M. et al. (1988) Proc. Natl Acad. Sci. USA 85, 8161–8165.
6. Del Porto, P. et al. (1995) Proc. Natl Acad. Sci. USA 92, 12105–12109.
7. Tunnacliffe, A. et al. (1987) EMBO J. 6, 2953–2957.
8. Tunnacliffe, A. et al. (1986) EMBO J. 5, 1245–1252.
9. Clevers, H.C. et al. (1988) Proc. Natl Acad. Sci. USA 85, 8156–8160.
10. **Davis, M.M. (1990) Annu. Rev. Biochem. 59, 475–496.**
11. Allison, J.P. and Havran, W.L. (1991) Annu. Rev. Immunol. 9, 679–705.
12. Chan, A.C. et al. (1994) Ann. Rev. Immunol. 12, 555–592.
13. **Malissen, B. and Malissen, M. (1996) Curr. Opin. Immunol. 8, 383–393.**
14. **Garcia, K.C. et al. (1996) Science 274, 209–219.**
15. **Garboczi, D.N. et al. (1996) Nature 384, 134–141.**
16. Fremont, D.H. et al. (1996) Curr. Opin. Immunol. 8, 93–100.
17. Weiss, A. and Littman, D.R. (1994) Cell 76, 263–274.
18. Wange, R. and Samelson, L.E. (1996) Immunity 5, 197–205.
19. Immunogenetics (1995) 42, 1–540.
20. Krissansen, G.W. et al. (1986) EMBO J. 5, 1799–1808.
21. van den Elsen, P. et al. (1984) Nature 312, 413–418.
22. Gold, D.P. et al. (1986) Nature 321, 431–434.
23. Weissman, A.M. et al. (1988) Proc. Natl Acad. Sci. USA 85, 9709–9713.
24. Jin, Y.-J. et al. (1990) Proc. Natl Acad. Sci. USA 87, 3319–3323.

CD4 T4, L3T4 (mouse), W3/25 (rat)

Molecular weights
Polypeptide   48 400

SDS-PAGE
  reduced   55 kDa
  unreduced   55 kDa

Carbohydrate
N-linked sites   2
O-linked   nil

Human gene location and size
12pter–p12; 33 kb [1]

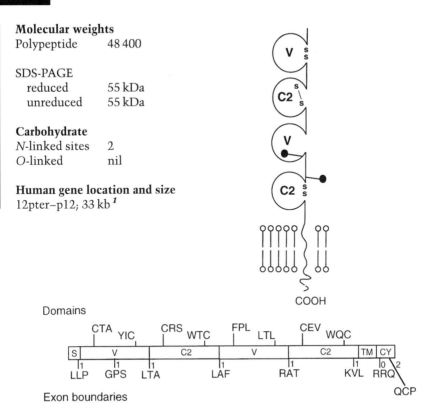

Domains

Exon boundaries

Tissue distribution

CD4 is expressed on most thymocytes and approximately two-thirds of peripheral blood T cells, which constitute the CD8⁻ cells [1]. In human and rat but not in mouse, CD4 is expressed on monocytes and macrophages [1].

Structure

The extracellular domain is made up of four IgSF domains. The structures of the N-terminal two domains and separately, the membrane-proximal two domains have been determined by X-ray crystallography, confirming that they are Ig-like [2,3]. Domain 2 is characterized by an unusual disulfide within one β sheet and domain 3 lacks a disulfide in the position conserved in most IgSF domains. Cat CD4 shows some unusual features with 17 residues inserted between domains 1 and 2 [4]. There is an additional Cys in domain 1 and the Cys in the unusual β strand C position in domain 2 is replaced with a Trp and there is an extra Cys in the β strand F [4]. The position of the N-terminus has been established for the rat homologue [5]. CD4 shows particularly close similarities in overall structure to the LAG-3 protein (see page 531). The cytoplasmic domain of CD4 is phosphorylated at Ser residues 408, 415, 431 when T cells are activated by antigen or phorbol esters [6].

Ligands and associated molecules

CD4 domains 1 and 2 bind to MHC Class II antigen[2,3]. There is evidence that CD4 domains 3 and 4 are involved in *cis* interactions with the CD3/TCR complex[7]. The cytoplasmic domain interacts with a lymphocyte-specific tyrosine kinase called Lck through a CXCP motif[2,8,9]. CD4 is a receptor for HIV-1 and the binding of the viral gp120 protein is to a region of the N-terminal domain[2,3].

Function

CD4 is an accessory molecule in the recognition of foreign antigens in association with MHC Class II antigens by T cells[1,2,3]. Interactions with MHC Class II and with Lck have been shown to have a role in CD4 function[7,10]. MAbs against CD4 inhibit T cell functions *in vivo* and *in vitro*[1].

Database accession numbers

	PIR	SWISSPROT	EMBL/GENBANK	REFERENCE
Human	A02109	P01730	M12807	1
Rat	A27449	P05540	M15768	5
Mouse	A02110	P06332	M13816	1

Amino acid sequence of human CD4

```
MNRGVPFRHL LLVLQLALLP AATQG                          -1
KKVVLGKKGD TVELTCTASQ KKSIQFHWKN SNQIKILGNQ GSFLTKGPSK  50
LNDRADSRRS LWDQGNFPLI IKNLKIEDSD TYICEVEDQK EEVQLLVFGL  100
TANSDTHLLQ GQSLTLTLES PPGSSPSVQC RSPRGKNIQG GKTLSVSQLE  150
LQDSGTWTCT VLQNQKKVEF KIDIVVLAFQ KASSIVYKKE GEQVEFSFPL  200
AFTVEKLTGS GELWWQAERA SSSKSWITFD LKNKEVSVKR VTQDPKLQMG  250
KKLPLHLTLP QALPQYAGSG NLTLALEAKT GKLHQEVNLV VMRATQLQKN  300
LTCEVWGPTS PKLMLSLKLE NKEAKVSKRE KAVWVLNPEA GMWQCLLSDS  350
GQVLLESNIK VLPTWSTPVQ PMALIVLGGV AGLLLFIGLG IFFCVRCRHR  400
RRQAERMSQI KRLLSEKKTC QCPHRFQKTC SPI                   433
```

References

1 Parnes, J.R. (1989) Adv. Immunol. 44, 265–311.
2 **Littman, D.R. (ed.) (1996) The CD4 Molecule. Curr. Top. Microbiol. Immunol. 205.**
3 Sakihama, T. et al. (1995) Immunol. Today 16, 581–587.
4 Norimine, J. et al. (1992) Immunology 75, 74–79.
5 Clark, S.J. et al. (1987) Proc. Natl Acad. Sci. USA 84, 1649–1653.
6 Shin, J. et al. (1990) EMBO J. 9, 425–434.
7 Vignali, D.A.A. et al. (1996) J. Exp. Med. 183, 2097–2107.
8 **Zamoyska, R. (1994) Immunity 1, 243–246.**
9 Turner, J.M. et al. (1990) Cell 60, 755–757.
10 Itano, A. et al. (1996) J. Exp. Med. 183, 731–741.

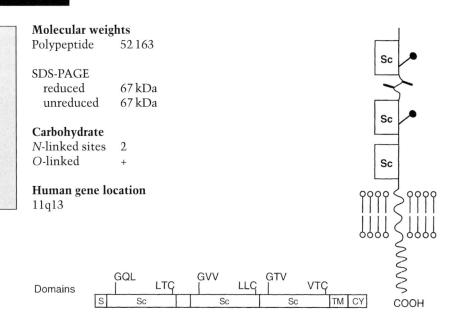

CD5   T1, Leu-1, Ly-1

Molecular weights
Polypeptide   52 163

SDS-PAGE
  reduced   67 kDa
  unreduced   67 kDa

Carbohydrate
N-linked sites   2
O-linked   +

Human gene location
11q13

Domains

GQL   LTC   GVV   LLC   GTV   VTC

S | Sc | Sc | Sc | TM | CY   COOH

Sc
Sc
Sc

Tissue distribution

CD5 is expressed on all mature T cells, most thymocytes [1,2] and on a subset of mature B cells [3].

Structure

The extracellular region consists of three scavenger receptor cysteine-rich domains [4]. Domain 1 is separated from domain 2 by a connecting peptide rich in Thr and Pro residues which contains O-linked carbohydrate (McAlister, M. et al., unpublished). The cytoplasmic domain contains an ITAM-like motif [5] (and see Chapter 3).

Ligands and associated molecules

CD5 coprecipitates with the TCR and, more directly, with Lck [5]. A report that CD5 purified from cells bound to CD72 has not been substantiated by functional experiments [6,7] or biochemical studies (Brown, M.H., unpublished).

Function

A role for CD5 in signal transduction is postulated based on stimulatory effects of mAbs [5,6]. CD5 is phosphorylated on tyrosine residues on T cell activation [5]. Thymocytes from CD5 knockout CD5$^{-/-}$ mice gave increased responses to receptor-mediated stimulation [6]. A role for CD5 in thymocyte selection is suggested by altered expression of TCR when CD5$^{-/-}$ mice were crossed with TCR transgenic mice [6]. Inhibition of T–B interaction by a mouse CD5 mAb is consistent with a role in cell–cell recognition [7].

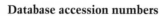

Database accession numbers

	PIR	*SWISSPROT*	*EMBL/GENBANK*	*REFERENCE*
Human	A26396	P06127	X04391	8
Mouse	A29079	P13379	M15177	1
Rat		P51882	D10728	2

Amino acid sequence of human CD5

```
MPMGSLQPLA TLYLLGMLVA SCLG                                  -1
RLSWYDPDFQ ARLTRSNSKC QGQLEVYLKD GWHMVCSQSW GRSSKQWEDP      50
SQASKVCQRL NCGVPLSLGP FLVTYTPQSS IICYGQLGSF SNCSHSRNDM     100
CHSLGLTCLE PQKTTPPTTR PPPTTTPEPT APPRLQLVAQ SGGQHCAGVV     150
EFYSGSLGGT ISYEAQDKTQ DLENFLCNNL QCGSFLKHLP ETEAGRAQDP     200
GEPREHQPLP IQWKIQNSSC TSLEHCFRKI KPQKSGRVLA LLCSGFQPKV     250
QSRLVGGSSI CEGTVEVRQG AQWAALCDSS SARSSLRWEE VCREQQCGSV     300
NSYRVLDAGD PTSRGLFCPH QKLSQCHELW ERNSYCKKVF VTCQDPNPAG     350
LAAGTVASII LALVLLVVLL VVCGPLAYKK LVKKFRQKKQ RQWIGPTGMN     400
QNMSFHRNHT ATVRSHAENP TASHVDNEYS QPPRNSRLSA YPALEGVLHR     450
SSMQPDNSSD SDYDLHGAQR L                                    471
```

References
1 Huang, H-J.S. et al. (1987) Proc. Natl Acad. Sci. USA 84, 204–208.
2 Murakami, T. and Matsuura, A. (1992) Sapporo Med. J. 61, 13–26.
3 Kantor, A.B. and Herzenberg, L.A. (1991) Annu. Rev. Immunol. 11, 501–538.
4 Resnick, D. et al. (1994) Trends Biochem. Sci. 19, 5–8.
5 Raab, M. et al. (1994) Mol. Cell. Biol. 14, 2862–2870.
6 **Tarakhovsky, A. et al. (1995) Science 269, 535–537.**
7 Muthukkumar, S. and Bondada, S. (1995) Int. Immunol. 7, 305–315.
8 Jones, N.H. et al. (1986) Nature 323, 346–349.

CD6 T12, Tp120

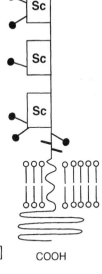

Molecular weights
Polypeptide   69 365

SDS-PAGE
  reduced   100–130 kDa
  unreduced   117 kDa

Carbohydrate
N-linked sites 8
O-linked   +

Human gene location
11

Domains

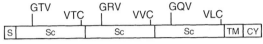

Tissue distribution

CD6 is expressed on peripheral blood T cells and medullary thymocytes[1]. It is also expressed by B cell chronic lymphocytic leukaemias and has been found in brain[1].

Structure

The extracellular region contains three scavenger receptor cysteine-rich domains and thus resembles another T cell molecule, CD5[2]. CD6 has a short membrane-proximal stalk[1] and contains polysulfated O-linked oligosaccharides[3]. The large cytoplasmic domain contains potential SH2, SH3, PKC and casein kinase-2 binding sites and may be alternatively spliced[4-6].

Ligands and associated molecules

The ligand for CD6 is CD166 or activated leucocyte cell adhesion molecule. CD166 contains five IgSF domains and is present on thymic epithelial cells and activated lymphocytes, monocytes and neural cells[7,8]. The interaction involves the N-terminal domain of CD166 and the membrane-proximal scavenger receptor cysteine-rich domain of CD6[8,9].

Function

Through its interaction with CD166 in the thymus, CD6 may have a role in T cell development. A role for CD6 in signal transduction is postulated based on stimulatory effects of mAbs[1,3,7]. CD6 is hyperphosphorylated on serine and phosphorylated on tyrosine residues on activation[3-5].

Database accession numbers

	PIR	SWISSPROT	EMBL/GENBANK	REFERENCE
Human	S26741	P30203	X60992	1,5
Mouse			U37543	4

Amino acid sequence of human CD6

```
MWLFFGITGL LTAALSGHPS PAPP                              -1
DQLNTSSAES ELWEPGERLP VRLTNGSSSC SGTVEVRLEA SWEPACGALW   50
DSRAAEAVCR ALGCGGAEAA SQLAPPTPEL PPPPAAGNTS VAANATLAGA  100
PALLCSGAEW RLCEVVEHAC RSDGRRARVT CAENRALRLV DGGGACAGRV  150
EMLEHGEWGS VCDDTWDLED AHVVCRQLGC GWAVQALPGL HFTPGRGPIH  200
RDQVNCSGAE AYLWDCPGLP GQHYCGHKED AGVVCSEHQS WRLTGGADRC  250
EGQVEVHFRG VWNTVCDSEW YPSEAKVLCQ SLGCGTAVER PKGLPHSLSG  300
RMYYSCNGEE LTLSNCSWRF NNSNLCSQSL AARVLCSASR SLHNLSTPEV  350
PASVQTVTIE SSVTVKIENK ESRELMLLIP SIVLGILLLG SLIFIAFILL  400
RIKGKYALPV MVNHQHLPTT IPAGSNSYQP VPITIPKEVF MLPIQVQAPP  450
PEDSDSGSDS DYEHYDFSAQ PPVALTTFYN SQRHRVTDEE VQQSRFQMPP  500
LEEGLEELHA SHIPTANPGH CITDPPSLGP QYHPRSNSES STSSGEDYCN  550
SPKSKLPPWN PQVFSSERSS FLEQPPNLEL AGTQPAFSAG PPADDSSSTS  600
SGEWYQNFQP PPQPPSEEQF GCPGSPSPQP DSTDNDDYDD ISAA        644
```

References

1 Aruffo, A. et al. (1991) J. Exp. Med. 174, 949–952.
2 Resnick, D. et al. (1994) Trends Biochem. Sci. 19, 5–8.
3 Swack, J.A. et al. (1991) J. Biol. Chem. 266, 7137–7143.
4 Robinson, W.H. et al. (1995) J. Immunol. 155, 4739–4748.
5 Robinson, W.H. et al. (1995) Eur. J. Immunol. 25, 2765–2769.
6 Whitney, G. et al. (1995) Mol. Immunol. 32, 89–92.
7 **Bowen, M.A. et al. (1995) J. Exp. Med. 181, 2213–2220.**
8 Whitney, G.S. et al. (1995) J. Biol. Chem. 270, 18187–18190.
9 Bajorath, J. et al. (1995) Protein Science 4, 1644–1647.

Molecular weights
Polypeptide   22 919

SDS-PAGE
  reduced   40 kDa
  unreduced   38 kDa

Carbohydrate
N-linked sites   2
O-linked   probable +

Human gene size and location
17q25.2–q25.3; 3.5 kb [1]

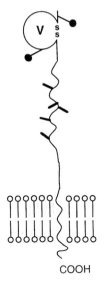

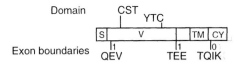

Domain   CST
                  YTC

| S | V | | TM | CY |

Exon boundaries
QEV   TEE TQIK   COOH

Tissue distribution

CD7 is the earliest marker antigen expressed in the T lineage, being found on T cell precursors in fetal liver and thorax prior to thymic colonization and in thymus and bone marrow [2,3]. CD7 is expressed on pluripotential haematopoietic cells, most human thymocytes and a major subset of peripheral blood T cells and NK cells [2,3]. CD7 is a marker for pluripotential stem cell leukaemias and T cell acute lymphocytic leukaemia [2].

Structure

A single IgSF domain is separated from the transmembrane sequence by four repeats containing a high proportion of Pro, Ser and Thr residues [4]. This region is likely to be O-glycosylated and to form an extended structure like that proposed for the CD8 hinge. The gene for CD7 is similar to the murine *Thy-1* gene which places it in a class of tissue-specific genes whose promoters lack a TATA element [1,3,5].

Ligands and associated molecules

No ligand for the extracellular region of CD7 has been identified. On crosslinking with mAb, CD7 associates with PI 3-kinase possibly through a YXXM motif in the cytoplasmic domain [7].

Function

The function of CD7 is unknown. A proposal that CD7 was an IgM receptor was not confirmed in expression studies using the cDNA clone [4]. CD7 mAbs co-stimulate T cell proliferation and induce second messengers [6,7]. Soluble recombinant CD7 has been reported to inhibit antigen-specific T cell proliferation and a mixed lymphocyte reaction[6].

Database accession numbers

	PIR	SWISSPROT	EMBL/GENBANK	REFERENCE
Human	S03520	P09564	X06180	4
Mouse		P50283	D10329	5

Amino acid sequence of human CD7

```
MAGPPRLLLL PLLLALARGL PGALA                                  -1
AQEVQQSPHC TTVPVGASVN ITCSTSGGLR GIYLRQLGPQ PQDIIYYEDG        50
VVPTTDRRFR GRIDFSGSQD NLTITMHRLQ LSDTGTYTCQ AITEVNVYGS       100
GTLVLVTEEQ SQGWHRCSDA PPRASALPAP PTGSALPDPQ TASALPDPPA       150
ASALPAALAV ISFLLGLGLG VACVLARTQI KKLCSWRDKN SAACVVYEDM       200
SHSRCNTLSS PNQYQ                                            215
```

References
1 Schanberg, L.E. et al. (1991) Proc. Natl Acad. Sci. USA 88, 603–607.
2 Haynes, B.F. et al. (1989) Immunol. Today 10, 87–91.
3 **Schanberg, L.E. et al. (1995) J. Immunol. 155, 2407–2418.**
4 Aruffo, A. and Seed, B. (1987) EMBO J. 6, 3313–3316.
5 Yoshikawa, K. et al. (1995) Immunogenetics 41, 159–161.
6 Leta, E. et al. (1995) Cell. Immunol. 165, 101–109.
7 Ward, S. et al. (1995) Eur. J. Immunol. 25, 502–507.

Molecular weights

Polypeptide α 23 552

               $\beta1$ 21 351

SDS-PAGE

   reduced α 32–34 kDa

                β 32–34 kDa

   unreduced   68 kDa plus higher multimers

Carbohydrate

N-linked sites α nil

                 β 1

O-linked α +

          β +

Human gene location and size

α chain: 2p12; 7 kb [1]

β chain: 2; >15 kb [1]

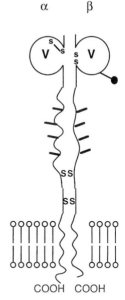

α β

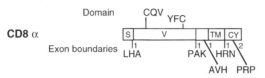

CD8 α

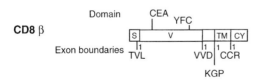

CD8 β

Tissue distribution

CD8 is expressed on most thymocytes and approximately one-third of peripheral blood T cells, which constitute the CD4⁻ cells [1]. CD8$\alpha\beta$ heterodimers are expressed only on TCR$\alpha\beta$ cells whereas CD8α homodimers can be expressed on $\alpha\beta$ and $\gamma\delta$ T cells and some NK cells [1-3].

Structure

CD8 is expressed as a heterodimer of CD8α and CD8β or as a CD8α homodimer [1-3]. CD8α is required for expression of CD8β [3]. The IgSF domains of CD8α and CD8β are separated from transmembrane sequences by hinge regions rich in Pro, Ser and Thr residues containing O-linked carbohydrate [1-4], with four sites identified in rat CD8α [4]. The N-terminus of the mature polypeptide has been established by protein sequencing [5]. Alternative splicing gives rise to a soluble form of CD8α [1] and a soluble form is predicted for CD8β[2]. An alternatively spliced form of mouse CD8α, called CD8α', has a shortened cytoplasmic domain[1]. Partial genomic structure of human CD8β shows it has a similar organization to the mouse CD8β gene[1]. The X-ray crystal structure of the IgSF domain of human CD8α did not contain the abnormal disulfide bond found in biochemical analysis of mouse and rat CD8[6]. In the mouse the genes for α and β chains are only 36 kb apart and are closely linked to the Igκ gene locus[1].

Ligands and associated molecules

The IgSF domain of CD8α binds to the α3 domain of MHC Class I[3]. Like CD4, a CXCP motif in the cytoplasmic domain of CD8α mediates binding to the tyrosine kinase Lck[3].

Function

CD8 acts as a co-receptor with MHC Class I-restricted TCRs in antigen recognition[1,3,7]. Analysis of mice lacking CD8α or CD8β show that the co-receptor function of CD8 is important for selection of MHC Class I-restricted CD8[+] T cells during development[3].

Database accession numbers

	PIR	SWISSPROT	EMBL/GENBANK	REFERENCE
Human α	A01999	P01732	M27161	5
Human β1	S01649	P10966	X13444	2
Human β2	S01873	P14860	X13445	2
Rat α	A24637	P07725	X03015	1
Rat β	A24184	P05541	X04310	1
Mouse α	A01998	P01731	M12825	1
Mouse β	A27619	P10300	X07698	1

Amino acid sequence of human CD8α

```
MALPVTALLL PLALLLHAAR P                                       -1
SQFRVSPLDR TWNLGETVEL KCQVLLSNPT SGCSWLFQPR GAAASPTFLL        50
YLSQNKPKAA EGLDTQRFSG KRLGDTFVLT LSDFRRENEG YYFCSALSNS       100
IMYFSHFVPV FLPAKPTTTP APRPPTPAPT IASQPLSLRP EACRPAAGGA       150
VHTRGLDFAC DIYIWAPLAG TCGVLLLSLV ITLYCNHRNR RRVCKCPRPV       200
VKSGDKPSLS ARYV                                              214
```

Amino acid sequence of human CD8β1

```
MRPRLWLLLA AQLTVLHGNS V                                       -1
LQQTPAYIKV QTNKMVMLSC EAKISLSNMR IYWLRQRQAP SSDSHHEFLA        50
LWDSAKGTIH GEEVEQEKIA VFRDASRFIL NLTSVKPEDS GIYFCMIVGS       100
PELTFGKGTQ LSVVDFLPTT AQPTKKSTLK KRVCRLPRPE TQKGPLCSPI       150
TLGLLVAGVL VLLVSLGVAI HLCCRRRRAR LRFMKQFYK                   189
```

References
1 Parnes, J.R. (1989) Adv. Immunol. 44, 265–311.
2 Norment, A.M. and Littman, D.R. (1988) EMBO J. 7, 3433–3439.
3 Zamoyska, R. (1994) Immunity 1, 243–246.

[4] Classon, B.J. et al. (1992) Int. Immunol. 4, 215–225.
[5] Littman, D.R. et al. (1985) Cell 40, 237–246.
[6] Leahy, D.J. et al. (1992) Cell 68, 1145–1162.
[7] Luescher, I.F. et al. (1995) Nature 373, 353–356.

Molecular weights
Polypeptide   25 277

SDS-PAGE
reduced   22–27 kDa
unreduced   22–27 kDa

Carbohydrate
N-linked sites   1
O-linked   nil

Human gene location
12p13; >20 kb [1]

NH$_2$

Tissue distribution

CD9 has a broad tissue distribution. Amongst haematopoietic cells, CD9 is mainly expressed by platelets, lymphoid progenitor cells and activated lymphocytes. CD9 is expressed to a lesser extent by eosinophils, granulocytes, monocytes and macrophages[2].

Structure

CD9 is a member of the TM4 superfamily and is predicted to have four trans-membrane regions, short cytoplasmic N- and C-termini, and two extracellular regions (reviewed in ref. 3). CD9 is highly conserved amongst vertebrates, the human CD9 protein sharing 65% and 59% sequence identity with the shark and hagfish CD9 homologues, respectively (Tomlinson, Flajnik and Barclay, unpublished).

Ligands and associated molecules

CD9 can associate in non-covalent complexes with the TM4SF molecules CD63 and CD81 and the integrins CD29/CD49c (VLA-3) and CD29/CD49f (VLA-6)[4]. In monkey kidney vero cells CD9 associates non-covalently with CD29/CD49c (VLA-3) and the membrane-anchored heparin-binding EGF-like growth factor at cell–cell contact sites[5]. CD9 associates non-covalently with the CD29 (β1) integrin subunit in a pre-B cell and a megakaryocytic cell line[6]. No extracellular ligand has been identified for CD9.

Function

A role for CD9 in cell adhesion through the regulation of integrin function and the activation of protein tyrosine kinases seems likely[5-9]. CD9 mAbs promote pre-B cell adhesion *in vitro* via the integrins CD29/CD49d (VLA-4) and CD29/CD49e (VLA-5)[7]. Studies using CD9-transfected cells showed that CD29 (β1) integrin-dependent motility of a B cell line was enhanced by CD9 expression and was dependent on protein tyrosine kinases, and another study showed that tumour cell motility and metastasis were suppressed by CD9 expression [3,8]. CD9 mAbs are potent activators of platelet aggregation and induce activation of the non-receptor protein tyrosine kinase Syk [9]. In mouse T cells, a CD9 mAb has been shown to deliver a potent co-stimulatory signal [10].

Database accession numbers

	PIR	SWISSPROT	EMBL/GENBANK	REFERENCE
Human	A40402	P21926	M38690	11,12
Rat	S39262	P40241	X76489	13
Mouse		P40240	L08115	14

Amino acid sequence of human CD9

```
MPVKGGTKSI KYLLFGFNFI FWLAGIAVLA IGLWLRFDSQ TKSIFEQETN    50
NNNSSFYTGV YILIGAAALM MLVGFLGCCG AVQESQCMLG LFFGFLLVIF   100
AIEIAAAIWG YSHKDEVIKE VQEFYKDTYN KLKTKDEPQR ETLKAIHYAL   150
NCCGLAGGVE QFISDICPKK DVLETFTVKS CPDAIKEVFD NKFHIIGAVG   200
IGIAVVMIFGM IFSMILCCAI RRNREMV                           228
```

References

1   Rubinstein, E. et al. (1993) Genomics 16, 132–138.
2   Jennings, L.K. et al. (1995) Leucocyte Typing V, 1249–1251.
3   **Wright, M.D. and Tomlinson, M.G. (1994) Immunol. Today 15, 588–594.**
4   Berditchevski, F. et al. (1996) Mol. Biol. Cell 7, 193–207.
5   Nakamura, K. et al. (1995) J. Cell Biol. 129, 1691–1705.
6   Rubinstein, E. et al. (1994) Eur. J. Immunol. 24, 3005–3013.
7   Masellis-Smith, A. and Shaw, A.R.E. (1994) J. Immunol. 152, 2768–2777.
8   Shaw, A.R.E. et al. (1995) J. Biol. Chem. 270, 24092–24099.
9   Ozaki, Y. et al. (1995) J. Biol. Chem. 270, 15119–15124.
10 Tai, X.-G. et al. (1996) J. Exp. Med. 184, 753–758.
11 Lanza, F. et al. (1991) J. Biol. Chem. 266, 10638–10645.
12 Boucheix, C. et al. (1991) J. Biol. Chem. 266, 117–122.
13 Kaprielian, Z. et al. (1995) J. Neurosci. 15, 562–573.
14 Rubinstein, E. et al. (1993) Thromb. Res. 71, 377–383.

CD10 Common acute lymphoblastic leukaemia antigen (CALLA)

Other names
Neutral endopeptidase (EC 3.4.24.11) (NEP)
Neprilysin
Enkephalinase
gp100

Molecular weights
Polypeptide   85 607

SDS-PAGE
  reduced   100 kDa
  unreduced   100 kDa

Carbohydrate
N-linked sites   6
O-linked   unknown

Human gene location and size
3q21–q27; >80 kb [1]

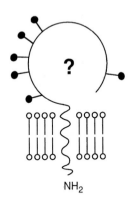

NH$_2$

Tissue distribution

Human CD10 is expressed on early B and T lymphoid precursors, B blasts, some granulocytes and bone marrow stromal cells. CD10 is also expressed on various epithelia (with especially high expression on brush border of kidney and gut), some smooth muscle and myoepithelial cells, brain and fibroblasts. CD10 is widely used as a marker of common (pre-B) acute lymphocytic leukaemias and certain lymphomas [2]. In contrast to the human, mouse CD10 is absent from B cells, T cells and granulocytes, but the expression pattern is similar to the human on bone marrow stromal cells and non-lymphoid tissues [3].

Structure

CD10 is a member of a group of type II membrane metalloproteases that includes the leucocyte antigens CD13, CD26, CD73 and BP-1 [2]. The CD10 glycoprotein has a short N-terminal cytoplasmic tail, a transmembrane region that functions as a signal peptide, and a large C-terminal extracellular region that contains six N-linked glycosylation sites. The extracellular domain also contains 12 cysteines which form disulfide bonds that are required for enzyme activity, and the characteristic pentapeptide motif (HEI/L/MXH) associated with zinc binding and catalytic activity in a number of zinc-dependent metalloproteases [2]. Other amino acids required for zinc binding, substrate binding and catalytic activity have been identified by alignment with the well-characterized bacterial metalloprotease thermolysin and by site-directed mutagenesis [2,4]. Exons 1 and 2, encoding the 5' untranslated region, can be alternatively spliced to yield three CD10 cDNAs with unique 5' untranslated sequences [5].

Function

CD10 is a zinc-binding metalloprotease which is thought to downregulate cellular responses to peptide hormones. By hydrolysing peptide bonds on the amino side of hydrophobic amino acids, CD10 reduces the local concentration of peptide available for receptor binding and signal transduction[2]. CD10 can cleave a variety of biologically active peptides including opioid enkephalins, fMLP, substance P, bombesin-like peptides, atrial natriuretic factor, endothelin, oxytocin, bradykinin and angiotensins I and II[2]. CD10 on neutrophils limits their inflammatory responses by degrading peptides such as fMLP, substance P and enkephalins[2]. CD10 on bone marrow stromal cells appears to regulate B cell development, since inhibition of CD10 enzyme activity *in vivo* enhances B cell maturation[6]. Targeted disruption of the gene for CD10 suggests a role in the modulation of septic shock, since CD10-deficient mice, which are otherwise grossly normal, exhibit enhanced lethality to endotoxin[7].

Database accession numbers

	PIR	SWISSPROT	EMBL/GENBANK	REFERENCE
Human	A41387	P08473	Y00811	8
Rat	A29295	P07861	M15944	9
Mouse			M81591	4

Amino acid sequence of human CD10

```
GKSESQMDIT DINTPKPKKK QRWTRLEISL SVLVLLLTII AVRMIALYAT    50
YDDGICKSSD CIKSAARLIQ NMDATTEPCR DFFKYACGGW LKRNVIPETS   100
SRYGNFDILR DELEVVLKDV LQEPKTEDIV AVQKAKALYR SCINESAIDS   150
RGGEPLLKLL PDIYGWPVAT ENWEQKYGAS WTAEKAIAQL NSKYGKKVLI   200
NLFVGTDDKN SVNHVIHIDQ PRLGLPSRDY YECTGIYKEA CTAYVDFMIS   250
VARLIRQEER LPIDENQLAL EMNKVMELEK EIANATAKPE DRNDPMLLYN   300
KMRLAQIQNN FSLEINGKPF SWLNFTNEIM STVNISITNE EDVVVYAPEY   350
LTKLKPILTK YSARDLQNLM SWRFIMDLVS SLSRTYKESR NAFRKALYGT   400
TSETATWRRC ANYVNGNMEN AVGRLYVEAA FAGESKHVVE DLIAQIREVF   450
IQTLDDLTWM DAETKKRAEE KALAIKERIG YPDDIVSNDN KLNNEYLELN   500
YKEDEYFENI IQNLKFSQSK QLKKLREKVD KDEWISGAAV VNAFYSSGRN   550
QIVFPAGILQ PPFFSAQQSN SLNYGGIGMV IGHEITHGFD DNGRNFNKDG   600
DLVDWWTQQS ASNFKEQSQC MVYQYGNFSW DLAGGQHLNG INTLGENIAD   650
NGGLGQAYRA YQNYIKKNGE EKLLPGLDLN HKQLFFLNFA QVWCGTYRPE   700
YAVNSIKTDV HSPGNFRIIG TLQNSAEFSE AFHCRKNSYM NPEKKCRVW    749
```

References
[1] D'Adamio, L. et al. (1989) Proc. Natl Acad. Sci. USA 86, 7103–7107.
[2] **Shipp, M.A. and Look, A.T. (1993) Blood 82, 1052–1070.**
[3] Kalled, S.L. et al. (1995) Eur. J. Immunol. 25, 677–687.
[4] Chen, C.-Y. et al. (1992) J. Immunol. 148, 2817–2825.
[5] Ishimaru, F. and Shipp, M.A. (1995) Blood 85, 3199–3207.
[6] Salles, G. et al. (1993) Proc. Natl Acad. Sci. USA 90, 7618–7622.
[7] **Lu, B. et al. (1995) J. Exp. Med. 181, 2271–2275.**
[8] Letarte, M. et al. (1988) J. Exp. Med. 168, 1247–1253.
[9] Malfroy, B. et al. (1987) Biochem. Biophys. Res. Commun. 144, 59–66.

CD11a

LFA-1 α subunit, integrin αL subunit

Molecular weights
Polypeptide   126 195

SDS-PAGE
  reduced   180 kDa
  unreduced   170 kDa

Carbohydrate
  N-linked sites   12
  O-linked sites   unknown

Human gene location and size
16 p11–13.1; >32 kb [1]

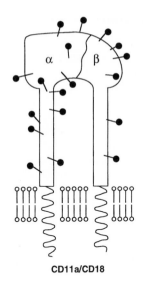

CD11a/CD18

Tissue distribution

CD11a is expressed on lymphocytes, granulocytes, monocytes and macrophages, with increased levels on memory T cells [1-4].

Structure

CD11a (integrin αL subunit) combines with CD18 (integrin β2 subunit) to form the integrin LFA-1 (αLβ2, CD11a/CD18). The αL subunit belongs to the subclass of integrin α subunits with an I-domain near the N-terminus [5]. A crystal structure of the I-domain has been obtained [6].

Ligands and associated molecules

The three ligands for LFA-1 are CD54 (ICAM-1), CD102 (ICAM-2) and CD50 (ICAM-3), each of which contains IgSF domains [7,8].

Function

CD11a/CD18 (LFA-1) was first described as an accessory molecule in cytotoxic lymphocyte killing [9]. It was subsequently found to mediate lymphocyte adhesion to many cells including endothelium [2-4,7,8]. The avidity of CD11a/CD18 to ligands is transiently upregulated on T cells upon activation. This may involve both aggregation of CD11a/CD18 on the cell surface and conformational change of the CD11a/CD18 antigen [8,10,11]. CD11a/CD18 has been shown to bind bacterial lipopolysaccharides [12]. The binding activity of CD11a/CD18 involves the I-domain of CD11a [13]. CD11a/CD18 is not expressed on leucocytes of patients with leucocyte adhesion deficiency (see **CD18**).

Database accession numbers

	PIR	SWISSPROT	EMBL/GENBANK	REFERENCE
Human	S03308	P20701	Y00796	5
Mouse		P24063	M60778	14

Amino acid sequence of human CD11a

```
MKDSCITVMA MALLSGFFFF APASS                                    -1
YNLDVRGARS FSPPRAGRHF GYRVLQVGNG VIVGAPGEGN STGSLYQCQS         50
GTGHCLPVTL RGSNYTSKYL GMTLATDPTD GSILACDPGL SRTCDQNTYL        100
SGLCYLFRQN LQGPMLQGRP GFQECIKGNV DLVFLFDGSM SLQPDEFQKI        150
LDFMKDVMKK LSNTSYQFAA VQFSTSYKTE FDFSDYVKWK DPDALLKHVK        200
HMLLLTNTFG AINYVATEVF REELGARPDA TKVLIIITDG EATDSGNIDA        250
AKDIIRYIIG IGKHFQTKES QETLHKFASK PASEFVKILD TFEKLKDLFT        300
ELQKKIYVIE GTSKQDLTSF NMELSSSGIS ADLSRGHAVV GAVGAKDWAG        350
GFLDLKADLQ DDTFIGNEPL TPEVRAGYLG YTVTWLPSRQ KTSLLASGAP        400
RYQHMGRVLL FQEPQGGGHW SQVQTIHGTQ IGSYFGGELC GVDVDQDGET        450
ELLLIGAPLF YGEQRGGRVF IYQRRQLGFE EVSELQGDPG YPLGRFGEAI        500
TALTDINGDG LVDVAVGAPL EEQGAVYIFN GRHGGLSPQP SQRIEGTQVL        550
SGIQWFGRSI HGVKDLEGDG LADVAVGAES QMIVLSSRPV VDMVTLMSFS        600
PAEIPVHEVE CSYSTSNKMK EGVNITICFQ IKSLYPQFQG RLVANLTYTL        650
QLDGHRTRRR GLFPGGRHEL RRNIAVTTSM SCTDFSFHFP VCVQDLISPI        700
NVSLNFSLWE EEGTPRDQRA QGKDIPPILR PSLHSETWEI PFEKNCGEDK        750
KCEANLRVSF SPARSRALRL TAFASLSVEL SLSNLEEDAY WVQLDLHFPP        800
GLSFRKVEML KPHSQIPVSC EELPEESRLL SRALSCNVSS PIFKAGHSVA        850
LQMMFNTLVN SSWGDSVELH ANVTCNNEDS DLLEDNSATT IIPILYPINI        900
LIQDQEDSTL YVSFTPKGPK IHQVKHMYQV RIQPSIHDHN IPTLEAVVGV        950
PQPPSEGPIT HQWSVQMEPP VPCHYEDLER LPDAAEPCLP GALFRCPVVF       1000
RQEILVQVIG TLELVGEIEA SSMFSLCSSL SISFNSSKHF HLYGSNASLA       1050
QVVMKVDVVY EKQMLYLYVL SGIGGLLLLL LIFIVLYKVG FFKRNLKEKM       1100
EAGRGVPNGI PAEDSEQLAS GQEAGDPGCL KPLHEKDSES GGGKD            1145
```

References

1. Larson, R.S. and Springer, T.A. (1990) Immunol. Rev. 114, 181–217.
2. Pigott, R. and Power, C. (1993) The Adhesion Molecule FactsBook. Academic Press, London.
3. Patarroyo, M. et al. (1990) Immunol. Rev. 114, 67–108.
4. Rieu, P. and Arnaout, M.A. (1995) In Adhesion Molecules and the Lung (Ward, P. and Lenfart, C., eds), vol. 89, pp. 1–42. Marcel Dekker, New York.
5. Larson, R.S. et al. (1989) J. Cell Biol. 108, 703–712.
6. Qu, A. and Leahy, D.J. (1995) Proc. Natl Acad. Sci. USA 92, 10277–10281.
7. **Springer, T.A. (1990) Nature 346, 425–433.**
8. **Springer, T.A. (1994) Cell 76, 301–314.**
9. Davignon, D. et al. (1981) Proc. Natl Acad. Sci. USA 78, 4535–4539.
10. Dustin, M.L. and Springer, T.A. (1991) Annu. Rev. Immunol. 9, 27–66.
11. **Lub, M. et al. (1995) Immunol. Today 16, 479–483.**
12. Wright, S.D. and Jong, M.T.C. (1986) J. Exp. Med. 164, 1876–1888.
13. Landis, R.C. et al. (1994) J. Cell Biol. 126, 529–537.
14. Kaufman, Y. et al. (1991) J. Immunol. 149, 369–374.

CD11b

Mac-1 (Mo-1, CR3) α subunit, integrin αM subunit

Molecular weights

Polypeptide   125 600

SDS-PAGE
- reduced   170 kDa
- unreduced   165 kDa

Carbohydrate
- N-linked sites   19
- O-linked sites   unknown

Human gene location

16 p11–13.1

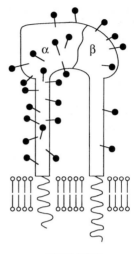

CD11b/CD18

Tissue distribution

CD11b is expressed mainly on myeloid and NK cells [1-4].

Structure

CD11b (integrin αM subunit) combines with CD18 (integrin β2 subunit) to form the integrin Mac-1 (αMβ2, CD11b/CD18). The αM subunit belongs to the subclass of integrin α subunits with an I-domain near the N-terminus [5-7]. Two crystal structures of the I-domain, possibly representing forms with active and an inactive conformations, have been obtained [8,9]. The N-terminal sequence of CD11b has been determined [10,11].

Ligands and associated molecules

Ligands reported for CD11b/CD18 include the complement fragment iC3b, CD54 (ICAM-1), fibrinogen, factor X, CD23, the neutrophil inhibitory factor (NIF) of canine hookworm, heparin, β-glucan, and bacterial lipopolysaccharide [12-19]. It has also been reported that CD11b/CD18 binds denatured proteins [14,20]. There is increasing evidence that CD11b/CD18 is associated with many membrane proteins at the cell surface including CD14, CD87 [21], and the Fcγ receptors CD16 and CD32 [21,22].

Function

CD11b/CD18 (Mac-1) is also known as the complement receptor type 3 (CR3) because of its binding to the iC3b complement fragment on opsonized targets [12,13]. It also mediates the subsequent ingestion process [23]. CD11b/CD18 is also important in the transendothelial migration of monocytes and neutrophils [24]. Its association with other membrane proteins may account

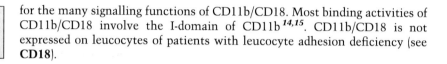

for the many signalling functions of CD11b/CD18. Most binding activities of CD11b/CD18 involve the I-domain of CD11b[14,15]. CD11b/CD18 is not expressed on leucocytes of patients with leucocyte adhesion deficiency (see **CD18**).

Database accession numbers

	PIR	SWISSPROT	EMBL/GENBANK	REFERENCE
Human	A31108	P11215	J03925	5
			M18044	6
			J04145	7
Mouse	S00551	P05555	X07640	25

Amino acid sequence of human CD11b

```
MALRVLLLTA LTLCHG                                                 -1
FNLDTENAMT FQENARGFGQ SVVQLQGSRV VVGAPQEIVA ANQRGSLYQC           50
DYSTGSCEPI RLQVPVEAVN MSLGLSLAAT TSPPQLLACG PTVHQTCSEN          100
TYVKGLCFLF GSNLRQQPQK FPEALRGCPQ EDSDIAFLID GSGSIIPHDF          150
RRMKEFVSTV MEQLKKSKTL FSLMQYSEEF RIHFTFKEFQ NNPNPRSLVK          200
PITQLLGRTH TATGIRKVVR ELFNITNGAR KNAFKILVVI TDGEKFGDPL          250
GYEDVIPEAD REGVIRYVIG VGDAFRSEKS RQELNTIASK PPRDHVFQVN          300
NFEALKTIQN QLREKIFAIE GTQTGSSSSF EHEMSQEGFS AAITSNGPLL          350
STVGSYDWAG GVFLYTSKEK STFINMTRVD SDMNDAYLGY AAAIILRNRV          400
QSLVLGAPRY QHIGLVAMFR QNTGMWESNA NVKGTQIGAY FGASLCSVDV          450
DSNGSTDLVL IGAPHYYEQT RGGQVSVCPL PRGQRARWQC DAVLYGEQGQ          500
PWGRFGAALT VLGDVNGDKL TDVAIGAPGE EDNRGAVYLF HGTSGSGISP          550
SHSQRIAGSK LSPRLQYFGQ SLSGGQDLTM DGLVDLTVGA QGHVLLLRSQ          600
PVLRVKAIME FNPREVARNV FECNDQVVKG KEAGEVRVCL HVQKSTRDRL          650
REGQIQSVVT YDLALDSGRP HSRAVFNETK NSTRRQTQVL GLTQTCETLK          700
LQLPNCIEDP VSPIVLRLNF SLVGTPLSAF GNLRPVLAED AQRLFTALFP          750
FEKNCGNDNI CQDDLSITFS FMSLDCLVVG GPREFNVTVT VRNDGEDSYR          800
TQVTFFFPLD LSYRKVSTLQ NQRSQRSWRL ACESASSTEV SGALKSTSCS          850
INHPIFPENS EVTFNITFDV DSKASLGNKL LLKANVTSEN NMPRTNKTEF          900
QLELPVKYAV YMVVTSHGVS TKYLNFTASE NTSRVMQHQY QVSNLGQRSL          950
PISLVFLVPV RLNQTVIWDR PQVTFSENLS STCHTKERLP SHSDFLAELR         1000
KAPVVNCSIA VCQRIQCDIP FFGIQEEFNA TLKGNLSFDW YIKTSHNHLL         1050
IVSTAEILFN DSVFTLLPGQ GAFVRSQTET KVEPFEVPNP LPLIVGSSVG         1100
GLLLLALITA ALYKLGFFKR QYKDMMSEGG PPGAEPQ                       1137
```

References

1. Pigott, R. and Power, C. (1993) The Adhesion Molecule FactsBook, Academic Press, London.
2. Larson, R.S. and Springer, T.A. (1990) Immunol. Rev. 114, 181–217.
3. Patarroyo, M. et al. (1990) Immunol. Rev. 114, 67–108.
4. Rieu, P. and Arnaout, M.A. (1995) In Adhesion Molecules and the Lung (Ward, P. and Lenfart, C., eds), vol. 89, pp. 1–42. Marcel Dekker, New York.
5. Corbi, A.L. et al. (1988) J. Biol. Chem. 263, 12403–12411.
6. Arnaout, M.A. et al. (1988) J. Cell Biol. 106, 2153–2158.
7. Hickstein, D.D. et al. (1989) Proc. Natl Acad. Sci. USA 86, 257–261.
8. Lee, J.O. et al. (1995) Cell 80, 631–638.
9. **Lee, J.O. et al. (1995) Structure 3, 1333–1340.**
10. Pierce, M.W. et al. (1986) Biochim. Biophys. Acta 87, 368–371.

[11] Miller, L.J. et al. (1987) J. Immunol. 138, 2381–2383.

[12] Beller, D.I. et al. (1982) J. Exp. Med. 156, 1000–1009.

[13] Wright, S.D. et al. (1983) Proc. Natl Acad. Sci. USA 80, 5699–5703.

[14] **Zhang, L. and Plow, E.F. (1996) J. Biol. Chem. 271, 18211–18216.**

[15] Diamond, M.S. et al. (1993) J. Cell Biol. 120, 1031–1043.

[16] Lecoanet-Henchoz, S. et al. (1995) Immunity 3, 119–125.

[17] Diamond, M.S. et al. (1995) J. Cell Biol. 130, 1473–1482.

[18] Thornton, B.P. et al. (1996) J. Immunol. 156, 1235–1246.

[19] Wright, S.D. and Jong, M.T.C. (1986) J. Exp. Med. 164, 1876–1888.

[20] **Davis, G.E. (1992) Exp. Cell Res. 200, 242–252.**

[21] **Petty, H.R. and Todd, R.F. III. (1996) Immunol. Today 17, 209–212.**

[22] Annendov, A. et al. (1996) Eur. J. Immunol. 26, 207–212.

[23] Gresham, H.D. et al. (1991) J. Clin. Invest. 88, 588–596.

[24] **Springer, T.A. (1994) Cell 76, 301–314.**

[25] Pytela, R. (1988) EMBO J. 7, 1371–1378.

CD11c

p150,95 α subunit, integrin αX subunit

Molecular weights

Polypeptide 125 897

SDS-PAGE
  reduced 150 kDa
  unreduced 145 kDa

Carbohydrate

N-linked sites 8
O-linked sites unknown

Human gene location and size
16p11–13.1; 25 kb [1]

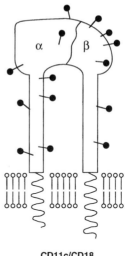

CD11c/CD18

Tissue distribution

CD11c is expressed mainly on myeloid cells with high levels on tissue macrophages. However, it is also found on NK cells, activated T cells and lymphoid cell lines including hairy cell leukaemias [1-4].

Structure

CD11c (integrin αX subunit) combines with CD18 (integrin β2 subunit) to form the integrin p150,95 (αXβ2, CD11c/CD18). The αX subunit belongs to the subclass of integrin α subunits with an I-domain near the N-terminus [5]. The N-terminal sequence of CD11c has been determined [6].

Ligands and associated molecules

CD11c/CD18 (p150,95) binds multiple ligands including the complement fragment iC3b, CD54 (ICAM-1), fibrinogen and bacterial lipopolysaccharide [7-12]. It has also been reported that CD11c/CD18 binds denatured proteins [13].

Function

CD11c/CD18 has been described to play important roles in cytotoxic T cell killing, and in neutrophil and monocyte adhesion to endothelium, although its ligands in these two cases have not been identified [14,15]. An antibody against rabbit CD11c/CD18 has been reported to induce T cell aggregation [16]. CD11c/CD18 is not expressed on leucocytes of patients with leucocyte adhesion deficiency (see **CD18**).

Database accession numbers

	PIR	SWISSPROT	EMBL/GENBANK	REFERENCE
Human	A36584	P20702	M81695	[5]
			Y00093	

Amino acid sequence of human CD11c

```
MTRTRAALLL FTALATSLG                                             -1
FNLDTEELTA FRVDSAGFGD SVVQYANSWV VVGAPQKITA ANQTGGLYQC           50
GYSTGACEPI GLQVPPEAVN MSLGLSLAST TSPSQLLACG PTVHHECGRN          100
MYLTGLCFLL GPTQLTQRLP VSRQECPRQE QDIVFLIDGS GSISSRNFAT          150
MMNFVRAVIS QFQRPSTQFS LMQFSNKFQT HFTFEEFRRT SNPLSLLASV          200
HQLQGFTYTA TAIQNVVHRL FHASYGARRD ATKILIVITD GKKEGDSLDY          250
KDVIPMADAA GIIRYAIGVG LAFQNRNSWK ELNDIASKPS QEHIFKVEDF          300
DALKDIQNQL KEKIFAIEGT ETTSSSSFEL EMAQEGFSAV FTPDGPVLGA          350
VGSFTWSGGA FLYPPNMSPT FINMSQENVD MRDSYLGYST ELALWKGVQS          400
LVLGAPRYQH TGKAVIFTQV SRQWRMKAEV TGTQIGSYFG ASLCSVDVDT          450
DGSTDLVLIG APHYYEQTRG GQVSVCPLPR GWRRWWCDAV LYGEQGHPWG          500
RFGAALTVLG DVNGDKLTDV VIGAPGEEEN RGAVYLFHGV LGPSISPSHS          550
QRIAGSQLSS RLQYFGQALS GGQDLTQDGL VDLAVGARGQ VLLLRTRPVL          600
WVGVSMQFIP AEIPRSAFEC REQVVSEQTL VQSNICLYID KRSKNLLGSR          650
DLQSSVTLDL ALDPGRLSPR ATFQETKNRS LSRVRVLGLK AHCENFNLLL          700
PSCVEDSVTP ITLRLNFTLV GKPLLAFRNL RPMLAALAQR YFTASLPFEK          750
NCGADHICQD NLGISFSFPG LKSLLVGSNL ELNAEVMVWN DGEDSYGTTI          800
TFSHPAGLSY RYVAEGQKQG QLRSLHLTCD SAPVGSQGTW STSCRINHLI          850
FRGGAQITFL ATFDVSPKAV LGDRLLLTAN VSSENNTPRT SKTTFQLELP          900
VKYAVYTVVS SHEQFTKYLN FSESEEKESH VAMHRYQVNN LGQRDLPVSI          950
NFWVPVELNQ EAVWMDVEVS HPQNPSLRCS SEKIAPPASD FLAHIQKNPV         1000
LDCSIAGCLR FRCDVPSFSV QEELDFTLKG NLSFGWVRQI LQKKVSVVSV         1050
AEITFDTSVY SQLPGQEAFM RAQTTTVLEK YKVHNPTPLI VGSSIGGLLL         1100
LALITAVLYK VGFFKRQYKE MMEEANGQIA PENGTQTPSP PSEK              1144
```

References

1 **Larson, R.S. and Springer, T.A. (1990) Immunol. Rev. 114, 181–217.**
2 Pigott, R. and Power, C. (1993) The Adhesion Molecule FactsBook. Academic Press, London.
3 Patarroyo, M. et al. (1990) Immunol. Rev. 114, 67–108.
4 Rieu, P. and Arnaout, M.A. (1995) In Adhesion Molecules and the Lung (Ward, P. and Lenfart, C., eds), vol. 89, pp. 1–42. Marcel Dekker, New York.
5 Corbi, A.L. et al. (1987) EMBO J. 6, 4023–4028.
6 Miller, L.J. et al. (1987) J. Immunol. 138, 2381–2383.
7 Myones, B.L. et al. (1988) J. Clin. Invest. 82, 640–651.
8 de Fougerolles, A.R. et al. (1995) Eur. J. Immunol. 25, 1008–1012.
9 Loike, J.D. et al. (1991) Proc. Natl Acad. Sci. USA 88, 1044–1048.
10 Postigo, A.A. et al. (1991) J. Exp. Med. 174, 1313–1322.
11 Wright, S.D. and Jong, M.T.C. (1986) J. Exp. Med. 164, 1876–1888.
12 Ingalls, R.R. and Golenbock, D.T. (1995) J. Exp. Med. 181, 1473–1479.
13 **Davis, G.E. (1992) Exp. Cell Res. 200, 242–252.**
14 Keizer, G.D. et al. (1987) J. Immunol. 138, 3130–3136.
15 Stacker, S.A. and Springer, T.A. (1991) J. Immunol. 146, 648–655.
16 Blackford, J. et al. (1996) Eur. J. Immunol. 26, 525–531.

Integrin αD subunit | CD11d

Molecular weights
Polypeptide   125 096

SDS-PAGE
    reduced   150 kDa

Carbohydrate
N-linked sites   10
O-linked sites   unknown

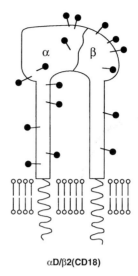

αD/β2(CD18)

Tissue distribution

The integrin αD subunit is expressed at moderate levels on peripheral blood leucocytes. It is expressed strongly on specialized cells in tissues, for example splenic red pulp macrophages and foamy macrophages in aortic fatty streaks [1].

Structure

The integrin αD subunit combines with CD18 (integrin β2 subunit) to form the integrin αDβ2. The αD subunit belongs to the subclass of integrin α subunits with an I-domain near the N-terminus [1]. The N-terminus has been determined by protein sequencing [1].

Ligands and associated molecules

The integrin αDβ2 binds CD50 (ICAM-3), but not CD54 (ICAM-1) or CD106 (VCAM-1) [1].

Database accession numbers

	PIR	SWISSPROT	EMBL/GENBANK	REFERENCE
Human			U37028	1

Amino acid sequence of human integrin αD subunit

```
MTFGTVLLLS VLASYHG                                              -1
FNLDVEEPTI FQEDAGGFGQ SVVQFGGSRL VVGAPLEVVA ANQTGRLYDC         50
AAATGMCQPI PLHIRPEAVN MSLGLTLAAS TNGSRLLACG PTLHRVCGEN        100
SYSKGSCLLL GSRWEIIQTV PDATPECPHQ EMDIVFLIDG SGSIDQNDFN        150
QMKGFVQAVM GQFEGTDTLF ALMQYSNLLK IHFTFTQFRT SPSQQSLVDP        200
IVQLKGLTFT ATGILTVVTQ LFHHKNGARK SAKKILIVIT DGQKYKDPLE        250
YSDVIPQAEK AGIIRYAIGV GHAFQGPTAR QELNTISSAP PQDHVFKVDN        300
FAALGSIQKQ LQEKIYAVEG TQSRASSSFQ HEMSQEGFST ALTMDGLFLG        350
AVGSFSWSGG AFLYPPNMSP TFINMSQENV DMRDSYLGYS TELALWKGVQ        400
NLVLGAPRYQ HTGKAVIFTQ VSRQWRKKAE VTGTQIGSYF GASLCSVDVD        450
SDGSTDLILI GAPHYYEQTR GGQVSVCPLP RGQRVQWQCD AVLRGEQGHP        500
WGRFGAALTV LGDVNEDKLI DVAIGAPGEQ ENRGAVYLFH GASESGISPS        550
HSQRIASSQL SPRLQYFGQA LSGGQDLTQD GLMDLAVGAR GQVLLLRSLP        600
VLKVGVAMRF SPVEVAKAVY RCWEEKPSAL EAGDATVCLT IQKSSLDQLG        650
DIQSSVRFDL ALDPGRLTSR AIFNETKNPT LTRRKTLGLG IHCETLKLLL        700
PDCVEDVVSP IILHLNFSLV REPIPSPQNL RPVLAVGSQD LFTASLPFEK        750
NCGQDGLCEG DLGVTLSFSG LQTLTVGSSL ELNVIVTVWN AGEDSYGTVV        800
SLYYPAGLSH RRVSGAQKQP HQSALRLACE TVPTEDEGLR SSRCSVNHPI        850
FHEGSNGTFI VTFDVSYKAT LGDRMLMRAS ASSENNKASS SKATFQLELP        900
VKYAVYTMIS RQEESTKYFN FATSDEKKMK EAEHRYRVNN LSQRDLAISI        950
NFWVPVLLNG VAVWDVVMEA PSQSLPCVSE RKPPQHSDFL TQISRSPMLD       1000
CSIADCLQFR CDVPSFSVQE ELDFTLKGNL SFGWVRETLQ KKVLVVSVAE       1050
ITFDTSVYSQ LPGQEAFMRA QMEMVLEEDE VYNAIPIIMG SSVGALLLLA       1100
LITATLYKLG FFKRHYKEML EDKPEDTATF SGDDFSCVAP NVPLS            1145
```

Reference
[1] Van der Vieren, M. et al. (1995) Immunity 3, 683–690.

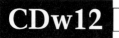
CDw12

Molecular weights

SDS-PAGE
reduced   90–120 kDa
unreduced   150–160 kDa

Tissue distribution

CDw12 is expressed on monocytes, granulocytes, NK cells and platelets [1-3].

Structure

Unknown.

Function

Unknown.

References
[1] Knapp, W. (1989) Leucocyte Typing IV, 781.
[2] Todd, R.F. (1995) Leucocyte Typing V, 771.
[3] van der Schoot, C.E. et al. (1989) Leucocyte Typing IV, 868–878.

CD13

Aminopeptidase N (EC 3.4.11.2), gp150, p161 (mouse)

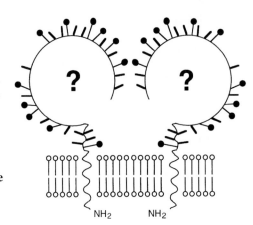

Molecular weights
Polypeptide   109 512

SDS-PAGE
  reduced   150–170 kDa
  unreduced   150–170 kDa

Carbohydrate
N-linked sites   11
O-linked   + abundant

Human gene location and size
15q25–q26; 20 kb [1]

Tissue distribution

CD13 is expressed by granulocytes and monocytes and their precursors. CD13 is a marker for most acute myeloid leukaemias and a smaller proportion of acute lymphoid leukaemias. Various non-haematopoietic cells express CD13, including epithelial cells from renal proximal tubules and intestinal brush border, endothelial cells, fibroblasts, brain cells, bone marrow stromal cells, osteoclasts and cells lining the biliary caniculae [2].

Structure

CD13 is a member of a group of type II integral membrane metalloproteases that includes the leucocyte antigens CD10, CD26, CD73 and BP-1 [2]. In common with CD10, the expression of CD13 appears to be controlled by distinct promoters in different cell types, and several CD13 transcripts have been identified that differ only in their 5′ untranslated region [2]. The CD13 glycoprotein has a short N-terminal cytoplasmic tail, a transmembrane region that functions as a signal peptide, and a large C-terminal extracellular region that contains 11 *N*-linked glycosylation sites and also *O*-linked glycosylation. The extracellular domain contains the characteristic pentapeptide motif (His-Glu-Ile/Leu/Met-Xaa-His) associated with zinc binding and catalytic activity in a number of zinc-dependent metalloproteases. CD13 is expressed as a non-covalently linked homodimer [2].

Ligands and associated molecules

CD13 is a receptor for coronaviruses, RNA viruses that cause respiratory disease in humans and several species of animals [2]. The binding site on CD13 for the swine coronavirus TGEV (transmissible gastroenteritis virus) is distinct from the enzymatic site [3].

Function

CD13 is a zinc-binding metalloprotease which plays a role in cell surface antigen presentation by trimming the N-terminal amino acids from MHC

Class II-bound peptides[4]. CD13 ectopeptidase activity is also thought to down-regulate cellular responses to peptide hormones by reducing the local concentration of peptide available for receptor binding[2]. Neutral amino acids are preferentially cleaved by CD13, although basic and acidic residues can also be removed. Peptide substrates for CD13 include opioid peptides and enkephalins in the brain, the phagocytosis-stimulating tetrapeptide tuftsin, and the neutrophil chemoattractant fMLP. CD13 appears to act in concert with another metalloprotease, CD10, in the hydrolysis of these peptides[2]. Unlike CD10, CD13 activity is inhibited by the peptide hormones substance P and bradykinin[5]. CD13 is upregulated by the anti-inflammatory cytokine IL-4, which suggests a possible indirect mechanism of IL-4 action through the modulation of cell surface antigen processing and/or bioactive peptides[6]. CD13 also appears to play a role, by a mechanism that is unclear, in the infection of cells by human cytomegalovirus (CMV), a herpesvirus[7].

Database accession numbers

	PIR	SWISSPROT	EMBL/GENBANK	REFERENCE
Human	S01658	P15144	X13276	8,9
Rat	A32852	P15684	M25073	10
Mouse			U77083	11

Amino acid sequence of human CD13

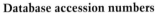

```
MAKGFYISKS LGILGILLGV AAVCTIIALS VVYSQEKNKN ANSSPVASTT    50
PSASATTNPA SATTLDQSKA WNRYRLPNTL KPDSYQVTLR PYLTPNDRGL   100
YVFKGSSTVR FTCKEATDVI IIHSKKLNYT LSQGHRVVLR GVGGSQPPDI   150
DKTELVEPTE YLVVHLKGSL VKDSQYEMDS EFEGELADDL AGFYRSEYME   200
GNVRKVVATT QMQAADARKS FPCFDEPAMK AEFNITLIHP KDLTALSNML   250
PKGPSTPLPE DPNWNVTEFH TTPKMSTYLL AFIVSEFDYV EKQASNGVLI   300
RIWARPSAIA AGHGDYALNV TGPILNFFAG HYDTPYPLPK SDQIGLPDFN   350
AGAMENWGLV TYRENSLLFD PLSSSSSNKE RVVTVIAHEL AHQWFGNLVT   400
IEWWNDLWLN EGFASYVEYL GADYAEPTWN LKDLMVLNDV YRVMAVDALA   450
SSHPLSTPAS EINTPAQISE LFDAISYSKG ASVLRMLSSF LSEDVFKQGL   500
ASYLHTFAYQ NTIYLNLWDH LQEAVNNRSI QLPTTVRDIM NRWTLQMGFP   550
VITVDTSTGT LSQEHFLLDP DSNVTRPSEF NYVWIVPITS IRDGRQQQDY   600
WLIDVRAQND LFSTSGNEWV LLNLNVTGYY RVNYDEENWR KIQTQLQRDH   650
SAIPVINRAQ IINDAFNLAS AHKVPVTLAL NNTLFLIEER QYMPWEAALS   700
SLSYFKLMFD RSEVYGPMKN YLKKQVTPLF IHFRNNTNNW REIPENLMDQ   750
YSEVNAISTA CSNGVPECEE MVSGLFKQWM ENPNNNPIHP NLRSTVYCNA   800
IAQGGEEEWD FAWEQFRNAT LVNEADKLRA ALACSKELWI LNRYLSYTLN   850
PDLIRKQDAT STIISITNNV IGQGLVWDFV QSNWKKLFND YGGGSFSFSN   900
LIQAVTRRFS TEYELQQLEQ FKKDNEETGF GSGTRALEQA LEKTKANIKW   950
VKENKEVVLQ WFTENSK                                       967
```

References
1 Look, A.T. et al. (1986) J. Clin. Invest. 78, 914–921.
2 **Shipp, M.A. and Look, A.T. (1993) Blood 82, 1052–1070.**
3 Delmas, B. et al. (1994) J. Virol. 68, 5216–5224.
4 **Larsen, S.L. et al. (1996) J. Exp. Med. 184, 183–189.**
5 Xu, Y. et al. (1995) Biochem. Biophys. Res. Commun. 208, 664–674.
6 van Hal, P.T.W. et al. (1994) J. Immunol. 153, 2718–2728.
7 Giugni, T.D. et al. (1996) J. Infect. Dis. 173, 1062–1071.

[8] Look, A.T. et al. (1989) J. Clin. Invest. 83, 1299–1307.
[9] Olsen, J. et al. (1988) FEBS Lett. 238, 307–314.
[10] Watt, V.M. and Yip, C.C. (1989) J. Biol. Chem. 264, 5480–5487.
[11] Chen, H. et al. (1996) J. Immunol. 157, 2593–2600.

CD14

Molecular weights
Polypeptide   35 773

SDS-PAGE
  reduced   53–55 kDa

Carbohydrate
N-linked sites   4
O-linked   unknown

Human gene location and size
5q31; 1.5 kb [1]

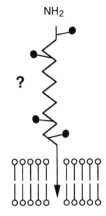

Tissue distribution

In human and mouse CD14 is predominantly expressed on cells of the myelomonocytic lineage including monocytes, macrophages and Langerhans cells [1-3]. CD14 is expressed at lower levels on neutrophils, but can be induced with certain cytokines or fMLP [4,5]. IFNγ or IL-13 treatment decreases monocyte expression. The antigen has also been detected, at low levels, on human B cells [6].

Structure

CD14 is a GPI-linked glycoprotein [7]. The extracellular region contains 10 repeats with some similarities to the leucine-rich glycoprotein (LRG) repeats [2]. However, they do not show the regular size nor enough of the sequence patterns characteristic of LRG repeats to be included in this family (see Chapter 3). Soluble forms of CD14 are present in normal serum and urine of nephrotic patients and culture media of cells expressing CD14 [7,8]. The N-terminus of the mature protein has been determined by amino acid sequence analysis [1,7].

Ligands and associated molecules

CD14 is a receptor for the complex of lipopolysaccharide (LPS) and the LPS-binding protein (LBP) [9].

Function

CD14 may be involved in the clearance of Gram-negative pathogens opsonized with LBP. TNFα synthesis induced by LPS in monocytes and macrophages can be blocked by anti-CD14 mAbs [9]. The interaction of CD14 with the LPS-LBP complex causes an increase in the adhesive activity of CR3 (CD11b/CD18) on neutrophils [5]. Transgenic mice overexpressing human CD14 show increased susceptibility to endotoxin shock [10], whereas CD14-deficient mice are highly resistant to either live Gram-negative bacteria or LPS [11]. CD14-deficient mice also show dramatically reduced levels of bacteraemia following *in vivo* challenge with *E. coli*, suggesting a role for CD14 in dissemination of Gram-negative bacteria.

Comments

The CD14 gene contains a single intron after the initiation codon [1,12]. CD14 maps within a chromosomal region containing other genes encoding growth factors (e.g. IL-3, IL-4, IL-5, IL-9, GM-CSF) and receptors (e.g. M-CSFR, PDGFR, α1- and β2-adrenergic receptors) [13]. Deletions in this region are frequently found in myeloid leukaemias [13].

Database accession numbers

	PIR	*SWISSPROT*	*EMBL/GENBANK*	*REFERENCE*
Human	A27637	P08571	X06882	12
Mouse	S03605	P10810	M34510	2

Amino acid sequence of human CD14

```
MERASCLLLL LLPLVHVSA                                          -1
TTPEPCELDD EDFRCVCNFS EPQPDWSEAF QCVSAVEVEI HAGGLNLEPF        50
LKRVDADADP RQYADTVKAL RVRRLTVGAA QVPAQLLVGA LRVLAYSRLK        100
ELTLEDLKIT GTMPPLPLEA TGLALSSLRL RNVSWATGRS WLAELQQWLK        150
PGLKVLSIAQ AHSPAFSYEQ VRAFPALTSL DLSDNPGLGE RGLMAALCPH        200
KFPAIQNLAL RNTGMETPTG VCAALAAAGV QPHSLDLSHN SLRATVNPSA        250
PRCMWSSALN SLNLSFAGLE QVPKGLPAKL RVLDLSCNRL NRAPQPDELP        300
EVDNLTLDGN PFLVPGTALP HEGSMNSGVV PAC                          333
ARSTLSVGVS GTLVLLQGAR GFA                                     +23
```

References
1   Goyert, S.M. et al. (1988) Science 239, 497–500.
2   Ferrero, E. et al. (1990) J. Immunol. 145, 331–336.
3   Gadd, S. (1989) Leucocyte Typing IV, 787–789.
4   Goyert, S.M. et al. (1989) Leucocyte Typing IV, 789–794.
5   Wright, S.D. et al. (1991) J. Exp. Med. 173, 1281–1286.
6   Labeta, M.O. et al. (1991) Mol. Immunol. 28, 115–122.
7   Haziot, A. et al. (1988) J. Immunol. 141, 547–552.
8   Bazil, V. and Strominger, J.L. (1991) J. Immunol. 147, 1567–1574.
9   **Wright, S.D. et al. (1990) Science 249, 1431–1433.**
10 Ferrero, E. et al. (1993) Proc. Natl Acad. Sci. USA 90, 2380–2384.
11 **Haziot, A. et al. (1996) Immunity 4, 407–414.**
12 Ferrero, E. and Goyert, S.M. (1988) Nucleic Acids Res. 16, 4173.
13 Le Beau, M.M. et al. (1993) Proc. Natl Acad. Sci. USA 90, 5484–5488.

Tissue distribution

CD15 is expressed on neutrophils, eosinophils and monocytes, but not platelets, lymphocytes or erythrocytes. It is also present in embryonic tissues and adenocarcinomas, myeloid leukemias and Reed–Sternberg cells [1,2].

Structure

CD15 antibodies recognize the terminal trisaccharide structure Galβ1→4[Fucα1→3]GlcNAc which is also referred to as the Lewis x (Le^x) antigen. This structure is found on a variety of glycoproteins and glycolipids at the cell surface [3–5]. For example, CD15 is carried by the CD11/CD18 and CD66 glycoproteins [1,6]. The majority of the CD15 antibodies are IgM, and they do not crossreact with the sialylated form of CD15 (CD15s, sLe^x) [2].

Function

CD15 antibodies have been shown to affect various cell activities. However, it is difficult to distinguish between effects on the CD15 structure itself and effects mediated by proteins which happen to carry the CD15 epitope [2,7]. CD15 antibodies can mediate complement activation and may have potential therapeutic value in the killing of CD15-expressing tumour cells [2].

References
[1] Stocks, S.C. et al. (1990) Biochem. J. 268, 275–280.
[2] Ball, E.D. (1995) Leucocyte Typing V, 790–794.
[3] Huang, L.C. et al. (1983) Blood 61, 1020–1023.
[4] Buescher, E.F. et al. (1984) Leucocyte Typing IV, 807–811.
[5] Spooncer, E. et al. (1984) J. Biol. Chem. 259, 4792–4801.
[6] Skubitz, K.M. and Snook, R.W. (1987) J. Immunol. 139, 1631–1639.
[7] Forsyth, K.D. et al. (1989) Eur. J. Immunol. 19, 1331–1334.

Tissue distribution

CD15s is expressed on neutrophils, basophils and monocytes, but its expression on lymphocytes is variable depending on the antibodies used for detection [1,2]. CD15s is also present on high-endothelium venules and subcapsular sinus cells in lymph nodes [3].

Structure

The CD15s antigen is the sialylated form of CD15 with the structure NeuAcα2 → 3Galβ1 → 4[Fucα1 → 3]GlcNAcβ. It is found at the non-reducing termini of N-linked or O-linked oligosaccharides on glycoproteins as well as on glycosphingolipids [4-6]. CD15s is not synthesized by the direct sialylation of CD15 but is instead synthesized by fucosylation of NeuAcα2 → 3Galβ1 → 4GlcNAcβ-R by the fucosyl transferase VII (FucT-VII). FucT-VII is distinct from FucT-IV which fucosylates Galβ1 → 4GlcNAcβ-R to yield CD15 [7].

Ligands and associated molecules

The selectins (CD62E, CD62P and CD62L) bind CD15s. However, although CD15s is carried by many glycoproteins, selectins appear to bind preferentially to a limited number of cell surface glycoproteins (see **CD62E, CD62L, CD62P**), suggesting either that recognition depends on the protein backbone or that these glycoproteins carry rare carbohydrate structures related to CD15s which are better ligands than CD15s itself [4-6,8].

Function

The importance of CD15s in health is illustrated by the disease leucocyte adhesion deficiency type II [9], in which a defect in fucosylation results in decreased levels of CD15s and CD15. Selectin-mediated cell adhesion is impaired in these patients [9,10]. Mice deficient in the enzyme FucT-VII exhibit leucocytosis, impaired leucocyte extravasation into inflamed tissues, and defective lymphocyte homing [7].

References

1. Kannagi, R. and Magnani, J.L. (1995) Leucocyte Typing V, 1529–1531.
2. Bochner, B.S. et al. (1996) J. Immunol. 157, 844–850.
3. Magnani, J.L. (1995) Leucocyte Typing V, 1524–1529.
4. Feizi, T. (1993) Curr. Opin. Struct. Biol. 3, 701–710.
5. **Varki, A. (1994) Proc. Natl Acad. Sci. USA 91, 7390–7397.**
6. Sears, P. and Wang, C.H. (1996) Proc. Natl Acad. Sci. USA 93, 12086–12093.
7. **Maly, P. et al. (1996) Cell 86, 643–653.**
8. Tu, L. et al. (1996) J. Immunol. 157, 3995–4004.
9. Etzioni, A. et al. (1992) New Engl. J. Med. 327, 301–314.
10. Phillips, M.L. et al. (1995) J. Clin. Invest. 2898–2906.

CD16 FcγRIII

Molecular weights

Polypeptide	TM form	27 268
	GPI-linked form	21 090

SDS-PAGE reduced		50–80 kDa

Carbohydrate

N-linked sites	TM form	5
	GPI-linked form	6
O-linked		unknown

Human gene location and size
Transmembrane form: 1q23; 9 kb [1,2]
GPI-linked form: 1q23; 9 kb [1,2]

TM form   GPI-linked form

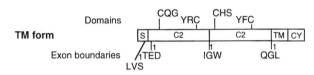

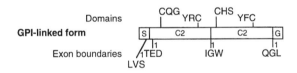

TM form

Domains: S | C2 | C2 | TM | CY

CQG YRC   CHS YFC

Exon boundaries: TED | IGW | QGL
LVS

GPI-linked form

Domains: S | C2 | C2 | G

CQG YRC   CHS YFC

Exon boundaries: TED | IGW | QGL
LVS

Tissue distribution

In humans the transmembrane (TM) form of CD16 is expressed on NK cells, macrophages and mast cells, whilst the GPI-linked form is expressed on neutrophils. In the mouse no GPI-linked form of CD16 has been identified and the transmembrane form is expressed on macrophages, NK cells, neutrophils, myeloid precursors and the majority of early CD4⁻CD8⁻TCR⁻ fetal thymocytes [3,4].

Structure

There are two distinct forms of human CD16 encoded by two linked genes: a transmembrane form with a 25 amino acid cytoplasmic tail and a glycosyl-phosphatidylinositol (GPI)-linked form [1,2,5]. Their extracellular sequences differ by only six amino acids and site-directed mutagenesis has shown that amino acid Ser186 (mature protein numbering) determines the attachment of the GPI anchor [3,6]. The extracellular region of CD16 comprises two C2-set IgSF domains [5].

Ligands and associated molecules

The transmembrane form is non-covalently associated with the FcεRI γ chain or the TCR ζ chain [6,7]. CD16 on mast cells is also associated with the β chain of the FcεRI [8].

Function

CD16 is a low-affinity receptor for aggregated IgG [3]. The transmembrane form binds IgG complexed to antigens and mediates phagocytosis and antibody-dependent cellular cytotoxicity. On NK cells, signal transduction by CD16 is mediated through the γ chain and crosslinking of CD16 with immune complexes or CD16-specific mAbs induces calcium mobilization and hydrolysis of membrane phosphoinositides [9]. In contrast the GPI-linked form on neutrophils binds to ligands but is unable to induce any signal or functional effect [3]. Targeted disruption of the mouse FcR γ chain common to CD16 and FcεRI results in immunocompromised mice [10].

Comments

CD16 (FcγRIII) has structural similarity to CD64 (FcγRI), CD32 (FcγRII) and FcεRIα [3]. The sequence LFAVDTGL is completely conserved in the transmembrane regions of CD16 and FcεRIα from human, mouse and rat [11]. A family of CD16 isoforms have been described in the rat [11]. Patients with paroxysmal nocturnal haemoglobinuria lack the GPI-linked form of CD16, and other GPI-linked cell surface molecules. This disease is characterized by the presence of circulating immune complexes and a susceptibility to bacterial infections [12].

Database accession numbers

	PIR	SWISSPROT	EMBL/GENBANK	REFERENCE
Human	JL0107	P08637	X16863, X52645	1
Mouse	S29360	P08508	M14215	13
Rat		P27645	M64368–M64370	11

Amino acid sequence of human CD16 TM form

```
MWQLLLPTAL LLLVSAG                                          -1
MRTEDLPKAV VFLEPQWYRV LEKDSVTLKC QGAYSPEDNS TQWFHNESLI      50
SSQASSYFID AATVDDSGEY RCQTNLSTLS DPVQLEVHIG WLLLQAPRWV     100
FKEEDPIHLR CHSWKNTALH KVTYLQNGKG RKYFHHNSDF YIPKATLKDS     150
GSYFCRGLFG SKNVSSETVN ITITQGLAVS TISSFFPPGY QVSFCLVMVL     200
LFAVDTGLYF SVKTNIRSST RDWKDHKFKW RKDPQDK                   237
```

Amino acid sequence of human CD16 GPI-linked form

```
MWQLLLPTAL LLLVSAG                                          -1
MRTEDLPKAV VFLEPQWYSV LEKDSVTLKC QGAYSPEDNS TQWFHNESLI      50
SSQASSYFID AATVNDSGEY RCQTNLSTLS DPVQLEVHIG WLLLQAPRWV     100
FKEEDPIHLR CHSWKNTALH KVTYLQNGKD RKYFHHNSDF HIPKATLKDS     150
GSYFCRGLVG SKNVSSETVN ITITQGLAVS TISSFS                    186
PPGYQVSFCL VMVLLFAVDT GLYFSVKTNI                          +30
```

There are two alleles of the GPI-linked form of CD16[3]. The sequence shown above represents the product of the NA-2 allele[1].

References

1. **Ravetch, J.V. and Perussia, B. (1989) J. Exp. Med. 170, 481–497.**
2. Qiu, W.Q. et al. (1990) Science 248, 732–735.
3. Ravetch, J.V. and Kinet, J.-P. (1991) Annu. Rev. Immunol. 9, 457–492.
4. Rodewald, H-R. et al. (1992) Cell 69, 139–150.
5. Simmons, D. and Seed, B. (1988) Nature 333, 568–570.
6. Hibbs, M.L. et al. (1989) Science 246, 1608–1611.
7. Lanier, L.L. et al. (1989) Nature 342, 803–806.
8. Kurosaki, T. et al. (1992) J. Exp. Med. 175, 447–451.
9. Wirthmueller, U. et al. (1992) J. Exp. Med. 175, 1381–1390.
10. **Takai, T. et al. (1994) Cell 76, 519–529.**
11. Farber, D.L. and Sears, D.W. (1991) J. Immunol. 146, 4352–4361.
12. Selvaraj, P. et al. (1988) Nature 333, 565–567.
13. Ravetch, J.V. et al. (1986) Science 234, 718–725.

CDw17　Lactosylceramide (LacCer)

Tissue distribution

CDw17 is expressed on human neutrophils, basophils, monocytes and platelets [1,2]. It is also found on post-proliferative granulocytes in the bone marrow [2]. Between 40 and 80% of CD19[+] peripheral B lymphocytes bind CDw17 mAbs, whereas other lymphocytes are negative [2]. CDw17 is also expressed on tonsillar CD45[+] dendritic cells, epithelial cells [2], and on endothelial cells within the intestinal epithelium [3].

Structure

CDw17 antibodies recognize the lactosyldisaccharide group (LacCer or $Gal\beta1\rightarrow4Glc\beta1\rightarrow1Cer$) of the glycosphingolipid lactosylceramide [4,5]. The antigen is not known to be associated with glycoproteins [1,2].

Ligands and associated molecules

The GM3 ganglioside on tumour cell lines has been shown to bind to CDw17-coated surfaces [6].

Function

CDw17 is the most abundant glycosphingolipid present on neutrophils [7]. The majority of LacCer on neutrophils is contained in intracellular granules, where it has been proposed to participate in the exocytosis or packaging of granule contents [1,8]. Surface expression of CDw17 is markedly decreased after activation with a number of stimuli. Downregulation is associated with membrane internalization and granule exocytosis, but not with superoxide production [1]. Treatment of neutrophils with CDw17 mAbs induces a moderate release of calcium ions into the cytoplasm and stimulates a strong oxidative burst, but has little effect on CD11b and CD67 surface expression [9]. However, upregulation of CDw17 expression is associated with the activation of platelets [10].

References
1　Symington, F.W. (1989) J. Immunol. 142, 2784–2790.
2　Thompson, J.S. and Lund-Johansen, F. (1995) Leucocyte Typing V, 822–823.
3　Karlsson, K. (1989) Annu. Rev. Biochem. 58, 309–350.
4　Symington, F.W. et al. (1984) J. Biol. Chem. 259, 6008–6012.
5　Kniep, B. et al. (1989) Leucocyte Typing IV, 877–879.
6　Kojima, N. and Hakomori, S. (1991) J. Biol. Chem. 266, 17552–17558.
7　Symington, F.W. et al. (1985) J. Immunol. 134, 2498–2506.
8　Symington, F.W. et al. (1987) J. Biol. Chem. 262, 11356–11363.
9　Lund-Johansen, F. et al. (1992) J. Immunol. 148, 3221–3229.
10　Michelson, A.D. et al. (1995) Leucocyte Typing V, 1207–1210.

CD18 Integrin β2 subunit

Molecular weights
Polypeptide   82 573

SDS-PAGE
  reduced   95 kDa
  non-reduced   90 kDa

Carbohydrate
N-linked sites   6
O-linked sites   unknown

Human gene location and size
21q22.3; ~40 kb [1]

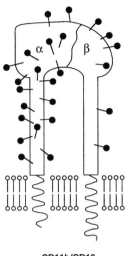

CD11b/CD18

Tissue distribution

CD18 is expressed on all leucocytes [2-5]. See entries for CD11 antigens and the integrin αD subunit for details of the expression of different CD18 (β2 integrin) complexes.

Structure

CD18 (integrin β2 subunit) combines with CD11a–c (αL, αM and αX) subunits, and the αD integrin subunit to form the integrins LFA-1 (αLβ2, CD11a/CD18), Mac-1 (αMβ2, CD11b/CD18), p150,95 (αXβ2, CD11c/CD18) and αDβ2. The N-terminus of CD18 is blocked [6,7].

Function

CD18 may be important in the regulation of ligand binding activities of various CD11/CD18 complexes. CD18 has been shown to interact with several cytoskeletal proteins including α-actinin [8] and filamin (ABP-280) [9], and the cytoplasmic regulatory molecule cytohesin-1 [10]. There are also a number of antibodies that promote the CD11/CD18 antigens to high affinity binding to ligands [11,12]. Leucocyte adhesion deficiency results from defects in the CD18 gene, leading to diminished expression of all CD18-containing integrins. The deficiency is very heterogeneous with varying degrees of clinical severity [13,14].

Database accession numbers

	PIR	SWISSPROT	EMBL/GENBANK	REFERENCE
Human	A25967	P05107	M15395	6
			X64072	7
Mouse	S04847	P11835	X14951	15

Amino acid sequence of human CD18

```
MLGLRPPLLA LVGLLSLGCV LS                              -1
QECTKFKVSS CRECIESGPG CTWCQKLNFT GPGDPDSIRC DTRPQLLMRG  50
CAADDIMDPT SLAETQEDHN GGQKQLSPQK VTLYLRPGQA AAFNVTFRRA 100
KGYPIDLYYL MDLSYSMLDD LRNVKKLGGD LLRALNEITE SGRIGFGSFV 150
DKTVLPFVNT HPDKLRNPCP NKEKECQPPF AFRHVLKLTN NSNQFQTEVG 200
KQLISGNLDA PEGGLDAMMQ VAACPEEIGW RNVTRLLVFA TDDGFHFAGD 250
GKLGAILTPN DGRCHLEDNL YKRSNEFDYP SVGQLAHKLA ENNIQPIFAV 300
TSRMVKTYEK LTEIIPKSAV GELSEDSSNV VHLIKNAYNK LSSRVFLDHN 350
ALPDTLKVTY DSFCSNGVTH RNQPRGDCDG VQINVPITFQ VKVTATECIQ 400
EQSFVIRALG FTDIVTVQVL PQCECRCRDQ SRDRSLCHGK GFLECGICRC 450
DTGYIGKNCE CQTQGRSSQE LEGSCRKDNN SIICSGLGDC VCGQCLCHTS 500
DVPGKLIYGQ YCECDTINCE RYNGQVCGGP GRGLCFCGKC RCHPGFEGSA 550
CQCERTTEGC LNPRRVECSG RGRCRCNVCE CHSGYQLPLC QECPGCPSPC 600
GKYISCAECL KFEKGPFGKN CSAACPGLQL SNNPVKGRTC KERDSEGCWV 650
AYTLEQQDGM DRYLIYVDES RECVAGPNIA AIVGGTVAGI VLIGILLLVI 700
WKALIHLSDL REYRRFEKEK LKSQWNNDNP LFKSATTTVM NPKFAES     747
```

References

1. Weitzman, J.B. et al. (1991) FEBS Lett. 294, 97–103.
2. Pigott, R. and Power, C. (1993) The Adhesion Molecule FactsBook. Academic Press, London.
3. **Larson, R.S. and Springer, T.A. (1990) Immunol. Rev. 114, 181–217.**
4. Patarroyo, M. et al. (1990) Immunol. Rev. 114, 67–108.
5. Rieu, P. and Arnaout, M.A. (1995) In Adhesion Molecules and the Lung (Ward, P. and Lenfart, C., eds), vol. 89, pp. 1–42. Marcel Dekker, New York.
6. Kishimoto, T.K. et al. (1987) Cell 48, 681–690.
7. Law, S.K.A. et al. (1987) EMBO J. 6, 915–919.
8. Pavalko, F.M. and LaRoche, S.M. (1993) J. Immunol. 151, 3795–3807.
9. Sharma, C.P. et al. (1995) J. Immunol. 154, 3461–3470.
10. Kolanus, W. et al. (1996) Cell 86, 233–242.
11. Ortlepp, S. et al. (1995) Eur. J. Immunol. 25, 637–643.
12. Petruzzelli, L. et al. (1995) J. Immunol. 155, 854–866.
13. **Kishimoto, T.K. et al. (1987) Cell 50, 193–202.**
14. **Arnaout, M.A. (1990) Immunol. Rev. 114, 145–180.**
15. Wilson, R.W. et al. (1989) Nucleic Acids Res. 17, 5397.

CD19

B4, Leu-12

Molecular weights
Polypeptide   59 154

SDS-PAGE
  reduced   95 kDa

Carbohydrate
N-linked sites   5
O-linked   unknown

Human gene location and size
16p11.2; 8 kb [1]

Encoded
by 9 exons

Tissue distribution

CD19 is expressed on B lineage cells with the exception of plasma cells. CD19 is also present on follicular dendritic cells [2].

Structure

The extracellular region of CD19 consists of two C2-set IgSF domains separated by a region of 67 residues with no significant sequence similarity to any known protein [3]. The large cytoplasmic domain is highly conserved between species [4] and contains several potential phosphorylation sites on Ser/Thr and Tyr residues [3]. Phosphorylation of tyrosine residues in the YEXM motifs creates binding motifs for the SH2 domains of phosphatidyl-inositol 3-kinase and non-receptor protein tyrosine kinases [5].

Ligands and associated molecules

CD19 is a component of the CD19/CD21/CD81/leu-13 signalling complex (reviewed in refs 2, 5 and 6). The CD19/CD21 interaction has a 1:1 stoi-chiometry and is mediated by both the extracellular and transmembrane regions of CD19, whereas the CD19/CD81 interaction involves the CD19 extracellular region only [5]. CD19 links this complex to cytoplasmic signal transduction pathways. The extensive cytoplasmic region of CD19 can associate with phosphatidylinositol 3-kinase, Vav and the Src family protein tyrosine kinases Lyn and Fyn (reviewed in refs 6 and 7).

Function

The CD19/CD21/CD81/leu-13 signalling complex modulates the threshold for the B cell antigen receptor[6,7]. The functions of CD81 and leu-13, the expression of which are not restricted to B cells, are not clear. However CD21 (complement receptor 2) binds fragments of C3 that have been covalently attached to glycoconjugates by complement activation. This enables CD19, plus associated intracellular signalling molecules, to be crosslinked to the B cell antigen receptor after preimmune recognition of an immunogen by the complement system, thus reducing the number of B cell receptor molecules which must be ligated to enable B cell activation[6,7]. This mechanism may be particularly important for the B cell during the primary immune response, prior to affinity maturation, when the low-affinity B cell antigen receptor must respond to low concentrations of antigen. This co-receptor role for CD19 is supported by data from CD19 knockout and transgenic mice[6,7].

Database accession numbers

	PIR	SWISSPROT	EMBL/GENBANK	REFERENCE
Human	JL0074	P15391	M28170	3
Mouse	B45808	P25918	M62542	4

Amino acid sequence of human CD19

```
MPPPRLLFFL LFLTPM                                             -1
EVRPEEPLVV KVEEGDNAVL QCLKGTSDGP TQQLTWSRES PLKPFLKLSL        50
GLPGLGIHMR PLASWLFIFN VSQQMGGFYL CQPGPPSEKA WQPGWTVNVE        100
GSGELFRWNV SDLGGLGCGL KNRSSEGPSS PSGKLMSPKL YVWAKDRPEI        150
WEGEPPCVPP RDSLNQSLSQ DLTMAPGSTL WLSCGVPPDS VSRGPLSWTH        200
VHPKGPKSLL SLELKDDRPA RDMWVMETGL LLPRATAQDA GKYYCHRGNL        250
TMSFHLEITA RPVLWHWLLR TGGWKVSAVT LAYLIFCLCS LVGILHLQRA        300
LVLRRKRKRM TDPTRRFFKV TPPPGSGPQN QYGNVLSLPT PTSGLGRAQR        350
WAAGLGGTAP SYGNPSSDVQ ADGALGSRSP PGVGPEEEEG EGYEEPDSEE        400
DSEFYENDSN LGQDQLSQDG SGYENPEDEP LGPEDEDSFS NAESYENEDE        450
ELTQPVARTM DFLSPHGSAW DPSREATSLG SQSYEDMRGI LYAAPQLHSI        500
RGQPGPNHEE DADSYENMDN PDGPDPAWGG GGRMGTWSTR                   540
```

References

[1] Zhou, L.-J. et al. (1992) Immunogenetics 35, 102–111.
[2] Tedder, T.F. et al. (1994) Immunol. Today 15, 437–442.
[3] Tedder, T.F. and Isaacs, C.M. (1989) J. Immunol. 143, 712–717.
[4] Zhou, L.-J. et al. (1991) J. Immunol. 147, 1424–1432.
[5] Fearon, D.T. and Carter, R.H. (1995) Annu. Rev. Immunol. 13, 127–149.
[6] **Doody, G.M. et al. (1996) Curr. Opin. Immunol. 8, 378–382.**
[7] DeFranco, A.L. (1996) Curr. Biol. 6, 548–550.

CD20   B1, Bp35, Ly-44 (mouse)

Molecular weights
Polypeptide   33 078

SDS-PAGE
  reduced   33–37 kDa

Carbohydrate
N-linked sites   nil
O-linked   nil

Human gene location and size
11q13; 16 kb [1]

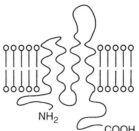

Tissue distribution

CD20 is expressed only on B lineage cells but is absent from plasma cells (reviewed in ref. 2).

Structure

CD20 is a member of the CD20/FcεRIβ superfamily of leucocyte surface antigens which also includes the β subunit of the high-affinity receptor for IgE (FcεRIβ) and HTm4. These molecules are predicted to have four trans-membrane regions, cytoplasmic N- and C-termini, and short extracellular loops [2,3]. The CD20/FcεRIβ superfamily shares no sequence similarity with another superfamily of four transmembrane molecules, the TM4SF. The gene for CD20 maps to the same region of the genome as FcεRIβ and HTm4 [4]. The cytoplasmic regions of CD20 are serine/threonine rich and contain multiple phosphorylation consensus sequences. Differential phosphorylation is responsible for the three forms of CD20 (33, 35 and 37 kDa), with activated B cells showing a relative increase in the phosphorylated 35 and 37 kDa forms [2].

Ligands and associated molecules

CD20 can exist in a multimolecular complex that includes the Src family tyrosine kinases Lyn, Fyn and Lck. This association may not be direct, since it is unaffected by deletion of a large proportion of the CD20 cytoplasmic regions [5]. This is consistent with flow cytometric energy transfer analyses which show that CD20 can exist in a complex with MHC Class I and II, and the TM4SF molecules CD53, CD81 and CD82 [6]. No extracellular ligand for CD20 has been identified.

Function

Indirect evidence suggests that CD20 functions as a B cell Ca^{2+} channel subunit, since the expression of CD20 in disparate cell types generates a quali-tatively similar channel activity to that found endogenously in B cells [7]. An ion channel function is consistent with reports that CD20 regulates cell cycle progression [8] and exists on the cell surface as a homo-oligomer [7].

Database accession numbers

	PIR	SWISSPROT	EMBL/GENBANK	REFERENCE
Human	A27400	P11836	X12530	9
Mouse	A30558	P19437	M62541	4

Amino acid sequence of human CD20

```
MTTPRNSVNG TFPAEPMKGP IAMQSGPKPL FRRMSSLVGP TQSFFMRESK      50
TLGAVQIMNG LFHIALGGLL MIPAGIYAPI CVTVWYPLWG GIMYIISGSL     100
LAATEKNSRK CLVKGKMIMN SLSLFAAISG MILSIMDILN IKISHFLKME     150
SLNFIRAHTP YINIYNCEPA NPSEKNSPST QYCYSIQSLF LGILSVMLIF     200
AFFQELVIAG IVENEWKRTC SRPKSNIVLL SAEEKKEQTI EIKEEVVGLT     250
ETSSQPKNEE DIEIIPIQEE EEEETETNFP EPPQDQESSP IENDSSP        297
```

References

1 Tedder, T.F. et al. (1989) J. Immunol. 142, 2560–2568.
2 **Tedder, T.F. and Engel, P. (1994) Immunol. Today 15, 450–454.**
3 Adra, C.N. et al. (1994) Proc. Natl Acad. Sci. USA 91, 10178–10182.
4 Tedder, T.F. et al. (1988) J. Immunol. 141, 4388–4394.
5 Deans, J.P. et al. (1995) J. Biol. Chem. 270, 22632–22638.
6 Szöllosi, J. et al. (1996) J. Immunol. 157, 2939–2946.
7 Bubien, J.K. et al. (1993) J. Cell Biol. 121, 1121–1132.
8 Kanzaki, M. et al. (1995) J. Biol. Chem. 270, 13099–13104.
9 Tedder, T.F. et al. (1988) Proc. Natl Acad. Sci. USA 85, 208–212.

CD21 CR2, EBV-receptor, C3d-receptor

Other names
Complement receptor type 2 (CR2)
C3d receptor
Epstein–Barr virus (EBV) receptor

Molecular weights
Polypeptide   16 CCP form   117 126
                 15 CCP form   110 929

SDS-PAGE
  reduced   145 kDa

Carbohydrate
N-linked sites   16 CCP form   12
                  15 CCP form   11
O-linked   unknown

Human gene location and size
1q32; ~30 kb [1,2]

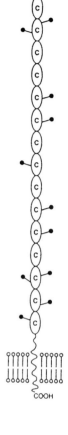

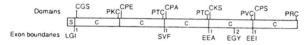

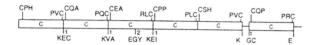

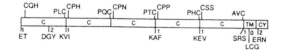

Tissue distribution

CD21 is expressed on mature B cells, follicular dendritic cells, and pharyngeal and cervical epithelial cells [3]. It is also expressed on fetal astrocytes [4].

Structure

The extracellular region consists of 15 or 16 complement control protein (CCP) domains, organized into four groups with a high degree of sequence identity between them [5,6]. The 11th CCP domain is absent in the 15 CCP domain isoform [3,5,6]. The CD21 gene is a member of the regulation of complement activation (RCA) gene cluster that encodes a family of C3/C4 binding proteins (see **CD35** and ref. 1). The cytoplasmic domain contains potential protein kinase C and tyrosine kinase phosphorylation sites [3,5,6].

Ligands and associated molecules

CD21 is a receptor for the C3 activation fragments iC3b and C3d [3]. It is also the receptor used by the Epstein–Barr virus to infect B lymphocytes [3,7]. CD21 has been shown to bind CD23 [8] and interferon α [9]. CD21 is one subunit in a multimeric complex on B cells which includes CD19 and CD81 [10]. CD21 is also associated with CD35 on B cells [11].

Function

When covalent antigen–complement complexes bind to the B cell antigen receptor (BCR, surface Ig), the simultaneous interaction of CD21 with the complement component C3d enhances signalling through the BCR. The CD21 signal, which is transduced through the associated molecules CD19 and CD81, very effectively lowers the activation threshold of the BCR [10]. Thus C3d may be considered as a molecular adjuvant [12] that directs the acquired immune response towards antigens recognized by the innate immune response [13]. Mice made defective in CD21 have an impaired immune response to T-dependent antigens [14,15]. The CD21/CD23 interaction may have a regulatory role in IgE production [8].

Database accession numbers

	PIR	SWISSPROT	EMBL/GENBANK	REFERENCE
Human	PL0009	P20023	M26004/M26016	2,5,6
Mouse	A43526	P19070	M35684	16,17

Amino acid sequence of human CD21

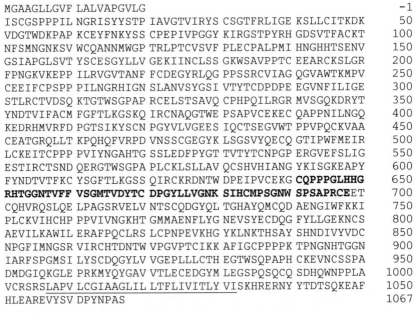

```
MGAAGLLGVF LALVAPGVLG                                          -1
ISCGSPPPIL NGRISYYSTP IAVGTVIRYS CSGTFRLIGE KSLLCITKDK         50
VDGTWDKPAP KCEYFNKYSS CPEPIVPGGY KIRGSTPYRH GDSVTFACKT        100
NFSMNGNKSV WCQANNMWGP TRLPTCVSVF PLECPALPMI HNGHHTSENV        150
GSIAPGLSVT YSCESGYLLV GEKIINCLSS GKWSAVPPTC EEARCKSLGR        200
FPNGKVKEPP ILRVGVTANF FCDEGYRLQG PPSSRCVIAG QGVAWTKMPV        250
CEEIFCPSPP PILNGRHIGN SLANVSYGSI VTYTCDPDPE EGVNFILIGE        300
STLRCTVDSQ KTGTWSGPAP RCELSTSAVQ CPHPQILRGR MVSGQKDRYT        350
YNDTVIFACM FGFTLKGSKQ IRCNAQGTWE PSAPVCEKEC QAPPNILNGQ        400
KEDRHMVRFD PGTSIKYSCN PGYVLVGEES IQCTSEGVWT PPVPQCKVAA        450
CEATGRQLLT KPQHQFVRPD VNSSCGEGYK LSGSVYQECQ GTIPWFMEIR        500
LCKEITCPPP PVIYNGAHTG SSLEDFPYGT TVTYTCNPGP ERGVEFSLIG        550
ESTIRCTSND QERGTWSGPA PLCKLSLLAV QCSHVHIANG YKISGKEAPY        600
FYNDTVTFKC YSGFTLKGSS QIRCKRDNTW DPEIPVCEKG CQPPPGLHHG        650
RHTGGNTVFF VSGMTVDYTC DPGYLLVGNK SIHCMPSGNW SPSAPRCEET        700
CQHVRQSLQE LPAGSRVELV NTSCQDGYQL TGHAYQMCQD AENGIWFKKI        750
PLCKVIHCHP PPVIVNGKHT GMMAENFLYG NEVSYECDQG FYLLGEKNCS        800
AEVILKAWIL ERAFPQCLRS LCPNPEVKHG YKLNKTHSAY SHNDIVYVDC        850
NPGFIMNGSR VIRCHTDNTW VPGVPTCIKK AFIGCPPPPK TPNGNHTGGN        900
IARFSPGMSI LYSCDQGYLV VGEPLLLCTH EGTWSQPAPH CKEVNCSSPA        950
DMDGIQKGLE PRKMYQYGAV VTLECEDGYM LEGSPQSQCQ SDHQWNPPLA       1000
VCRSRSLAPV LCGIAAGLIL LTFLIVITLY VISKHRERNY YTDTSQKEAF       1050
HLEAREVYSV DPYNPAS                                          1067
```

The 11th CCP domain (in **bold**) is only found in the 16 CCP form.

References

1 Hourcade, D. et al. (1992) Genomics 12, 289–300.
2 Fujisaku, A. et al. (1990) J. Biol. Chem. 264, 2118–2125.
3 **Ahearn, J.M. and Fearon, D.T. (1989) Adv. Immunol. 46, 183–219.**
4 Gasque, P. et al. (1996) J. Immunol. 156, 2247–2255.
5 Weis, J.J. et al. (1989) J. Exp. Med. 167, 1047–1066.
6 Moore, M.D. et al. (1987) Proc. Natl Acad. Sci. USA 84, 9194–9198.
7 Tanner, J. et al. (1987) Cell 50, 203–213.
8 Aubry, J.P. et al. (1992) Nature 358, 505–507.
9 Delcayre, A.X. et al. (1991) EMBO J. 10, 919–926.
10 **Doody, G.M. et al. (1996) Curr. Opin. Immunol. 8, 378–382.**
11 Tuvenson, D.A. et al. (1991) J. Exp. Med. 173, 1083–1089.
12 Dempsey P.W. et al. (1996) Science 271, 348–350.
13 **Fearon, D.T. and Locksley, R.M. (1996) Science 272, 50–54.**
14 Molina, H. et al. (1996) Proc. Natl Acad. Sci. USA 93, 3357–3361.
15 Ahearn, J.M. et al. (1996) Immunity 4, 251–262
16 Fingeroth, J.D. et al. (1989) Proc. Natl Acad. Sci. USA 86, 242–246.
17 Molina, H. et al. (1990) J. Immunol. 145, 2974–2983.

CD22

BL-CAM, Leu-14, Lyb-8

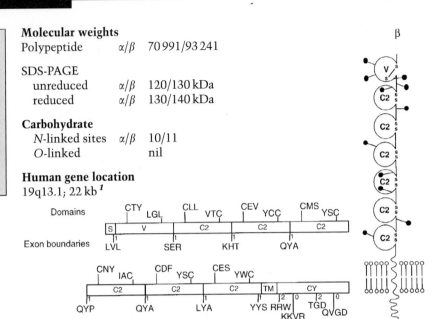

Molecular weights

Polypeptide $\quad \alpha/\beta \quad$ 70 991/93 241

SDS-PAGE
    unreduced $\quad \alpha/\beta \quad$ 120/130 kDa
    reduced $\quad\quad \alpha/\beta \quad$ 130/140 kDa

Carbohydrate
    N-linked sites $\quad \alpha/\beta \quad$ 10/11
    O-linked $\quad\quad\quad$ nil

Human gene location
19q13.1; 22 kb [1]

Tissue distribution

CD22 is detected in the cytoplasm early in B cell development (late pro-B cell stage), appears on the cell surface simultaneously with surface IgD, and is found on most mature B cells, where expression is closely correlated with surface IgD [2]. Expression is lost with terminal differentiation of B cells and is absent on plasma cells. Activation of B cells via surface Ig increases CD22 expression.

Structure

CD22 is a member of a structurally related group of IgSF domain-containing sialic acid binding proteins called the sialoadhesin family, which includes sialoadhesin, CD33, and myelin-associated glycoprotein (MAG) [3]. Members of this family share ~35% identity between their 2–4 membrane-distal IgSF domains. Like other members of the sialoadhesin family, CD22 is predicted to have an unusual disulphide bond between β strands B and E in domain 1 and a disulphide bond between domains 1 and 2 [3]. The predominant form of CD22 in humans (CD22β) [4] and the only identified form in the mouse [5] contains seven IgSF domains in the extracellular region. A human cDNA clone has been identified which encodes a variant (CD22α) lacking IgSF domains 3 and 4 and with a truncated cytoplasmic domain [6]. At least three CD22 alleles have been identified in the mouse [7,8]. The exon structure of the CD22 gene indicates that CD22α represents an alternatively spliced transcript of the CD22 gene [1]. CD22β is the predominant form detected by immunoprecipitation experiments but a smaller protein has been detected which may correspond to CD22α [9]. The cytoplasmic region contains six tyrosines, four of which are in SH2-binding YxxL motifs.

Ligands and associated molecules

The CD22 binds to sialoglycoconjugate NeuAcα2 $\rightarrow$ 6Galβ1 $\rightarrow$ 4GlcNAc which is widely present on *N*-linked carbohydrates[10]. The binding site lies on the GFCC'C" β sheet of the membrane-distal IgSF domain and includes an arginine (residue 101) conserved in all sialoadhesin family proteins[8]. CD22 forms a loose complex with the B cell antigen receptor (BCR)[2]. The cytoplasmic domain is tyrosine phosphorylated upon ligation of the BCR and associates, via SH2 domains, with the tyrosine phosphatase SHP-1, the tyrosine kinase Syk, and phospholipase C-γ1[11,12]. The tyrosine kinase Lck and phosphatidylinositol 3-kinase have also been reported to bind to the cytoplasmic domain[13].

Function

CD22 down-modulates the B cell activation threshold, presumably through its association with SHP-1 and other signalling molecules[2,11]. Mice deficient in CD22 show exaggerated antibody responses to antigen and have raised levels of autoantibodies[14]. CD22 can also mediate cell adhesion through its interaction with cell surface molecules bearing the appropriate sialoglyco-conjugates[2], but only when the cells expressing CD22 do not themselves carry these sialoglycoconjugates[10]. Although the significance of sialic acid binding by CD22 is not known, ligation-induced restribution of CD22 on B cells decreases the BCR activation threshold, providing a plausible link between the adhesion and signalling functions[11].

Database accession numbers

	PIR	SWISSPROT	EMBL/GENBANK	REFERENCE
Human CD22β	JH0371	Q01665	X59350	4
Human CD22α (short)	A35648	P20273	X52785	6
Mouse CD22β				
DBA/2J		P35329	L16928	7
BALB/c	A46512	P35329	L02844	5

Amino acid sequence of human CD22β

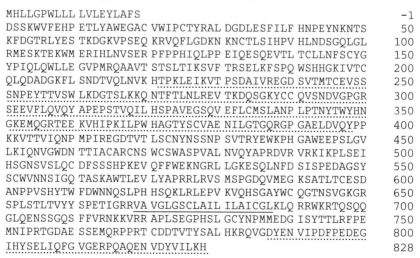

```
MHLLGPWLLL LVLEYLAFS                                           -1
DSSKWVFEHP ETLYAWEGAC VWIPCTYRAL DGDLESFILF HNPEYNKNTS         50
KFDGTRLYES TKDGKVPSEQ KRVQFLGDKN KNCTLSIHPV HLNDSGQLGL         100
RMESKTEKWM ERIHLNVSER PFPPHIQLPP EIQESQEVTL TCLLNFSCYG         150
YPIQLQWLLE GVPMRQAAVT STSLTIKSVF TRSELKFSPQ WSHHGKIVTC         200
QLQDADGKFL SNDTVQLNVK HTPKLEIKVT PSDAIVREGD SVTMTCEVSS         250
SNPEYTTVSW LKDGTSLKKQ NTFTLNLREV TKDQSGKYCC QVSNDVGPGR         300
SEEVFLQVQY APEPSTVQIL HSPAVEGSQV EFLCMSLANP LPTNYTWYHN         350
GKEMQGRTEE KVHIPKILPW HAGTYSCVAE NILGTGQRGP GAELDVQYPP         400
KKVTTVIQNP MPIREGDTVT LSCNYNSSNP SVTRYEWKPH GAWEEPSLGV         450
LKIQNVGWDN TTIACARCNS WCSWASPVAL NVQYAPRDVR VRKIKPLSEI         500
HSGNSVSLQC DFSSSHPKEV QFFWEKNGRL QKESQLNFD SISPEDAGSY          550
SCWVNNSIGQ TASKAWTLEV LYAPRRLRVS MSPGDQVMEG KSATLTCESD         600
ANPPVSHYTW FDWNNQSLPH HSQKLRLEPV KVQHSGAYWC QGTNSVGKGR         650
SPLSTLTVYY SPETIGRRVA VGLGSCLAIL ILAICGLKLQ RRWKRTQSQQ         700
GLQENSSGQS FFVRNKKVRR APLSEGPHSL GCYNPMMEDG ISYTTLRFPE         750
MNIPRTGDAE SSEMQRPPRT CDDTVTYSAL HKRQVGDYEN VIPDFPEDEG         800
IHYSELIQFG VGERPQAQEN VDYVILKH                                 828
```

The amino acid sequence of human CD22α is as above with dotted underlined areas (encoded by exons 6, 7 and 15) deleted and the cytoplasmic domain terminating with the sequence TMRTSFQIF QKMRGFITQS.

References
1   Wilson, G.L. et al. (1993) J. Immunol. 150, 5013–5024.
2   Law, C.L. et al. (1994) Immunol. Today 15, 442–449.
3   Crocker, P.R. et al. (1996) Biochem. Soc. Trans. 24, 150–156.
4   Wilson, G.L. et al. (1991) J. Exp. Med. 173, 137–146.
5   Torres, R.M. et al. (1992) J. Immunol. 149, 2641–2649.
6   Stamenkovic, I. and Seed, B. (1990) Nature 345, 74–77.
7   Law, C.L. et al. (1993) J. Immunol. 151, 175–187.
8   van der Merwe, P.A. et al. (1996) J. Biol. Chem. 271, 9273–9280.
9   Schwartz-Albiez, R. et al. (1991) Int. Immunol. 3, 623–33.
10 **Powell, L.D. and Varki, A. (1995) J. Biol. Chem. 270, 14243–14246.**
11 Doody, G.M. et al. (1996) Curr. Opin. Immunol. 8, 378–382.
12 Law, C.L. et al. (1996) J. Exp. Med. 183, 547–560.
13 Tuscano, J.M. et al. (1996) Eur. J. Immunol. 26, 1246–1252.
14 **O'Keefe, T.L. et al. (1996) Science 274, 798–801.**

Molecular weights
Polypeptide   FcεRIIa   36 468

SDS-PAGE
   reduced   45 kDa
   non-reduced   45 kDa

Carbohydrate
N-linked sites   1
O-linked   probable +

Human gene location and size
19p13.3; 13 kb [1]

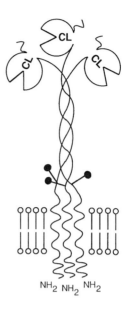

Tissue distribution

CD23 is expressed on B cells and monocytes, and more weakly on a variety of other haematopoietic cells including T cells, follicular dendritic cells, eosinophils, NK cells, Langerhans cells and platelets. On B cells, CD23 expression is restricted to mIgM⁺mIgD⁺ cells and is lost upon differentiation into plasma cells [2]. CD23 on B cells is upregulated following B cell activation, CD40 ligation, or in response to IL-4 or IL-13 [3].

Structure

CD23 is a type II membrane protein. The extracellular region contains a C-terminal C-type lectin domain and three membrane-proximal repeats of 21 amino acids. These repeats form an α-helical coiled-coil stalk that results in trimer formation [4]. Two alternatively spliced forms called FcεRIIa and FcεRIIb, differing in the first nine amino acids of the N-terminal cytoplasmic region, are expressed on different cell types. FcεRIIa is restricted to resting B cells, whereas FcεRIIb is expressed by other cell types and is induced upon B cell activation [2]. Proteolytic cleavage of the membrane-bound form generates a soluble product of 37 kDa, which can be further degraded into 33 kDa, 29 kDa, 25 kDa and 16 kDa fragments that retain their lectin head groups [4].

Ligands and associated molecules

The Fc region of IgE, CD21, and the integrin α chains CD11b and CD11c are ligands for CD23. In each case the C-type lectin domain of CD23 is responsible for ligand binding. IgE binding to CD23 is a protein–protein interaction that involves the third constant domain of the IgE heavy chain [4]. CD23 interacts with two sites on CD21. One site (CCP domains 5–8) is a lectin–carbohydrate type of interaction whereas the other (CCP domains 1–2) is a protein–protein interaction (reviewed in ref. 3). CD23 binds to the integrins CD11b/CD18 and CD11c/CD18, but not CD11a/CD18. This interaction is at least partly dependent on lectin–carbohydrate binding (reviewed in ref. 5). CD23 has been shown to associate non-covalently with MHC Class II in B cells, by co-immunoprecipitation analyses in weak detergent[2].

Function

CD23 is involved in the regulation of IgE synthesis. Following binding of IgE and IgE-containing immune complexes, CD23 exerts a negative feedback signal that reduces IgE synthesis[3,6,7]. Consistent with this function, mice rendered deficient for CD23 have one major phenotype, namely high serum IgE levels and increased specific IgE responses in response to T cell-dependent antigens[6]. Transgenic mice that overexpress CD23 show impaired IgE responses[6]. The *in vivo* role of soluble CD23 (sCD23) is not clear, but it is proposed that sCD23 can function as a cytokine that enhances IgE synthesis, probably through binding to surface membrane IgE and CD21[3]. The role of CD23 as a cell–cell adhesion molecule is also not clear; the CD23 interaction with CD21 may be important in enhancing IgE synthesis, in B cell homotypic adhesion and in the rescue of germinal centre B cells from apoptosis[3]. The ligand pairing of CD23 with the integrins CD11b/CD18 and CD11c/CD18 is thought to play a role in monocyte activation[5,8]. The two forms of CD23 have been implicated in different signalling pathways and specific functions. The Tyr (amino acid 6) of FcεRIIa is involved in endocytosis and the Asp-Pro motif (amino acids 2–3) of FcεRIIb is associated with phagocytosis[6]. CD23 is cleaved from the cell surface by *Der p* I, the group I protease allergen of the house dust mite *Dermatophagoides pteronyssinus*. Loss of surface CD23 and increase of sCD23 may combine to enhance IgE synthesis, providing a mechanism by which the dust mite induces an atopic condition in some individuals[9].

Database accession numbers

	PIR	SWISSPROT	EMBL/GENBANK	REFERENCE
Human	A26067	P06734	M15059	10
Mouse	A43518	P20693	M99371	11

Amino acid sequence of human CD23

FcεRIIa

```
MEEGQYSEIE ELPRRRCCRR GTQIVLLGLV TAALWAGLLT LLLLWHWDTT    50
QSLKQLEERA ARNVSQVSKN LESHHGDQMA QKSQSTQISQ ELEELRAEQQ   100
RLKSQDLELS WNLNGLQADL SSFKSQELNE RNEASDLLER LREEVTKLRM   150
ELQVSSGFVC NTCPEKWINF QRKCYYFGKG TKQWVHARYA CDDMEGQLVS   200
IHSPEEQDFL TKHASHTGSW IGLRNLDLKG EFIWVDGSHV DYSNWAPGEP   250
TSRSQGEDCV MMRGSGRWND AFCDRKLGAW VCDRLATCTP PASEGSAESM   300
GPDSRPDPDG RLPTPSAPLH S                                 321
```

FceRIIb

```
MNPPSQEIEE                                              10
```

The sequence differences between FcεRIIa and FcεRIIb reside within the first nine amino acids. The sequence downstream of this region is identical in both forms.

References
1. Suter, U. et al. (1987) Nucleic Acids Res. 15, 7295–7308.
2. Sarfati, M. et al. (1995) Leucocyte Typing V, 530–533.
3. **Bonnefoy, J.-Y. et al. (1995) Curr. Opin. Immunol. 7, 355–359.**
4. Sutton, B.J. and Gould, H.J. (1993) Nature 366, 421–428.
5. **Bonnefoy, J.-Y. et al. (1996) Immunol. Today 17, 418–420.**
6. **Lamers, M.C. and Yu, P. (1995) Immunol. Rev. 148, 71–95.**
7. Mudde, G.C. et al. (1995) Immunol. Today 16, 380–383.
8. Dugas, B. et al. (1995) Immunol. Today 16, 574–580.
9. Hewitt, C.R.A. et al. (1995) J. Exp. Med. 182, 1537–1544.
10. Ikuta, K. et al. (1987) Proc. Natl Acad. Sci. USA 84, 819–823.
11. Bettler, B. et al. (1989) Proc. Natl Acad. Sci. USA 86, 7566–7570.

Molecular weights
Polypeptide   3128

SDS-PAGE
   reduced   35–45 kDa

Carbohydrate
N-linked sites   2
O-linked   probable +

Human gene location
6q21

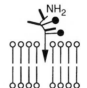

Tissue distribution

Human CD24 is expressed on B cells, but decreases on activation and is lost at the plasma cell stage. The antigen is also present on granulocytes, a small number of thymocytes (2%) and normal epithelium [1-5]. Mouse CD24 is present at all stages of B cell development and on most thymocytes [6,7]. The absence of expression from mature T cells is closely associated with their maturation from CD4⁺CD8⁺CD24⁺ thymocytes to either CD4⁺CD8⁻CD24⁻ or CD4⁻CD8⁺CD24⁻ T cells. The antigen is also expressed on mouse monocytes, granulocytes, Langerhans cells and erythrocytes [6,8]. Rat CD24 expression has been detected, using *in situ* hybridization, in the developing central nervous system and in the epithelium of developing non-neural tissues [9].

Structure

CD24 is a GPI-linked sialoglycoprotein. The mature protein is predicted to be only 33 amino acids long and has a high content (48%) of Ser and Thr residues that may be the site of O-linked glycosylation [4]. Different CD24 mAbs recognize epitopes that are dependent on sialic acid [10]. The precursor forms of mouse and rat CD24 show 62.5% and 65% amino acid identity to the human sequence. However, the mature form of the molecule shows only 33% (mouse/human) and 42% (rat/human) sequence identity [4,9,11]. It is possible that the rodent sequences are not CD24 homologues but members of a closely related family.

Ligands and associated molecules

CD24 has been reported to be a P-selectin ligand (see **CD62P**) [12].

Function

CD24 may play a role in regulation of B cell proliferation and differentiation. CD24 mAbs have been shown to inhibit human B cell differentiation into antibody-secreting cells [13] and synergize with phorbol esters in triggering B cell proliferation [14]. Crosslinking of CD24 induces an increase in intracellular calcium levels in B cells and the production of hydrogen peroxide in granulocytes[5]. In the mouse, CD24 can provide costimulatory activity for CD4[+] T cell activation and is involved in the aggregation of LPS-activated splenic B cells[15,16].

Comments

Multiple CD24 genes have been identified and mapped in both human and mouse[17,18]. In addition to the human CD24 gene on chromosome 6q21, the human CD24 cDNA hybridized to sequences on chromosome 15q21–22 and Yq11 but these genes have not been shown to be functional. Mouse CD24 genes have been mapped to chromosomes 10 (*Cd24a*), 8 (*Cd24b*) and 14 (*Cd24c*)[19]. The *Cd24a* gene has a single intron and encodes the CD24 mRNA. Both the *Cd24b* and *Cd24c* genes lack the intron, are not expressed in adult mouse tissues and may have arisen by retropositioning.

Database accession numbers

	PIR	SWISSPROT	EMBL/GENBANK	REFERENCE
Human		P25063	M58664, L33930	4
Mouse		P24807	M58661	11
Rat		Q07490	Z11663	9

Amino acid sequence of human CD24

```
MGRAMVARLG LGLLLLALLL PTQIYS                    -1
SETTTGTSSN SSQSTSNSGL APNPTNATTK AAG            33
GALQSTASLF VVSLSLLHLY S                        +21
```

References

1 Kemshead, J.T. et al. (1982) Hybridoma 1, 109–123.
2 Hsu, S-M. and Jaffe, E.S. (1984) Am. J. Pathol. 114, 387–395.
3 Jackson, D. et al. (1992) Cancer Res. 52, 5264–5270.
4 **Kay, R. et al. (1991) J. Immunol. 147, 1412–1416.**
5 Fischer, G.F. et al. (1990) J. Immunol. 144, 638–641.
6 Takei, F. et al. (1981) Immunology 42, 371–378.
7 Crispe, I.N. and Bevan, M.J. (1987) J. Immunol. 138, 2013–2018.
8 Enk, A.H. and Katz, S.I. (1994) J. Immunol. 152, 3264–3270.
9 Shirasawa, T. et al. (1993) Dev. Dyn. 198, 1–13.
10 Larkin, M. et al. (1991) Clin. Exp. Immunol. 85, 536–541.
11 Kay, R. et al. (1990) J. Immunol. 145, 1952–1959.
12 **Aigner, S. et al. (1995) Int. Immunol. 7, 1557–1565.**
13 de Rie, M.A. et al. (1987) Leucocyte Typing III, 402-405.
14 Rabinovitch, P.S. et al. (1987) Leucocyte Typing III, 435–439.
15 Liu, Y. et al. (1992) J. Exp. Med. 175, 437–445.
16 **Kadmon, G. et al. (1992) J. Cell Biol. 118, 1245–1258.**
17 Hough, M.R. et al. (1994) Genomics 22, 154–161.
18 Wenger, R.H. et al. (1991) Eur. J. Immunol. 21, 1039–1046.
19 Wenger, R.H. et al. (1993) J. Biol. Chem. 268, 23345–23352.

CD26

Dipeptidyl peptidase IV (EC 3.4.14.5)

Other names
Tp103
Adenosine deaminase binding protein
Thymocyte-activating molecule (THAM) (mouse)

Molecular weights
Polypeptide   88 319

SDS-PAGE
    reduced   110 kDa
    unreduced   110, 140 kDa

Carbohydrate
N-linked sites   9
O-linked   unknown

Human gene location and size
2q24.3; 70 kb [1]

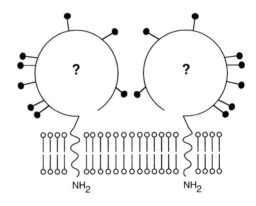

Tissue distribution

CD26 is expressed by a variety of haematopoietic and non-haematopoietic cell types. On leucocytes, CD26 is expressed primarily on mature thymocytes in the medulla. Expression is weak on mature T cells and is restricted to memory T cells, although CD26 is upregulated on T cell activation. On non-haematopoietic cells, CD26 is found on epithelial cells of the intestine, kidney proximal tubule, bile duct and prostate gland (reviewed in refs 2 and 3).

Structure

CD26 is a type II integral membrane dipeptidylpeptidase with a short N-terminal cytoplasmic tail, a transmembrane region and a large C-terminal extracellular region that contains nine N-glycosylation sites. CD26 is a member of the polyoligo peptidase family. The C-terminal region contains the putative catalytic site, consisting of Gly-Trp-Ser-Tyr-Gly motif (amino acids 628–632), Asp708 and His740, in the reverse order of the serine protease family. CD26 is expressed as a non-covalently linked homodimer [2,3].

Ligands and associated molecules

CD26 associates non-covalently with adenosine deaminase (ADA), the deficiency of which results in severe combined immunodeficiency in humans. This interaction is mediated by the extracellular region of CD26 and is not dependent on catalytic activity (reviewed in ref. 2). CD26 co-immunoprecipitates and co-modulates with CD45 on T cells [2]. A ligand for CD26 is the extracellular matrix protein collagen. This interaction does not require CD26 catalytic activity and mAb blocking studies indicate that the binding site is within residues 236–491 [4].

Function

CD26 is proposed to perform three distinct functions, as a membrane bound protease, a T cell co-stimulatory molecule and a cell adhesion molecule[2]. CD26 has a unique specificity amongst cell surface serine proteases: dipeptides are cleaved from the N-terminus of polypeptides if proline is at the penultimate position. This enzymatic activity is responsible for the intestinal digestion and renal transport of proline-containing polypeptides. Indeed, the Fischer 344 rat strain lacks functional CD26, resulting in impaired renal absorption of proline-containing peptides[2]. CD26 also functions as a T cell co-stimulatory molecule. Expression of the T cell receptor (TCR) complex is required for CD26 signalling, in which the TCR ζ chain is necessary but not sufficient[5]. The mechanism for CD26 signalling is not known, but may be related to the association of CD26 with CD45 and ADA[2]. In particular, ADA binding to CD26 on T cells is proposed to reduce the local concentration of adenosine, a nucleoside which inhibits T cell proliferation[6]. It is not clear whether catalytic activity is required for CD26 signalling[2]. However, the cell adhesion role of CD26, in binding to the extra-cellular matrix via collagen, does not depend on catalytic activity[4].

Comments

CD26 is associated with human immunodeficiency virus (HIV) disease progression, which is a feature of many other T cell molecules. There is some correlation between CD26 expression and HIV entry, replication and cytopathicity. In addition, CD26 is downregulated as the disease progresses. However, CD26 is clearly not a co-receptor for HIV, as was originally reported (reviewed in ref. 7).

Dipeptidyl peptidase IV activity has been measured in serum, but this does not appear to be the result of CD26 cleavage from the cell surface. Instead, a novel 175 kDa T cell antigen DPPT-L, related to CD26, is thought to be responsible[8].

Database accession numbers

	PIR	SWISSPROT	EMBL/GENBANK	REFERENCE
Human	S24313	P27487	X60708	9
Rat	A33315	P14740	J04591	10
Mouse	S23752	P28843	X58384	11

Amino acid sequence of human CD26

```
MKTPWKILLG LLGAAALVTI ITVPVVLLNK GTDDATADSR KTYTLTDYLK    50
NTYRLKLYSL RWISDHEYLY KQENNILVFN AEYGNSSVFL ENSTFDEFGH   100
SINDYSISPD GQFILLEYNY VKQWRHSYTA SYDIYDLNKR QLITEERIPN   150
NTQWVTWSPV GHKLAYVWNN DIYVKIEPNL PSYRITWTGK EDIIYNGITD   200
WVYEEEVFSA YSALWWSPNG TFLAYAQFND TEVPLIEYSF YSDESLQYPK   250
TVRVPYPKAG AVNPTVKFFV VNTDSLSSVT NATSIQITAP ASMLIGDHYL   300
CDVTWATQER ISLQWLRRIQ NYSVMDICDY DESSGRWNCL VARQHIEMST   350
TGWVGRFRPS EPHFTLDGNS FYKIISNEEG YRHICYFQID KKDCTFITKG   400
TWEVIGIEAL TSDYLYYISN EYKGMPGGRN LYKIQLIDYT KVTCLSCELN   450
PERCQYYSVS FSKEAKYYQL RCSGPGLPLY TLHSSVNDKG LRVLEDNSAL   500
```

```
DKMLQNVQMP SKKLDFIILN ETKFWYQMIL PPHFDKSKKY PLLLDVYAGP    550
CSQKADTVFR LNWATYLAST ENIIVASFDG RGSGYQGDKI MHAINRRLGT    600
FEVEDQIEAA RQFSKMGFVD NKRIAIWGWS YGGYVTSMVL GSGSGVFKCG    650
IAVAPVSRWE YYDSVYTERY MGLPTPEDNL DHYRNSTVMS RAENFKQVEY    700
LLIHGTADDN VHFQQSAQIS KALVDVGVDF QAMWYTDEDH GIASSTAHQH    750
IYTHMSHFIK QCFSLP                                        766
```

References
1 Abbott, C.A. et al. (1994) Immunogenetics 40, 331–338.
2 **Fleischer, B. (1994) Immunol. Today 15, 180–184.**
3 Shipp, M.A. and Look, A.T. (1993) Blood 82, 1052–1070.
4 Loster, K. et al. (1995) Biochem. Biophys. Res. Commun. 217, 341–348.
5 Mittrucker, H.-W. et al. (1995) Eur. J. Immunol. 25, 295–297.
6 Dong, R.-P. et al. (1996) J. Immunol. 156, 1349–1355.
7 Dalgleish, A. (1995) Nature Med. 1, 881–882.
8 Duke-Cohan, J.S. et al. (1996) J. Immunol. 156, 1714–1721.
9 Misumi, Y. et al. (1992) Biochim. Biophys. Acta 1131, 333–336.
10 Ogata, S. et al. (1989) J. Biol. Chem. 264, 3596–3601.
11 Marguet, D. et al. (1992) J. Biol. Chem. 267, 2200–2208.

CD27

Molecular weights
Polypeptide   26 898

SDS-PAGE
  reduced   50–55 kDa
  unreduced   120 kDa

Carbohydrate
N-linked sites   1
O-linked   +++

Human gene location and size
12p13 [1]; 7 kb [1]

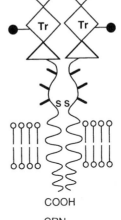

COOH

Domains		CPE		CIP		CRN			

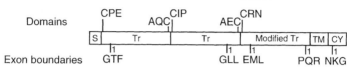

Exon boundaries   GTF   GLL EML   PQR NKG

Tissue distribution

CD27 protein is present on T cells of both CD4$^+$ and CD8$^+$ subsets and on medullary thymocytes, some B cells and NK cells [2–4]. Expression on T cells is upregulated on activation and is higher on CD45RA$^+$ than CD45RO$^+$ cells [2,4].

Structure

CD27 is a member of the TNFR superfamily, with two full cysteine-rich repeats and one half repeat in the extracellular domain of the protein [2,5,6]. The 70 amino acid membrane-proximal region contains sites for O-linked glycosylation [7]. Extensive O-glycosylation has been established by studies on biosynthesis and effect of N- and O-glycanases [7]. The protein is found on the surface of T cells as a disulfide-linked homodimer [6]. Soluble CD27 is released probably by proteolytic cleavage on activation [4].

Ligands and associated molecules

CD27 binds a ligand CD27L also called CD70, a type II membrane protein which is a member of the TNF superfamily [2–4].

Function

Cells expressing CD70 can interact via CD27 to co-stimulate T cell proliferation, generate cytotoxic T cells and enhance cytokine production [2,3]. CD70 binding to CD27 on B cells co-stimulates B cell proliferation and immunoglobulin production [3]. CD27 is phosphorylated on serine residues and hyperphosphorylated with T cell activation [8]. No tyrosine phosphorylation is observed.

Database accession numbers

	PIR	SWISSPROT	EMBL/GENBANK	REFERENCE
Human	A46517	P26842	M63928	[6]
Mouse	A49053	P41272	L24495	[9]

Amino acid sequence of human CD27

```
MARPHPWWLC VLGTLVGLSA                                        -1
TPAPKSCPER HYWAQGKLCC QMCEPGTFLV KDCDQHRKAA QCDPCIPGVS       50
FSPDHHTRPH CESCRHCNSG LLVRNCTITA NAECACRNGW QCRDKECTEC      100
DPLPNPSLTA RSSQALSPHP QPTHLPYVSE MLEASTAGHM QTLADFRQLP      150
ARTLSTHWPP QRSLCSSDFI RILVIFSGMF LVFTLAGALF LHQRRKYRSN      200
KGESPVEPAE PCRYSCPREE EGSTIPIQED YRKPEPACSP                 240
```

References
[1] Loenen, W.A.M. et al. (1992) J. Immunol. 149, 3937–3943.
[2] Gruss, H.-J. and Dower, S.K. (1995) Blood 85, 3378–3404.
[3] Kobata, T. et al. (1995) Proc. Natl Acad. Sci. USA 92, 11249–11253.
[4] Hintzen, R.Q. et al. (1994) Immunol. Today 15, 307–311.
[5] Armitage, R.J. (1994) Curr. Opin. Immunol. 6, 407–413.
[6] Camerini, D. et al. (1991) J. Immunol. 147, 3165–3169.
[7] Loenen, W.A.M. et al. (1992) Eur. J. Immunol. 22, 447–456.
[8] De Jong, R. et al. (1991) J. Immunol. 146, 2488–2494.
[9] Gravestein, L.A. et al. (1993) Eur. J. Immunol. 23, 943–950.

Molecular weights

Polypeptide   23 085

SDS-PAGE
   reduced   44 kDa
   unreduced   90 kDa

Carbohydrate
N-linked sites   5
O-linked   unknown

Human gene location and size
2q33; 36 kb [1,2]

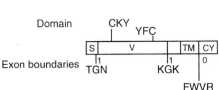

Tissue distribution

CD28 is constitutively expressed on most T lineage cells and plasma cells [3,4]. Mature thymocytes have higher levels of CD28 than the immature cells and among peripheral T cells, all $CD4^+$ cells and ~50% of human $CD8^+$ cells are positive. In general, activation of T cells leads to enhanced CD28 expression but ligation of CD28 leads to its transient downregulation [4].

Structure

CD28 is disulfide-linked homodimer with a single IgSF domain in its extracellular portion [3]. It is structurally similar to CD152 (CTLA-4, 31% identity), binds the same ligands (see below), and the two genes are less than 150 kb apart [5], suggesting that they share a common ancestor in evolution.

Ligands and associated molecules

Like CD152, CD28 binds both CD80 and CD86 using a highly conserved motif (MYPPPY) in the CDR3-like loop [6]. CD28 binds CD80 with a low affinity (K_d 4 μM) and dissociates very rapidly ($k_{off} \geq 1.6\,s^{-1}$) [7]. Binding to CD86 may be even weaker [8]. The cytoplasmic domain interacts with phosphatidylinositol 3-kinase (PI 3-kinase), the complex between GRB-2 and the guanine nucleotide exchange protein SOS (GRB-2/SOS), and the tyrosine kinase ITK [9,10]. SH2 domains in PI 3-kinase and GRB-2/SOS mediate binding to the CD28 motif YMNMT, after it has been phosphoryled by Lck and Fyn [9,10].

Function

Studies *in vitro* suggested that ligation of CD28 on T cells by CD80 and CD86 on antigen presenting cells provides a co-stimulatory signal required for T cell activation[3]. However, mice lacking CD28[11] are able to mount effective T cell responses and are mainly defective in T cell-dependent antibody responses, suggesting that CD28 is mainly important for T cell–B cell interactions and humoral immunity[4]. Ligation of CD28 activates several signal-transduction pathways, including PI 3-kinase[9], and inhibits degradation of cytokine mRNA[12].

Database accession numbers

	PIR	SWISSPROT	EMBL/GENBANK	REFERENCE
Human	A39983	P10747	J02988	13
Mouse	A43523	P31041	M34563	14
Rat	S24413	P31042	X55288	15

Amino acid sequence of human CD28

```
MLRLLLALNL FPSIQVTG                                          -1
NKILVKQSPM LVAYDNAVNL SCKYSYNLFS REFRASLHKG LDSAVEVCVV        50
YGNYSQQLQV YSKTGFNCDG KLGNESVTFY LQNLYVNQTD IYFCKIEVMY       100
PPPYLDNEKS NGTIIHVKGK HLCPSPLFPG PSKPFWVLVV VGGVLACYSL       150
LVTVAFIIFW VRSKRSRLLH SDYMNMTPRR PGPTRKHYQP YAPPRDFAAY       200
RS                                                          202
```

References

1 Lafage–Pochitaloff, M. et al. (1990) Immunogenetics 31, 198–201.
2 Lee, K.P. et al. (1990) J. Immunol. 145, 344–352.
3 Linsley, P.S. and Ledbetter, J.A. (1993) Annu. Rev. Immunol. 11, 191–211.
4 **Lenschow, D.J. et al. (1996) Annu. Rev. Immunol. 14, 233–258.**
5 Buonavista, N. et al. (1992) Genomics 13, 856–861.
6 Peach, R.J. et al. (1994) J. Exp. Med. 180, 2049–2058.
7 van der Merwe, P.A. et al., (1997) J. Exp. Med. 185, 394–403.
8 Greene, J.L. et al. (1996) J. Biol. Chem. 271, 26762–26771.
9 June, C.H. et al. (1994) Immunol. Today 15, 321–331.
10 Raab, M. et al. (1995) Proc. Natl Acad. Sci. USA 92, 8891–8895.
11 Shahinian, A. et al. (1993) Science 261, 609–612.
12 June, C.H. et al. (1990) Immunol. Today 11, 211–216.
13 Aruffo, A. and Seed, B. (1987) Proc. Natl Acad. Sci. USA 84, 8573–8577.
14 Gross, J.A. et al. (1990) J. Immunol. 144, 3201–3210.
15 Clark, G.J. and Dallman, M.J. (1992) Immunogenetics 35, 54–57.

CD29

Integrin β1 subunit

Molecular weights

Polypeptides
A isoform	86 242
B isoform	85 273
C isoform	89 446
D isoform	86 710

SDS-PAGE (A isoform)
reduced	130 kDa
unreduced	115 kDa

Carbohydrate
N-linked sites	12
O-linked sites	unknown

Human gene location
10p11.2

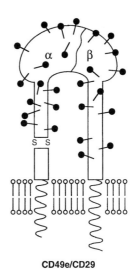

CD49e/CD29

Tissue distribution

CD29 is expressed on most cells. It is expressed on all leucocytes, although only at low levels on granulocytes [1,2]. On T cells, CD29 is expressed at higher levels on memory than naive cells [1,2].

Structure

CD29 forms heterodimers with many integrin α subunits including the CD49a–f (α1–α6) and CD51 (αV) antigens and, in non-lymphoid tissues, α7–α9 [3-6]. The CD49a–f/CD29 heterodimers are also termed the very late antigens (VLA-1 to VLA-6) because two of them (VLA-1 and -2) appear on lymphocytes several weeks after stimulation. Four CD29 isoforms (A–D) with different cytoplasmic domains are generated by alternative splicing [7-10]. The B isoform (β1³'ᵛ) is found in the placenta and is expressed on human umbilical vein endothelial cells (HUVECs) as well as lymphoma, neuroblastoma and hepatoma cell lines [8]. The C isoform (β1s) is expressed on platelets and a number of haematopoietic cell lines but not detected on peripheral blood lymphocytes or HUVECs [9]. The D isoform is exclusively expressed in skeletal and cardiac muscle [10].

Ligands and associated molecules

Integrins which include CD29 bind to several cell surface and extracellular matrix molecules (see **CD49a–f** and **CD51**).

Function

Integrin heterodimers containing CD29 mediate cell–cell and cell–matrix adhesion (see **CD49a–f** and **CD51**). The adhesive properties of CD29 heterodimers on T cells can be regulated by cell activation [11], possibly through interactions between the cytoplasmic domain of CD29 and the cytoskeleton[2,12]. The different cytoplasmic domains in the A–D isoforms may allow interactions with different intracellular elements [7-10].

Database accession numbers

	PIR	SWISSPROT	EMBL/GENBANK	REFERENCE
Human A form	B27079	P05556	X07979	7
Human B form			U33879	8
Human C form			U33882	9
Human D form			U33880	10
Mouse	PL0104	P09055	X15202	13
	S01659		Y00769	14

Amino acid sequence of human CD29

```
MNLQPIFWIG LISSVCCVFA                                         -1
QTDENRCLKA NAKSCGECIQ AGPNCGWCTN STFLQEGMPT SARCDDLEAL        50
KKKGCPPDDI ENPRGSKDIK KNKNVTNRSK GTAEKLKPED IHQIQPQQLV       100
LRLRSGEPQT FTLKFKRAED YPIDLYYLMD LSYSMKDDLE NVKSLGTDLM       150
NEMRRITSDF RIGFGSFVEK TVMPYISTTP AKLRNPCTSE QNCTTPFSYK       200
NVLSLTNKGE VFNELVGKQR ISGNLDSPEG GFDAIMQVAV CGSLIGWRNV       250
TRLLVFSTDA GFHFAGDGKL GGIVLPNDGQ CHLENNMYTM SHYYDYPSIA       300
HLVQKLSENN IQTIFAVTEE FQPVYKELKN LIPKSAVGTL SANSSNVIQL       350
IIDAYNSLSS EVILENGKLS EGVTISYKSY CKNGVNGTGE NGRKCSNISI       400
GDEVQFEISI TSNKCPKKDS DSFKIRPLGF TEEVEVILQY ICECECQSEG       450
IPESPKCHEG NGTFECGACR CNEGRVGRHC ECSTDEVNSE DMDAYCRKEN       500
SSEICSNNGE CVCGQCVCRK RDNTNEIYSG KFCECDNFNC DRSNGLICGG       550
NGVCKCRVCE CNPNYTGSAC DCSLDTSTCE ASNGQICNGR GICECGVCKC       600
TDPKFQGQTC EMCQTCLGVC AEHKECVQCR AFNKGEKKDT CTQECSYFNI       650
TKVESRDKLP QPVQPDPVSH CKEKDVDDCW FYFTYSVNGN NEVMVHVVEN       700
PECPTGPDII PIVAGVVAGI VLIGLALLLI WKLLMIIHDR REFAKFEKEK       750
MNAKWDT                                                      757
```

The A–D isoforms terminate as follows:

```
A: GENPIYKSAV TTVVNPKYEG K                                   778
B: VSYKTSKKQS GL                                             769
C: SLSVAQPGVQ WCDISSLQPL TSRQQFSCLS LPSTWDYRVK ILFIRVP       804
D: QENPIYKSPI NNFKNPNYGR KAGL                                781
```

References

1 Pigott, R. and Power, C. (1993) The Adhesion Molecule FactsBook. Academic Press, London.

2 **Hemler, M.E. (1990) Annu. Rev. Immunol. 114, 365–400.**

3 Song, W.K. et al. (1992) J. Cell Biol. 117, 643–657.

4 Ziober, B.L. et al. (1993) J. Biol. Chem. 268, 26773–26783.

5 Bossy, B. et al. (1991) EMBO J. 10, 2375–2385.

6 Palmer, E.L. et al. (1993) J. Cell Biol. 123, 1289–1297.

7 Argraves, W.S. et al. (1987) J. Cell Biol. 105, 1183–1190.

8 Balzac, F. et al. (1993) J. Cell Biol. 121, 171–178

9 Languino, R.L. and Ruoslahti, E. (1992) J. Biol. Chem. 267, 7116–7120.
10 Belkin, A.M. et al. (1996) J. Cell Biol. 132, 211–216.
11 Shimizu, Y. et al. (1990) Nature 345, 250–253.
12 **Schwartz, M.A. et al. (1995) Annu. Rev. Cell Dev. Biol. 11, 549–599.**
13 Holers, V.M. et al. (1989) J. Exp. Med. 169, 1589–1605.
14 Tominaga, S.I. (1988) FEBS Lett. 138, 315–319.

Molecular weights
Polypeptide   61 893

SDS-PAGE
  reduced   105–120 kDa
  unreduced   105–120 kDa

Carbohydrate
N-linked sites   2
O-linked   ++++

Human gene location
1p36 [1]

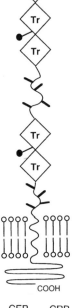

COOH

Domains

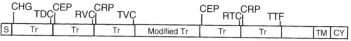

Tissue distribution

CD30 antigen is not found on resting lymphocytes or monocytes, but is expressed on mitogen-activated B and T cells[1]. In normal tissue the antigen is found on large lymphoid cells in sections of lymph node, tonsil, and thymus[1]. CD30 is present on Reed–Sternberg cells of Hodgkin's lymphoma and many other malignant cell lines[1].

Structure

CD30 is a member of the TNFR superfamily with five clearly identifiable Cys-rich repeats[2-4]. The five repeats are interrupted after repeat 3 by a hinge sequence of about 60 amino acids that may have derived from the central region of another TNFR repeat. This is argued because there are two Cys residues at the end of this region which are surrounded by sequence patterns typical of TNFR repeats. Repeats 2 and 5 show particular sequence similarities, suggesting that CD30 may have evolved by gene duplication of a precursor structure with three repeats[2,3]. Biochemical analysis of CD30 revealed the presence of *O*-linked sugars accounting for 4 kDa on SDS-PAGE[5]. It is likely that both the central hinge region and the membrane-proximal region are sites for *O*-glycosylation by virtue of the high content of Ser, Thr, and Pro residues. In cell lines, CD30 is phosphorylated on serine and tyrosine residues[5].

Ligands and associated molecules

CD30 binds to CD153, a member of the TNF superfamily.

Function

The CD153–CD30 interaction co-stimulates T cell proliferation[1,3] and upregulates expression of adhesion molecules and cytokine release[1]. A role for the CD153–CD30 interaction in deletion of thymocytes is suggested from studies with CD30-deficient mice[6]. CD30+ T cell clones produce T_H2-type cytokines. A role for the CD153–CD30 interaction in T_H2-type autoimmune disease has been suggested[1,7].

Comments

Truncated CD30 protein is released from the cell surface and found as a soluble protein in the serum of some patients with adult T cell leukaemia or other CD30+ lymphomas[1]. Levels of soluble CD30 correlated with disease[1].

Database accession numbers

	PIR	SWISSPROT	EMBL/GENBANK	REFERENCE
Human	A42086	P28908	M83554	8
Mouse			U25416	2

Amino acid sequence of human CD30

```
MRVLLAALGL LFLGALRA                                           -1
FPQDRPFEDT CHGNPSHYYD KAVRRCCYRC PMGLFPTQQC PQRPTDCRKQ         50
CEPDYYLDEA DRCTACVTCS RDDLVEKTPC AWNSSRVCEC RPGMFCSTSA        100
VNSCARCFFH SVCPAGMIVK FPGTAQKNTV CEPASPGVSP ACASPENCKE        150
PSSGTIPQAK PTPVSPATSS ASTMPVRGGT RLAQEAASKL TRAPDSPSSV        200
GRPSSDPGLS PTQPCPEGSG DCRKQCEPDY YLDEAGRCTA CVSCSRDDLV        250
EKTPCAWNSS RTCECRPGMI CATSATNSCA RCVPYPICAA ETVTKPQDMA        300
EKDTTFEAPP LGTQPDCNPT PENGEAPAST SPTQSLLVDS QASKTLPIPT        350
SAPVALSSTG KPVLDAGPVL FWVILVLVVV VGSSAFLLCH RRACRKRIRQ        400
KLHLCYPVQT SQPKLELVDS RPRRSSTQLR SGASVTEPVA EERGLMSQPL        450
METCHSVGAA YLESLPLQDA SPAGGPSSPR DLPEPRVSTE HTNNKIEKIY        500
IMKADTVIVG TVKAELPEGR GLAGPAEPEL EEELEADHTP HYPEQETEPP        550
LGSCSDVMLS VEEEGKEDPL PTAASGK                                577
```

References
1 Gruss, H.-J. and Dower, S.K. (1995) Blood 85, 3378–3404.
2 van Kooten, C. and Banchereau, J. (1996) Adv. Immunol. 61, 1–77.
3 Smith, C.A. et al. (1993) Cell 73, 1349–1360.
4 Armitage, R.J. (1994) Curr. Opin. Immunol. 6, 407–413.
5 Nawrocki, J.F. et al. (1988) J. Immunol. 141, 672–680.
6 Amakawa, R. et al. (1996) Cell 84, 551–562.
7 Del Prete, G. et al. (1995) Immunol. Today 16, 76–80.
8 Durkop, H. et al. (1992) Cell 68, 421–427.

Molecular weights
Polypeptide   79 579

SDS-PAGE
  reduced   130–140 kDa
  unreduced   130–140 kDa

Carbohydrate
N-linked sites   9
O-linked   unknown

Human gene location and size
17q23–ter; 65 kb [1]

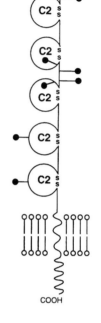

Domains

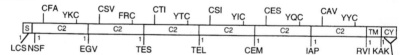

Tissue distribution

CD31 is present on virtually all monocytes, platelets and granulocytes. Approximately 50% of resting PBL are CD31[+2]. CD31 expression changes on maturation of CD4[+] T cells[3]. CD31 is highly expressed on endothelial cells and concentrated at the junctions between them[2].

Structure

CD31 contains six IgSF C2-set domains with sequence similarity with the carcinoembryonic antigen (CD66), NCAM (CD56) and CD32[4–6]. It is possible that there is a disulfide bond between domains 4 and 5.

Ligands and associated molecules

CD31 interacts homotypically in cell adhesion assays[7]. In addition it interacts heterotypically with the integrin $\alpha v \beta 3$[8,9] and glycosaminoglycans[10]. Several domains seem to be involved in the homotypic interaction whereas domain

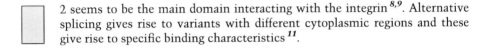

2 seems to be the main domain interacting with the integrin [8,9]. Alternative splicing gives rise to variants with different cytoplasmic regions and these give rise to specific binding characteristics [11].

Function

MAbs and recombinant CD31 proteins can inhibit neutrophil migration through blood vessels by blocking at the stage of interaction with the basement membrane [12].

Comments

A Leu to Val polymorphism in CD31 (residue 98 in mature protein below) is a minor transplantation antigen where matching provides a significantly lower risk of graft-versus-host disease in bone marrow transplants [13].

Database accession numbers

	PIR	SWISSPROT	EMBL/GENBANK	REFERENCE
Human	A40096	P16284	M28526, M37780	4–6
Mouse		Q08481	L06039	14

Amino acid sequence of human CD31

```
MQPRWAQGAT MWLGVLLTLL LCSSLEG                            -1
QENSFTINSV DMKSLPDWTV QNGKNLTLQC FADVSTTSHV KPQHQMLFYK    50
DDVLFYNISS MKSTESYFIP EVRIYDSGTY KCTVIVNNKE KTTAEYQLLV   100
EGVPSPRVTL DKKEAIQGGI VRVNCSVPEE KAPIHFTIEK LELNEKMVKL   150
KREKNSRDQN FVILEFPVEE QDRVLSFRCQ ARIISGIHMQ TSESTKSELV   200
TVTESFSTPK FHISPTGMIM EGAQLHIKCT IQVTHLAQEF PEIIIQKDKA   250
IVAHNRHGNK AVYSVMAMVE HSGNYTCKVE SSRISKVSSI VVNITELFSK   300
PELESSFTHL DQGERLNLSC SIPGAPPANF TIQKEDTIVS QTQDFTKIAS   350
KSDSGTYICT AGIDKVVKKS NTVQIVVCEM LSQPRISYDA QFEVIKGQTI   400
EVRCESISGT LPISYQLLKT SKVLENSTKN SNDPAVFKDN PTEDVEYQCV   450
ADNCHSHAKM LSEVLRVKVI APVDEVQISI LSSKVVESGE DIVLQCAVNE   500
GSGPITYKFY REKEGKPFYQ MTSNATQAFW TKQKASKEQE GEYYCTAFNR   550
ANHASSVPRS KILTVRVILA PWKKGLIAVV IIGVIIALLI IAAKCYFLRK   600
AKAKQMPVEM SRPAVPLLNS NNEKMSDPNM EANSHYGHND DVRNHAMKPI   650
NDNKEPLNSD VQYTEVQVSS AESHKDLGKK DTETVYSEVR KAVPDAVESR   700
YSRTEGSLDG T                                            711
```

References
1 Kirschbaum, N. et al. (1994) Blood 84, 4028–4037.
2 DeLisser, H.M. et al. (1994) Immunol. Today 15, 490–495.
3 Demeure, C.E. et al. (1996) Immunology 88, 110–115.
4 Newman, P.J. et al. (1990) Science 247, 1219–1222.
5 Simmons, D.L. et al. (1990) J. Exp. Med. 171, 2147–2152.
6 Stockinger, H. et al. (1990) J. Immunol. 145, 3889–3897.
7 Fawcett, J. et al. (1995) J. Cell Biol. 128, 1229–1241.
8 Piali, L. et al. (1995) J. Cell Biol. 130, 451–460.
9 Buckley, C.D. et al. (1996) J. Cell Sci. 109, 437–445.
10 DeLisser, H.M. et al. (1993) J. Biol. Chem. 268, 16037–16046.

11 Yan, H.C. et al. (1995) J. Biol. Chem. 270, 23672–23680.
12 **Wakelin, M.W. et al. (1996) J. Exp. Med. 184, 229–239.**
13 Behar, E. et al. (1996) New Engl. J. Med. 334, 286–291.
14 Xie, Y. and Muller, W.A. (1993) Proc. Natl Acad. Sci. USA 90, 5569–5573.

Molecular weights

Polypeptides:		
	A form	31 049
	B1 form	29 206
	B2 form	27 107
	B3 form	29 206
	C form	30 757

SDS-PAGE	
reduced	40 kDa

Carbohydrate

N-linked sites	2
O-linked sites	nil

A isoform

Human gene location and size

There are three genes in 1q23–24 in the order of A–C–B in which the C gene is likely to have arisen from an unequal crossover between A and B; each gene is ~15–19 kb. The CD32 genes are intercalated with those of CD16 in a complex locus [1-3].

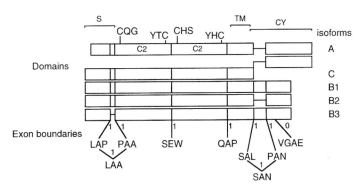

Tissue distribution

CD32 isoforms are expressed on a range of leucocytes including monocytes, macrophages, Langerhans cells, granulocytes, B cells, and platelets, as well as on endothelial cells of the placenta [3,4]. All isoforms are expressed on monocytes, the B isoforms are present on B lymphocytes, and the A and C isoforms are found on neutrophils.

Structure

CD32 contains two extracellular C2-set IgSF domains. There are six isoforms of CD32 derived from three genes. The C isoform is a hybrid between the A and B isoforms; it is identical to the B isoforms at the N-terminal (extracellular domain) but identical to the A isoform at the C-terminal (transmembrane and cytoplasmic segments). Three gene products are derived from the B gene. An exon is omitted in each of the B2 and B3 transcripts, leading to the B2 isoform with 19 residues deleted from the cytoplasmic domain and the B3 isoform having a shortened leader sequence[2-5]. A soluble variant of the A isoform has also been described (sequence not shown) that is generated by the alternative splicing of the mRNA[3,6].

Ligands and associated molecules

CD32 is a low-affinity Fcγ receptor and only binds polymeric or aggregated IgG[3]. The isotype preference for CD32 is IgG3 > IgG1 > IgG2 = IgG4[3,4]. The A isoform has been shown to associate with CD11b/CD18 but not CD11c/CD18[7]. The cytoplasmic portion of the B1 isoform associates with the tyrosine phosphatase SHP-1 and the inositol-5'-phosphatase (SHIP)[14-16] via a phosphorylated IxYxxL motif[11-16].

Function

Occupation of CD32 can trigger IgG-mediated phagocytosis and an oxidative burst in neutrophils and monocytes, possibly in coordination with the ligation of other receptors such as CD26 and CD11b/CD18[4,8-10]. Co-ligation of membrane Ig with the B1 isoform of CD32 inhibits signalling through membrane Ig[11-16]. As a result there is a dampening of the B cell response to antigen for which an IgG already exists. Co-ligation of CD32 B1 with membrane Ig leads to phosphorylation of Tyr247 in the IxYxxL motif which then binds SHP-1 and SHIP, leading to the inhibition of inositol phosphate production and Ca^{2+} entry into the cell[11-16]. CD32 expression on placental epithelia may indicate a role in transport of IgG[17].

Database accession numbers

		PIR	SWISSPROT	EMBL/GENBANK	REFERENCE
Human	A	JL0118	P12318	M31932	5
		S02297		Y00644	18
Human	B1	JL0119	P31994	M31935	5
Human	B2			M31934	5
				X17653	17
		A43543		X52473	19
Human	B3			M31933	5
Human	C	S06946	P31995	X17652	17
Mouse	b1	S29361	P08101	M16367	20
				M17515	21
Mouse	b2	B40071	P08102	M14216	20,22
		A93384		X04648	23

Amino acid sequences of human CD32

```
A          M AMETQMSQNV CPRNLWLLQP LTVLLLLASA DSQAA          -1
           *  * ******* * ******** * ** *  ** ****
C  MGILSFLPVL ATESDWADCK SPQPWGHMLL WTAVLFLAPV AGTPA          -1
B1 .......... ........--- ---------- ---------- -----          -1
B2 ---------- ---------- ---------- ---------- -----          -1
B3 ---------- ---------- ---------- -------... ....-          -1

A  APPKAVLKLE PPWINVLQED SVTLTCQGAR SPESDSIQWF HNGNLIPTHT     50
            *                * **
C  APPKAVLKLE PQWINVLQED SVTLTCRGTH SPESDSIQWF HNGNLIPTHT     50
B1 ---------- ---------- ---------- ---------- ----------     50
B2 ---------- ---------- ---------- ---------- ----------     50
B3 ---------- ---------- ---------- ---------- ----------     50

A  QPSYRFKANN NDSGEYTCQT GQTSLSDPVH LTVLSEWLVL QTPHLEFQEG    100
C  QPSYRFKANN NDSGEYTCQT GQTSLSDPVH LTVLSEWLVL QTPHLEFQEG    100
B1 ---------- ---------- ---------- ---------- ----------    100
B2 ---------- ---------- ---------- ---------- ----------    100
B3 ---------- ---------- ---------- ---------- ----------    100

A  ETIMLRCHSW KDKPLVKVTF FQNGKSQKFS RLDPTFSIPQ ANHSHSGDYH    150
        *                    *      *      *
C  ETIVLRCHSW KDKPLVKVTF FQNGKSKKFS RSDPNFSIPQ ANHSHSGDYH    150
B1 ---------- ---------- ---------- ---------- ----------    150
B2 ---------- ---------- ---------- ---------- ----------    150
B3 ---------- ---------- ---------- ---------- ----------    150

A  CTGNIGYTLF SSKPVTITVQ VPSMGSSSPM GIIVAVVIAT AVAAIVAAVV    200
                *  ***            ***
C  CTGNIGYTLY SSKPVTITVQ AP...SSSPM GIIVAVVTGI AVAAIVAAVV    197
B1 ---------- ---------- --...----- ---------- ----------    197
B2 ---------- ---------- --...----- ---------- ----------    197
B3 ---------- ---------- --...----- ---------- ----------    197

A  ALIYCRKKRI S                                             211
C  ALIYCRKKRI S                                             208
B1 ---------- -                                             208
B2 ---------- -                                             208
B3 ---------- -                                             208

A  ..................A NSTDPVKAAQ FEPPGRQMIA IRKRQLEETN    242
C  ..................- ---------- ---------- -----P----    239

B1 ALPGYPECRE MGETLPEKPA NPTNPDEADK VGAENTITYS LLMHPDALEE    258
B2 .......... ........-- ---------- ---------- ----------    239
B3 ---------- ---------- ---------- ---------- ----------    258

A  NDYETADGGY MTLNPRAPTD DDKNIYLTLP PNDHVNSNN               281
C  ---------- ---------- ---------- ---------               278

B1 PDDQNRI                                                  265
B2 -------                                                  246
B3 -------                                                  265
```

The C isoform is a hybrid of the A and B isoforms, and is listed between them. The B and C sequences are grouped until C residue 208, and are marked with an asterisk when different from the A isoform. A and C are grouped from C residue 209. Residues identical to the top sequence within the group are marked with dashes. The dotted stretches denote gaps. These result from exon omissions except for three additional residues (173–175) in isoform A. The IxYxxL motif is in bold.

References
1 Qiu, W.Q. et al. (1990) Science 248, 732–735.
2 Warmerdam, P.A.M. et al. (1993) J. Biol. Chem. 268, 7346–7349.
3 **van de Winkel, J.G.J. and Capel, P.J.A. (1993) Immunol. Today 14, 215–221.**
4 Ravetch, J.V. and Kinet, J.P. (1991) Annu. Rev. Immunol. 9, 457–492.
5 **Brooks, D.G. et al. (1989) J. Exp. Med. 170, 1369–1385.**
6 Warmerdam, P.A.M. et al. (1992) J. Exp. Med. 172, 19–25.
7 Annendov, A. (1996) Eur. J. Immunol. 26, 207–212.
8 Huizinga, T.W.J. et al. (1989) J. Immunol. 142, 2365–2369.
9 Brown, E.J. (1991) Curr. Opin. Immunol. 3, 76–82.
10 Zhou, M.J. and Brown, E.J. (1994) J. Cell Biol. 125, 1407–1416.
11 Muta, T. et al. (1994) Nature 368, 70–73.
12 Choquet, D. et al. (1993) J. Cell Biol. 121, 355–363.
13 D'Ambrosia, D. et al. (1995) Science 268, 293–297.
14 Bijsterbosch, M.K. and Klaus, G.G. (1985) J. Exp. Med. 162, 1825–1836.
15 Doody, G.M. et al. (1996) Curr. Opin. Immunol. 8, 378–382.
16 Scharenberg, A. M. and Kinet, J. -P (1996) Cell 87, 961–964
17 Stuart, S. G. et al. (1989) EMBO J. 8, 3657–3666.
18 Stuart, S. G. (1987) J. Exp. Med. 166, 1668–1684.
19 Engelhart, R. et al. (1990) Eur. J. Immunol. 20, 1367–1377.
20 Ravetch, J.V. et al. (1986) Science 234, 718–725.
21 Hogarth, P.M. et al. (1987) Immunogenetics 26, 161–168.
22 Hogarth, P.M. et al. (1991) J. Immunol. 146, 369–376.
23 Lewis, V.A. et al. (1986) Nature 324, 372–375.

CD33

Molecular weights
Polypeptide   37 908

SDS-PAGE
    reduced   67 kDa

Carbohydrate
N-linked sites 5
O-linked   nil

Human gene location and size
19q13.3; <35 kb [1]

Domains

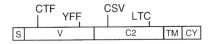

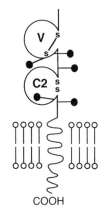

Tissue distribution

CD33 is absent from pluripotential stem cells but appears on myelomonocytic precursors after CD34 [2]. It then continues to be expressed in both the myeloid and monocyte lineages although it is absent on granulocytes [3]. CD33 is an important marker for distinguishing myeloid from lymphoid leukaemias [3].

Structure

CD33 is the smallest member of a structurally related group of IgSF domain-containing sialic acid-binding proteins called the sialoadhesin family, which includes sialoadhesin, CD22, and myelin-associated glycoprotein (MAG) [4]. The genes for CD22, CD33 and MAG lie in the region 19q13.1–3 [1,4]. Like other members of the Sialoadhesin family, CD33 is predicted to have an unusual disulfide bond between β strands B and E in domain 1 and a disulfide bond between domains 1 and 2 [4]. Two CD33 cDNA clones have been isolated in the mouse encoding CD33 isoforms with different cytoplasmic domains [5].

Ligands and associated molecules

Like sialoadhesin, CD33 binds to the sialoglycoconjugates NeuAcα2 → 3Galβ1 → 3(4)GlcNAc and NeuAcα2 → 3Galβ1 → 3GalNAc on glyco-proteins [3].

Function

May mediate cell–cell adhesion. Cells expressing CD33 require desialylation before they can bind cells bearing the appropriate sialoglycoconjugate [3], suggesting that inhibitory cis-interactions may regulate or block any adhesion function [3].

Database accession numbers

	PIR	SWISSPROT	EMBL/GENBANK	REFERENCE
Human	A30521	P20138	M23197	6
Mouse			S71345/S71403	5

Amino acid sequence of human CD33

```
MPLLLLLPLL WAGALAM                                              -1
DPNFWLQVQE SVTVQEGLCV LVPCTFFHPI PYYDKNSPVH GYWFREGAII          50
SGDSPVATNK LDQEVQEETQ GRFRLLGDPS RNNCSLSIVD ARRRDNGSYF         100
FRMERGSTKY SYKSPQLSVH VTDLTHRPKI LIPGTLEPGH SKNLTCSVSW         150
ACEQGTPPIF SWLSAAPTSL GPRTTHSSVL IITPRPQDHG TNLTCQVKFA         200
GAGVTTERTI QLNVTYVPQN PTTGIFPGDG SGKQETRAGV VHGAIGGAGV         250
TALLALCLCL IFFIVKTHRR KAARTAVGRN DTHPTTGSAS PKHQKKSKLH         300
GPTETSSCSG AAPTVEMDEE LHYASLNFHG MNPSKDTSTE YSEVRTQ            347
```

References

1 Peiper, S.C. et al. (1988) Blood 72, 314–321.
2 Andrews, R.G. et al. (1989) J. Exp. Med. 169, 1721–1731.
3 **Freeman, S.D. et al. (1995) Blood 85, 2005–2012.**
4 Crocker, P.R. et al. (1996) Biochem. Soc. Trans. 24, 150–156.
5 Tchilian, E.Z. et al. (1994) Blood 83, 3188–3198.
6 Simmons, D. and Seed, B. (1988) J. Immunol. 141, 2797–2800.

CD34 Sgp90

Molecular weights
Polypeptide   37319

SDS-PAGE
  reduced   90–120 kDa
  unreduced   90–120 kDa

Carbohydrate
N-linked sites   9
O-linked   +++

Human gene location and size
1q32; ~26 kb [1]

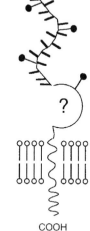

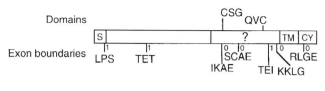

Domains

CSG QVC

S ? TM CY

Exon boundaries
LPS   TET   SCAE   RLGE
IKAE   TEI KKLG

COOH

Tissue distribution

CD34 is expressed on a small subpopulation (1–4%) of bone marrow cells which includes haematopoietic stem cells (HSC). It is also present on bone marrow stromal cells and on most endothelial cells [1,2]. Although a marker for primitive HSC in humans, CD34 has been reported to be absent from these cells in the mouse [3,4].

Structure

CD34 is a highly glycosylated type I transmembrane glycoprotein. The first 130 amino acids are predicted to be heavily O-glycosylated and have a mucin-like structure [2]. This is followed by a sequence of about 100 amino acids that can be expected to have a globular structure, based on the presence of six Cys residues [2]. The cytoplasmic domain contains two sites for protein kinase C phosphorylation (and is phosphorylated following PKC activation [5]) and one site for tyrosine phosphorylation [2]. A splice-variant of CD34 encodes a truncated protein lacking most of the cytoplasmic domain [6,7].

Ligands and associated molecules

CD62L (L-selectin) binds to sialoglycoconjugates present on a subpopulation of CD34 glycoforms; this binding requires sulfation and probably fucosylation of CD34 [8,9]. CD62E (E-selectin) can also bind CD34 [10].

Function

The ability of CD34 to bind the selectins CD62L and CD62E and its expression on endothelium suggests a role in leucocyte-endothelial interactions [11]. In support of this, CD34 is the major CD62L ligand in tonsillar high-endothelial venules and can mediate attachment and rolling of leucocytes *in vitro* [10]. Curiously, CD34-deficient mice exhibit no detectable abnormality in neutrophil or lymphocyte trafficking but show decreased eosinophil accumulation in the lung following inhalation of allergen [12]. Only minor haematopoietic defects have been reported in CD34-deficient mice [12,13].

Database accession numbers

	PIR	SWISSPROT	EMBL/GENBANK	REFERENCE
Human	A38078	P28906	M81104	2
Mouse			S69293	14

Amino acid sequence of human CD34

```
MPRGWTALCL LSLLPSGFM                                           -1
SLDNNGTATP ELPTQGTFSN VSTNVSYQET TTPSTLGSTS LHPVSQHGNE         50
ATTNITETTV KFTSTSVITS VYGNTNSSVQ SQTSVISTVF TTPANVSTPE        100
TTLKPSLSPG NVSDLSTTST SLATSPTKPY TSSSPILSDI KAEIKCSGIR        150
EVKLTQGICL EQNKTSSCAE FKKDRGEGLA RVLCGEEQAD ADAGAQVCSL        200
LLAQSEVRPQ CLLLVLANRT EISSKLQLMK KHQSDLKKLG ILDFTEQDVA        250
SHQSYSQKTL IALVTSGALL AVLGITGYFL MNRRSWSPTG ERLGEDPYYT        300
ENGGGQGYSS GPGTSPEAQG KASVNRGAQK NGTGQATSRN GHSARQHVVA        350
DTEL                                                         354
```

References
1 Satterthwaite, A.B. et al. (1992) Genomics 12, 788–794.
2 Simmons, D.L. et al. (1992) J. Immunol. 148, 267–271.
3 Andrews, R.G. et al. (1990) J. Exp. Med. 172, 355–358.
4 Osawa, M. et al. (1996) Science 273, 242–245.
5 Fackler, M.J. et al. (1990) J. Biol. Chem. 265, 11056–11061.
6 Nakamura, Y. et al. (1993) Exp. Hematol. 21, 236–242.
7 Fackler, M.J. et al. (1995) Blood 85, 3040–3047.
8 Baumhueter, S. et al. (1993) Science 262, 436–438.
9 Rosen, S.D. and Bertozzi, C.R. (1996) Curr. Biol. 6, 261–264.
10 Puri, K.D. et al. (1995) J. Cell. Biol. 131, 261–270.
11 Lasky, L.A. (1995) Annu. Rev. Biochem. 64, 113–139.
12 **Suzuki, A. et al. (1996) Blood 87, 3550–3562.**
13 **Cheng, J. et al. (1996) Blood 87, 479–490.**
14 Brown, J. et al. (1991) Int. Immunol. 3, 175–184.

Molecular weights
Polypeptide (A or F allotype): 219 638

SDS-PAGE
reduced	250 kDa
unreduced	190 kDa

Carbohydrate
N-linked sites	20
O-linked sites	unknown

Human gene location and size
1q32; 140 kb [1]

A allotype

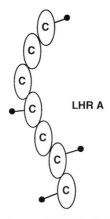

LHR A

3 more LRHs (B, C & D)

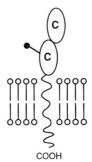

COOH

		CNA	DRC	CRN	PIC	CGL	PQC	CTP	PSC	CQP	PTC	CDD	PVC	CPS	PRC
Domains LHR-A	S	C		C		C		C		C		C		C	

	CQA	DVC	CKT	PJC	CGL	PQC	CTP	PSC	CQP	PTC	CDD	PVC	CPS	PRC
Domains LHR-B	C		C		C		C		C		C		C	

	CQA	DVC	CKT	PIC	CGL	PQC	CTP	PSC	CQP	PRC	CDD	PVC	CPN	PKC
Domains LHR-C	C		C		C		C		C		C		C	

	CKT	DNC	CGP	PIC	CEP	PRC	CTA	PHC	CQP	PRC	CDA	PVC	CPN	PRC
Domains LHR-D	C		C		C		C		C		C		C	

	CPH	HYC	CSF	AKC			
Domains	C		C		TM	CY

Tissue distribution

CD35 is found on erythrocytes, B cells, a subset of T cells, monocytes, neutrophils, eosinophils, follicular dendritic cells and kidney glomerular podocytes [1,2].

Structure

Four CD35 allotypes (A (or F), B (or S), C and D) have been identified in humans. The extracellular domain of the most common (82%) A allotype is composed of 30 complement control protein (CCP) domains. Sequence comparisons show that its first 28 CCP domains are arranged in four long homologous repeats (LHR-A, -B, -C, and -D) each of which contains seven CCP domains. The B allotype (18%) has five LHRs. The C and D allotypes are rare (<0.01%) and from protein size estimates are presumed to have three and six LHRs, respectively [1–5].

Ligands and associated molecules

CD35 binds the complement components C3b and C4b.

Function

CD35 mediates neutrophil and monocyte phagocytosis of particles coated with C3b and/or C4b. This interaction also enhances phagocytosis mediated by the Fc receptors. Expression of CD35 is important for clearance of complement-containing immune complexes by the liver and spleen [1,2]. CD35 is a complex receptor with one binding site for C4b in LHR-A and two binding sites for C3b in LHR-B and LHR-C. In each case, the binding site is located in the first four CCP domains within each LHR [6,7]. CD35 is also a regulator of both the classical and alternative complement pathways. It accelerates the dissociation of the C3-convertase complexes (also mediated by the decay accelerating factor CD55), and acts as a cofactor for the factor I-mediated cleavage of C3b and C4b (also mediated by CD46) [1,2].

Comments

The CD35 gene is located within the regulators of complement activation (RCA) gene complex on chromosome 1q32 which also contains the genes for CD21, CD35, CD46, CD55, factor H, and the two subunits of the C4 binding protein, all of which contain CCP domains [8]. This region appears to have evolved rapidly in mammals because in many cases homologues of these genes have not been identified in other species. Furthermore, those homologues identified often differ in structure, expression, and function. For example, the most abundant form of CD35 on chimpanzee erythrocytes has only one LHR (equivalent to LHR-A) and binds both C3b and C4b [9–11]. Mice lack a structural equivalent of human CD35 but instead have a single gene that codes for both CR1 and CR2 [12–14]. Mouse CR2 has 15 CCP domains and CR1 contains an additional six CCP at its N-terminus. These additional CCP domains confer C3b binding activity. A related mouse gene Crry encodes a membrane protein with five CCP domains. The sequence of the first four CCP domains of Crry are most similar to the first four CCP domains of human CD35. However, Crry can mediate both decay accelerating activity (like CD55) and cofactor activity (like CD46) for both the classical and alternative complement activation pathways[15]. The CR1/Crry regulatory proteins of the rat are different yet again[16-18].

Database accession numbers

	PIR	SWISSPROT	EMBL/GENBANK	REFERENCE
Human	S03843	P17927	Y00816	3,4
	A28507		X05309	
Mouse (Crry)	A43519		M34164–74	12
Mouse (CR1)			M36470	13

Amino acid sequence of human CD35

```
MGASSPRSPE PVGPPAPGLP FCCGGSLLAV VVLLALPVAW G            -1
QCNAPEWLPF ARPTNLTDEF EFPIGTYLNY ECRPGYSGRP FSIICLKNSV    50
WTGAKDRCRR KSCRNPPDPV NGMVHVIKGI QFGSQIKYSC TKGYRLIGSS   100
SATCIISGDT VIWDNETPIC DRIPCGLPPT ITNGDFISTN RENFHYGSVV   150
TYRCNPGSGG RKVFELVGEP SIYCTSNDDQ VGIWSGPAPQ CIIPNKCTPP   200
NVENGILVSD NRSLFSLNEV VEFRCQPGFV MKGPRRVKCQ ALNKWEPELP   250
SCSRVCQPPP DVLHAERTQR DKDNFSPGQE VFYSCEPGYD LRGAASMRCT   300
PQGDWSPAAP TCEVKSCDDF MGQLLNGRVL FPVNLQLGAK VDFVCDEGFQ   350
LKGSSASYCV LAGMESLWNS SVPVCEQIFC PSPPVIPNGR HTGKPLEVFP   400
FGKAVNYTCD PHPDRGTSFD LIGESTIRCT SDPQGNGVWS SPAPRCGILG   450
HCQAPDHFLF AKLKTQTNAS DFPIGTSLKY ECRPEYYGRP FSITCLDNLV   500
WSSPKDVCKR KSCKTPPDPV NGMVHVITDI QVGSRINYSC TTGHRLIGHS   550
SAECILSGNA AHWSTKPPIC QRIPCGLPPT IANGDFISTN RENFHYGSVV   600
TYRCNPGSGG RKVFELVGEP SIYCTSNDDQ VGIWSGPAPQ CIIPNKCTPP   650
NVENGILVSD NRSLFSLNEV VEFRCQPGFV MKGPRRVKCQ ALNKWEPELP   700
SCSRVCQPPP DVLHAERTQR DKDNFSPGQE VFYSCEPGYD LRGAASMRCT   750
PQGDWSPAAP TCEVKSCDDF MGQLLNGRVL FPVNLQLGAK VDFVCDEGFQ   800
LKGSSASYCV LAGMESLWNS SVPVCEQIFC PSPPVIPNGR HTGKPLEVFP   850
FGKAVNYTCD PHPDRGTSFD LIGESTIRCT SDPQGNGVWS SPAPRCGILG   900
HCQAPDHFLF AKLKTQTNAS DFPIGTSLKY ECRPEYYGRP FSITCLDNLV   950
WSSPKDVCKR KSCKTPPDPV NGMVHVITDI QVGSRINYSC TTGHRLIGHS  1000
SAECILSGNT AHWSTKPPIC QRIPCGLPPT IANGDFISTN RENFHYGSVV  1050
TYRCNLGSRG RKVFELVGEP SIYCTSNDDQ VGIWSGPAPQ CIIPNKCTPP  1100
NVENGILVSD NRSLFSLNEV VEFRCQPGFV MKGPRRVKCQ ALNKWEPELP  1150
SCSRVCQPPP EILHGEHTPS HQDNFSPGQE VFYSCEPGYD LRGAASLHCT  1200
PQGDWSPEAP RCAVKSCDDF LGQLPHGRVL FPLNLQLGAK VSFVCDEGFR  1250
LKGSSVSHCV LVGMRSLWNN SVPVCEHIFC PNPPAILNGR HTGTPSGDIP  1300
YGKEISYTCD PHPDRGMTFN LIGESTIRCT SDPHGNGVWS SPAPRCELSV  1350
RAGHCKTPEQ FPFASPTIPI NDFEFPVGTS LNYECRPGYF GKMFSISCLE  1400
NLVWSSVEDN CRRKSCGPPP EPFNGMVHIN TDTQFGSTVN YSCNEGFRLI  1450
GSPSTTCLVS GNNVTWDKKA PICEIISCEP PPTISNGDFY SNNRTSFHNG  1500
TVVTYQCHTG PDGEQLFELV GERSIYCTSK DDQVGVWSSP PPRCISTNKC  1550
TAPEVENAIR VPGNRSFFSL TEIIRFRCQP GFVMVGSHTV QCQTNGRWGP  1600
```

```
KLPHCSRVCQ PPPEILHGEH TLSHQDNFSP GQEVFYSCEP SYDLRGAASL   1650
HCTPQGDWSP EAPRCTVKSC DDFLGQLPHG RVLLPLNLQL GAKVSFVCDE   1700
GFRLKGRSAS HCVLAGMKAL WNSSVPVCEQ IFCPNPPAIL NGRHTGTPFG   1750
DIPYGKEISY ACDTHPDRGM TFNLIGESSI RCTSDPQGNG VWSSPAPRCE   1800
LSVPAACPHP PKIQNGHYIG GHVSLYLPGM TISYTCDPGY LLVGKGFIFC   1850
TDQGIWSQLD HYCKEVNCSF PLFMNGISKE LEMKKVYHYG DYVTLKCEDG   1900
YTLEGSPWSQ CQADDRWDPP LAKCTSRAHD ALIVGTLSGT IFFILLIIFL   1950
SWIILKHRKG NNAHENPKEV AIHLHSQGGS SVHPRTLQTN EENSRVLP     1998
```

References

1   Fearon, D.T. and Ahearn, J.M. (1989) Curr. Topics Microbiol. Immunol. 155, 83–98.
2   **Ahearn, J.M. and Fearon, D.T. (1989) Adv. Immunol. 46, 183–219.**
3   Klickstein, L.B. et al. (1987) J. Exp. Med. 165, 1095–1112.
4   Klickstein, L.B. et al. (1988) J. Exp. Med. 168, 1699–1717.
5   Wong, W.W. et al. (1989) J. Exp. Med. 169, 847–863.
6   Krych, M. et al. (1991) Proc. Natl Acad. Sci. USA 88, 4353–4357.
7   Kalli, D.R. et al. (1991) J. Exp. Med. 174, 1451–1460.
8   Hourcade, D. et al. (1992) Genomics 12, 289–300.
9   Birmingham, D.J. et al. (1994) J. Immunol. 153, 691–700.
10 Nickells, M.W. et al. (1995) J. Immunol. 154, 2829–2837.
11 **Subramanian, V.B. et al. (1996) J. Immunol. 157, 1242–1247.**
12 Paul, M.S. et al. (1990) J. Immunol. 144, 1988–1996.
13 Kurtz, C.B. et al. (1990) J. Immunol. 144, 3581–3591.
14 Molina, H. et al. (1992). J. Exp. Med. 175, 121–129.
15 **Kim, Y.U. et al. (1995) J. Exp. Med. 151–159.**
16 Funabashi, K. et al. (1994) Immunology 81, 444–451.
17 Takizawa, H. et al. (1994) J. Immunol. 152, 3032–3038.
18 Quigg, R.I. and Holers, V.M. (1995) J. Immunol. 155, 1481–1488.

CD36

Platelet glycoprotein IV, FAT (rat)

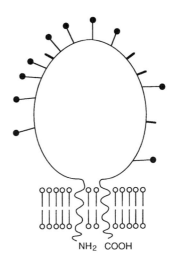

Molecular weights
Polypeptide   53 053

SDS-PAGE
  reduced   88 kDa
  unreduced   88 kDa

Carbohydrate
N-linked sites   10
O-linked   +

Human gene location and size
7q11.2; >32 kb [1]

NH₂ COOH

Tissue distribution

CD36 expression is restricted to platelets, monocytes, macrophages, erythrocyte precursors, adipocytes, activated keratinocytes, and some endothelial and epithelial cells (reviewed in ref. 2). In the mouse, CD36 is expressed in B cells [3].

Structure

CD36 is thought to have two transmembrane regions, short N- and C-terminal cytoplasmic tails, and a heavily glycosylated extracellular region [2,4]. This model is controversial, since an extracellular location for the N-terminus has also been proposed [5]. However, recent data has shown both N- and C-termini to be palmitoylated at cysteine residues 3, 7, 464 and 466, and the N-terminus to be membrane anchored [4]. CD36 is a member of a superfamily that includes the receptor for high-density lipoprotein SR-BI (also known as CLA-1), the lysosomal protein LIMP II, and the *Drosophila* epithelial molecule Emp (see ref. 4). CD36 mRNA exhibits considerable size heterogeneity as a result of alternate splicing of 5'-untranslated and 3'-untranslated exons. In addition, skipping of coding exons 4 and 5, in an erythroleukaemia cell line, generates a CD36 isoform of 57 kD that lacks amino acids 41–143 in the extracellular region [6]. CD36 has been proposed as a candidate gene through which the transcription factor Oct-2 could affect B cell differentiation in the mouse [3].

Ligands and associated molecules

A number of different ligands have been identified for CD36: the extracellular matrix components collagen [2] and thrombospondin [7]; oxidized low-density lipoprotein [8]; fatty acids [9]; anionic phospholipids [10]; and *Plasmodium falciparum* erythrocyte membrane protein 1 (PfEMP1) [11]. CD36 associates non-covalently with the Src family protein tyrosine kinases Fyn, Lyn and Yes [2].

Function

CD36 is a multifunctional glycoprotein that has roles as a cell adhesion molecule, a scavenger receptor, a signal transducer and in the pathogenesis of malaria. CD36 on macrophages functions in the phagocytic clearance of apoptotic cells, which is thought to involve an interaction of CD36 with thrombospondin [7]. An interaction between CD36 and anionic phospholipids in the outer leaflet of the plasma membrane may contribute to the recognition of apoptotic cells by macrophages [10]. CD36 is also a macrophage scavenger receptor for oxidized low-density lipoprotein, and is therefore predicted to play a part in atherogenesis [8]. CD36 has a role in platelet function as a receptor for collagen [2]. CD36 appears to transduce signals through its associated Src family protein tyrosine kinases. Following ligand binding, a signal transduction cascade is initiated which can activate platelets and lead to an oxidative burst in platelets and macrophages [2]. On adipocytes, CD36 is involved in the binding and transport into the cell of long-chain fatty acids [9]. CD36 has a direct role in *Plasmodium falciparum* malaria pathogenesis as an endothelial cell receptor for PfEMP1, a large antigenically variant malarial protein expressed on the surface of parasitized erythrocytes [11].

Database accession numbers

	PIR	SWISSPROT	EMBL/GENBANK	REFERENCE
Human	A30989	P16671	M24795	12
Rat		Q07969	L19658	13
Mouse		Q08857	L23108	14

Amino acid sequence of human CD36

```
MGCDRNCGLI AGAVIGAVLA VFGGILMPVG DLLIQKTIKK QVVLEEGTIA    50
FKNWVKTGTE VYRQFWIFDV QNPQEVMMNS SNIQVKQRGP YTYRVRFLAK   100
ENVTQDAEDN TVSFLQPNGA IFEPSLSVGT EADNFTVLNL AVAAASHIYQ   150
NQFVQMILNS LINKSKSSMF QVRTLRELLW GYRDPFLSLV PYPVTTTVGL   200
FYPYNNTADG VYKVFNGKDN ISKVAIIDTY KGKRNLSYWE SHCDMINGTD   250
AASFPPFVEK SQVLQFFSSD ICRSIYAVFE SDVNLKGIPV YRFVLPSKAF   300
ASPVENPDNY CFCTEKIISK NCTSYGVLDI SKCKEGRPVY ISLPHFLYAS   350
PDVSEPIDGL NPNEEEHRTY LDIEPITGFT LQFAKRLQVN LLVKPSEKIQ   400
VLKNLKRNYI VPILWLNETG TIGDEKANMF RSQVTGKINL LGLIEMILLS   450
VGVVMFVAFM ISYCACRSKT IK                                472
```

References

1 Armesilla, A.L. and Vega, M.A. (1994) J. Biol. Chem. 269, 18985–18991.
2 **Greenwalt, D.E. et al. (1992) Blood 80, 1105–1115.**
3 König, H. et al. (1995) Genes Dev. 9, 1598–1607.
4 **Tao, N. et al. (1996) J. Biol. Chem. 271, 22315–22320.**
5 Pearce, S.F.A. et al. (1994) Blood 84, 384–389.
6 Tang, Y. et al. (1994) J. Biol. Chem. 269, 6011–6015.
7 Navazo, M.D.P. et al. (1996) J. Biol. Chem. 271, 15381–15385.
8 Nozaki, S. et al. (1995) J. Clin. Invest. 96, 1859–1865.
9 Ibrahimi, A. et al. (1996) Proc. Natl Acad. Sci. USA 93, 2646–2651.
10 Rigotti, A. et al. (1995) J. Biol. Chem. 270, 16221–16224.

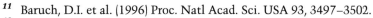

[11] Baruch, D.I. et al. (1996) Proc. Natl Acad. Sci. USA 93, 3497–3502.
[12] Oquendo, P. et al. (1989) Cell 58, 95–101.
[13] Abumrad, N.A. et al. (1993) J. Biol. Chem. 268, 17665–17668.
[14] Endemann, G. et al. (1993) J. Biol. Chem. 268, 11811–11816.

CD37

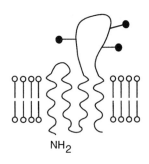

Molecular weights
Polypeptide   31 703

SDS-PAGE
reduced   40–52 kDa

Carbohydrates
N-linked sites   3
O-linked   nil

Human gene location
19p13–q13.4

NH$_2$

Tissue distribution

CD37 was originally defined as an antigen of mature B lymphocytes. It is highly expressed on mature B cells, but not on pre-B cells or plasma cells. There is low expression on T cells, neutrophils, monocytes and some myelomonocytic leukaemia cells. CD37 is not expressed by NK cells, platelets or erythrocytes. Immunoelectron microscopy has shown that a large proportion of CD37 protein is present in intracellular vesicles [1].

Structure

CD37 is a member of the TM4 superfamily and is predicted to have four trans-membrane regions, short cytoplasmic N- and C-termini, and two extracellular regions (reviewed in ref. 2). CD37 is heavily glycosylated at three N-linked sites but there is no O-linked carbohydrate [1]. Gene mapping data suggest that CD37 and CD53 have evolved by gene duplication and divergence from a common ancestral gene [3].

Ligands and associated molecules

CD37 on B cells associates non-covalently with MHC Class II, CD19, CD21 and the TM4SF molecules CD53, CD81 and CD82 [4]. No extracellular ligand has been identified for CD37.

Function

Unknown.

Database accession numbers

	PIR	SWISSPROT	EMBL/GENBANK	REFERENCE
Human	A47629	P11049	X14046	5,6
Rat	B47629	P31053	X53517	5,6
Mouse			U18367–U18372	7

Amino acid sequence of human CD37

```
MSAQESCLSL IKYFLFVFNL FFFVLGSLIF CFGIWILIDK TSFVSFVGLA      50
FVPLQIWSKV LAISGIFTMG IALLGCVGAL KELRCLLGLY FGMLLLLFAT     100
QITLGILIST QRAQLERSLR DVVEKTIQKY GTNPEETAAE ESWDYVQFQL     150
RCCGWHYPQD WFQVLILRGN GSEAHRVPCS CYNLSATNDS TILDKVILPQ     200
LSRLGHLARS RHSADICAVP AESHIYREGC AQGLQKWLHN NLISIVGICL     250
GVGLLELGFM TLSIFLCRNL DHVYNRLARY R                         281
```

References

1. Schwartz-Albiez, R. et al. (1988) J. Immunol. 140, 905–914.
2. **Wright, M.D. and M.G. Tomlinson (1994) Immunol. Today 15, 588–594.**
3. Wright, M.D. et al. (1993) Int. Immunol. 5, 209–216.
4. Angelisova, P. et al. (1994) Immunogenetics 39, 249–256.
5. Classon, B.J. et al. (1989) J. Exp. Med. 169, 1497–1502.
6. Classon, B.J. et al. (1990) J. Exp. Med. 172, 1007.
7. Tomlinson, M.G. and Wright, M.D. (1996) Mol. Immunol. 33, 867–872.

CD38 T10

Other names
ADP-ribosyl cyclase
Cyclic ADP-ribose hydrolase

Molecular weights
Polypeptide   34 301

SDS-PAGE
  reduced   46 kDa
  unreduced   46 kDa

Carbohydrate
N-linked sites   4
O-linked   unknown

Human gene location
4p15

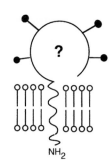

Tissue distribution

CD38 is found on immature cells of the B and T cell lineages, but not on most mature resting peripheral lymphocytes. It is also present on thymocytes, pre-B cells, germinal centre B cells, mitogen-activated T cells, Ig-secreting plasma cells, monocytes, NK cells, erythroid and myeloid progenitors in the bone marrow and brain cells [1-4]. In the mouse, CD38 has been used to subdivide TcR+CD4−CD8− thymocytes, with CD38+ cells biased towards Vβ8.2 expression and capable of producing large amounts of IL-4 following stimulation [5].

Structure

CD38 is a type II membrane glycoprotein, with the transmembrane sequence near the N-terminus [1].

Ligands and associated molecules

The Moon-1 mAb blocks CD38-mediated binding of several cell lines to human vein endothelial cells. Moon-1 recognizes a molecule (120 kDa) expressed by endothelium, monocytes, platelets, NK cells, T cells and B cells [6].

Function

CD38 is a bifunctional enzyme that can synthesize cyclic ADP-ribose (cADPR) from nicotinamide adenine dinucleotide (NAD+) as well as hydrolyse cADPR to ADP-ribose [4]. As such, CD38 might mediate ADP-ribosylation of an as yet uncharacterized physiologic target molecule [7]. Antibodies to human and mouse CD38 have a wide range of biological effects, including the induction of B and T cell proliferation, protection of B cells from apoptosis, inhibition of B lymphopoiesis and enhancement of macrophage APC function [4].

Signalling through CD38 results in Tyr phosphorylation, and activation of the protein kinase Syk, the c-*cbl* proto-oncogene and Bruton Tyr kinase [8-10].

Database accession numbers

	PIR	SWISSPROT	EMBL/GENBANK	REFERENCE
Human	A43521	P28907	M34461	1
Mouse	I49586		L11332	11
Rat	JC2410		D30795	12

Amino acid sequence of human CD38

```
MANCEFSPVS GDKPCCRLSR RAQLCLGVSI LVLILVVVLA VVVPRWRQTW    50
SGPGTTKRFP ETVLARCVKY TEIHPEMRHV DCQSVWDAFK GAFISKHPCN   100
ITEEDYQPLM KLGTQTVPCN KILLWSRIKD LAHQFTQVQR DMFTLEDTLL   150
GYLADDLTWC GEFNTSKINY QSCPDWRKDC SNNPVSVFWK TVSRRFAEAA   200
CDVVHVMLNG SRSKIFDKNS TFGSVEVHNL QPEKVQTLEA WVIHGGREDS   250
RDLCQDPTIK ELESIISKRN IQFSCKNIYR PDKFLQCVKN PEDSSCTSEI   300
```

References
1   Jackson, D.G. and Bell, J. I. (1990) J. Immunol. 144, 2811–2815.
2   Alessio, M. et al. (1990) J. Immunol. 145, 878–884.
3   Mizuguchi, M. et al. (1995) Brain Res. 697, 235–240.
4   **Lund, F. et al. (1995) Immunol. Today 16, 469–473.**
5   Bean, A.G. et al. (1995) Int. Immunol. 7, 213–221.
6   Deaglio, S. et al. (1996) J. Immunol. 156, 727–734.
7   Grimaldi, J.C. et al. (1995) J. Immunol. 155, 811–817.
8   Silvennoinen, O. et al. (1996) J. Immunol. 156, 100–107.
9   Kontani, K. et al. (1996) J. Biol. Chem. 271, 1534–1537.
10 Kikuchi, Y. et al. (1995) Proc. Natl Acad. Sci. USA 92, 11814–11818.
11 Harada, N. et al. (1993) J. Immunol. 151, 3111–3118.
12 Li, Q. et al. (1994) Biochem. Biophys. Res. Commun. 202, 629–636.

CD39

Molecular weights
Polypeptides   57 965

SDS-PAGE
  reduced   78 kDa

Carbohydrate
N-linked sites   4
O-linked sites   unknown

Human gene location
10q23.1–24.1

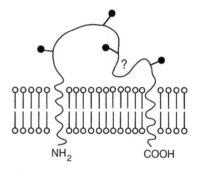

Tissue distribution

CD39 was originally identified on Epstein–Barr virus-transformed B cells [1] and subsequently shown to be present on activated B and NK cells, and subsets of activated T cells. It is not expressed by resting lymphoid cells. CD39 expression in lymphoid tissues is limited to the mantle zone and paracortical lymphocytes, macrophages, dendritic cells and Langerhans cells and is absent from germinal centres [2,3].

Structure

The derived amino acid sequence contains three hydrophobic segments. However the N-terminal segment may be an unusual signal sequence and the central segment may not be membrane-spanning since it is short and contains a Gln and an Asp residue [4]. There is experimental evidence that the C-terminal segment traverses the membrane and is orientated as shown in the figure. However the topology of the remainder of the molecule is not known and the figure shown is a model proposed in ref. 4.

Function

CD39 can mediate B cell homotypic adhesion [2]. The primary sequence of CD39 contains four segments that are characteristic of ecto-apyrase from plants and yeast [5] and transfection of CD39 cDNA into COS cells induces ecto-apyrase activity [6]. ATP, which leaks from damaged cells (e.g. lysed target cells), could be toxic to the lymphocytes. Molecules such as CD39 may protect activated lymphocytes through hydrolysis of extracellular ATP [6].

Database accession numbers

	PIR	SWISSPROT	EMBL/GENBANK	REFERENCE
Human	I56242	P49961	S73813	4

Amino acid sequence of human CD39

```
MEDTKESNVK TFCSKNILAI LGFSSIIAVI ALLAVGLTQN KALPENVKYG      50
IVLDAGSSHT SLYIYKWPAE KENDTGVVHQ VEECRVKGPG ISKFVQKVNE     100
IGIYLTDCME RAREVIPRSQ HQETPVYLGA TAGMRLLRME SEELADRVLD     150
VVERSLSNYP FDFQGARIIT GQEEGAYGWI TINYLLGKFS QKTRWFSIVP     200
YETNNQETFG ALDLGGASTQ VTFVPQNQTI ESPDNALQFR LYGKDYNVYT     250
HSFLCYGKDQ ALWQKLAKDI QVASNEILRD PCFHPGYKKV VNVSDLYKTP     300
CTKRFEMTLP FQQFEIQGIG NYQQCHQSIL ELFNTSYCPY SQCAFNGIFL     350
PPLQGDFGAF SAFYFVMKFL NLTSEKVSQE KVTEMMKKFC AQPWEEIKTS     400
YAGVKEKYLS EYCFSGTYIL SLLLQGYHFT ADSWEHIHFI GKIQGSDAGW     450
TLGYMLNLTN MIPAEQPLST PLSHSTYVFL MVLFSLVLFT VAIIGLLIFH     500
KPSYFWKDMV                                               510
```

References
[1] Rowe, M. et al. (1982) Int. J. Cancer 29, 373–381.
[2] Kansas, G.S. et al. (1991) J. Immunol. 146, 2235–2244.
[3] Goutefangeas, C. et al. (1992) Eur. J. Immunol. 22, 2681–2685.
[4] **Maliszewski, C.R. et al. (1994) J. Immunol. 153, 3574–3583.**
[5] Handa, M. and Guidotti, G. (1996) Biochem. Biophys. Res. Comm. 218, 916–923.
[6] **Wang, T.F. and Guidotti, G. (1996) J. Biol. Chem. 271, 9898–9901.**

CD40

Molecular weights
Polypeptide   26 989

SDS-PAGE
  reduced   48 kDa
  unreduced   48 kDa

Carbohydrate
N-linked sites   2
O-linked   nil

Human gene location
20q12–q13.2 [1,2]

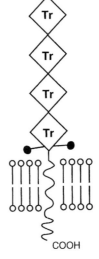

| | CRE | | CGE | | CEE | | CPV | | VVC | | |
| | | TEC | | TIC | | TIC | | | | | |
Domains | S | Tr | | Tr | | Tr | | Tr | | TM | CY |

Tissue distribution

CD40 is found on all mature B lymphocytes but is absent from plasma cells [1,2]. It is also present on some epithelium including thymus and on some endothelial cells [1,2]. It is expressed on lymphoid interdigitating and follicular dendritic cells and activated monocytes [1,2].

Structure

CD40 antigen is a member of the TNFR superfamily and contains four cysteine-rich repeats [1].

Ligands and associated molecules

CD40 binds to CD154, a type II membrane protein of the TNF superfamily. The cytoplasmic domain of CD40 binds to CRAF-1, a member of the TRAF (TNFR-associated proteins) family. Binding is dependent on Thr234 which is an essential residue for signal transduction via CD40 [1]. A novel 23 kDa protein co-precipitates specifically with CD40 [3].

Function

CD154 binding to CD40 on B cells is required for secondary immune responses and germinal centre formation [1,2,4]. Mutations in CD154 which abolish binding to CD40 cause the immunodeficiency disease hyper-IgM syndrome, which is characterized by lack of isotype switching in Ig production and lack of germinal centres [1,2,4]. There is evidence for a role for the CD154–CD40 interaction in negative selection and peripheral tolerance [1,2,4]. Mice deficient in CD40 or CD154 have increased susceptibility to parasite infection [5].

Database accession numbers

	PIR	SWISSPROT	EMBL/GENBANK	REFERENCE
Human	S04460	P25942	X60592	6
Mouse	A46476	P27512	M83312	7

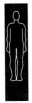

Amino acid sequence of human CD40

```
MVRLPLQCVL WGCLLTAVHP                                      -1
EPPTACREKQ YLINSQCCSL CQPGQKLVSD CTEFTETECL PCGESEFLDT     50
WNRETHCHQH KYCDPNLGLR VQQKGTSETD TICTCEEGWH CTSEACESCV    100
LHRSCSPGFG VKQIATGVSD TICEPCPVGF FSNVSSAFEK CHPWTSCETK    150
DLVVQQAGTN KTDVVCGPQD RLRALVVIPI IFGILFAILL VLVFIKKVAK    200
KPTNKAPHPK QEPQEINFPD DLPGSNTAAP VQETLHGCQP VTQED         245
```

References
1   van Kooten, C. and Banchereau, J. (1996) Adv. Immunol. 61, 1–77.
2   Gruss, H.-J. and Dower, S.K. (1995) Blood 85, 3378–3404.
3   Morio, T. et al. (1995) Proc. Natl Acad. Sci. USA 92, 11633–11636.
4   Foy, T.M. et al. (1996) Annu. Rev. Immunol. 14, 591–617.
5   Noelle, R.J. (1996) Immunity 4, 415–419.
6   Stamenkovic, I. et al. (1989) EMBO J. 8, 1403–1410.
7   Torres, R.M. and Clark, E.A. (1992) J. Immunol. 148, 620–626.

CD41 | GPIIb of the GPIIb/IIIa complex, integrin αIIb subunit

Molecular weights
Polypeptides   110 005

SDS-PAGE
  reduced   125 + 22 kDa
  unreduced   140 kDa

Carbohydrates
N-linked sites   5
O-linked sites   unknown

Human gene location and size
17q21.32; 17 kb [1]

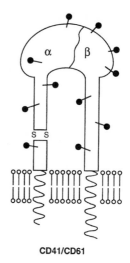

CD41/CD61

Tissue distribution

CD41 is expressed on platelets and megakaryocytes [1,2].

Structure

CD41 is the integrin αIIb subunit that is expressed as a heterodimer non-covalently associated with the integrin β3 subunit CD61 [1,2]. The association between CD41 and CD61 is calcium dependent [3,4]. CD41 is post-translationally cleaved into large (125 kDa) N-terminal and small (22 kDa) fragments which are disulfide-linked [1,2]. The transmembrane sequence is in the smaller fragment. The N-terminal sequences of both fragments have been determined [5,6]. Whereas the N-terminus of the small fragment is usually at residue Gln891, a fragment with the N-terminus at Leu902 has also been detected. Alternatively spliced mRNA which lacks sequence from an exon encoding the 34 residues Arg917–Gln950 has been reported in megakaryotes [7]. The significance of this alternatively spliced mRNA is unclear since this deletion interferes with surface expression of the protein [8]. Intramolecular disulfide bonds are formed between neighbouring cysteines along the primary sequence, beginning at Cys56 [9]. Electron microscopy of purified CD41/CD61 has provided a structural model for all integrins [10].

Ligands and associated proteins

The ligands for CD41/CD61 include fibrinogen, von Willebrand factor, fibronectin, vitronectin, and thrombospondin [11,12]. Binding to these ligands depends on the activation state of the platelets. Unstimulated platelets only bind immobilized fibrinogen. Binding to soluble fibrinogen and other ligands requires stimulation of platelets by agonists such as thrombin, ADP and collagen [11,13]. Binding usually involves an RGD motif on ligands [11-13] but CD41/CD61 also binds to the HHLGGAKQAGDV sequence in the γ chain of

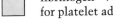

fibrinogen [14]. CD41/CD61 binding to multiple sites on fibrinogen is important for platelet adhesion [15].

Function

CD41/CD61 is the major integrin on platelets and is important for platelet adhesion and aggregation [12]. Three missense mutations (G242D, R327H and G418D – numbered as in the mature protein) have been identified which result in the disease Glanzmann thrombasthenia [16]. Glanzmann thrombasthenia can also be caused by defects in the integrin $\beta3$ subunit (see **CD61**). Mutations of CD41 at Ile843 give rise to the HPA-3 alloantigenic polymorphism [17]. The HPA-3B allele (Ser843) forms an additional O-glycosylation site [17], and is associated with neonatal alloimmune thrombocytopenia [18].

Database accession numbers

	PIR	SWISSPROT	EMBL/GENBANK	REFERENCE [19]
Human	A29522	P08514	J02764	

Amino acid sequence of human CD41

```
MARALCPLQA LWLLEWVLLL LGPCAAPPAW A                      -1
LNLDPVQLTF YAGPNGSQFG FSLDFHKDSH GRVAIVVGAP RTLGPSQEET   50
GGVFLCPWRA EGGQCPSLLF DLRDETRNVG SQTLQTFKAR QGLGASVVSW  100
SDVIVACAPW QHWNVLEKTE EAEKTPVGSC FLAQPESGRR AEYSPCRGNT  150
LSRIYVENDF SWDKRYCEAG FSSVVTQAGE LVLGAPGGYY FLGLLAQAPV  200
ADIFSSYRPG ILLWHVSSQS LSFDSSNPEY FDGYWGYSVA VGEFDGDLNT  250
TEYVVGAPTW SWTLGAVEIL DSYYQRLHRL RAEQMASYFG HSVAVTDVNG  300
DGRHDLLVGA PLYMESRADR KLAEVGRVYL FLQPRGPHAL GAPSLLLTGT  350
QLYGRFGSAI APLGDLDRDG YNDIAVAAPY GGPSGRGQVL VFLGQSEGLR  400
SRPSQVLDSP FPTGSAFGFS LRGAVDIDDN GYPDLIVGAY GANQVAVYRA  450
QPVVKASVQL LVQDSLNPAV KSCVLPQTKT PVSCFNIQMC VGATGHNIPQ  500
KLSLNAELQL DRQKPRQGRR VLLLGSQQAG TTLNLDLGGK HSPICHTTMA  550
FLRDEADFRD KLSPIVLSLN VSLPPTEAGM APAVVLHGDT HVQEQTRIVL  600
DSGEDDVCVP QLQLTASVTG SPLLVGADNV LELQMDAANE GEGAYEAELA  650
VHLPQGAHYM RALSNVEGFE RLICNQKKEN ETRVVLCELG NPMKKNAQIG  700
IAMLVSVGNL EEAGESVSFQ LQIRSKNSQN PNSKIVLLDV PVRAEAQVEL  750
RGNSFPASLV VAAEEGEREQ NSLDSWGPKV EHTYELHNNG PGTVNGLHLS  800
IHLPGQSQPS DLLYILDIQP QGGLQCFPQP PVNPLKVDWG LPIPSPSPIH  850
PAHHKRDRRQ IFLPEPEQPS RLQDPVLVSC DSAPCTVVQC DLQEMARGQR  900
AMVTVLAFLW LPSLYQRPLD QFVLQSHAWF NVSSLPYAVP PLSLPRGEAQ  950
VWTQLLRALE ERAIPIWWVL VGVLGGLLLL TILVLAMWKV GFFKRNRPPL 1000
EEDDEEGE                                              1008
```

References

1 **Kieffer, N. and Phillips, D.R. (1990)** Annu. Rev. Cell Biol. 6, 334–357.
2 Pigott, R. and Power, C. (1993) The Adhesion Molecule FactsBook. Academic Press, London.
3 Jennings, L.K. and Phillips, D.R. (1982) J. Biol. Chem. 257, 10458–10466.
4 Weisel, J.W. et al. (1992) J. Biol. Chem. 267, 16637–16643.
5 Charo, I.F. et al. (1986) Proc. Natl Acad. Sci. USA 83, 8351–8355.
6 Loftus, J.C. et al. (1988) J. Biol. Chem. 263, 11025–11028.

7 Bray, P.F. et al. (1990) J. Biol. Chem. 265, 9587–9590.

8 Kolodziej, M.A. et al. (1992) Blood 78, 2344–2353.

9 Calvette, J.J. et al. (1989) Biochem. J. 261, 561–568.

10 Carrell, N.A. et al. (1985) J. Biol. Chem. 260, 1743–1749.

11 **Phillips, D.R. et al. (1991) Cell 65, 359–362.**

12 Du, X. et al. (1991) Cell 65, 409–416.

13 Ginsberg, M.H. et al. (1993) Thromb. Haemost. 70, 87–93.

14 D'Souza, S.E. et al. (1991) Nature 350, 66–68.

15 Savage, B. et al. (1995) J. Biol. Chem. 270, 28812–28817.

16 Bray, P.F. (1994) Thromb. Haemost. 72, 492–502.

17 Calvette, J.J. and Muniz-Diaz, E. (1993) FEBS Lett. 328, 30–34.

18 Lymen, S. et al. (1990) Blood 75, 2343–2348.

19 Poncz, M. et al. (1987) J. Biol. Chem. 262, 8476–8482.

CD42a, b   GPIX (CD42a), GPIB (CD42b)

Molecular weights

Polypeptides	CD42a	17 259
	CD42bα	67 193
	CD42bβ	19 320

SDS-PAGE

unreduced	CD42a	22 kDa
	CD42b	160–170 kDa
reduced	CD42a	17–22 kDa
	CD42bα	135–145 kDa
	CD42bβ	22–25 kDa

Carbohydrate

N-linked sites	CD42a	1
	CD42bα	4
	CD42bβ	1
O-linked	CD42bα	
		+ abundant

Human gene location and size
CD42bα: 17pter–p12; ~3.4 kb [1]

Tissue distribution

Restricted to platelets and megakaryocytes. Red blood cells, granulocytes, T cells and thymocytes do not express CD42a,b. The CD42a,b complex is a major component of the platelet surface (25 000 copies per platelet) [2].

Structure

Each polypeptide starts with a region of about 30 amino acids that shares sequence similarities among the chains. This is followed by a region of Leu-rich repeats (LRR) [3]. There is one in each of the CD42a and CD42bβ chains and seven in the CD42bα chain. Following the LRR repeats is another region of about 60 amino acids in each chain that shows sequence similarities and is likely to have a globular structure as deduced from the presence of four conserved Cys residues. For CD42a and CD42bβ the transmembrane sequence then follows whereas in CD42bα a region of about 150 amino acids containing a high level of Ser, Thr and Pro residues precedes the transmembrane sequence. This is likely to be heavily O-glycosylated and can be deduced to be about 35 nm in length as revealed by electron micrographs[4]. The diagram shown is based on the electron micrographs of the CD42 complex which show two globular regions 9 nm and 16 nm in diameter separated by a narrow stalk 35 nm in length[4]. The small globular region is presumed to consist of the region of CD42bα that shows sequence similarity to the CD42a and CD42bβ chains. CD42bα and CD42bβ are disulfide linked[2,3]. CD42a, CD42bα and CD42bβ together with GPV form a multimeric complex at the cell surface[2,3]. CD42a and GPV, another LRR-containing polypeptide, associate with the complex non-covalently[2,3]. The protein sequence of CD42bα is encoded by a single exon[1].

Ligands and associated molecules

CD42bα binds to von Willebrand factor[3]. The binding site on CD42bα lies in a hinge region between the LRR motifs and the stalk[3]. Snake venom proteins bind to CD42b and inhibit binding of von Willebrand factor[5]. CD42b is also a receptor for thrombin, possibly only when the CD42–GP V complex is highly multimeric as there are only 50 sites per platelet[6].

Function

Binding of CD42b to von Willebrand factor bound to exposed subendothelial surfaces is essential for platelet adhesion at sites of injury[3]. A bleeding disorder, Bernard–Soulier syndrome, is characterized by defects in CD42a,b expression[3].

Database accession numbers

	PIR	SWISSPROT	EMBL/GENBANK	REFERENCE
CD42a	A33731	P14770	X52997	7
CD42bα	A27075	P07359	J02940	8
CD42bβ	B26864	P13224	J03259	9

Amino acid sequence of human CD42a

```
MPAWGALFLL WATAEA                                              -1
TKDCPSPCTC RALETMGLWV DCRGHGLTAL PALPARTRHL LLANNSLQSV         50
PPGAFDHLPQ LQTLDVTQNP WHCDCSLTYL RLWLEDRTPE ALLQVRCASP        100
SLAAHGPLRL TGYQLGSCGW QLQASWVRPG VLWDVALVAV AALGLALLAG        150
LLCATTEALD                                                    160
```

Amino acid sequence of human CD42b α chain

```
MPLLLLLLLL PSPLHP                                            -1
HPICEVSKVA SHLEVNCDKR NLTALPPDLP KDTTILHLSE NLLYTFSLAT       50
LMPYTRLTQL NLDRCELTKL QVDGTLPVLG TLDLSHNQLQ SLPLLGQTLP       100
ALTVLDVSFN RLTSLPLGAL RGLGELQELY LKGNELKTLP PGLLTPTPKL       150
EKLSLANNNL TELPAGLLNG LENLDTLLLQ ENSLYTIPKG FFGSHLLPFA       200
FLHGNPWLCN CEILYFRRWL QDNAENVYVW KQGVDVKAMT SNVASVQCDN       250
SDKFPVYKYP GKGCPTLGDE GDTDLYDYYP EEDTEGDKVR ATRTVVKFPT       300
KAHTTPWGLF YSWSTASLDS QMPSSLHPTQ ESTKEQTTFP PRWTPNFTLH       350
MESITFSKTP KSTTEPTPSP TTSEPVPEPA PNMTTLEPTP SPTTPEPTSE       400
PAPSPTTPEP TPIPTIATSP TILVSATSLI TPKSTFLTTT KPVSLLESTK       450
KTIPELDQPP KLRGVLQGHL ESSRNDPFLH PDFCCLLPLG FYVLGLFWLL       500
FASVVLILLL SWVGHVKPQA LDSGQGAALT TATQTTHLEL QRGRQVTVPR       550
AWLLFLRGSL PTFRSSLFLW VRPNGRVGPL VAGRRPSALS QGRGQDLLST       600
VSIRYSGHSL                                                   610
```

Amino acid sequence of human CD42b β chain

```
MGSGPRGALS LLLLLLAPPS RPAAG                                  -1
CPAPCSCAGT LVDCGRRGLT WASLPTAFPV DTTELVLTGN NLTALPPGLL       50
DALPALRTAH LGANPWRCDC RLVPLRAWLA GRPERAPYRD LRCVAPPALR       100
GRLLPYLAED ELRAACAPGP LCWGALAAQL ALLGLGLLHA LLLVLLLCRL       150
RRLRARARAR AAARLSLTDP LVAERAGTDE S                           181
```

References
1 Wenger, R.H. et al. (1988) Biochem. Biophys. Res. Commun. 156, 389–395.
2 Lopez, J.A. et al. (1996) J. Biol. Chem. 269, 23716–23721.
3 **Roth, G.J. (1992) Immunol. Today, 13, 100–105.**
4 Fox, J.E.B. et al. (1988) J. Biol. Chem. 263, 4882–4890.
5 Kawasaki, T. et al. (1996) J. Biol. Chem. 271, 10635–10639.
6 Greco, N.J. et al. (1996) Biochemistry 35, 906–914.
7 Hickey, M.J. et al. (1989) Proc. Natl Acad. Sci. USA 86, 6773–6777.
8 Lopez, J.A. et al. (1987) Proc. Natl Acad. Sci. USA 84, 5615–5619.
9 Lopez, J.A. et al. (1988) Proc. Natl Acad. Sci. USA 85, 2135–2139.

CD43 | Leukosialin, sialophorin, Ly-48 (mouse), W3/13 (rat)

Molecular weights
Polypeptide   38 801

SDS-PAGE
   reduced   neutrophils and platelets   115–135 kDa
              T cells and thymocytes   95–115 kDa

Carbohydrate
N-linked sites   1
O-linked   + abundant

Human gene location and size
16p11.2; 4.6 kb [1]

COOH

Tissue distribution

CD43 is the major sialoglycoprotein on thymocytes, T cells and neutrophils [2,3]. It is also present on activated (but not resting) B cells, plasma cells, NK cells, granulocytes, monocytes, macrophages, platelets, and bone marrow haematopoietic stem cells [1]. Activation of neutrophils leads to downregulation of CD43 as a result of proteolytic cleavage [4]. A soluble form of CD43, called galactoglycoprotein, is present in human serum [5].

Structure

The CD43 extracellular domain of 239 amino acids is mucin-like with a high content of Ser and Thr residues that carry 70–85 O-linked oligosaccharides [6]. It has an extended structure, approximately 45 nm in length, and contains four repeats of an 18 amino acid sequence [6,7]. The molecular weight of the molecule and its antigenicity varies, depending on the nature of the O-glycans [7]. The cytoplasmic domain is highly conserved between species and is constitutively phosphorylated on Ser residues, probably by protein kinase C [8]. The coding sequence of CD43 is contained within a single exon [1].

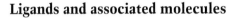

Ligands and associated molecules

The extracellular domain has been reported to interact with CD54, but this is controversial[9]. An interaction with albumin has also been reported[3]. The membrane-proximal portion of the cytoplasmic domain mediates an association with the cytoskeleton[10].

Function

CD43, which is both abundant and very large, appears to function as an anti-adhesion molecule, inhibiting T cell interactions, including T cell killing, and increasing the threshold for T cell activation[9]. Antibodies to CD43 have a co-stimulatory effect on T cell activation[11] and can induce cell clustering[12], but the physiological significance of these effects is not clear. Cells infected with HIV express CD43 with altered glycosylation, and autoantibodies to this form of CD43 are detectable in all HIV-infected individuals[13].

Database accession numbers

	PIR	SWISSPROT	EMBL/GENBANK	REFERENCE
Human	A39822	P16150	J04168	6
Rat	S00842	P13838	Y00090	14
Mouse	A43545	P15702	X17018	15

Amino acid sequence of human CD43

```
MATLLLLLGV LVVSP                                             -1
DALGSTTAVQ TPTSGEPLVS TSEPLSSKMY TTSITSDPKA DSTGDQTSAL       50
PPSTSINEGS PLWTSIGAST GSPLPEPTTY QEVSIKMSSV PQETPHATSH      100
PAVPITANSL GSHTVTGGTI TTNSPETSSR TSGAPVTTAA SSLETSRGTS      150
GPPLTMATVS LETSKGTSGP PVTMATDSLE TSTGTTGPPV TMTTGSLEPS      200
SGASGPQVSS VKLSTMMSPT TSTNASTVPF RNPDENSRGM LPVAVLVALL      250
AVIVLVALLL LWRRRQKRRT GALVLSRGGK RNGVVDAWAG PAQVPEEGAV      300
TVTVGGSGGD KGSGFPDGEG SSRRPTLTTF FGRRKSRQGS LAMEELKSGS      350
GPSLKGEEEP LVASEDGAVD APAPDEPEGG DGAAP                      385
```

References

1 Shelley, C.S. et al. (1990) Biochem. J. 270, 569–576.
2 Brown, W.R.A. et al. (1981) Nature 289, 456–460.
3 Nathan, C. et al. (1993) J. Cell Biol. 122, 243–256.
4 Rieu, P. et al. (1992) Eur. J. Immunol. 22, 3021–3026.
5 Schmid, K. et al. (1992) Proc. Natl Acad. Sci. USA 89, 663–667.
6 Pallant, A. et al. (1989) Proc. Natl Acad. Sci. USA 86, 1328–1332.
7 **Cyster, J.G. et al. (1991) EMBO J. 10, 893–902.**
8 Piller, V. et al. (1989) J. Biol. Chem. 264, 18824–18831.
9 **Manjunath, N. et al. (1995) Nature 377, 535–538.**
10 Yonemura, S. et al. (1993) J. Cell Biol. 120, 437–449.
11 Sperling, A.I. et al. (1995) J. Exp. Med. 182, 139–146.
12 Cyster, J.G. and Williams, A.F. (1992) Eur. J. Immunol. 22, 2565–2572.
13 Giordanengo, V. et al. (1995) Blood 86, 2302–2311.
14 Killeen, N. et al. (1987) EMBO J. 6, 4029–4034.
15 Cyster, J. et al. (1990) Eur. J. Immunol. 20, 875–881.

Other names
Lymphocyte homing receptor
Hermes antigen
In(Lu)-related p80
Extracellular matrix receptor
  type III (ECMRIII)
Hutch-1
Ly-24 (mouse)
p85
HCAM

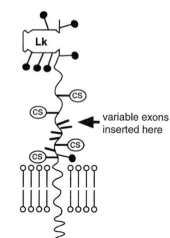

CD44H

variable exons
inserted here

COOH

Molecular weights

Polypeptide	CD44H	37 237
	CD44v	variable

SDS gel		
reduced	CD44H without glycosaminoglycans	80–95 kDa
	Other CD44 variants	110–250 kDa

Carbohydrate

N-linked sites	CD44H	7
O-linked	CD44H	++
	CD44v	+++/++++
Glycosaminoglycans [1]	Chondroitin sulfate (CS) (CD44H and CD44v)	
	Heparan sulfate (CD44v only)	

Human gene location and size
11pter–p13 [2]; 50 kb [3]

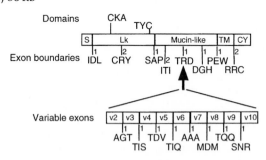

Tissue distribution

The standard form of CD44 without variable exons (CD44H or CD44s) is very widely expressed on haematopoeitic and non-haematopoeitic cells, being present on epithelial, endothelial, mesothelial and mesenchymal cells, and in the nervous system [4]. CD44H is the major isoform expressed on lymphoid, myeloid and erythroid cells[4,5]. Expression is increased on activated and memory/effector T cells[4]. CD44 isoforms encoded by additional variable exons (CD44v) are widely expressed on epithelial cells but are only present at low levels on leucocytes, with the exception of a subpopulation of bone marrow plasma cells[6]. Activation of lymphocytes and monocytes leads to a transient increase in the expression of CD44v isoforms[6]. Soluble forms of CD44 can be detected in body fluids[4]. They are generated by proteolytic shedding and perhaps also by alternative splicing to exons containing stop codons[7].

Structure

Alternative splicing of the CD44 gene can generate a large number of CD44 isoforms, all of which are heavily glycosylated[4]. The standard isoform (CD44H) comprises a membrane-distal link module[8], a membrane-proximal mucin-like region, a transmembrane segment, and a 70 residue cytoplasmic domain. In humans, all other CD44 isoforms (CD44v) are generated by the insertion of various combinations of at least nine exons units (v2–v10) after Thr202 in the mucin-like region, adding up to 380 residues to the extracellular portion[9]. These variable exons also encode mucin-like sequences (~30% Ser/Thr residues)[9]. In addition to carrying O- and N-linked oligosaccharides, proteoglycan isoforms of CD44 have been identified with the covalently linked glycosaminoglycans (GAGs) chondroitin sulfate (CS) and heparan sulfate (HS). One or more of the partial consensus sequences for GAG-modification (SG) in CD44H are modified by CS on lymphocytes[1,4]. However a full consensus sequence (SGxG) encoded by the v3 exon appears to be the primary site for HS modification in CD44v isoforms[1]. The cytoplasmic domain is phosphorylated on serine/threonine residues[4]. Two alleles of CD44 differing at a single residue constitute the India (In) blood group antigens In^a (Arg26) and In^b (Pro26)[10].

Ligands and associated molecules

The membrane-distal link module of CD44 binds the extracellular matrix (ECM) GAG hyaluronan (HA). The ability of CD44 to bind HA is highly regulated[4]. For example, leucocytes expressing CD44 do not bind HA constitutively but are able to bind following activation[4,11]. Molecular mechanism implicated in regulating binding include clustering, altered glycosylation, differential use of exons, and interactions with the cytoskeleton[4]. CD44 has also been reported to bind the ECM proteins collagen, fibronectin and laminin; these interactions are probably mediated by CS carried by CD44[4]. Similarly, CD44 molecules carrying HS can bind growth factors such as basic fibroblast growth factor[12]. HS may also mediate reported interactions between CD44 and chemokines such as macrophage inflammatory protein 1β. CD44 is a receptor for the chemotactic cytokine osteopontin[13]. The cytoplasmic domain interacts with the actin cytoskeleton through associations with ankyrin[14] and members of the ERM (ezrin, radixin and moesin) family[15]. CD44 also associates with (and may activate) the cytoplasmic tyrosine kinase Lck[16].

Function

CD44 contributes to the adhesion of leucocytes to endothelial cells [4,17], stromal cells and ECM [4,18]. These interactions appear to be mediated by CD44 binding to HA associated with cells and ECM [17,18], although alternative ligands may exist [4]. CD44 appears to mediate extravasation of activated and memory/effector lymphocytes (rather than naive lymphocytes) into sites of inflammation (rather than to primary or secondary lymphoid tissues) [4,17,19]. Expression of the v6 exon in the rat confers metastatic potential on tumour cell lines [4]. The same exon is expressed in activated lymphocytes *in vivo* and antibodies specific for this exon inhibit the immune response *in vivo* [4]. Expression of the v3 exon in human B lymphoma cells increases their metastatic potential [20]. This effect does not appear to result from enhanced HA adhesion [20] but does requires an intact HS GAG consensus sequence (SGxG), consistent with a role for growth factor or chemokine binding to HS (D. Jackson, personal communication). CD44 may transduce signals to cells following interactions with ECM [4] or with soluble ligands such as osteopontin [13].

Database accession numbers

	PIR	SWISSPROT	EMBL/GENBANK	REFERENCE
Human CD44H			M33827	21
Human CD44 gene			M69215	3
			L05407–L05424	
Mouse CD44H	A34424	P15379	M27129	22
Rat CD44H		P26051	M61875	23

Amino acid sequence of human CD44H

```
MDKFWWHAAW GLCLVPLSLA                                  -1
QIDLNITCRF AGVFHVEKNG RYSISRTEAA DLCKAFNSTL PTMAQMEKAL  50
SIGFETCRYG FIEGHVVIPR IHPNSICAAN NTGVYILTYN TSQYDTYCFN  100
ASAPPEEDCT SVTDLPNAFD GPITITIVNR DGTRYVQKGE YRTNPEDIYP  150
SNPTDDDVSS GSSSERSSTS GGYIFYTFST VHPIPDEDSP WITDSTDRIP  200
ATRDQDTFHP SGGSHTTHGS ESDGHSHGSQ EGGANTTSGP IRTPQIPEWL  250
IILASLLALA LILAVCIAVN SRRRCGQKKK LVINSGNGAV EDRKPSGLNG  300
EASKSQEMVH LVNKESSETP DQFMTADETR NLQNVDMKIG V           341
```

Notes

1 CD44v isoforms are generated by insertion of additional sequences after Thr202 (bold and underlined).
2 Partial consensus GAG linkage sites (SG) are underlined with dotted lines.

Sequence encoded by variable exons

```
TLMSTSATAT ETATKRQETW DWFSWLFLPS ESKNHLHTTT QMAGTSSNTI  50
SAGWEPNEEN EDERDRHLSF SGSGIDDDED FISSTISTTP RAFDHTKQNQ  100
DWTQWNPSHS NPEVLLQTTT RMTDVDRNGT TAYEGNWNPE AHPPLIHHEH  150
HEEEETPHST STIQATPSST TEETATQKEQ WFGNRWHEGY RQTPREDSHS  200
TTGTAAASAH TSHPMQGRTT PSPEDSSWTD FFNPISHPMG RGHQAGRRMD  250
MDSSHSTTLQ PTANPNTGLV EDLDRTGPLS MTTQQSNSQS FSTSHEGLEE  300
DKDHPTTSTL TSSNRNDVTG GRRDPNHSEG STTLLEGYTS HYPHTKESRT  350
FIPVTSAKTG SFGVTAVTVG DSNSNVNRSL S                      381
```

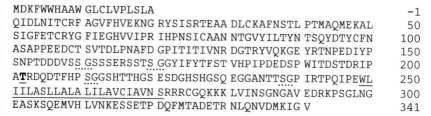

Notes

1 Sequence encoded by exons v2–v10 is shown [9]. In humans exon v1 contains an in-frame stop codon and is probably not used. The underlined residues span the exon splice junctions and can vary with different exon combinations.

2 A full consensus GAG linkage site (SGxG) is underlined with dotted lines.

References

[1] **Jackson, D.G. et al. (1995) J. Cell. Biol. 128, 673–685.**

[2] Forsberg, U.H. et al. (1989) Immunogenetics 29, 405–407.

[3] Screaton, G.R. et al. (1992) Proc. Natl Acad. Sci. USA 89, 12160–12164.

[4] **Lesley, J. et al. (1993) Adv. Immunol. 54, 271–335.**

[5] Schlossman, S.F. et al. (eds) (1995) Leucocyte Typing V: white cell differentiation antigens. Oxford University Press, Oxford.

[6] Mackay, C.R. et al. (1994) J. Cell. Biol. 124, 71–82.

[7] Yu, Q. and Toole, B.P. (1996) J. Biol. Chem. 271, 20603–20607.

[8] Kohda, D. et al. (1996) Cell 86, 767–775.

[9] Screaton, G.R. et al. (1993) J. Biol. Chem. 268, 12235–12238.

[10] Telen, M.J. et al. (1996) J. Biol. Chem. 271, 7147–7153.

[11] Lesley, J. et al. (1994) J. Exp. Med. 180, 383–387.

[12] Bennett, K.L. et al. (1995) J. Cell. Biol. 128, 687–698.

[13] Weber, G.F. et al. (1996) Science 271, 509–512.

[14] Lokeshwar, V.B. et al. (1994) J. Cell. Biol. 126, 1099–1109.

[15] Tsukita, S. et al. (1994) J. Cell. Biol. 126, 391–401.

[16] Taher, T.E.I. et al. (1996) J. Biol. Chem. 271, 2863–2867.

[17] DeGrendele, H.C. et al. (1996) J. Exp. Med. 183, 1119–1130.

[18] Clark, R.A. et al. (1996) J. Cell Biol. 134, 1075–1087.

[19] Butcher, E.C. and Picker, L.J. (1996) Science 272, 60–66.

[20] Bartolazzi, A. et al. (1995) J. Cell Sci. 108, 1723–1733.

[21] Stamenkovic, I. et al. (1989) Cell 56, 1057–1062.

[22] Nottenburg, C. et al. (1989) Proc. Natl Acad. Sci. USA 86, 8521–8525.

[23] Gunthert, U. et al. (1991) Cell 65, 13–24.

Molecular weights

| Polypeptide | 127 438 (0) |
| | 145 590 (ABC) |

SDS-PAGE

reduced	180–240 kDa
B cells	240 kDa
thymocytes	180 kDa
T cells	multiple bands

Carbohydrate

| N-linked sites | 11–16 |
| O-linked | + abundant (especially on isoforms expressing A, B, C exon products) |

Human gene location and size

1 q31–q32; 120 kb [1]

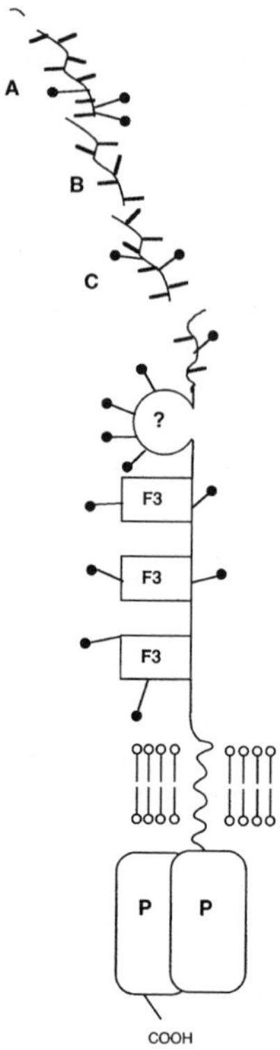

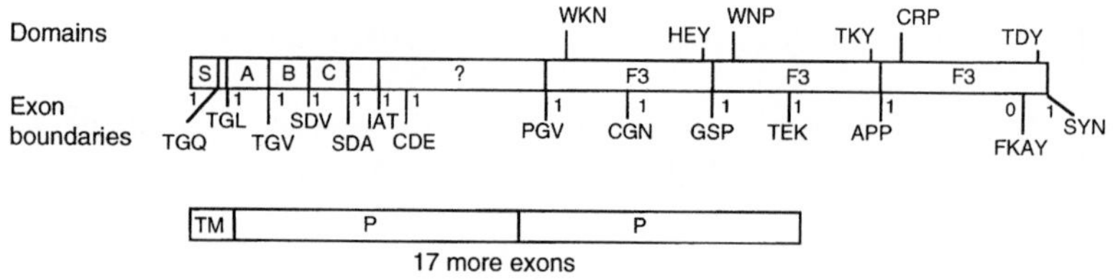

| Domains | WKN | HEY | WNP | TKY | CRP | TDY |

17 more exons

Tissue distribution

CD45 proteins are found on all cells of haematopoietic origin, except erythrocytes[2]. Various isoforms of CD45 are generated by alternative splicing of three exons that can be inserted immediately after an N-terminal sequence of eight amino acids found on all isoforms. Of the eight possible combinations of exons, seven have been found at the mRNA level[2,3]. The isoforms are expressed differentially on leucocytes and their expression can be followed with mAbs specific for protein encoded by the alternate exons or by an mAb that recognizes the junction of the eight amino acid N-terminal conserved sequence and the rest of the conserved part of the protein. These epitopes are termed CD45RA, CD45RB, CD45RC and CD45R0 respectively. Other mAbs react with the common part of the structure and recognize all CD45 isoforms. B cells express a single isoform, including the A, B and C exon encoded sequences. Among peripheral CD4+ T cells various combinations including one or two of the alternate exons are found. This differential expression has been of use in defining subsets of CD4+ T cells, in which naive T cells express forms of CD45 including these exons, whereas activated cells and most memory cells express forms including these exons at low levels and label with mAbs specific for the CD45R0 epitope. Thymocytes express primarily the low M_r isoform of CD45.

Structure

The extracellular domain of CD45 is from 391 to 552 amino acids long with 11–16 N-linked carbohydrate attachment sites. Protein sequence coded by exons 3–8 is rich in Ser, Thr and Pro and has multiple O-linked carbohydrates[2,4]. Binding of several mAbs recognizing the ABC segments is affected by glycosylation although in most cases the mAb can react with the unglycosylated protein backbone[5]. The rest of the extracellular domain contains 16 cysteine residues which are largely conserved between mouse, rat and human[2]. Three putative fibronectin type III domains have been identified; these are unusual because of their high Cys content[6,7]. CD45 has been shown to be sulfated[8]. The cytoplasmic domain is large (700 amino acids) and contains two PTPase (phosphotyrosine phosphatase) domains[9]. The membrane-proximal domain has enzymatic activity[10] but is dependent on the second domain[11,12]. The intracellular domain is phosphorylated on Ser, in response to PKC activation[2].

Ligands and associated molecules

CD45 has been reported to be associated at the cell surface with several cell surface antigens such as CD4, TCR, CD2, Thy-1 and CD26[12]. CD22 can bind CD45 and other glycoproteins through sialic acid residues[13]. The cytoplasmic part of CD45 is associated with fodrin[2]. CD45 associates with a lymphocyte-specific protein termed lymphocyte phosphatase-associated phosphoprotein (LPAP) or CD45-associated protein (CD45-AP) through an interaction involving the transmembrane region of CD45[14,15]. CD45 is also associated with a phosphorylated glycoprotein of M_r 116 kDa present in all haematopoietic cells[16].

Function

Expression of CD45 is necessary for signalling through the T cell receptor[17]. Gene deletion experiments indicate a role for CD45 in the selection of both T and B lymphocytes[18,19]. The variants in the extracellular region correlate with functional subpopulations of lymphocytes and may affect threshold of activation[20].

Database accession numbers

	PIR	SWISSPROT	EMBL/GENBANK	REFERENCE
Human (ABC)		P08575	Y00638	3
Rat (ABC)	A02247	P04157	Y00065	21
Mouse (0)	A29381	P06800	M14342	22

Amino acid sequence of human CD45

```
MYLWLKLLAF GFAFLDTEVF VTG                                     -1
QSPTPSPT                                                       8
GLTTAKMPSW PLSSDPLPTH TTAFSPASTF ERENDFSETT TSLSPDNTST
QVSPDSLDNA SAFNTT                                             74A
GVSSVQTPHL PTHADSQTPS AGTDTQTFSG SAANAKLNPT PGSNAIS          121B
DVPGERSTAS TFPTDPVSPL TTTLSLAHHS SAALPARTSN TTITANTS         169C
DAYLNASETT TLSPSGSAVI STTTIATTPS KPTCDEKYAN ITVDYLYNKE        219
TKLFTAKLNV NENVECGNNT CTNNEVHNLT ECKNASVSIS HNSCTAPDKT        269
LILDVPPGVE KFQLHDCTQV EKADTTICLK WKNIETFTCD TQNITYRFQC        319
GNMIFDNKEI KLENLEPEHE YKCDSEILYN NHKFTNASKI IKTDFGSPGE        369
PQIIFCRSEA AHQGVITWNP PQRSFHNFTL CYIKETEKDC LNLDKNLIKY        419
DLQNLKPYTK YVLSLHAYII AKVQRNGSAA MCHFTTKSAP PSQVWNMTVS        469
MTSDNSMHVK CRPPRDRNGP HERYHLEVEA GNTLVRNESH KNCDFRVKDL        519
QYSTDYTFKA YFHNGDYPGE PFILHHSTSY NSKALIAFLA FLIIVTSIAL        569
LVVLYKIYDL HKKRSCNLDE QQELVERDDE KQLMNVEPIH ADILLETYKR        619
KIADEGRPFL AEFQSIPRVF SKFPIKEARK PFNQNKNRYV DILPYDYNRV        669
ELSEINGDAG SNYINASYID GFKEPRKYIA AQGPRDETVD DFWRMIWEQK        719
ATVIVMVTRC EEGNRNKCAE YWPSMEEGTR AFGDVVVKIN QHKRCPDYII        769
QKLNIVNKKE KATGREVTHI QFTSWPDHGV PEDPHLLLKL RRRVNAFSNF        819
FSGPIVVHCS AGVGRTGTYI GIDAMLEGLE AENKVDVYGY VVKLRRQRCL        869
MVQVEAQYIL IHQALVEYNQ FGETEVNLSE LHPYLHNMKK RDPPSEPSPL        919
EAEFQRLPSY RSWRTQHIGN QEENKSKNRN SNVIPYDYNR VPLKHELEMS        969
KESEHDSDES SDDDSDSEEP SKYINASFIM SYWKPEVMIA AQGPLKETIG       1019
DFWQMIFQRK VKVIVMLTEL KHGDQEICAQ YWGEGKQTYG DIEVDLKDTD       1069
KSSTYTLRVF ELRHSKRKDS RTVYQYQYTN WSVEQLPAEP KELISMIQVV       1119
KQKLPQKNSS EGNKHHKSTP LLIHCRDGSQ QTGIFCALLN LLESAETEEV       1169
VDIFQVVKAL RKARLGMVST FEQYQFLYDV IASTYPAQNG QVKKNNHQED       1219
KIEFDNEVDK VKQDANCVNP LGAPEKLPEA KEQAEGSEPT SGTEGPEHSV       1269
NGPASPALNQ GS                                               1281
```

References

1 Fernandez-Luna, J. et al. (1991) Genomics 10, 754–764.
2 **Thomas, M.L. (1989) Annu. Rev. Immunol. 7, 339–369.**
3 Streuli, M. et al. (1987) J. Exp. Med. 166, 1548–1566.
4 Jackson, D.I. and Barclay, A.N. (1989) Immunogenetics 29, 281–287.
5 Cyster, J.G. et al. (1994) Int. Immunol. 6, 1875–1881.
6 Bork, P. and Doolittle, R.F. (1993) Protein Sci. 2, 1185–1187.
7 Okumura, M. et al. (1996) J. Immunol. 157, 1569–1575.
8 Giordanengo, V. et al. (1995) Eur. J. Immunol. 25, 274–278.
9 Tonks, N.K. et al. (1988) Biochemistry 27, 8695–8701.
10 Streuli, M. et al. (1990) EMBO J. 9, 2399–2407.
11 Johnson, P. et al. (1992) J. Biol. Chem. 267, 8035–8041.
12 **Trowbridge, I.S. and Thomas, M.L. (1994) Annu. Rev. Immunol. 12, 85–116.**
13 Sgroi, D. et al. (1993) J. Biol. Chem. 268, 7011–7018.
14 Bruyns, E. et al. (1995) J. Biol. Chem. 270, 31372–31376.
15 McFarland, E.D.C. and Thomas, M.L. (1995) J. Biol. Chem. 270, 28103–28107.
16 Arendt, C.W. and Ostergaard, H.L. (1995) J. Biol. Chem. 270, 2313–2319.
17 Pingel, J.T. and Thomas, M.L. (1989) Cell 58, 1055–1065.

[18] Byth, K.F. et al. (1996) J. Exp. Med. 183, 1707–1718.

[19] Cyster, J.G. et al. (1996) Nature 381, 325–328.

[20] Leitenberg, D. et al. (1996) J. Exp. Med. 183, 249–259.

[21] Barclay, A.N. et al. (1987) EMBO J. 6, 1259–1264.

[22] Saga, Y. et al. (1986) Proc. Natl Acad. Sci. USA 83, 6940–6944.

Molecular weights
Polypeptides　　　　　　　　　　37 018–40 387
(multiple splicing variants)

SDS-PAGE
　reduced　　　　　　　　　　　51–68 kDa
　unreduced　　　　　　　　　　46–63 kDa

Carbohydrate
N-linked sites　　　　　　　　　3
O-linked sites　　　　　　　　　+/++
(depending on slicing variant)

Human gene location and size
1q 32; >43 kb [1,2].

Tissue distribution

CD46 is expressed on all peripheral blood cells and platelets but not erythrocytes [1,2]. CD46 is also expressed on fibroblasts, endothelial and epithelial cells, and tissues of the reproductive system, including fallopian tube, uterine endometrium, placenta and sperm. CD46 is not expressed on unfertilized oocytes but appears at the 6–8 cell stage embryo [1-4].

Structure

CD46 is a type I membrane protein with four complement control protein (CCP) domains, a Ser/Thr/Pro rich (STP) region, and a further 13 residues in the extracellular portion [5]. The N-terminal protein sequence has been determined [6]. There are six CD46 variants determined from cDNA clones, derived from the combination of three variants in the STP region and two variants in the cytoplasmic domain. The three variants in the STP region express both STP^A and STP^B exons, only STP^B, or neither exon. The two cytoplasmic variants are the consequence of the presence or absence of the exon CY1 [1,5]. Thus the six isoforms are designated ABC1, ABC2, BC1, BC2, C1 and C2; A, B and C indicate the expression of the STP^A, STP^B and STP^C exons, and 1 and 2 denote the cytoplasmic exons expressed. However, the two isoforms ABC1 and ABC2 have not been observed in peripheral blood cells or cell lines [5]. Most cells of a given individual express the same ratio of the four remaining isoforms, although selective expression of certain isoforms has been noted in the brain, kidney and salivary gland [5,7].

Ligands and associated molecules

CD46 binds the complement components C3b and C4b [1,2], and is a receptor for the measles virus [8] and for *Streptococcus pyogenes* [9].

Function

CD46 is a member of the regulator of complement activation (RCA) family of proteins [2]. It acts as a cofactor which binds to C3b and C4b, thereby permitting factor I, a serine protease of the complement system, to convert C3b and C4b into fragments that cannot support further complement activation [1,2]. Of the variants that have different STP regions, the BC isoforms are found to be more efficient than the C isoforms in the regulation of C4b activity, although both sets of isoforms have similar regulatory activities on C3b [10]. CD46 with cytoplasmic tail type 1 (CY1) has been shown to be processed four times faster into its mature forms [11]. The complement regulatory proteins CD46, CD55 and CD59 are likely to be important in protecting the sperm and fetus from rejection by the maternal immune system [2,12]. Transgenic pigs are being produced which express human complement regulatory proteins in order to prevent complement-mediated hyperacute rejection – a major problem in xenotransplantation of pig organs to humans [13].

Database accession numbers

		PIR	SWISSPROT	EMBL/GENBANK	REFERENCE
Human	BC1	I54479	P15529	M58050	5,14
	BC2	S01896		Y00651	5,6,15
	C2			S51940	5,16

Amino acid sequence of human CD46

```
MEPPGRRECP FPSWRFPGLL LAAMVLLLYS FSDA                    -1
CEEPPTFEAM ELIGKPKPYY EIGERVDYKC KKGYFYIPPL ATHTICDRNH   50
TWLPVSDDAC YRETCPYIRD PLNGQAVPAN GTYEFGYQMH FICNEGYYLI  100
GEEILYCELK GSVAIWSGKP PICEKVLCTP PPKIKNGKHT FSEVEVFEYL  150
DAVTYSCDPA PGPDPFSLIG ESTIYCGDNS VWSRAAPECK VVKCRFPVVE  200
NGKQISGFGK KFYYKATVMF ECDKGFYLDG SDTIVCDSNS TWDPPVPKCL  250

ABC KVLPPSSTKP PALSHSVSTS STTKSPASSA SGPRPTYKPP VSNYPGYPKP 300
-BC K......... .......VSTS STTKSPASSA SGPRPTYKPP VSNYPGYPKP 285
--C K......... .......... .......... .GPRPTYKPP VSNYPGYPKP 270

All EEGILDSLDV WVIAVIVIAI VVGVAVICVV PYRYLQRRKK KG 342/327/312

CY1 TYLTDETHRE VKFTSL                              358/343/328
CY2 KADGGAEYAT YQTKSTTPAE QRG                      365/350/335
```

To represent the six isoforms, all possible sequences in the variable STP and cytoplasmic regions are shown, including the residue numbering. Residues missing due to exon deletion are marked with dots.

References

1 Liszewski, M.K. et al. (1991) Annu. Rev. Immunol. 9, 431–455.
2 **Liszewski, M.K. et al. (1996) Adv. Immunol. 61, 201–283.**
3 Fenichel, P. et al. (1995) Am. J. Reprod. Immunol. 33, 155–164.
4 Jensen, T.S. et al. (1995) Am. J. Reprod. Immunol. 34, 1–9.
5 **Post, T.W. et al. (1991) J. Exp. Med. 174, 93–102.**
6 Lublin, D.M. et al. (1988) J. Exp. Med. 168, 181–194.
7 Johnstone, R.W. et al. (1993) Mol. Immunol. 30, 1231–1241.
8 Manchester, M. et al. (1994) Proc. Natl Acad. Sci. USA 91, 2161–2165.
9 Okada, N. et al. (1995) Proc. Natl Acad. Sci. USA 92, 2489–2493.
10 Liszewski, M.K. and Atkinson, J.P. (1996) J. Immunol. 156, 4415–4421.
11 Liszewski, M.K. et al. (1994) J. Biol. Chem. 269, 10776–10779.
12 **Rooney, I.A. et al. (1993) Immunol. Res. 12, 276–294.**
13 **Cozzi, E. and White, D.J.G. (1995) Nature Med. 1, 964–966.**
14 Purcell, D.F. et al. (1991) Immunogenetics 33, 335–344.
15 Purcell, D.F. et al. (1990) Immunogenetics 31, 21–28.
16 Cervoni, F. et al. (1993) Mol. Reprod. Dev. 34, 107–113.

Molecular weights
Polypeptide 35 213

SDS-PAGE
  reduced 47–52 kDa
  unreduced 43–50.5, 110 kDa

Carbohydrate
N-linked sites 6
O-linked unknown

Human gene location
3q13.1–q13.2

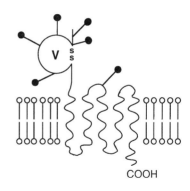

COOH

Tissue distribution

CD47 has a broad tissue distribution with expression on virtually all haemato-poietic cells, including thymocytes, T cells, B cells, monocytes, platelets and erythrocytes, as well as on epithelial cells, endothelial cells, fibroblasts, sperm, and tumour cell lines. CD47 is part of the Rh complex on erythrocytes and is not expressed on Rh_{null} erythrocytes [1].

Structure

The CD47 structure is unusual in combining an IgSF domain with a multipass transmembrane mode of attachment to the cell membrane. CD47 is predicted to have five membrane-spanning regions, an N-terminal IgSF V-set domain and short cytoplasmic regions. Immunofluorescence microscopy has proved the C-terminal tail to be cytoplasmic [2]. Four alternatively spliced forms of the C-terminus have been identified [3]. These are generated by the variable usage of three short exons. Two predominant splice variants have been demonstrated *in vivo* and these have distinct tissue expression patterns. The form with the shorter cytoplasmic tail is expressed by bone marrow-derived cells, endothelial cells and fibroblasts, whereas the longer form is expressed mainly by neural tissue [3].

Ligands and associated molecules

The CD47 molecule associates non-covalently with the CD61 (β3) integrins CD51/CD61 (αvβ3) and CD41/CD61 (αIIbβ3) [2]. The IgSF domain of CD47 is thought to mediate these interactions [4]. A ligand for CD47 is the C-terminal cell binding domain of thrombospondin, an extracellular adhesion molecule which regulates motility and proliferation in many cell types [5].

Function

CD47 plays a role in the chemotactic and adhesive interactions of leucocytes with endothelial cells. The mechanism of action is not entirely understood, but is thought to involve the modulation of the function of integrins, with which CD47 is physically and functionally linked, and its binding to thrombospondin [5-7]. The binding of thrombospondin to CD47 on endothelial cells *in vitro* induces a chemotactic response that is inhibited by a CD47 mAb [5]. CD47 mAbs also inhibit neutrophil migration across endothelium and epithelium, without affecting CD11b/CD18 integrin-mediated neutrophil adhesion to epithelium [6,7]. Human cells that lack CD47 are deficient in some CD51 integrin ligand binding functions [4]. CD47 knockout mice show increased susceptibility to bacterial infections due to granulocyte defects in CD61 integrin function, activation of oxidative burst and phagocytosis [8].

Comments

CD47 species homologues have been identified in the poxviruses vaccinia and variola major [9]. The vaccinia virus A38L gene product is a 33 kDa membrane glycoprotein with 28% sequence identity to mammalian CD47. Proteolysis studies of A38L translated *in vitro* in microsomal membranes are consistent with the proposed membrane topology of human CD47. The A38L protein is expressed at a low level in infected cells *in vivo* but its function is not clear, since deletion of the A38L gene does not affect virus particle production or virulence [9].

Database accession numbers

	PIR	SWISSPROT	EMBL/GENBANK	REFERENCE
Human		Q08722	Z25521	2
Mouse			Z25524	2
Vaccinia	S29922	P24763	X57318	10

Amino acid sequence of human CD47

```
MWPLVAALLL GSACCGSA                                          -1
QLLFNKTKSV EFTFCNDTVV IPCFVTNMEA QNTTEVYVKW KFKGRDIYTF        50
DGALNKSTVP TDFSSAKIEV SQLLKGDASL KMDKSDAVSH TGNYTCEVTE       100
LTREGETIIE LKYRVVSWFS PNENILIVIF PIFAILLFWG QFGIKTLKYR       150
SGGMDEKTIA LLVAGLVITV IVIVGAILFV PGEYSLKNAT GLGLIVTSTG       200
ILILLHYYVF STAIGLTSFV IAILVIQVIA YILAVVGLSL CIAACIPMHG       250
PLLISGLSIL ALAQLLGLVY MKFVASNQKT IQPPRKAVEE PLNAFKESKG       300
MMNDE                                                       305
```

References

1 Hadam, M.R. (1989) Leucocyte Typing IV, 658–660.
2 Lindberg, F.P. et al. (1993) J. Cell Biol. 123, 485–496.
3 Reinhold, M.I. et al. (1995) J. Cell Sci. 108, 3419–3425.
4 Lindberg, F.P. et al. (1996) J. Cell Biol. 134, 1313–1322.
5 Gao, A.-G. et al. (1996) J. Biol. Chem. 271, 21–24.
6 Cooper, D. et al. (1995) Proc. Natl Acad. Sci. USA 92, 3978–3982.
7 Parkos, C.A. et al. (1996) J. Cell Biol. 132, 437–450.
8 **Lindberg, F.P. et al. (1996) Science 274, 795–798.**
9 Parkinson, J.E. et al. (1995) Virology 214, 177–188.
10 Smith, G.L. et al. (1991) J. Gen. Virol. 72, 1349–1376.

Molecular weights
Polypeptide   22 344

SDS-PAGE
  reduced   40–47 kDa

Carbohydrate
N-linked sites   6
O-linked   unknown

Human gene location and size
1q21–q23; >28 kb [1]

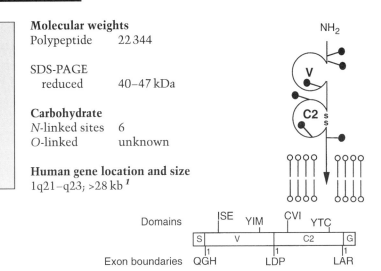

Tissue distribution

Widely expressed on haematopoetic cells with the exception of granulocytes (but some on eosinophils), platelets and erythrocytes[2,3]. Expression is increased following activation of T and B cells. Rat CD48 (OX-45) is more widely expressed, being present on erythrocytes, endothelium and some connective tissue[4].

Structure

CD48 contains two IgSF domains and is a member of the CD2 family of molecules which includes CD58, Ly-9, 2B4 and CD150[5]. Within this group CD48 is most similar to CD58, which is a ligand for human CD2[5]. Like one splice variant of CD58, CD48 possesses a glycosyl-phosphatidylinositol (GPI) membrane anchor. The site of GPI attachment is shown as Ser194 on the basis of homology with the rat sequence[6]. The CD48 gene lies close to the Ly-9 and 2B4 genes in the mouse[7–9] and within 410 kb of the putative human Ly-9 gene[9]. These genes are likely to have arisen in a series of gene duplication events, and duplication of this entire chromosomal region is likely to have given rise to the region encoding CD2 and CD58[7,9].

Ligands and associated molecules

Human CD48 has been reported to bind CD2 but with an affinity considerably (>100-fold) lower than CD58, the major CD2 ligand[5]. In mice and rats CD48 appears to be the major CD2 ligand[5]. Rat CD48 binds CD2 with an affinity of K_d 60–90 μM and dissociates with a very fast dissociation rate constant ($k_{off} \geq 6\,s^{-1}$). The CD2 binding site lies on the GFCC'C'' β sheet of the V-set domain and CD2 binds CD48 in a head-to-head orientation[5]. Immuno-precipitation studies suggest associations with the cytoplasmic tyrosine kinases Lck and Fyn[10].

Function

In the mouse and the rat CD48 is the major CD2 ligand and so may contribute to T cell antigen recognition [5]. CD48 antibodies suppress the immune response in mice but the precise role of the CD48–CD2 interaction is unclear since no abnormality has been detected in CD2-deficient mice [5].

Database accession numbers

	PIR	SWISSPROT	EMBL/GENBANK	REFERENCE
Human	A53244	P09326	M37766	[11]
Rat	S01299	P10252	X13016	[6]
Mouse	JL0143	P18181	X17501	[7]

Amino acid sequence of human CD48

```
MWSRGWDSCL ALELLLLPLS LLVTSI                          -1
QGHLVHMTVV SGSNVTLNIS ESLPENYKQL TWFYTFDQKI VEWDSRKSKY  50
FESKFKGRVR LDPQSGALYI SKVQKEDNST YIMRVLKKTG NEQEWKIKLQ 100
VLDPVPKPVI KIEKIEDMDD NCYLKLSCVI PGESVNYTWY GDKRPFPKEL 150
QNSVLETTLM PHNYSRCYTC QVSNSVSSKN GTVCLSPPCT LARS       194
FGVEWIASWL VVTVPTILGL LLT                             +23
```

References

1 Fisher, R.C. and Thorley-Lawson, D.A. (1991) Mol. Cell. Biol. 11, 1614–1623.
2 Hadam, M.R. (1989) in Leucocyte Typing IV, Knapp, W. et al. (ed.). Oxford University Press, Oxford, pp. 661–667.
3 Vaughan, H.A. et al. (1983) Transplantation 36, 446–450.
4 Arvieux, J. et al. (1986) Mol. Immunol. 23, 983–990.
5 **Davis, S.J. and van der Merwe, P.A. (1996) Immunol. Today 17, 177–187.**
6 Killeen, N. et al. (1988) EMBO J. 7, 3087-3091.
7 Wong, Y.W. et al. (1990) J. Exp. Med. 171, 2115–2130.
8 Mathew, P.A. et al. (1993) J. Immunol. 151, 5328–5337.
9 Kingsmore, S.F. et al. (1995) Immunogenetics 42, 59–62.
10 Garnett, D. et al. (1993) Eur. J. Immunol. 171, 2115–2130.
11 Staunton, D.E. and Thorley-Lawson, D.A. (1987) EMBO J. 6, 3695–3701.

CD49a

Other names
α1 integrin subunit
VLA-1 α subunit

Molecular weights
Polypeptides   127 839

SDS-PAGE
  reduced   210 kDa
  unreduced   200 kDa

Carbohydrate
N-linked sites   26
O-linked sites   unknown

Human gene location
5

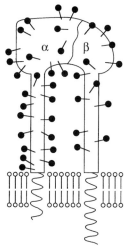

CD49a/CD29

Tissue distribution

CD49a is expressed on monocytes and at low levels on resting T cells [1,2]. Its expression on T cells is increased upon prolonged stimulation *in vitro* [2,3]. It is also found at increased levels on T lymphocytes in synovial joints of patients with rheumatoid arthritis; however, its expression is reduced following phytohaemagglutinin stimulation [4]. CD49a expression on NK cells is upregulated by IL-2 [5].

Structure

CD49a is the α1 integrin subunit which forms a non-covalent heterodimer with CD29, the β1 integrin subunit. CD49a belongs to the integrin α subclass which contains an I-domain [6]. The N-terminal sequence has been determined [7].

Ligands and associated molecules

CD49a/CD29 binds laminin and collagen through different binding sites [2,5].

Function

The integrin CD49a/CD29 on choriocarcinoma and melanoma cells binds collagen and the E1 fragment of laminin [8,9]. Solubilized CD49a/CD29 complexes have been shown to bind collagen [6,8]. However, collagen binding is not mediated by CD49a/CD29 on cultured T lymphoyctes [10].

Database accession numbers

	PIR	SWISSPROT	EMBL/GENBANK	REFERENCE
Human			X68742	6
Rat	A35854	P18614	X52140	11

Amino acid sequence of human CD49a

```
MVPRRPASLE VTVACIWLLT VILGFCVS                                  -1
FNVDVKNSMT FSGPVEDMFG YTVQQYENEE GKWVLIGSPL VGQPKNRTGD          50
VYKCPVGRGE SLPCVKLDLP VNTSIPNVTE VKENMTFGST LVTNPNGGFL         100
ACGPLYAYRC GHLHYTTGIC SDVSPTFQVV NSIAPVQECS TQLDIVIVLD         150
GSNSIYPWDS VTAFLNDLLK RMDIGPKQTQ VGIVQYGENV THEFNLNKYS         200
STEEVLVAAK KIVQRGGRQT MTALGTDTAR KEAFTEARGA RRGVKKVMVI         250
VTDGESHDNH RLKKVIQDCE DENIQRFSIA ILGSYNRGNL STEKFVEEIK         300
SIASEPTEKH FFNVSDELAL VTIVKTLGER IFALEATADQ SAASFEMEMS         350
QTGFSAHYSQ DWVMLGAVGA YDWNGTVVMQ KASQIIIPRN TTFNVESTKK         400
NEPLASYLGY TVNSATASSG DVLYIAGQPR YNHTGQVIIY RMEDGNIKIL         450
QTLSGEQIGS YFGSILTTTD IDKDSNTDIL LVGAPMYMGT EKEEQGKVYV         500
YALNQTRFEY QMSLEPIKQT CCSSRQHNSC TTENKNEPCG ARFGTAIAAV         550
KDLNLDGFND IVIGAPLEDD HGGAVYIYHG SGKTIRKEYA QRIPSGGDGK         600
TLKFFGQSIH GEMDLNGDGL TDVTIGGLGG AALFWSRDVA VVKVTMNFEP         650
NKVNIQKKNC HMEGKETVCI NATVCFEVKL KSKEDTIYEA DLQYRVTLDS         700
LRQISRSFFS GTQERKVQRN ITVRKSECTK HSFYMLDKHD FQDSVRITLD         750
FNLTDPENGP VLDDSLPNSV HEYIPFAKDC GNKEKCISDL SLHVATTEKD         800
LLIVRSQNDK FNVSLTVKNT KDSAYNTRTI VHYSPNLVFS GIEAIQKDSC         850
ESNHNITCKV GYPFLRRGEM VTFKILFQFN TSYLMENVTI YLSATSDSEE         900
PPETLSDNVV NISIPVKYEV GLQFYSSASE YHISIAANET VPEVINSTED         950
IGNEINIFYL IRKSGSFPMP ELKLSISFPN MTSNGYPVLY PTGLSSSENA        1000
NCRPHIFEDP FSINSGKKMT TSTDHLKRGT ILDCNTCKFA TITCNLTSSD        1050
ISQVNVSLIL WKPTFIKSYF SSLNLTIRGE LRSENASLVL SSSNQKRELA        1100
IQISKDGLPG RVPLWVILLS AFAGLLLLML LILALWKIGF FKRPLKKKME        1150
K                                                            1151
```

References
1 Pigott, R. and Power, C. (1993) The Adhesion Molecule FactsBook. Academic Press, London.
2 **Hemler, M.E. (1990) Annu. Rev. Immunol. 114, 365–400.**
3 Hemler, M.E. et al. (1984) J. Immunol. 132, 3011–3018.
4 Hemler, M.E. et al. (1986) J. Clin. Invest. 78, 696–702.
5 Perez-Villar, J.J. et al. (1996) Eur. J. Immunol. 26, 2023–2029.
6 **Briesewitz, R. et al. (1993) J. Biol. Chem. 268, 2989–2996.**
7 Takada, Y. et al. (1987) Proc. Natl Acad. Sci. USA 84, 3239–3243.
8 Kramer, R.H. and Marks, N. (1989) J. Biol. Chem. 264, 4684–4688.
9 Hall, D.E. et al. (1990) J. Cell Biol. 110, 2175–2184.
10 Goldman, R. et al. (1992) Eur. J. Immunol. 22, 1109–1114.
11 Ignatius, M.J. et al. (1990) J. Cell Biol. 111, 709–720.

CD49b

Other names
Integrin α2 subunit
VLA-2 α subunit
Ia subunit of platelet GP Ia–IIa

Molecular weights
Polypeptides   126 378

SDS-PAGE
  reduced   165 kDa
  unreduced   160 kDa

Carbohydrates
N-linked sites   10
O-linked sites   unknown

Human gene location
5q23–31

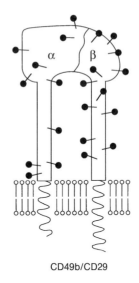

CD49b/CD29

Tissue distribution

CD49b is expressed on monocytes, platelets, B and T lymphocytes, and NK cells[1-4]. The level of expression on T cells is elevated upon prolonged culture[2]. Like CD49a/CD29, CD49b/CD29 is also found on lymphocytes in the synovial joints of rheumatoid patients. In contrast to CD49a/CD29, CD49b/CD29 is further upregulated on stimulation with phytohaem-agglutinin[5].

Structure

CD49b is the α2 integrin subunit which forms a non-covalently associated heterodimer with CD29 (β1 integrin subunit). CD49b belongs to the integrin α subclass which contains an I-domain[6]. The N-terminal sequence of CD49b has been determined[6]. A polymorphism at residue 505 gives rise to the platelet alloantigenic Br^a (Lys) and Br^b (Glu) variants[7].

Ligands and associated molecules

CD49b/CD29 binds collagen and laminin[2]. Binding to both ligands can be inhibited by peptides containing the DGEA sequence[8]. The I-domain of CD49b is involved in collagen binding[9].

Function

CD49b/CD29 mediates the Mg^{2+}-dependent adhesion of platelets to collagen[8,10]. It is also a collagen receptor on leucocytes[11,12] and fibroblasts[13]. CD49b/CD29 may be utilized by fibroblasts for the reorganization of the collagen matrix during wound healing[14,15]. The upregulation of CD49b/CD29 may also be used by tumour cells to remodel the collagen matrix during tumor growth, invasion and metastasis [15-17]. CD49b/CD29 can act as a laminin receptor in certain cell lines but not in platelets or fibroblasts [12]. CD49b/CD29 integrin is a receptor for echovirus-1 [18].

Database accession numbers

	PIR	SWISSPROT	EMBL/GENBANK	REFERENCE
Human	A33998	P17301	X17033	6
Cattle			L25886	9

Amino acid sequence of human CD49b

```
MGPERTGAAP LPLLLVLALS QGILNCCLA                               -1
YNVGLPEAKI FSGPSSEQFG YAVQQFINPK GNWLLVGSPW SGFPENRMGD        50
VYKCPVDLST ATCEKLNLQT STSIPNVTEM KTNMSLGLIL TRNMGTGGFL       100
TCGPLWAQQC GNQYYTTGVC SDISPDFQLS ASFSPATQPC PSLIDVVVVC       150
DESNSIYPWD AVKNFLEKFV QGLDIGPTKT QVGLIQYANN PRVVFNLNTY       200
KTKEEMIVAT SQTSQYGGDL TNTFGAIQYA RKYAYSAASG GRRSATKVMV       250
VVTDGESHDG SMLKAVIDQC NHDNILRFGI AVLGYLNRNA LDTKNLIKEI       300
KAIASIPTER YFFNVSDEAA LLEKAGTLGE QIFSIEGTVQ GGDNFQMEMS       350
QVGFSADYSS QNDILMLGAV GAFGWSGTIV QKTSHGHLIF PKQAFDQILQ       400
DRNHSSYLGY SVAAISTGES THFVAGAPRA NYTGQIVLYS VNENGNITVI       450
QAHRGDQIGS YFGSVLCSVD VDKDTITDVL LVGAPMYMSD LKKEEGRVYL       500
FTIKKGILGQ HQFLEGPEGI ENTRFGSAIA ALSDINMDGF NDVIVGSPLE       550
NQNSGAVYIY NGHQGTIRTK YSQKILGSDG AFRSHLQYFG RSLDGYGDLN       600
GDSITDVSIG AFGQVVQLWS QSIADVAIEA SFTPEKITLV NKNAQIILKL       650
CFSAKFRPTK QNNQVAIVYN ITLDADGFSS RVTSRGLFKE NNERCLQKNM       700
VVNQAQSCPE HIIYIQEPSD VVNSLDLRVD ISLENPGTSP ALEAYSETAK       750
VFSIPFHKDC GEDGLCISDL VLDVRQIPAA QEQPFIVSNQ NKRLTFSVTL       800
KNKRESAYNT GIVVDFSENL FFASFSLPVD GTEVTCQVAA SQKSVACDVG       850
YPALKREQQV TFTINFDFNL QNLQNQASLS FQALSESQEE NKADNLVNLK       900
IPLLYDAEIH LTRSTNINFY EISSDGNVPS IVHSFEDVGP KFIFSLKVTT       950
GSVPVSMATV IIHIPQYTKE KNPLMYLTGV QTDKAGDISC NADINPLKIG      1000
QTSSSVSFKS ENFRHTKELN CRTASCSNVT CWLKDVHMKG EYFVNVTTRI      1050
WNGTFASSTF QTVQLTAAAE INTYNPEIYV IEDNTVTIPL MIMKPDEKAE      1100
VPTGVIIGSI IAGILLLLAL VAILWKLGFF KRKYEKMTKN PDEIDETTEL      1150
SS                                                         1152
```

References

1. Pigott, R. and Power, C. (1993) The Adhesion Molecule FactsBook. Academic Press, London.
2. **Hemler, M.E. (1990) Annu. Rev. Immunol. 114, 365–400.**
3. Hemler, M.E. et al. (1984) J. Immunol. 132, 3011–3018.
4. Perez-Villar, J.J. et al. (1996) Eur. J. Immunol. 26, 2023–2029.
5. Hemler, M.E. et al. (1986) J. Clin. Invest. 78, 696–702.
6. **Takada, Y. and Hemler, M.E. (1989) J. Cell Biol. 109, 397–407.**
7. Santoso, S. et al. (1993) J. Clin. Invest. 92, 2427–2432.
8. Staatz, W.D. et al. (1991) J. Biol. Chem. 266, 7363–7367.
9. Kamata, T. et al. (1994) J. Biol. Chem. 269, 9659–9663.
10. Staatz, W.D. et al. (1989) J. Cell Biol. 108, 1917–1924.
11. Goldman, R. et al. (1992) Eur. J. Immunol. 22, 1109–1114.
12. Elices, M.J. and Hemler, M.E. (1989) Proc. Natl Acad. Sci. USA 86, 9906–9910.

[13] Wayner, E.A. and Carter, W.G. (1987) J. Cell Biol. 105, 1873–1884.

[14] Schiro, J.A. et al. (1991) Cell 67, 403–410.

[15] Klein, C.E. et al. (1991) J. Cell Biol. 115, 1427–1436.

[16] Chan, B.M.C. et al. (1991) Science 251, 1600–1602.

[17] Chen, F.A. et al. (1991) J. Exp. Med. 173, 1111–1119.

[18] Bergelson, J.M. et al. (1992) Science 255, 1718–1720.

CD49c

Other names
Integrin α3 subunit
VLA-3 α subunit

Molecular weights
Polypeptides   113 343

SDS-PAGE
    reduced   130 + 25 kDa
    unreduced   150 kDa

Carbohydrate
N-linked sites   14
O-linked sites   unknown

Human gene location
17q

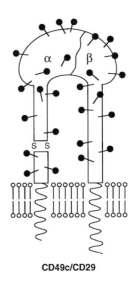

CD49c/CD29

Tissue distribution

CD49c is expressed at low levels on monocytes, and B and T lymphocytes [1,2]. It is expressed on most cultured adherent cell lines but not on lymphoid cell lines [3].

Structure

CD49c is the α3 integrin subunit which forms non-covalently associated heterodimers with CD29 (β1 integrin subunit). It belongs to the integrin α subclass which does not contain an I-domain and is cleaved into large N-terminal and small C-terminal chains which remain disulfide linked [2,4]. The N-terminal sequence of CD49c has been determined [5].

Ligands and associated molecules

The integrin CD49c/CD29 has been shown to bind many ligands, but its affinity for these ligands depends on the cell type on which it is expressed, divalent cation concentrations, and the presence of other integrin heterodimers on the cell [6,7]. Thus, CD49c/CD29 binds fibronectin at the RGD sites but this binding is only detectable on cells that do not express the CD49e/CD29 integrin [6]. CD49c/CD29 also binds collagen and laminin, but this binding is not inhibited by the RGD-containing peptides [6,7]. CD49c/CD29 has been shown to mediate the binding of cells to epiligrin, an extra-cellular matrix protein on epithelial basement membranes [8].

Function

K562 cells (which do not express any endogenous CD49 antigens) failed to bind fibronectin, collagen or laminin when transfected with CD49c cDNA, but showed binding to epiligrin, suggesting a role for CD49c/CD29 in mediating cell adhesion to the epithelial basement membranes [8,9]. CD49c/CD29 has been found at contact sites between cultured cells and so may have a role in cell–cell as well as cell–matrix adhesion [10].

Database accession numbers

	PIR	SWISSPROT	EMBL/GENBANK	REFERENCE
Human	A40021	P26006	M59911	4
Hamster	A35761	P17852	J05281	11

Amino acid sequence of human CD49c

```
MGPGPSRAPR APAPRLMLCA LALMVAAGGC VVSA            -1
FNLDTRFLVV KEAGNPGSLF GYSVALHRQT ERQQRYLLLA GAPRELAVPD   50
GYTNRTGAVY LCPLTAHKDD CERMNITVKN DPGHHIIEDM WLGVTVASQG  100
PAGRVLVCAH RYTQVLWSGS EDQRRMVGKC YVRGNDLELD SSDDWQTYHN  150
EMCNSNTDYL ETGMCQLGTS GGFTQNTVYF GAPGAYNWKG NSYMIQRKEW  200
DLSEYSYKDP EDQGNLYIGY TMQVGSFILH PKNITIVTGA PRHRHMGAVF  250
LLSQEAGGDL RRRQVLEGSQ VGAYFGSAIA LADLNNDGWQ DLLVGAPYYF  300
ERKEEVGGAI YVFMNQAGTS FPAHPSLLLH GPSGSAFGLS VASIGDINQD  350
GFQDIAVGAP FEGLGKVYIY HSSSKGLLRQ PQQVIHGEKL GLPGLATFGY  400
SLSGQMDVDE NFYPDLLVGS LSDHIVLLRA RPVINIVHKT LVPRPAVLDP  450
ALCTATSCVQ VELCFAYNQS AGNPNYRRNI TLAYTLEADR DRRPPRLRFA  500
GSESAVFHGF FSMPEMRCQK LELLLMDNLR DKLRPIIISM NYSLPLRMPD  550
RPRLGLRSLD AYPILNQAQA LENHTEVQFQ KECGPDNKCE SNLQMRAAFV  600
SEQQQKLSRL QYSRDVRKLL LSINVTNTRT SERSGEDAHE ALLTLVVPPA  650
LLLSSVRPPG ACQANETIFC ELGNPFKRNQ RMELLIAFEV IGVTLHTRDL  700
QVQLQLSTSS HQDNLWPMIL TLLVDYTLQT SLSMVNHRLQ SFFGGTVMGE  750
SGMKTVEDVG SPLKYEFQVG PMGEGLVGLG TLVLGLEWPY EVSNGKWLLY  800
PTEITVHGNG SWPCRPPGDL INPLNLTLSD PGDRPSSPQR RRRQLDPGGG  850
QGPPPVTLAA AKKAKSETVL TCATGRAHCV WLECPIPDAP VVTNVTVKAR  900
VVWNSTFIEDY RDFDRVRVNG WATLFLRTSI PTINMENKTT WFSVDIDSEL  950
VEELPAEIEL WLVLVAVGAG LLLLGLIILL LWKCGFFKRA RTRALYEAKR 1000
QKAEMKSQPS ETERLTDD                                   1018
```

References

1 Pigott, R. and Power, C. (1993) The Adhesion Molecule FactsBook. Academic Press, London.
2 **Hemler, M.E. (1990) Annu. Rev. Immunol. 114, 365–400.**
3 Rettig, W.J. and Old, L.J. (1992) Annu. Rev. Immunol. 7, 481–511.
4 Takada, Y. et al. (1991) J. Cell Biol. 115, 257–266.
5 Takada, Y. et al. (1987) Proc. Natl Acad. Sci. USA 84, 3239–3243.
6 Elices, M.J. et al. (1991) J. Cell Biol. 112, 169–181.
7 Gehlsen, K.R. et al. (1989) J. Biol. Chem. 264, 19034–19038.
8 **Carter, W.G. et al. (1991) Cell 65, 599–610.**
9 **Weitzman, J.B. et al. (1993) J. Biol. Chem. 268, 8651–8657.**
10 Kaufmann, R. et al. (1989) J. Cell Biol. 109, 1807–1815.
11 Tsuji, T. et al. (1990) J. Biol. Chem. 265, 7016–7021.

CD49d

Other names
Integrin α4 subunit
VLA-4 α subunit

Molecular weights
Polypeptides   111 228

SDS-PAGE
  reduced   150 kDa
  unreduced   180 kDa
  unreduced variant   150 kDa

Carbohydrates
N-linked sites   11
O-linked sites   unknown

Human gene location
2q31–q32

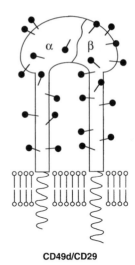

CD49d/CD29

Tissue distribution

CD49d is the α4 integrin subunit which can combine with CD29 (the β1 integrin subunit), to form the integrin CD49d/CD29 (α4β1, VLA-4), or with the β7 integrin subunit, to form the integrin α4β7. CD49d/CD29 is expressed on most leucocytes, with the possible exception of neutrophils and platelets [1-3]. α4β7 is expressed on most lymph node T and B cells, NK cells and eosinophils [3,4]. CD49d/CD29 is also expressed in non-lymphoid tissues [5].

Structure

CD49d does not belong to either of the two main groups of integrin α subunits: it contains neither an I-domain, nor a cleavage site to yield the characteristic N-terminal 125 kDa and C-terminal 30 kDa disulfide-linked peptides [6]. Instead, it contains a variably used cleavage site which yields two non-disulfide-linked fragments of 80 and 70 kDa [7]. CD49d migrates at either 150 kDa or 180 kDa in non-reducing SDS-PAGE. The 180 kDa form requires unoxidized cysteines and divalent cations and is likely to be the functionally more important form of the molecule [8,9]. The N-terminal sequence of CD49d has been determined [10].

Ligands and associated molecules

Both CD49d/CD29 (VLA-4) and the α4β7 integrin bind VCAM-1 as well as an alternatively spliced form of fibronectin which contains the peptide CS-1 [2,11]. The α4β7 integrin also binds the mucosal addressin MAdCAM-1 [2,3,12].

Function

CD49d/CD29 is involved in the migration of leucocytes from blood to tissues at sites of inflammation. In addition, CD49d/CD29-mediated binding has been shown to provide a co-stimulatory signal to T cells for activation and proliferation [13]. The α4β7 integrin is responsible for the homing of α4β7+ lymphocytes to the gut through recognition of MAdCAM-1 on mucosal high endothelial venules [3,12] (see the entry Integrin β7 subunit). Unlike the β2 integrins, which require selectin-mediated tethering and rolling of leucocytes before they can mediate arrest and firm adhesion to endothelium [14], CD49d/CD29 [15] and α4β7 [16] can mediate both the initial tethering/rolling as well as the subsequent firm adhesion.

Database accession numbers

	PIR	SWISSPROT	EMBL/GENBANK	REFERENCE
Human	S06046	P13612	X16983	5,17
Mouse	A41131	Q00651	X53176	18

Amino acid sequence of human CD49d

```
MFPTESAWLG KRGANPGPEA AVRETVMLLL CLGVPTGRP               -1
YNVDTESALL YQGPHNTLFG YSVVLHSHGA NRWLLVGAPT ANWLANASVI   50
NPGAIYRCRI GKNPGQTCEQ LQLGSPNGEP CGKTCLEERD NQWLGVTLSR   100
QPGENGSIVT CGHRWKNIFY IKNENKLPTG GCYGVPPDLR TELSKRIAPC   150
YQDYVKKFGE NFASCQAGIS SFYTKDLIVM GAPGSSYWTG SLFVYNITTN   200
KYKAFLDKQN QVKFGSYLGY SVGAGHFRSQ HTTEVVGGAP QHEQIGKAYI   250
FSIDEKELNI LHEMKGKKLG SYFGASVCAV DLNADGFSDL LVGAPMQSTI   300
REEGRVFVYI NSGSGAVMNA METNLVGSDK YAARFGESIV NLGDIDNDGF   350
EDVAIGAPQE DDLQGAIYIY NGRADGISST FSQRIEGLQI SKSLSMFGQS   400
ISGQIDADNN GYVDVAVGAF RSDSAVLLRT RPVVIVDASL SHPESVNRTK   450
FDCVENGWPS VCIDLTLCFS YKGKEVPGYI VLFYNMSLDV NRKAESPPRF   500
YFSSNGTSDV ITGSIQVSSR EANCRTHQAF MRKDVRDILT PIQIEAAYHL   550
GPHVISKRST EEFPPLQPIL QQKKEKDIMK KTINFARFCA HENCSADLQV   600
SAKIGFLKPH ENKTYLAVGS MKTLMLNVSL FNAGDDAYET TLHVKLPVGL   650
YFIKILELEE KQINCEVTDN SGVVQLDCSI GYIYVDHLSR IDISFLLDVS   700
SLSRAEEDLS ITVHATCENE EEMDNLKHSR VTVAIPLKYE VKLTVHGFVN   750
PTSFVYGSND ENEPETCMVE KMNLTFHVIN TGNSMAPNVS VEIMVPNSFS   800
PQTDKLFNIL DVQTTTGECH FENYQRVCAL EQQKSAMQTL KGIVRFLSKT   850
DKRLLYCIKA DPHCLNFLCN FGKMESGKEA SVHIQLEGRP SILEMDETSA   900
LKFEIRATGF PEPNPRVIEL NKDENVAHVL LEGLHHQRPK RYFTIVIISS   950
SLLLGLIVLL LISYVMWKAG FFKRQYKSIL QEENRRDSWS YINSKSNDD    999
```

References

1 Pigott, R. and Power, C. (1993) The Adhesion Molecule FactsBook. Academic Press, London.

2 **Lobb, R.R. and Hemler, M.E. (1994) J. Clin. Invest. 94, 1722–1728.**

3 Rott, L.S. et al. (1996) J. Immunol. 156, 3727–3736.

4 Erle, D.J. et al. (1994) J. Immunol. 153, 517–528.

5 Rosen, G.D. et al. (1992) Cell 69, 1107–1119.

6 Takada, Y. et al. (1989) EMBO J. 8, 1361–1368.

7 Hemler, M.E. et al. (1987) J. Biol. Chem. 262, 11478–11485.

8 Parker C.M. et al. (1990) J. Biol. Chem. 268, 7028–7035.

9 Pujades, C. et al. (1996) Biochem. J. 313, 899–908.

10 Takada, Y. et al. (1987) Proc. Natl Acad. Sci. USA 84, 3239–3243.

11 Kilger, G. et al. (1995) J. Biol. Chem. 270, 5979–5984.

12 Berlin, C. et al. (1993) Cell 74, 185–195.

[13] Shimizu, Y. et al. (1990) J. Immunol. 145, 59–67.
[14] Springer, T.A. (1994) Cell 76, 301–314.
[15] **Alon, R. et al. (1995) J. Cell Biol. 128, 1243–1253.**
[16] **Berlin, C. et al. (1995) Cell 80, 413–422.**
[17] Rubio, M. et al. (1992) Eur. J. Immunol. 22, 1099–1102.
[18] Neuhaus, H. et al. (1991) J. Cell Biol. 115, 1149–1158.

CD49e

Other names
Integrin α5 subunit
VLA-5 (fibronectin receptor) α subunit
Ic subunit of GPIc–IIa

Molecular weights
Polypeptides   110 012

SDS-PAGE
    reduced   135 + 25 kDa
    unreduced   155 kDa

Carbohydrate
N-linked sites   14
O-linked sites   unknown

Human gene location
12q11–q13

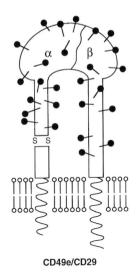

CD49e/CD29

Tissue distribution

CD49e is expressed on thymocytes, T cells, monocytes and platelets[1,2]. Expression is increased on activated and memory T cells[2,3]. It is also expressed on very early B cells and on activated B cells[4].

Structure

CD49e associates with CD29 to form the CD49e/CD29 integrin (α5β1, VLA-5). CD49e does not have an I-domain[5,6]. It is cleaved at one site to yield 135 kDa N-terminal and 25 kDa C-terminal disulfide-linked peptides. The N-terminal sequence of CD49e has been determined[7]. Electron microscopy of purified CD49e/CD29 has provided the structural model for all integrins[8].

Ligands and associated molecules

CD49e/CD29 is the fibronectin receptor and binds to the RGD sequence of fibronectin[2,9]. CD49e/CD29 has been shown to bind the neural adhesion molecule L1, which is also expressed on some leucocytes[10].

Function

CD49e/CD29-mediated binding to fibronectin provides a co-stimulatory signal to T cells[11]. It also enhances Fcγ receptor- and complement receptor-mediated phagocytosis[12,13], and VLA-2-mediated binding of monocytes to collagen[14]. CD49e/CD29 is involved in monocyte migration into extracellular tissues[15].

Database accession numbers

	PIR	SWISSPROT	EMBL/GENBANK	REFERENCE
Human	A27079	P08648	X06256	5,6
Mouse	PL0103	P11688	X15203	16

Amino acid sequence of human CD49e

```
MGSRTPESPL HAVQLRWGPR RRPPLVPLLL LLVPPPPRVG G          -1
FNLDAEAPAV LSGPPGSFFG FSVEFYRPGT DGVSVLVGAP KANTSQPGVL  50
QGGAVYLCPW GASPTQCTPI EFDSKGSRLL ESSLSSSEGE EPVEYKSLQW  100
FGATVRAHGS SILACAPLYS WRTEKEPLSD PVGTCYLSTD NFTRILEYAP  150
CRSDFSWAAG QGYCQGGFSA EFTKTGRVVL GGPGSYFWQG QILSATQEQI  200
AESYYPEYLI NLVQGQLQTR QASSIYDDSY LGYSVAVGEF SGDDTEDFVA  250
GVPKGNLTYG YVTILNGSDI RSLYNFSGEQ MASYFGYAVA ATDVNGDGLD  300
DLLVGAPLLM DRTPDGRPQE VGRVYVYLQH PAGIEPTPTL TLTGHDEFGR  350
FGSSLTPLGD LDQDGYNDVA IGAPFGGETQ QGVVFVFPGG PGGLGSKPSQ  400
VLQPLWAASH TPDFFGSALR GGRDLDGNGY PDLIVGSFGV DKAVVYRGRP  450
IVSASASLTI FPAMFNPEER SCSLEGNPVA CINLSFCLNA SGKHVADSIG  500
FTVELQLDWQ KQKGGVRRAL FLASRQATLT QTLLIQNGAR EDCREMKIYL  550
RNESEFRDKL SPIHIALNFS LDPQAPVDSH GLRPALHYQS KSRIEDKAQI  600
LLDCGEDNIC VPDLQLEVFG EQNHVYLGDK NALNLTFHAQ NVGEGGAYEA  650
ELRVTAPPEA EYSGLVRHPG NFSSLSCDYF AVNQSRLLVC DLGNPMKAGA  700
SLWGGLRFTV PHLRDTKKTI QFDFQILSKN LNNSQSDVVS FRLSVEAQAQ  750
VTLNGVSKPE AVLFPVSDWH PRDQPQKEED LGPAVHHVYE LINQGPSSIS  800
QGVLELSCPQ ALEGQQLLYV TRVTGLNCTT NHPINPKGLE LDPEGSLHHQ  850
QKREAPSRSS ASSGPQILKC PEAECFRLRC ELGPLHQQES QSLQLHFRVW  900
AKTFLQREHQ PFSLQCEAVY KALKMPYRIL PRQLPQKERQ VATAVQWTKA  950
EGSYGVPLWI IILAILFGLL LLGLLIYILY KLGFFKRSLP YGTAMEKAQL  1000
KPPATSDA                                               1008
```

References

1. Pigott, R. and Power, C. (1993) The Adhesion Molecule FactsBook. Academic Press, London.
2. **Hemler, M.E. (1990) Annu. Rev. Immunol. 114, 365–400.**
3. Shimizu, Y. et al. (1990) Nature 345, 250–253.
4. Ballard, L.L. et al. (1991) Clin. Exp. Immunol. 84, 336–346.
5. Argraves, W.S. et al. (1986) J. Cell Biol. 105, 1183–1190.
6. Fitzgerald, L.A. et al. (1987) Biochemistry 26, 8158–8165.
7. Takada, Y. et al. (1987) Proc. Natl Acad. Sci. USA 84, 3239–3243.
8. **Nermut, M.N. et al. (1988) EMBO J. 7, 4093–4099.**
9. **Hynes, R.O. (1992) Cell 69, 11–25.**
10. Ruppert, M. et al. (1995) J. Cell Biol. 131, 1881–1891.
11. Shimizu, Y. et al. (1990) J. Immunol. 145, 59–67.
12. Wright, S.D. et al. (1984) J. Cell Biol. 99, 336–339.
13. Pommier, C.G. et al. (1983) J. Exp. Med. 157, 1844–1854.
14. Pacifici, R. et al. (1994) J. Immunol. 153, 2222–2233.
15. Weber, C. et al. (1996) J. Cell Biol. 134, 1063–1073.
16. Holers, V.M. et al. (1989) J. Exp. Med. 169, 1589–1605.

CD49f

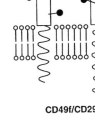

CD49f/CD29

Tissue distribution

CD49f is the α6 integrin subunit which can combine with CD29 (the β1 integrin subunit) to form the integrin VLA-6 (CD49f/CD29), which is expressed on thymocytes, T lymphocytes and monocytes [1,2]. Increased expression is found on activated and memory T cells [2,3]. CD49f also combines with CD104 to form the α6β4 integrin. Both CD49f/CD29 and CD49f/CD104 are widely expressed on epithelia in non-lymphoid tissues [4] (see **CD104**).

Structure

CD49f does not have an I-domain [5,6]. It is cleaved at one site to yield 120 kDa N-terminal and 30 kDa C-terminal peptides which remain disulfide-linked. The N-terminal sequence of CD49f has been determined [7,8]. Two alternatively spliced forms of CD49f cDNA have been described with different cytoplasmic domains [6,9]. The A form alone is expressed in the lung, liver, spleen and cervix, whereas only the B form is seen in the brain, ovary and kidney. Both forms are detected in other tissues [9].

Ligands and associated molecules

CD49f/CD29 (α6β1 integrin) is the laminin receptor on platelets [10], monocytes [11] and T lymphocytes [3,12].

Function

CD49f/CD29-mediated T cell binding to laminin provides a co-stimulatory signal to T cells for activation and proliferation [12].

Database accession numbers

	PIR	SWISSPROT	EMBL/GENBANK	REFERENCE
Human	B36429	P23229	X53586	5
			X59512	6

Amino acid sequence of human CD49f

```
MAAAGQLCLL YLSAGLLSRL GAA                               -1
FNLDTREDNV IRKYGDPGSL FGFSLAMHWQ LQPEDKRLLL VGAPRGEALP   50
LQRANRTGGL YSCDITARGP CTRIEFDNDA DPTSESKEDQ WMGVTVQSQG  100
PGGKVVTCAH RYEKRQHVNT KQESRDIFGR CYVLSQNLRI EDDMDGGDWS  150
FCDGRLRGHE KFGSCQQGVA ATFTKDFHYI VFGAPGTYNW KGIVRVEQKN  200
NTFFDMNIFE DGPYEVGGET EHDESLVPVP ANSYLGFSLD SGKGIVSKDE  250
ITFVSGAPRA NHSGAVVLLK RDMKSAHLLP EHIFDGEGLA SSFGYDVAVV  300
DLNKDGWQDI VIGAPQYFDR DGEVGGAVYV YMNQQGRWNN VKPIRLNGTK  350
DSMFGIAVKN IGDINQDGYP DIAVGAPYDD LGKVFIYHGS ANGINTKPTQ  400
VLKGISPYFG YSIAGNMDLD RNSYPDVAVG SLSDSVTIFR SRPVINIQKT  450
ITVTPNRIDL RQKTACGAPS GICLQVKSCF EYTANPAGYN PSISIVGTLE  500
AEKERRKSGL SSRVQFRNQG SEPKYTQELT LKRQKQKVCM EETLWLQDNI  550
RDKLRPIPIT ASVEIQEPSS RRRVNSLPEV LPILNSDEPK TAHIDVHFLK  600
EGCGDDNVCN SNLKLEYKFC TREGNQDKFS YLPIQKGVPE LVLKDQKDIA  650
LEITVTNSPS NPRNPTKDGD DAHEAKLIAT FPDTLTYSAY RELRAFPEKQ  700
LSCVANQNGS QADCELGNPF KRNSNVTFYL VLSTTEVTFD TPYLDINLKL  750
ETTSNQDNLA PITAKAKVVI ELLLSVSGVA KPSQVYFGGT VVGEQAMKSE  800
DEVGSLIEYE FRVINLGKPL TNLGTATLNI QWPKEISNGK WLLYLVKVES  850
KGLEKVTCEP QKEINSLNLT ESHNSRKKRE ITEKQIDDNR KFSLFAERKY  900
QTLNCSVNVN CVNIRCPLRG LDSKASLILR SRLWNSTFLE EYSKLNYLDI  950
LMRAFIDVTA AAENIRLPNA GTQVRVTVFP SKTVAQYSGV PWWIILVAIL 1000
AGILMLALLV FILWKCGFFK RNKKDHYDAT YHKAEIHAQP SDKERLTSDA 1050
```

The above sequence is the A form. In the B form the sequence in **bold** is replaced with:

```
            CGFFK RSRYDDSVPR YHAVRIRKEE REIKDEKYID 1050
NLEKKQWITK WNRNESYS                                  1068
```

References

1. Pigott, R. and Power, C. (1993) The Adhesion Molecule FactsBook. Academic Press, London.
2. **Hemler, M.E. (1990) Annu. Rev. Immunol. 114, 365–400.**
3. Shimizu, Y. et al. (1990) Nature 345, 250–253.
4. Natali, P.G. et al. (1992) J. Cell Sci. 103, 1243–1247.
5. Tamura, R.N. et al. (1990) J. Cell Biol. 111, 1593–1604.
6. Hogervorst, F. et al. (1991) Eur. J. Biochem. 199, 425–433.
7. Hemler, M.E. et al. (1989) J. Biol. Chem. 264, 6529–6535.
8. Kajiji, S. et al. (1989) EMBO J. 8, 673–680.
9. **Tamura, R.N. et al. (1991) Proc. Natl Acad. Sci. USA 88, 10183–10187.**
10. Sonnenberg, A. et al. (1988) Nature 336, 487–489.
11. Tobias, J.W. et al. (1987) Blood 69, 1265–1268.
12. Shimizu, Y. et al. (1990) J. Immunol. 145, 59–67.

Molecular weights

Polypeptide   56 255

SDS-PAGE
  reduced   120–160 kDa (neutrophils)
                  110–130 kDa (T lymphocytes)

Carbohydrate
N-linked sites 15
O-linked   probably nil

Human gene location
19p13.3–13.2 [1]

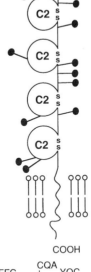

COOH

Domains	CST		CQV		CTL		CMA		CQA			
		ILC		FSC		IVC		FFC		YQC		
S	C2		C2		C2		C2		C2		TM	CY

Tissue distribution

CD50 is constitutively expressed at high levels on leucocytes, including resident epidermal dendritic Langerhans cells [2]. CD50 is generally not found on endothelia but has been detected on blood vessels within some lymphomas [3]. CD50 is released from activated lymphocytes and neutrophils, probably by proteolytic cleavage, and soluble forms of CD50 are detectable in the blood [4,5].

Structure

CD50 is a heavily and variably [6] glycosylated cell surface glycoprotein closely related to CD54 (ICAM-1) whose gene is also located in the region 19p13.3–13.2 [7–9]. Both proteins have five C2-set IgSF domains in their extracellular regions with 52% identity. The two membrane-distal IgSF domains of CD50 share ~37% identity with the extracellular portion of CD102 (ICAM-2). Electron microscopy studies suggest that CD50 is a straight rod approximately 15 nm in length [10]. The CD50 cytoplasmic domain, which is poorly conserved in CD54 and CD102, is phosphorylated on tyrosine and serine residues following cell activation [11].

Ligands and associated molecules

CD50, like CD54 and CD102, is a ligand for the leucocyte integrin LFA-1 (CD11a/CD18) [7–9]. Residues on the GFC β-sheet of the N-terminal domain interact with CD11a I domain [10,12]. Optimal LFA-1 binding to CD50 (as well as CD54 and CD102) requires activation of the cells expressing LFA-1 [13]. Unlike CD54, CD50 does not bind the integrins CD11b/CD18 (Mac-1) or CD11c/CD18 (p150,95). Crosslinked CD50 antibodies co-precipitate the tyrosine kinases Fyn and Lck [14].

Function

CD50 mediates adhesion between leucocytes. It is constitutively expressed on resting antigen-presenting cells, including dendritic cells, and appears to be important in the initial interactions between T cells and dendritic cells leading to T cell activation [2]. Extensive crosslinking of CD50 on T cells with mAbs can mobilize intracellular Ca^{2+} [14], activate tyrosine phosphorylation, and stimulate T cell adhesion and proliferation [14,15], but the functional significance of these observations is unclear.

Database accession numbers

	PIR	SWISSPROT	EMBL/GENBANK	REFERENCE
Human	S28904	P32942	X69711	7–9

Amino acid sequence of human CD50

```
MATMVPSVLW PRACWTLLVC CLLTPGVQG                         -1
QEFLLRVEPQ NPVLSAGGSL FVNCSTDCPS SEKIALETSL SKELVASGMG   50
WAAFNLSNVT GNSRILCSVY CNGSQITGSS NITVYGLPER VELAPLPPWQ  100
PVGQNFTLRC QVEGGSPRTS LTVVLLRWEE ELSRQPAVEE PAEVTATVLA  150
SRDDHGAPFS CRTELDMQPQ GLGLFVNTSA PRQLRTFVLP VTPPRLVAPR  200
FLEVETSWPV DCTLDGLFPA SEAQVYLALG DQMLNATVMN HGDTLTATAT  250
ATARADQEGA REIVCNVTLG GERREARENL TVFSFLGPIV NLSEPTAHEG  300
STVTVSCMAG ARVQVTLDGV PAAAPGQPAQ LQLNATESDD GRSFFCSATL  350
EVDGEFLHRN SSVQLRVLYG PKIDRATCPQ HLKWKDKTRH VLQCQARGNP  400
YPELRCLKEG SSREVPVGIP FFVNVTHNGT YQCQASSSRG KYTLVVVMDI  450
EAGSSHFVPV FVAVLLTLGV VTIVLALMYV FREHQRSGSY HVREESTYLP  500
LTSMQPTEAM GEEPSRAE                                     518
```

References

1 Bossy, D. et al. (1994) Genomics 23, 712–713.
2 Starling, G.C. et al. (1995) Eur. J. Immunol. 25, 2528–2532.
3 Cordell, J.L. et al. (1994) J. Clin. Pathol. 47, 143–147.
4 Del Pozo, M.A. et al. (1994) Eur. J. Immunol. 24, 2586–2594.
5 Pino-Otin, M.R. et al. (1995) J. Immunol. 154, 3015–3024.
6 de Fougerolles, A.R. et al. (1995) Eur. J. Immunol. 25, 1008–1012.
7 de Fougerolles, A.R. et al. (1993) J. Exp. Med. 177, 1187–1192.
8 Fawcett, J. et al. (1992) Nature 360, 481–484.
9 Vazeux, R. et al. (1992) Nature 360, 485–488.
10 Sadhu, C. et al. (1994) Cell Adhesion Commun. 2, 429–440.
11 Skubitz, K.M. et al. (1995) J. Immunol. 154, 2888–2895.
12 Van Kooyk, Y. et al. (1996) J. Exp. Med. 183, 1247–1252.
13 **de Fougerolles, A.R. et al. (1994) J. Exp. Med. 179, 619–629.**
14 Juan, M. et al. (1994) J. Exp. Med. 179, 1747–1756.
15 Hernandez-Caselles, T. et al. (1993) Eur. J. Immunol. 23, 2799–2806.

CD51 α subunit of vitronectin receptor, integrin αV subunit

Molecular weights
Polypeptide   121 716

SDS-PAGE
  reduced   125 + 24 kDa
  unreduced   150 kDa

Carbohydrate
N-linked sites   13
O-linked sites   unknown

Human gene location
2q31–q32

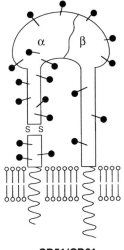

CD51/CD61

Tissue distribution

CD51 in combination with CD61 (αVβ3 integrin) is expressed on platelets but at a lower level than the integrin CD41/CD61 [1,2]. It is expressed on endothelial cells, certain activated leucocytes, NK cells, macrophages and neutrophils [3,4]. It is also expressed on other tissues including smooth muscle cells and osteoclasts [3]. CD51 is the most promiscuous integrin α subunit; it can form heterodimers with the β1 (CD29), β3 (CD61), β5, β6, and β8 integrin subunits in various tissues [5].

Structure

CD51 (integrin αV subunit) falls into the α subclass with no I-domain. It is processed into a large N-terminal chain and a small C-terminal chain which remain disulfide linked [6]. The N-terminal sequences of both chains have been determined [7].

Ligands and associated molecules

CD51/CD61 is also known as the vitronectin receptor. It mediates binding of platelets to immobilized vitronectin without prior activation. Other ligands for CD51/CD61 include RGD-containing proteins such as fibrinogen, fibronectin, von Willebrand factor, laminin and thrombospondin [2,8] and the neural adhesion molecule L1, which is expressed on certain leucocytes [9]. CD51/CD61 also mediates cell–cell adhesion via an interaction with CD31 [10,11]. It has been shown to associate on the cell surface with CD47 [4,12,13].

Function

CD51/CD61 acts as an activation-independent receptor for platelet attachment and spreading on vitronectin and other RGD-containing proteins, including matrix components [2,8]. It mediates leucocyte–endothelial cell adhesion via interaction with CD31 [10,11]. It has also been shown to initiate bone resorption by mediating the adhesion of osteoclasts to osteopontin [14], and it may play a role in angiogenesis [3]. Antagonists of CD51/CD61 have been shown to inhibit tumour growth by disrupting angiogenesis [15].

Database accession numbers

	PIR	SWISSPROT	EMBL/GENBANK	REFERENCE
Human	A27421	P06756	M14648	6,7
Mouse		P43406	U14135	16

Amino acid sequence of human CD51

```
MAFPPRRRLR LGPRGLPLLL SGLLLPLCRA                                -1
FNLDVDSPAE YSGPEGSYFG FAVDFFVPSA SSRMFLLVGA PKANTTQPGI          50
VEGGQVLKCD WSSTRRCQPI EFDATGNRDY AKDDPLEFKS HQWFGASVRS          100
KQDKILACAP LYHWRTEMKQ EREPVGTCFL QDGTKTVEYA PCRSQDIDAD          150
GQGFCQGGFS IDFTKADRVL LGGPGSFYWQ GQLISDQVAE IVSKYDPNVY          200
SIKYNNQLAT RTAQAIFDDS YLGYSVAVGD FNGDGIDDFV SGVPRAARTL          250
GMVYIYDGKN MSSLYNFTGE QMAAYFGFSV AATDINGDDY ADVFIGAPLF          300
MDRGSDGKLQ EVGQVSVSLQ RASGDFQTTK LNGFEVFARF GSAIAPLGDL          350
DQDGFNDIAI AAPYGGEDKK GIVYIFNGRS TGLNAVPSQI LEGQWAARSM          400
PPSFGYSMKG ATDIDKNGYP DLIVGAFGVD RAILYRARPV ITVNAGLEVY          450
PSILNQDNKT CSLPGTALKV SCFNVRFCLK ADGKGVLPRK LNFQVELLLD          500
KLKQKGAIRR ALFLYSRSPS HSKNMTISRG GLMQCEELIA YLRDESEFRD          550
KLTPITIFME YRLDYRTAAD TTGLQPILNQ FTPANISRQA HILLDCGEDN          600
VCKPKLEVSV DSDQKKIYIG DDNPLTLIVK AQNQGEGAYE AELIVSIPLQ          650
ADFIGVVRNN EALARLSCAF KTENQTRQVV CDLGNPMKAG TQLLAGLRFS          700
VHQQSEMDTS VKFDLQIQSS NLFDKVSPVV SHKVDLAVLA AVEIRGVSSP          750
DHIFLPIPNW EHKENPETEE DVGPVVQHIY ELRNNGPSSF SKAMLHLQWP          800
YKYNNNTLLY ILHYDIDGPM NCTSDMEINP LRIKISSLQT TEKNDTVAGQ          850
GERDHLITKR DLALSEGDIH TLGCGVAQCL KIVCQVGRLD RGKSAILYVK          900
SLLWTETFMN KENQNHSYSL KSSASFNVIE FPYKNLPIED ITNSTLVTTN          950
VTWGIQPAPM PVPVWVIILA VLAGLLLLAV LVFVMYRMGF FKRVRPPQEE          1000
QEREQLQPHE NGEGNSET                                            1018
```

References
1 Pigott, R. and Power, C. (1993) The Adhesion Molecule FactsBook. Academic Press, London.
2 **Keiffer, N. and Phillips, D.R. (1990) Annu. Rev. Cell Biol. 6, 329–357.**
3 Varner, J.A. et al. (1995) Cell Adhes. Comm. 3, 367–374.
4 Hendey, B. et al. (1996) Blood 87, 2038–2048.
5 Busk, M. et al. (1992) J. Biol. Chem. 267, 5790–5796.
6 Suzuki, S. et al. (1987) J. Biol. Chem. 262, 14080–14085.
7 Suzuki, S. et al. (1986) Proc. Natl Acad. Sci. USA 83, 8614–8618.
8 **Ginsberg, M.H. et al. (1993) Thromb. Haemost. 70, 87–93.**
9 Ebeling, O. et al. (1996) Eur. J. Immunol. 26, 2508–2516.
10 Piali, L. et al. (1995) J. Cell Biol. 130, 451–460.
11 Buckley, C.D. et al. (1996) J. Cell Sci. 109, 437–455.
12 Lindberg, F.P. et al. (1996) J. Cell Biol. 134, 1313–1322.

¹³ Gao, A.G. et al. (1996) J. Cell Biol. 135, 533–544.

¹⁴ Ross, F.P. et al. (1993) J. Biol. Chem. 268, 9901–9907.

¹⁵ Varner, J.A. and Cheresh, D.A. (1996) Curr. Opin. Cell Biol. 8, 724–730.

¹⁶ Wada, J. et al. (1996) J. Cell Biol. 132, 1161–1176.

Molecular weights
Polypeptide   1208

SDS-PAGE
   reduced   21–28 kDa
   unreduced   21–28 kDa

Carbohydrate
N-linked sites   1
O-linked   Nil

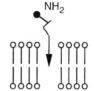

Tissue distribution

CD52 is expressed at high levels (5×10^5 molecules per cell) on lymphocytes and monocytes, but not on plasma cells, platelets or erythrocytes. In non-lymphoid tissues, CD52 is expressed by the epithelial cells of the epididymis and seminal vesicle. These cells appear to secrete the antigen into seminal plasma, where it can be taken up by sperm which are CD52 positive but do not express CD52 mRNA [1].

Structure

CD52 is an unusually short glycoprotein bearing a GPI anchor. The cDNA encodes a leader sequence of 24 amino acids followed by a 12 amino acid N-terminal sequence and a C-terminal GPI signal sequence [2]. The major component of the molecule is a large sialylated, polylactosamine-containing core-fucosylated tetraantennary *N*-linked oligosaccharide [3]. Two subclasses of CD52 have been identified, CD52-I and CD52-II, differing only in the PI moiety of the GPI anchor [3]. The functional relevance of the two subclasses is not known. The N-terminus and GPI anchor attachment site have been determined biochemically [1,2]. CD52 species homologues have been identified in the monkey [4], dog [5], rat [6] and mouse [7]. Although these molecules share little amino acid sequence homology within the short peptide core, significant sequence identities are apparent in the leader and GPI signal sequences (see below). Where tissue expression data are available, the expression patterns of the CD52 species homologues are similar to that of the human [4–7]. Moreover, the similarities in gene structure and promoter sequence of human CD52 and the predicted mouse homologue, B7(2), strongly support their classification as species homologues (M. Tone, personal communication).

Function

The function of CD52 is unknown. However, CD52 is an exceptionally good target for complement-mediated cell lysis and antibody-mediated cellular cytotoxicity [8]. CD52 mAbs are very effective *in vivo* for lymphocyte depletion and a humanized CD52 mAb (CAMPATH-1H [9]) is giving promising results in clinical studies as a treatment of malignant lymphomas and rheumatoid arthritis (e.g. see ref. 10). CD52 may be such a good target for serotherapy because the CAMPATH-1 epitope lies close to the plasma membrane, within the C-terminal tripeptide and the GPI anchor, thus facilitating complement lysis [8].

Database accession numbers

	PIR	SWISSPROT	EMBL/GENBANK	REFERENCE
Human	S18766	P31358	X62466	2
Monkey	S27152	P32763	X67495	4
Dog			S77412	5
Rat	S40081		X76697	6
Mouse			M55561	7

Amino acid sequences of CD52

```
Rat      MNTFL.LLLT ISLLVVVQIQ TGDL                                          -1
Mouse    MKSFL.LFLT IILLVVIQIQ TGSL                                          -1
Human    MKRFLFLLLT ISLLVMVQIQ TGLS                                          -1
Monkey   MKRFLFLLLT ISLLVMVQIQ TGVT                                          -1
Dog      MKGFLFLLLT ISLLVMIQIQ TGVL                                          -1


Rat      GQNSTAVTTP ANKAATTAAA TTKAAATTAT KTTTAVRKTP GKPPKAG   47
Mouse    GQ........ ....ATTAAS GTNKNSTSTK KT........ ..PLKSG   25
Human    GQNDTSQTSS PS........ .......... .......... ........   12
Monkey   QNATSQ.SS PS........ .......... .......... .......   11
Dog      GNSTTPRMTT KKVKSATPA. .......... .......... .......   19


Rat      ASSITDVGAC TFLFF.ANTL MCLFYLS                           73
Mouse    ASSIIDAGAC SFLFF.ANTL MCLFYLS                           51
Human    ASSNI.SG.G IFLFFVANAI IHLFCFS                           37
Monkey   ASSNL.SG.G GFLFFVANAI IHLFYFS                           36
Dog      LSSL..GG.G SVLLFLANTL IQLFYLS                           43
```

References

1 Taylor, V. and Hale, G. (1995) Leucocyte Typing V, 235–237.
2 Xia, M.-Q. et al. (1991) Eur. J. Immunol. 21, 1677–1684.
3 **Treumann, A. et al. (1995) J. Biol. Chem. 270, 6088–6099.**
4 Perry, A.C.F. et al. (1992) Biochim. Biophys. Acta 1171, 122–124.
5 Ellerbrock, K. et al. (1994) Int. J. Androl. 17, 314–323.
6 Kirchhoff, C. (1994) Biol. Reprod. 50, 896–902.
7 Kubota, H. et al. (1990) J. Immunol. 145, 3924–3931.
8 Xia, M.-Q. et al. (1993) Mol. Immunol. 30, 1089–1096.
9 Riechmann, L. et al. (1988) Nature 332, 323–327.
10 Osterborg, A. et al. (1996) Br. J. Haematol. 93, 151–153.

CD53 OX-44 (rat)

Molecular weights
Polypeptide   24 341

SDS-PAGE
    reduced   35–42 kDa
    unreduced   35–42 kDa

Carbohydrate
N-linked sites   2
O-linked   nil

Human gene location
1p21–p13.3; >26 kb [1]

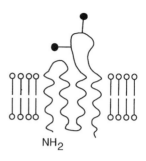

Tissue distribution

CD53 is expressed by T and B cells, monocytes, macrophages, granulocytes, dendritic cells, osteoblasts and osteoclasts. It is absent from platelets and erythrocytes (reviewed in ref. 2). In the rat and mouse, CD53 is expressed on only about 12% of thymocytes and is largely absent from the CD4+CD8+ population [3]. CD53 expression on thymocytes is induced by T cell receptor engagement during repertoire selection [3].

Structure

CD53 is a member of the TM4 superfamily and is predicted to have four transmembrane regions, short cytoplasmic N- and C-termini, and two extracellular regions (reviewed in ref. 2). Epitope mapping of anti-rat CD53 mAbs has proved the major hydrophilic region to be extracellular, which is consistent with the proposed topology of TM4SF molecules [2]. Gene mapping data suggest that CD37 and CD53 have evolved by gene duplication and divergence from a common ancestral gene [4].

Ligands and associated molecules

Co-immunoprecipitation and flow cytometric energy transfer studies have shown that CD53 associates non-covalently with a number of other molecules: CD2 in rat NK and T cells [2]; the integrin CD29/CD49d (VLA-4) in a human T cell line [5]; MHC Class I and II, CD19, CD20, CD21, CD37, CD81 and CD82 in human B cells [6]; and a protein tyrosine phosphatase in rat lymph node cells [7]. No extracellular ligand has been identified for CD53.

Function

In vitro experiments using mAbs suggest that CD53 can transduce signals in human B cells, monocytes and granulocytes, and in rat macrophages, NK and T cells [2].

Database accession numbers

	PIR	SWISSPROT	EMBL/GENBANK	REFERENCE
Human	A37243	P19397	M37033	8,9
Rat	A39574	P24485	M57276	10
Mouse			X97227	4

Amino acid sequence of human CD53

```
MGMSSLKLLK YVLFFFNLLF WICGCCILGF GIYLLIHNNF GVLFHNLPSL    50
TLGNVFVIVG SIIMVVAFLG CMGSIKENKC LLMSFFILLL IILLAEVTLA   100
ILLFVYEQKL NEYVAKGLTD SIHRYHSDNS TKAAWDSIQS FLQCCGINGT   150
SDWTSGPPAS CPSDRKVEGC YAKARLWFHS NFLYIGIITI CVCVIEVLGM   200
SFALTLNCQI DKTSQTIGL                                     219
```

References

1. Korinek, V. and Horejsi, V. (1993) Immunogenetics 38, 272–279.
2. **Wright, M.D. and Tomlinson, M.G. (1994) Immunol. Today 15, 588–594.**
3. Tomlinson, M.G. et al. (1995) Eur. J. Immunol. 25, 2201–2206.
4. Wright, M.D. et al. (1993) Int. Immunol. 5, 209–216.
5. Mannion, B.A. et al. (1996) J. Immunol. 157, 2039–2047.
6. Szöllosi, J. et al. (1996) J. Immunol. 157, 2939–2946.
7. Carmo, A.M. and Wright, M.D. (1995) Eur. J. Immunol. 25, 2090–2095.
8. Amiot, M. (1990) J. Immunol. 145, 4322–4325.
9. Angelisova, P. et al. (1990) Immunogenetics 32, 281–285.
10. Bellacosa, A. et al. (1990) Mol. Cell Biol. 11, 2864–2872.

CD54   ICAM-1

Molecular weights
Polypeptide   55 402

SDS-PAGE
  reduced   85–110 kDa

Carbohydrate
N-linked sites   8
O-linked   unknown

Human gene location and size
19p13.3–13.2 [1]; 12 kb [2]

COOH

Domains

| S | C2 | C2 | C2 | C2 | C2 | TM | CY |

CST PMC   CQV FSC   CSL LTC   CEA FSC   CQA YLC

| 1 | 1 | 1 | 1 | 1 | 1 |

PGP   YWT   FVL   YSF   LYG   LSP

Exon boundaries

Tissue distribution

CD54 has a wide tissue distribution, being expressed on both haematopoietic and non-haematopoietic cells [3]. Expression on resting leucocytes is low but is upregulated on activation [4,5]. Similarly, expression on endothelium and other non-haematopoietic cells is strongly upregulated by inflammatory mediators [4,5]. A soluble form of ICAM-1 is detectable in the blood [6].

Structure

CD54 is closely related to CD50 (ICAM-3) whose gene is also located in the region 19p13.3–13.2. Both proteins have five C2-set IgSF domains in their extracellular regions with 52% identity. The two membrane-distal IgSF domains of CD54 also share ~34% identity with the extracellular portion of CD102 (ICAM-2). Electron microscopy studies suggest that CD54 is a bent rod, 18.7 nm in length [7]. Cell surface CD54 may exist as a non-covalent linked dimer [8]. A number of alternatively spliced forms of CD54 are expressed in the mouse [9]. These isoforms, which have a more restricted pattern of expression, lack combinations of domains 2–4, but most still bind LFA-1.

Ligands and associated molecules

CD54, like CD50 and CD102, is a ligand for the leucocyte integrin CD11a/CD18 (LFA-1) [7]. CD54 also binds the related integrins CD11b/CD18

(Mac-1)[10] and CD11c/CD18 (p150,95)[11] and has been reported to bind hyaluronan[12] and fibrinogen[13]. CD54 is a receptor for the major group of rhinoviruses[7] and is one of the receptors on endothelium (others include CD36 and thrombospondin) for *Plasmodium falciparum*-infected erythrocytes[14]. The LFA-1 binding site lies on the GFC β sheet of the membrane-distal domain (domain 1)[7]. Rhinoviruses bind an overlapping site on domain 1 (and possibly 2)[7] whereas Mac-1 binds to domain 3[10].

Function

Endothelial CD54 contributes to the extravasation of leucocytes from blood vessels, particularly in areas of inflammation[15]. CD54 on antigen-presenting cells contributes to antigen-specific T cell activation, presumably by enhancing interactions between T cells and antigen-presenting cells[15].

Database accession numbers

	PIR	SWISSPROT	EMBL/GENBANK	REFERENCE
Human	A29849	P05362	X06990	16
Mouse	A45815	P13597	X52264	17
Rat			D00913	18

Amino acid sequence of human CD54

```
MAPSSPRPAL PALLVLLGAL FPGPG                            -1
NAQTSVSPSK VILPRGGSVL VTCSTSCDQP KLLGIETPLP KKELLLPGNN  50
RKVYELSNVQ EDSQPMCYSN CPDGQSTAKT FLTVYWTPER VELAPLPSWQ 100
PVGKNLTLRC QVEGGAPRAN LTVVLLRGEK ELKREPAVGE PAEVTTTVLV 150
RRDHHGANFS CRTELDLRPQ GLELFENTSA PYQLQTFVLP ATPPQLVSPR 200
VLEVDTQGTV VCSLDGLFPV SEAQVHLALG DQRLNPTVTY GNDSFSAKAS 250
VSVTAEDEGT QRLTCAVILG NQSQETLQTV TIYSFPAPNV ILTKPEVSEG 300
TEVTVKCEAH PRAKVTLNGV PAQPLGPRAQ LLLKATPEDN GRSFSCSATL 350
EVAGQLIHKN QTRELRVLYG PRLDERDCPG NWTWPENSQQ TPMCQAWGNP 400
LPELKCLKDG TFPLPIGESV TVTRDLEGTY LCRARSTQGE VTREVTVNVL 450
SPRYEIVIIT VVAAAVIMGT AGLSTYLYNR QRKIKKYRLQ QAQKGTPMKP 500
NTQATPP                                               507
```

References

1 Trask, B. et al. (1993) Genomics 15, 133–145.
2 Voraberger, G. et al. (1991) J. Immunol. 147, 2777–2786.
3 Smith, M.E.F. and Thomas, J.A. (1990) J. Clin. Pathol. 43, 893–900.
4 Springer, T.A. (1990) Nature 346, 425–434.
5 Dustin, M.L. and Springer, T.A. (1991) Annu. Rev. Immunol. 9, 27–66.
6 Gearing, A.J.H. and Newman, W. (1993) Immunol. Today 14, 506–512.
7 Staunton, D.E. et al. (1990) Cell 61, 243–254.
8 **Miller, J. et al. (1995) J. Exp. Med. 182, 1231–1241.**
9 King, P.D. et al. (1995) J. Immunol. 154, 6080–6093.
10 Diamond, M.S. et al. (1991) Cell 65, 961–971.
11 de Fourgerolles, A.R. et al. (1995) Eur. J. Immunol. 25, 1008–1012.
12 McCourt, P.A.G. et al. (1994) J. Biol. Chem. 269, 30081–30084.
13 Languino, L.R. et al. (1993) Cell 73, 1423–1434.
14 Berendt, A.R. et al. (1992) Cell 68, 71–81.

[15] Xu, H. et al. (1994) J. Exp. Med. 180, 95–109.
[16] Simmons, D. et al. (1988) Nature 331, 624–627.
[17] Ballantyne, C.M. et al. (1989) Nucleic Acids Res. 17, 5853.
[18] Kita, Y. et al. (1992) Biochim. Biophys. Acta 1131, 108–110.

Molecular weights

Polypeptides   34 964

SDS-PAGE
  reduced   60–70 kDa
  unreduced   64–73 kDa

Carbohydrate

N-linked sites   1
O-linked sites   abundant

Human gene location and size

1q32; ~40 kb [1,2]

Tissue distribution

CD55 is expressed on all cells in contact with serum, including all haematopoietic cells and the vascular endothelium. It is widely expressed on epithelia in the gastointestinal and genitourinary tracts and the central nervous system. A soluble form of CD55 is present in plasma and body fluids [2].

Structure

The N-terminal region of the extracellular portion of CD55 consists of four complement control protein (CCP) domains attached to a Ser- and Thr-rich segment that is heavily O-glycosylated [1-4]. It has been proposed that this segment serves as a spacer to project the functional CCP domains from the cell surface [2]. CD55 expressed on a Chinese hamster ovary cell line defective in O-glycosylation is rapidly degraded, suggesting that the carbohydrate structures serve to protect CD55 from proteolysis [5]. The N-terminus of CD55 has been determined by protein sequencing [6]. The glycoprotein is GPI-anchored at Ser319 [7]. A minor form of CD55 mRNA arises from alternate splicing of an additional exon, but a corresponding protein has not been identified [1-3]. A covalently linked homodimeric form has been described [8].

Ligands and associated molecules

CD55 interacts with complement components (see below) and CD97, a seven-transmembrane domain protein which also contains three extracellular EGF domains [9].

Function

CD55 is a member of the regulator of complement activation (RCA) family of proteins[2] (see **CD35**). It accelerates the dissociation of the components of the C3-convertases, namely C2a from C4b in the C4b2a complex (the C3-convertase of the classical pathway), and factor Bb from the C3bBb complex (the C3-convertase of the alternative pathway). CD55 expression increases upon T cell activation and antibodies to CD55 are mitogenic in the presence of phorbol esters[10]. CD55 and the two other complement regulatory proteins, CD46 and CD59, have received much attention in their role in reproduction and xenotransplantaion (see **CD46**).

Comments

The mouse has two genes for CD55, one codes for a GPI-anchored protein and the other for a transmembrane protein[11]. Analysis of mRNA expression showed that the GPI-anchored form is detected in most tissues, whereas the transmembrane form is highly expressed in the testes, and is also detected in bone marrow, lymph nodes, lung and liver. CD55 expressed on mouse erythrocytes is resistant to phosphatidylinositol-specific phospholipase C treatment whereas CD55 on the surface of spleen and PBMCs is removed by phospholipase C, suggesting that the two forms of CD55 are expressed on different cell types[12]. This is another example of the lack of conservation between species of genes in the RCA complex (see **CD35**).

Database accession numbers

	PIR	SWISSPROT	EMBL/GENBANK	REFERENCE
Human	A26359	P08174	M35156	3,4
		P09679		
Human Alt-form			M30142	1,3
Mouse GPI-form			L41366	11
Mouse TM-form			L41365	11

Amino acid sequence of human CD55

```
MTVARPSVPA ALPLLGELPR LLLLVLLCLP AVWG                   -1
DCGLPPDVPN AQPALEGRTS FPEDTVITYK CEESFVKIPG EKDSVICLKG   50
SQWSDIEEFC NRSCEVPTRL NSASLKQPYI TQNYFPVGTV VEYECRPGYR  100
REPSLSPKLT CLQNLKWSTA VEFCKKKSCP NPGEIRNGQI DVPGGILFGA  150
TISFSCNTGY KLFGSTSSFC LISGSSVQWS DPLPECREIY CPAPPQIDNG  200
IIQGERDHYG YRQSVTYACN KGFTMIGEHS IYCTVNNDEG EWSGPPPECR  250
GKSLTSKVPP TVQKPTTVNV PTTEVSPTSQ KTTTKTTTPN AQATRSTPVS  300
RTTKHFHETT PNKGSGTTS                                    319
GTTRLLSGHT CFTLTGLLGT LVTMGLLT                          +28
```

References
1 Post, T.W. et al. (1990) J. Immunol. 144, 740–744.
2 **Liszewski, M.K. et al. (1996) Adv. Immunol. 61, 201–283.**
3 Caras, I.W. et al. (1987) Nature 325, 545–549.
4 Medof, M.E. et al. (1987) Proc. Natl. Acad. Sci. USA 84, 2007–2011.
5 Reddy, P. et al. (1989) J. Biol. Chem. 264, 17329–17336.

[6] Davitz, M.A. et al. (1987) J. Immunol. Methods 97, 71–76.

[7] Moran, P. et al. (1991) J. Biol. Chem. 266, 1250–1257.

[8] Nickells, M.W. et al. (1994) J. Immunol. 152, 676–685.

[9] Hamann, J. et al. (1996) J. Exp. Med. 184, 1185–1189.

[10] Davis, L.S. et al. (1988) J. Immunol. 141, 2246–2252.

[11] Spicer, A.P. et al. (1995) J. Immunol. 155, 3079–3091.

[12] Kameyoshi, Y. et al. (1989) Immunology 68, 439–444.

Other names
NKH-1 antigen
Leu-19 antigen
Fasciclin II (*Drosophila*)
apCAM (Mollusc)

Molecular weights

SDS-PAGE
  reduced or unreduced
      180 kD (long cytoplasmic domain form)
      140 kD (short cytoplasmic domain form)
      120 kD (GPI-linked form)

Carbohydrate
N-linked sites   6
O-linked   unknown

Human gene location
11q23.1

Domains		CQV YKC		CDV YRC		CDA YIC		CEA YIC		CEV YNC		FDE TTY		LSP RHY		
	S	C2		C2		C2		C2		C2		F3		F3	TM	CY

Tissue distribution

On human haematopoietic cells CD56 is restricted to NK cells and a subpopulation of T lymphocytes. CD56 is not expressed on mouse or rat haematopoietic cells. Amongst both human and murine non-haematopoietic tissues, CD56 is expressed in adult neural tissue and muscle, and in many embryonic tissues. A number of tumour cell types are positive for CD56, including some myeloid leukaemias, myelomas, neuroblastomas, Wilms' tumours and small cell lung carcinomas (reviewed in refs 1 and 2).

Structure

CD56 is an isoform of the neural cell adhesion molecule (NCAM) that is virtually identical to the 140 kDa brain isoform. Various NCAMs, including soluble and GPI-anchored isoforms, arise by alternative splicing from a single gene and are post-translationally modified by glycosylation, acylation, sulfation and phosphorylation. The extracellular domain of NCAM consists of five C2-set IgSF domains and two fibronectin type III domains. Electron microscopy of the purified protein suggests that these domains are tandemly arranged to form a flexible rod-like structure projecting from the cell surface (reviewed in ref. 1). The three-dimensional structure of the N-terminal IgSF domain has a high similarity to domain 1 of VCAM-1 [3].

Ligands and associated molecules

CD56 has a clear function in homotypic binding to CD56 molecules on other cells. All five IgSF domains appear to be involved, and these pair up in an antiparallel alignment such that domain 1 binds to domain 5, domain 2 to 4, and domain 3 with itself[4]. NCAM on neuronal cells can bind to chondroitin sulfate proteoglycans of the cell matrix. The result of this interaction is the inhibition of neurite outgrowth[5]. NCAM *cis*-interactions with other molecules have not been defined, although indirect evidence suggests a potential association of NCAM with the related neural cell adhesion molecule L1, and with the fibroblast growth factor receptor through which NCAM may transduce signals (reviewed in refs 6 and 7).

Function

The significance of CD56 expression on NK cells is not clear and remains controversial[2]. However, the role of NCAM as a homotypic cell adhesion molecule on neuronal cells has been well studied (reviewed in refs 7 and 8). *In vitro* data suggest that NCAM functions in the control of neuronal development by regulating cell migration, neurite outgrowth, selective fasciculation and axon sorting, target recognition, and synaptic plasticity[8]. NCAM knockout mice appear grossly normal, but do have subtle defects in neuronal guidance and connectivity. Moreover, these animals exhibit deficient spatial learning which implicates NCAM in synaptic plasticity[8]. NCAM gene targeting to produce mice that express only a secreted NCAM results in a dominant embryonic lethality. This suggests a role for NCAM in heterophilic interactions, in addition to its relatively well characterized function in homotypic adhesion[9]. The capacity of NCAM for cell adhesion can be down-modulated by post-translational attachment of a large polysialic acid (PSA) moiety to the fifth IgSF domain. PSA expression is regulated by neuronal activity at the synapse and is required for the induction of synaptic plasticity by NCAM[10].

Comment

NCAM is highly conserved between species, the murine homologue sharing 24% and 26% amino acid identity with the insect and mollusc homologues, respectively[11]. The *Drosophila* homologue (fasciclin II) functions in selective fasciculation and axon sorting[8], and the mollusc *Aplysia* homologue (apCAM) has a role in synaptic plasticity[11].

Database accession numbers for some NCAM isoforms

	PIR	SWISSPROT	EMBL/GENBANK	REFERENCE
Human	A26883	P13592	X16841	12
Rat	S00846	P13596	X06564	13
Mouse	A29673	P13595	Y00051	14
Chicken	A25435	P13590	M15861	15
Xenopus	S09600	P16170	M25696	16
Drosophila	B41054	P34082	M77166	17
Mollusc	C42632		M89648	11

Amino acid sequence of NK cell CD56 (ref. 18)

```
MLQTKDLIWT LFFLGTAVS                                            -1
LQVDIVPSQG EISVGESKFF LCQVAGDAKD KDISWFSPNG EKLTPNQQRI          50
SVVWNDDSSS TLTIYNANID DAGIYKCVVT GEDGSESEAT VNVKIFQKLM         100
FKNAPTPQEF REGEDAVIVC DVVSSLPPTI IWKHKGRDVI LKKDVRFIVL         150
SNNYLQIRGI KKTDEGTYRC EGRILARGEI NFKDIQVIVN VPPTIRARQN         200
IVNATANLGQ SVTLVCDAER FPEPTMSWTK DGEQIEQEED DEKYIFSDDS         250
SQLTIKKVDK NDEAEYICIA ENKAGEQDAT IHLKVFAKPK ITYVENQTAM         300
ELEEQVTLTC EASGDPIPSI TWRTSTRNIS SEEKASWTRP EKQETLDGHM         350
VVRSHARVSS LTLKSIQYTD AGEYICTASN TIGQDSQSMY LEVQYAPKLQ         400
GPVAVYTWEG NQVNITCEVF AYPSATISWF RDGQLLPSSN YSNIKIYNTP         450
SASYLEVTPD SENDFGNYNC TAVNRIGQES FEFILVQADT PSSPSIDQVE         500
PYSSTAQVQF DEPEATGGVP ILKYKAEWRA VGEEVWHSKW YDAKEASMEG         550
IVTIVGLKPE TTYAVRLAAL NGKGLGEISA ASEFKTQPVQ GEPSAPKLEG         600
QMGEDGNSIK VNLIKQDDGG SPIRHYLVRY RALSSEWKPE IRLPSGSDHV         650
MLKSLDWNAE YEVYVVAENQ QGKSKAAHFV FRTSAQPTAI PANGSPTSGL         700
STGAIVGILI VIFVLLLVVV DITCYFLNKC GLFMCIAVNL CGKAGPGAKG         750
KDMEEGKAAF SKDESKEPIV EVRTEEERTP NHDGGKHTEP NETTPLTEPE         800
KGPVEAKPEC QETETKPAPA EVKTVPNDAT QTKENESKA                     839
```

References

1. Goridis, C. and Brunet, J.-F. (1992) Semin. Cell Biol. 3, 189–197.
2. Lanier, L.L. and Hemperly, J.J. (1995) Leucocyte Typing V, 1398–1400.
3. Thomsen, N.K. et al. (1996) Nat. Struct. Biol. 3, 581–585.
4. Ranheim, T.S. et al. (1996) Proc. Natl Acad. Sci. USA 93, 4071–4075.
5. Friedlander, D.R. et al. (1994) J. Cell. Biol. 125, 669–680.
6. Feizi, T. (1994) Trends Biochem. Sci. 19, 233–234.
7. Baldwin, T.J. et al. (1996) J. Cell. Biochem. 61, 502–513.
8. Goodman, C.S. (1996) Annu. Rev. Neurosci. 19, 341–377.
9. **Rabinowitz, J.E. et al. (1996) Proc. Natl Acad. Sci. USA 93, 6421–6424.**
10. **Muller, D. et al. (1996) Neuron 17, 413–422.**
11. Mayford, M. et al. (1992) Science 256, 638–644.
12. Barton, C.H. et al. (1988) Development 104, 165–173.
13. Small, S.J. et al. (1987) J. Cell Biol. 105, 2335–2345.
14. Santoni, M.-J. et al. (1987) Nucleic Acids Res. 15, 8621–8641.
15. Cunningham, B.A. et al. (1987) Science 236, 799–806.
16. Krieg, P.A. et al. (1989) Gene 17, 10321–10335.
17. Grenningloh, G. et al. (1991) Cell 67, 45–57.
18. Hemperly, J.J. et al. (1990) J. Mol. Neurosci. 2, 71–78.

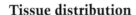

CD57 HNK-1, Leu-7 antigen

Tissue distribution

CD57 is present on a subset of NK cells and of T lymphocytes [1]. Red blood cells, granulocytes, monocytes and platelets do not express CD57 [1]. The antigen is expressed on receptors in the nervous system [2,3]. In chicken, CD57 has been identified on integrins [2-4].

Structure

CD57 is an oligosaccharide antigenic determinant present on a variety of polypeptides, lipids and chondroitin sulfate proteoglycans depending on the tissue examined [2,3]. The polypeptides associated with the antigen on leucocytes have not been characterized in detail. The structure of CD57 as carried by a glycolipid is a 3'-sulfated glucuronic acid and the COOH of the glucuronic acid is important for the epitope [3]. The antigen is conserved across species [2-4].

Ligands and associated molecules

CD57 binds to L- and P- but not E-selectin in a Ca^{2+}-dependent manner and is involved in homophilic interactions of P0 [2-4]. CD57 binds to the second globular domain of the E8 fragment of laminin [2-4].

Function

The function of CD57 is unknown. Myelinating Schwann cells associating with motor but not sensory axons express CD57 on myelin-associated glycoprotein (MAG) [2-4].

References
1. Schubert, J. et al. (1989) In Leucocyte Typing IV (Knapp, W., ed.) Oxford University Press, Oxford, pp. 711–714.
2. Schachner, M. et al. (1995) Prog. Brain Res. 105, 183–188.
3. Jungalwala, F. B. (1994) Neurochem. Res. 19, 945–957.
4. **Schachner, M. and Martini, R. (1995) Trends Neurosci. 18, 183–191.**

CD58　LFA-3

Molecular weights
Polypeptide
　　Transmembrane form　25 339

SDS-PAGE
　　reduced　　　　　　45–70 kDa
　　unreduced　　　　　45–70 kDa

Carbohydrate
N-linked sites　　　　　6
O-linked　　　　　　　unknown

Human gene location
1p13.1 [1,2]

V

C2 ^s_s　OR

COOH

Domains

	FHV		CMI		
		YEM		IQC	
S	V		C2	TM	CY

Tissue distribution

CD58 is expressed on most haematopoietic cells (including erythrocytes) and on various non-haematopoietic cells, such as fibroblasts, endothelium and epithelia [3,4]. It is expressed on about half of peripheral blood B and T cells and at high levels on monocytes [3]. Expression is particularly high on memory T cells [3] and dendritic cells [5]. In lymphoid tissues CD58 is expressed on all dendritic cells and macrophages, and on germinal centre B cells, medullary thymocytes and medullary (but not cortical) thymic epithelial cells [4]. The sheep CD58 homologue binds human CD2 and mediates the phenomenon of sheep erythrocyte rosetting on human T cells [1].

Structure

CD58 contains a membrane-distal V-set and a membrane-proximal C2-set IgSF domain, and is a member of the CD2 family of molecules, which includes CD48, Ly-9, 2B4, and CD150. Within this group CD58 is most similar to CD48, which is the major CD2 ligand in the mouse and rat [6]. Alternative splicing gives rise to either transmembrane- or glycosyl-phosphatidyl-inositol-anchored forms [7]. The N-terminus of the mature polypeptide has been established by protein sequencing [8].

Ligands and associated molecules

The extracellular portion of CD58 binds to CD2 [1,7] on the GFCC'C'' β sheet of the V-set domain [6]. CD2 binds CD58 in solution with a very low affinity (K_d 9–22 μM) as a result of a very fast dissociation rate constant ($k_{off} \geq 4\,s^{-1}$) [6]. Membrane-attached (GPI-anchored) CD58 binds half-maximally to cell surface CD2 at a surface density of ~20 molecules/μm^2 and there is rapid exchange of bound and free CD58 at the adhesion interface [9].

Function

CD58 expressed on antigen-presenting cells and target cells enhances T cell antigen recognition through binding to CD2 on T cells [1,6,10]. This is partly a consequence of improved adhesion but signals transmitted through the CD2 may also contribute [1,10,11]. Structural studies suggest that the CD2-mediated adhesion may optimize the inter-membrane distance for antigen recognition by the T cell receptor [6].

Database accession numbers

	PIR	SWISSPROT	EMBL/GENBANK	REFERENCE
Human	A28564	P19256	Y00636	8
Human (GPI)	S01269		X06296	12

Amino acid sequence of human CD58

```
MLRLLLALNL FPSIQVTGNK ILVKQSPM                              -1
FSQQIYGVVY GNVTFHVPSN VPLKEVLWKK QKDKVAELEN SEFRAFSSFK      50
NRVYLDTVSG SLTIYNLTSS DEDEYEMESP NITDTMKFFL YVLESLPSPT     100
LTCALTNGSI EVQCMIPEHY NSHRGLIMYS WDCPMEQCKR NSTSIYFKME     150
NDLPQKIQCT LSNPLFNTTS SIILTTCIPS SGHSRHRYAL IPIPLAVITT     200
CIVLYMNGIL KCDRKPDRTN SN                                   222
```

GPI-anchored form (Ser180 is a potential site for GPI attachment):

```
SGHSRHRYAL IPIPLAVITT CIVLYMNVL                            209
```

References
1. Moingeon, P. et al. (1989) Immunol. Rev. 111, 111–144.
2. Mitchell, E.L.D. et al. (1995) Cytogenet. Cell Genet. 70, 183–185.
3. Sanders, M.E. et al. (1988) J. Immunol. 140, 1401–1407.
4. Smith, M.E.F. and Thomas, J.A. (1990) J. Clin. Pathol. 43, 893–900.
5. Freudenthal, P.S. and Steinman, R.M. (1990) Proc. Natl Acad. Sci. USA 87, 7698–7702.
6. **Davis, S.J. and van der Merwe, P.A. (1996) Immunol. Today 17, 177–187.**
7. Dustin, M.L. and Springer, T.A. (1991) Annu. Rev. Immunol. 9, 27–66.
8. Wallner, B.P. et al. (1987) J. Exp. Med. 166, 923–932.
9. Dustin, M.L. et al. (1996) J. Cell. Biol. 132, 465–474.
10. Bierer, B.E. and Burakoff, S.J. (1989) Immunol. Rev. 111, 267–294.
11. Beyers, A.D. et al. (1989) Immunol. Rev. 111, 59–77.
12. Seed, B. (1987) Nature. 329, 840–842.

CD59

Complement protectin, MIRL, H19, MACIF, HRF20, P-18

Molecular weights
Polypeptide   8961

SDS-PAGE
  reduced   19 kDa
  non-reduced   19 kDa

Carbohydrate
N-linked sites   1
O-linked sites   unknown

Human gene location and size
11p13; >27 kb [1,2]

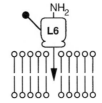

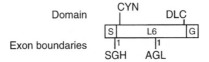

Domain

Exon boundaries

Tissue distribution

CD59 is expressed on leucocytes, erythrocytes, platelets, a variety of endothelial and epithelial cells, placenta and spermatozoa. It is also found in a number of bodily fluids including blood plasma, saliva, amniotic fluid, seminal fluid and urine [2-4].

Structure

CD59 contains a single Ly-6 domain and it attaches to the cell surface via a GPI anchor [5,6]. The N-terminal residue has been determined by protein sequencing [8], and the GPI attachment sites has been shown to be Asn77 [7]. The disulfide bond pattern has been established to be Cys3-Cys26, Cys6-Cys13, Cys19-Cys39, Cys45-Cys63, and Cys64-Cys69 [7-9]. The three-dimensional structure has been determined by NMR [8,9] and shown to be similar to the snake venom neurotoxins.

Ligands and associated molecules

CD59 binds complement components C8 and C9 (see below). A proposed interaction with CD2 has not been confirmed [10].

Function

CD59 restricts the cytolytic activity of homologous complement by binding to C8 and C9 and blocking assembly of the membrane attack complex [2,3,11]. It does not block the lytic activity of perforin in cell-mediated cytotoxicity [12]. It is unlikely that CD59 is synthesized by all cells on which it is expressed. CD59 can be transferred between cells via fluid phase vesicles (prostasomes) and other non-membranous complexes, which also explains its presence in many body fluids [4,13]. Paroxysmal noctural hemoglobinuria (PNH) is likely to be the direct consequence of the absence of CD59 on the cell surface, although, in most cases, it results from defects in the synthesis of GPI anchors [14,15]. CD59 and the two other complement regulatory proteins, CD46 and CD55, have received much attention for their role in reproduction and xenotransplantation (see **CD46**).

Database accession numbers

	PIR	SWISSPROT	EMBL/GENBANK	REFERENCE
Human	A46252	P13987	X16447	5
Rat	S53340	P27274	U48255	16

Amino acid sequence of human CD59

```
MGIQGGSVLF GLLLVLAVFC HSGHS                              -1
LQCYNCPNPT ADCKTAVNCS SDFDACLITK AGLQVYNKCW KFEHCNFNDV   50
TTRLRENELT YYCCKKDLCN FNEQLEN                            77
GGTSLSEKTV LLLVTPFLAA AWSLHP                            +26
```

References

1 Tone, M. et al. (1992) J. Mol. Biol. 227, 971–976.
2 **Liszewski, M.K. et al. (1996) Adv. Immunol. 61, 201–283.**
3 Davies, A. and Lachmann, P.J. (1993) Immunol. Res. 12, 258–275.
4 Rooney, I.A. et al. (1993) J. Exp. Med. 177, 1409–1420.
5 Davies, A. et al. (1989) J. Exp. Med. 170, 637–654.
6 Stefanova, I. et al. (1989) Mol. Immunol. 26, 153–161.
7 Sugita, Y. et al. (1993) J. Biochem. 114, 473–477.
8 Fletcher, C.M. et al. (1994) Structure 2, 185–199.
9 Kieffer, B. et al. (1994) Biochemistry 33, 4471–4482.
10 van der Merwe P.A. et al. (1994) Biochemistry 33, 10149–10160.
11 **Lachmann, P.J. (1991) Immunol. Today 12, 312–315.**
12 Meri, S. et al. (1990) J. Exp. Med. 172, 367–370.
13 Rooney, I.A. et al. (1996) J. Clin. Invest. 97, 1675–1686.
14 Yamashina, M. et al. (1990) New Engl. J. Med. 323, 1184–1189.
15 Bessler, M. et al. (1994) EMBO J. 13, 110–117.
16 Rushmere, N.K. et al. (1994) Biochem. J. 304, 595–601.

CD60 UM4D4

Tissue distribution

CD60 is expressed on 25–45% of T cells and on platelets [1]. Smaller proportions of leucocytes from other lineages also express the antigen. Red blood cells do not express CD60.

Structure

The minimal CD60 epitope consists of the trisaccharide NeuAc2 → 8NeuAc2 → 3Galβ1 → 4 [2]. Four mAbs to CD60 have been shown to recognize mainly acetylated forms of the ganglioside GD3. Antibody binding is reduced or abolished following O-deacetylation of the antigen [3].

Ligands and associated molecules

The NeuAc2 → 8NeuAc2 → 3Galβ1 → 4 epitope is present on some gangliosides and is immunoprecipitated in association with polypeptides whose molecular weights vary with the tissue examined [2,4]. It remains to be determined whether the oligosaccharide/glycolipid is covalently associated with these polypeptides.

Function

CD60 antibodies deliver co-stimulatory signals in the presence of accessory cells or low doses of phorbol esters [5], and augment signalling via CD3 [4]. CD60$^+$ T cells within the CD4 and CD8 subsets provide B cell help and secrete higher levels of IL-4, whereas CD60$^-$CD8$^+$ cells perform cytotoxic and suppressor functions and are a major source of IFNγ [4,6].

Comment

The CD60 antigen is expressed at high levels on 75% of T cells from the synovial fluid of arthritic patients [7], and on 75% of T cells from cutaneous psoriatic lesions [8], and may have a role in the pathogenesis of these diseases.

References
[1] Rieber, E.P. (1989) Leucocyte Typing IV, 361.
[2] Kniep, B. et al. (1989) Leucocyte Typing IV, 362–364.
[3] Kniep, B. et al. (1992) Biochem. Biophys. Res. Commun. 187, 1343–1349.
[4] Rieber, E.P. et al. (1989) Leucocyte Typing IV, 366–368.
[5] Higgs, J.B. et al. (1988) J. Immunol. 140, 3758–3765.
[6] **Rieber, E.P. and Rank, G. (1994) J. Exp. Med. 179, 1385–1390.**
[7] Fox, D.A. et al. (1990) J. Clin. Invest. 86, 1124–1136.
[8] Baadsgaard, O. et al. (1990) J. Invest. Dermatol. 95, 275–282.

CD61 Integrin β3 subunit

Molecular weights
Polypeptide   84 390
   variant   83 445

SDS-PAGE
   reduced   105 kDa
   unreduced   90 kDa

Carbohydrates
   N-linked sites   6
   O-linked sites   unknown

Human gene location and size
17q21.3; ~65kb [1,2]

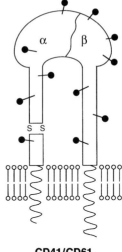

CD41/CD61

Tissue distribution

CD61 is expressed on platelets, megakaryocytes, monocytes, macrophages and endothelial cells [1,3].

Structure

CD61 is the integrin β3 subunit. The N-terminus of CD61 has been determined [4]. An alternative cytoplasmic domain of CD61 has been detected at the mRNA level in human placental tissue and two human cell lines [5]. An intramolecular disulfide bond map has been proposed [6].

Ligands and associated molecules

CD61 combines with CD41 to form the platelet glycoprotein IIb/IIIa (integrin αIIbβ3) and with CD51 to form the vitronectin receptor (integrin αVβ3). The cytoplasmic tail of CD61 has been shown to interact with the molecule β3-endonexin [7].

Function

See **CD41** and **CD51** for the functions of the CD41/CD61 and CD51/CD61 complexes respectively [8]. Variations in the CD61 sequence are associated with platelet-specific alloantigens: L33P (HPA-1A/B); R143Q (HPA-4A/B); P407A (MO+); R489Q (CA+) and R636C (SR[a] +) (see SWISSPROT entry). Five missense mutations of CD61 have been associated with Glanzmann thrombasthenia (residue locations are given according to the sequence of the mature protein as shown below): D119Y, R214Q and R214W lead to the loss of ligand binding activities of CD41/CD61 complexes [9–11]; C374Y results in the diminished expression of CD41/CD61 on platelets although ligand binding specificities appear to remain intact [12]; and S752P in the cytoplasmic domain renders the CD41/CD61 non-responsive to platelet activation [13]. Other mutations, including deletions and erroneous splicing, have been described [14].

Database accession numbers

	PIR	SWISSPROT	EMBL/GENBANK	REFERENCE
Human	A26547	P05106	J02703	15
			M20311	16

Amino acid sequence of human CD61

```
MRARPRPRPL WVTVLALGAL AGVGVG                               -1
GPNICTTRGV SSCQQCLAVS PMCAWCSDEA LPLGSPRCDL KENLLKDNCA     50
PESIEFPVSE ARVLEDRPLS DKGSGDSSQV TQVSPQRIAL RLRPDDSKNF    100
SIQVRQVEDY PVDIYYLMDL SYSMKDDLWS IQNLGTKLAT QMRKLTSNLR    150
IGFGAFVDKP VSPYMYISPP EALENPCYDM KTTCLPMFGY KHVLTLTDQV    200
TRFNEEVKKQ SVSRNRDAPE GGFDAIMQAT VCDEKIGWRN DASHLLVFTT    250
DAKTHIALDG RLAGIVQPND GQCHVGSDNH YSASTTMDYP SLGLMTEKLS    300
QKNINLIFAV TENVVNLYQN YSELIPGTTV GVLSMDSSNV LQLIVDAYGK    350
IRSKVELEVR DLPEELSLSF NATCLNNEVI PGLKSCMGLK IGDTVSFSIE    400
AKVRGCPQEK EKSFTIKPVG FKDSLIVQVT FDCDCACQAQ AEPNSHRCNN    450
GNGTFECGVC RCGPGWLGSQ CECSEEDYRP SQQDECSPRE GQPVCSQRGE    500
CLCGQCVCHS SDFGKITGKY CECDDFSCVR YKGEMCSGHG QCSCGDCLCD    550
SDWTGYYCNC TTRTDTCMSS NGLLCSGRGK CECGSCVCIQ PGSYGDTCEK    600
CPTCPDACTF KKECVECKKF DRGALHDENT CNRYCRDEIE SVKELKDTGK    650
DAVNCTYKNE DDCVVRFQYY EDSSGKSILY VVEEPECPKG PDILVVLLSV    700
MGAILLIGLA ALLIWKLLIT IHDRKEFAKF EEERARAKWD T             741

ANNPLYKEAT STFTNITYRG T                                   762
VRDGAGRFLK SLV                                            754
                                                   (variant)
```

References
1 **Kieffer, N. and Phillips, D.R. (1990) Annu. Rev. Cell Biol. 6, 334–357.**
2 Lanza, F. et al. (1990) J. Biol. Chem. 18098–18103.
3 Pigott, R. and Power, C. (1993) The Adhesion Molecule FactsBook. Academic Press, London.
4 Charo, I.F. et al. (1986) Proc. Natl Acad. Sci. USA 83, 8351–8355.
5 van Kuppevelt, T.H.M.S.M. et al. Proc. Natl Acad. Sci. USA 86, 5415–5418.
6 Calvette, J.J. et al. (1991) Biochem. J. 274, 63–71.
7 Shattil, S.J. et al. (1995) J. Cell Biol. 131, 807–816.
8 **Ginsberg, M.H. et al. (1993) Thromb. Haemost. 70, 87–93.**
9 Loftus, J.C. et al. (1990) Science 249, 915–918.
10 Bajt, M.L. et al. (1992) J. Biol. Chem. 267, 3789–3794.
11 Lanza, F. et al. (1992) J. Clin. Invest. 89, 1995–2004.
12 Grimaldi, C.M. et al. (1996) Blood 88, 1666–1675.
13 Chen, Y.P. et al. (1992) Proc. Natl Acad. Sci. USA 89, 10169–10173.
14 **Bray, P.F. (1994) Thromb. Haemost. 72, 492–502.**
15 Fitzgerald, L.A. et al. (1987) J. Biol. Chem. 262, 3936–3939.
16 Zimrin, A.B. et al. (1988) J. Clin. Invest. 81, 1470–1475.

CD62E ELAM-1, E-selectin

Molecular weights
Polypeptide   64 467

SDS-PAGE
  reduced   97 and 107–115 kDa

Carbohydrate
N-linked sites   11
O-linked   unknown

Human gene location and size
1 q23-25; ~13 kb [1,2]

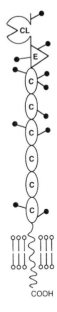

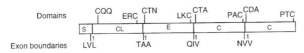

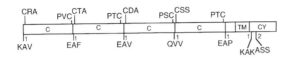

Tissue distribution

CD62E is expressed on endothelial cells at sites of inflammation [3]. It is not expressed on leucocytes. Various inflammatory mediators induce expression of CD62E on cultured endothelial cells [3]. Soluble forms of CD62E are present in plasma [4].

Structure

CD62E is a member of the selectin family of cell surface molecules (along with CD62L and CD62P) [3]. The genes encoding these protein lie within 300 kb of each [2,5]. CD62E consists of an N-terminal C-type lectin domain, an EGF-like domain, six complement control protein domains, an eight amino acid spacer, a transmembrane sequence and a cytoplasmic domain [6]. The crystal structure of a fragment comprising the C-type lectin and EGF domains has been solved, revealing that these two domains are not intimately associated [7].

Ligands and associated molecules

Like CD62L and CD62P, CD62E binds with low affinity to oligosaccharide sequences related to sialylated Lewis x (sLe^x, CD15s) through its C-type lectin domain [8]. The carbohydrate binding site on this domain has been localized to a region surrounding the Ca^{2+} binding site [7]. CD62E binds particularly well to 3-sialyl di-Le^x (comprising sLe^x followed by an additional Le^x unit), which is an unusual structure found only on N-glycans [9]. One glycoprotein ligand for CD62E is a particular glycoform of the ubiquitous

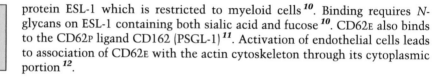

protein ESL-1 which is restricted to myeloid cells [10]. Binding requires *N*-glycans on ESL-1 containing both sialic acid and fucose [10]. CD62E also binds to the CD62P ligand CD162 (PSGL-1) [11]. Activation of endothelial cells leads to association of CD62E with the actin cytoskeleton through its cytoplasmic portion [12].

Function

Like other selectins, CD62E is an adhesion molecule that contributes to the initial tethering and rolling of leucocytes on endothelial surfaces, a prerequisite for leucocyte extravasation into tissues [3]. CD62E (like CD62L) contributes to the later stages of leucocyte influx into inflamed tissues. Although no abnormality has been detected in CD62E-deficient mice, these mice are unusually susceptible to blocking of CD62P, suggesting overlapping but complementary roles for these molecules [3]. In support of this, mice deficient in both CD62E and CD62P have severe defects in leucocyte recruitment to inflammatory sites and are susceptible to opportunistic bacterial infections [13].

Database accession numbers

	PIR	SWISSPROT	EMBL/GENBANK	REFERENCE
Human	A32606	P16581	M30640	6
Mouse		Q00690	M80778	14
Rat		P98105	L25527	unpublished

Amino acid sequence of human CD62E

```
MIASQFLSAL TLVLLIKESG A                                   -1
WSYNTSTEAM TYDEASAYCQ QRYTHLVAIQ NKEEIEYLNS ILSYSPSYYW     50
IGIRKVNNVW VWVGTQKPLT EEAKNWAPGE PNNRQKDEDC VEIYIKREKD    100
VGMWNDERCS KKKLALCYTA ACTNTSCSGH GECVETINNY TCKCDPGFSG    150
LKCEQIVNCT ALESPEHGSL VCSHPLGNFS YNSSCSISCD RGYLPSSMET    200
MQCMSSGEWS APIPACNVVE CDAVTNPANG FVECFQNPGS FPWNTTCTFD    250
CEEGFELMGA QSLQCTSSGN WDNEKPTCKA VTCRAVRQPQ NGSVRCSHSP    300
AGEFTFKSSC NFTCEEGFML QGPAQVECTT QGQWTQQIPV CEAFQCTALS    350
NPERGYMNCL PSASGSFRYG SSCEFSCEQG FVLKGSKRLQ CGPTGEWDNE    400
KPTCEAVRCD AVHQPPKGLV RCAHSPIGEF TYKSSCAFSC EEGFELHGST    450
QLECTSQGQW TEEVPSCQVV KCSSLAVPGK INMSCSGEPV FGTVCKFACP    500
EGWTLNGSAA RTCGATGHWS GLLPTCEAPT ESNIPLVAGL SAAGLSLLTL    550
APFLLWLRKC LRKAKKFVPA SSCQSLESDG SYQKPSYIL                589
```

References

1 Collins, T. et al. (1991) J. Biol. Chem. 266, 2466–2473.
2 Watson, M.L. et al. (1990) J. Exp. Med. 172, 263–272.
3 **Tedder, T.F. et al. (1995) FASEB J. 9, 866–873.**
4 Gearing, A.J.H. and Newman, W. (1993) Immunol. Today 14, 506–512.
5 Oakey, R.J. et al. (1992) Hum. Mol. Genet. 1, 613–620.
6 Bevilacqua, M.P. et al. (1989) Science 243, 1160–1165.
7 **Graves, B.J. et al. (1994) Nature 367, 532–538.**
8 Varki, A. (1994) Proc. Natl Acad. Sci. USA 91, 7390–7397.
9 Patel, T.P. et al. (1994) Biochemistry 33, 14815–14824.

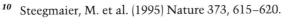
[10] Steegmaier, M. et al. (1995) Nature 373, 615–620.

[11] McEver, R.P. et al. (1995) J. Biol. Chem. 270, 11025–11028.

[12] Yoshida, M. et al. (1996) J. Cell Biol. 133, 445–455.

[13] Frenette, P.S. et al. (1996) Cell 84, 563–574.

[14] Weller, A. et al. (1992) J. Biol. Chem. 267, 15176–15183.

CD62L

LECAM-1, LAM-1, L-selectin

Other names
Lymph node homing receptor
MEL-14 antigen
Leu-8
TQ1

Molecular weights
Polypeptide   37 402

SDS-PAGE
   reduced   74 kDa (lymphocytes)
             95 kDa (neutrophils)
   unreduced 65 kDa (lymphocytes)

Carbohydrate
N-linked sites   7
O-linked   nil

Human gene location and size
1 q23-25; >30 kb [1]

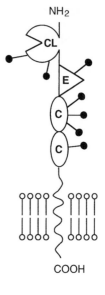

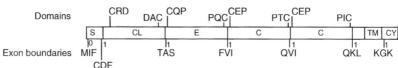

Tissue distribution

Most haematopoietic cells express CD62L at some stage of differentiation[2]. The majority of B and naive T cells express CD62L but only subpopulations of memory T and NK cells are CD62L positive. Subpopulations of immature and mature thymocytes express CD62L. Most monocytes, neutrophils and eosinophils express CD62L. CD62L is rapidly lost upon activation of lymphocytes and neutrophils as a result of proteolytic cleavage[2]. A soluble form of CD62L is present at high levels in the blood[3].

Structure

CD62L is a member of the selectin family of cell surface molecules (which includes CD62E and CD62P[2]). Its gene lies between the CD62P and CD62E genes, and all three loci are within 300 kb of each other[4,5]. It consists of an N-terminal lectin C-type domain, an EGFSF domain, two CCP domains, a 15 amino acid spacer containing the proteolytic cleavage site (between Lys283 and Ser284), a transmembrane sequence and a short cytoplasmic domain. The short cytoplasmic domain bears no sequence similarity to the cytoplasmic domains of CD62P or CD62E but is highly conserved across species. The N-terminus of mature murine CD62L has been determined by protein sequencing.

Ligands and associated molecules

Like CD62E and CD62P, CD62L binds with low affinity to anionic oligo-saccharide sequences related to sialylated Lewis x (sLe^x, CD15s) through its C-type lectin domain[6]. CD62P and CD62L also bind various structurally unrelated anionic carbohydrates such as heparan sulfate and sulfatides[6]. CD62L binds particularly well to carbohydrates present on certain glycoforms of CD34, GlyCAM-1 and MAdCAM-1[2,7,8]. The precise nature of these high-affinity carbohydrate ligands is not known but binding requires fucosylation, sialylation and sulfation, suggesting a role for structures related to sulfated sLe^x[8]. CD62L also binds CD162 (PSGL-1)[9]. The 11 C-terminal residues of the 17 amino acid cytoplasmic domain, which are essential for CD62L adhesion, mediate association with a complex of cytoskeletal proteins which includes α-actinin[10]. These residues are not required for localization of CD62L to microvilli (see below).

Function

Like other selectins, CD62L mediates the initial tethering and rolling of leucocytes on endothelial surfaces, which is a prerequisite for leucocyte extravasation from the blood into tissues[2]. More specifically, CD62L is important for the homing of naive lymphocytes via high endothelial venules to peripheral lymph nodes and Peyer's patches[11]. CD62L also contributes, along with other selectins, to the recruitment of leucocytes from the blood to areas of inflammation[2]. Unlike CD62P, CD62L contributes mainly to the later recruitment (after 1 h), presumably due to delay in the induction of suitable endothelial ligands[2]. The localization of CD62L to the tips of surface microvilli is required for optimal CD62L-mediated attachment and rolling under flow[12]. CD62L can also mediate neutrophil–neutrophil interactions through recognition of CD162[9]. Ligation of CD62L can stimulate its proteolytic release from the cell, which may be important for high rolling velocities[13]. Ligation of CD62L on T cells with soluble GlyCAM-1 stimulates adhesion through β2 (CD18) integrins[14].

Database accession numbers

	PIR	SWISSPROT	EMBL/GENBANK	REFERENCE
Human	A33912	P14151	M25280	1
Mouse	A32375	P18337	M36005	7
Rat	S23936	P30836	D10831	15

Amino acid sequence of human CD62L

```
MIFPWKCQST QRDLWNIFKL WGWTMLCCDF LAHHGTDC               -1
WTYHYSEKPM NWQRARRFCR DNYTDLVAIQ NKAEIEYLEK TLPFSRSYYW   50
IGIRKIGGIW TWVGTNKSLT EEAAENWGDGE PNNKKNKEDC VEIYIKRNKD  100
AGKWNDDACH KLKAALCYTA SCQPWSCSGH GECVEIINNY TCNCDVGYYG   150
PQCQFVIQCE PLEAPELGTM DCTHPLGNFS FSSQCAFSCS EGTNLTGIEE   200
TTCGPFGNWS SPEPTCQVIQ CEPLSAPDLG IMNCSHPLAS FSFTSACTFI   250
CSEGTELIGK KKTICESSGI WSNPSPICQK LDKSFSMIKE GDYNPLFIPV   300
AVMVTAFSGL AFIIWLARRL KKGKKSKRSM NDPY                   334
```

References

[1] Ord, D.C. et al. (1990) J. Biol. Chem. 265, 7760–7767.

[2] Tedder, T.F. et al. (1995) FASEB J. 9, 866–873.

[3] Gearing, A.J.H. and Newman, W. (1993) Immunol. Today 14, 506–512.

[4] Watson, M.L. et al. (1990) J. Exp. Med. 172, 263–272.

[5] Oakey, R.J. et al. (1992) Hum. Mol. Genet. 1, 613–620.

[6] Varki, A. (1994) Proc. Natl Acad. Sci. USA 91, 7390–7397.

[7] **Lasky, L.A. (1995) Annu. Rev. Biochem. 64, 113–139.**

[8] Rosen, S.D. and Bertozzi, C.R. (1996) Curr. Biol. 6, 261–264.

[9] Walcheck, B. et al. (1996) J. Clin. Invest. 98, 1081–1087.

[10] Pavalko, F.M. et al. (1995) J. Cell Biol. 129, 1155–1164.

[11] Butcher, E.C. and Picker, L.J. (1996) Science 272, 60–66.

[12] von Andrian, U.H. et al. (1995) Cell 82, 989–999.

[13] Walcheck, B. et al. (1996) Nature 380, 720–723.

[14] Hwang, S.T. et al. (1996) J. Exp. Med. 184, 1343–1348.

[15] Watanabe, T. et al. (1992) Biochim. Biophys. Acta 1131, 321–324.

Molecular weights
Polypeptide   86 244

SDS-PAGE
  reduced   140 kDa
  non-reduced   140 kDa

Carbohydrate
N-linked sites   12
O-linked   unknown

Human gene location
1q21–q24 [1]; >50 kb [2]

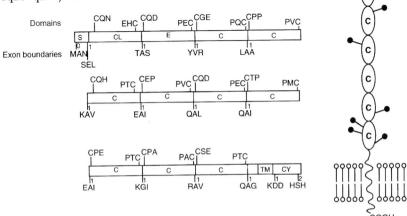

Tissue distribution

CD62P is present on megakaryocytes, activated platelets and activated endothelial cells. It is stored in secretory granules in platelets and endothelial cells and is rapidly translocated to the plasma membrane upon activation of these cells[3]. Expression is transient as CD62P is rapidly internalized and then degraded in lysosomes[3]. Soluble forms of CD62P originating from alternative splicing and possibly proteolytic cleavage are detectable in plasma at levels of 0.1–1 µg/mL[4].

Structure

CD62P is a member of the selectin family of cellular adhesion molecules which includes CD62E (E-selectin) and CD62L (L-selectin)[3,5]. The extracellular region contains an N-terminal C-type lectin domain, followed by an EGF domain and nine CCP domains[6]. Alternative splicing results in variants lacking the seventh CCP domain or encoding a soluble, secreted form of CD62P[2,3]. The extracellular portion forms an extended rod approximately 48 nm long[7]. The short cytoplasmic domain, which bears no homology to the CD62E or CD62L cytoplasmic domains, is phosphorylated on Ser, Thr, Tyr and His residues following platelet activation[8]. The N-terminus of CD62 has been determined by protein sequencing[6].

Ligands and associated molecules

Like CD62E and CD62L, CD62P binds with low affinity to anionic oligosaccharide sequences related to sialylated Lewis x (sLe^x, CD15s) through its C-type lectin domain[9]. CD62P and CD62L also bind various structurally unrelated anionic carbohydrates such as heparan sulfate and sulfatides[9]. The major CD62P ligand on neutrophils is the mucin-like cell surface glycoprotein CD162 (PSGL-1). Optimal binding to CD162 requires O-linked sLe^x-like structures as well as sulfated NH$_2$-terminal tyrosines[10]. The conserved EGF domain of P-selectin is required for optimal binding, and it has been suggested that it may contain a second binding site which interacts with the sulfotyrosine-containing region on CD162[10]. Mouse CD62P has been reported to bind certain glycoforms of the mucin CD24[11].

Function

Endothelial CD62P mediates the rolling of neutrophils on activated endothelium, a prerequisite for recruitment of neutrophils into areas of inflammation. CD62P appears to be particularly important early on (within minutes) with other selectins contributing at later stages[12]. Endothelial CD62P also mediates rolling of platelets and some T lymphocyte subsets. CD62P on adherent platelets promotes leucocyte accumulation in thrombi[12]. Platelet CD62P can also contribute indirectly to T lymphocyte homing to high endothelial venules (HEVs); activated CD62P$^+$ platelets attached to lymphocytes can mediate lymphocyte rolling through an interaction between platelet CD62P and endothelial peripheral node addressin[13]. Mice deficient in CD62P show reduced neutrophil rolling and delayed recruitment into inflamed tissues[12]. CD62P and CD62E have overlapping roles since mice deficient in both CD62P and CD62E show much more severe defects in leucocyte extravasation and are susceptible to opportunistic infections[14].

Database accession numbers

	PIR	SWISSPROT	EMBL/GENBANK	REFERENCE
Human	A30359	P16109	M25322	6
Mouse	A42755	Q01102	M87861	15
Rat		P98106	L23088	16

Amino acid sequence of human CD62

```
MANCQIAILY QRFQRVVFGI SQLLCFSALI SELTNQKEVA A              -1
WTYHYSTKAY SWNISRKYCQ NRYTDLVAIQ NKNEIDYLNK VLPYYSSYYW      50
IGIRKNNKTW TWVGTKKALT NEAENWADNE PNNKRNNEDC VEIYIKSPSA     100
PGKWNDEHCL KKKHALCYTA SCQDMSCSKQ GECLETIGNY TCSCYPGFYG     150
PECEYVRECG ELELPQHVLM NCSHPLGNFS FNSQCSFHCT DGYQVNGPSK     200
LECLASGIWT NKPPQCLAAQ CPPLKIPERG NMICLHSAKA FQHQSSCSFS     250
CEEGFALVGP EVVQCTASGV WTAPAPVCKA VQCQHLEAPS EGTMDCVHPL     300
TAFAYGSSCK FECQPGYRVR GLDMLRCIDS GHWSAPLPTC EAISCEPLES     350
```

```
PVHGSMDCSP SLRAFQYDTN CSFRCAEGFM LRGADIVRCD NLGQWTAPAP    400
VCQALQCQDL PVPNEARVNC SHPFGAFRYQ SVCSFTCNEG LLLVGASVLQ    450
CLATGNWNSV PPECQAIPCT PLLSPQNGTM TCVQPLGSSS YKSTCQFICD    500
EGYSLSGPER LDCTRSGRWT DSPPMCEAIK CPELFAPEQG SLDCSDTRGE    550
FNVGSTCHFS CNNGFKLEGP NNVECTTSGR WSATPPTCKG IASLPTPGLQ    600
CPALTTPGQG TMYCRHHPGT FGFNTTCYFG CNAGFTLIGD STLSCRPSGQ    650
WTAVTPACRA VKCSELHVNK PIAMNCSNLW GNFSYGSICS FHCLEGQLLN    700
GSAQTACQEN GHWSTTVPTC QAGPLTIQEA LTYFGGAVAS TIGLIMGGTL    750
LALLRKRFRQ KDDGKCPLNP HSHLGTYGVF TNAAFDPSP               789
```

Two alternatively spliced variants are shown. One variant lacks exon 11 which encodes the seventh CCP domain (shown in italics). The other variant lacks exon 14 (shown in bold) and encodes a soluble form of CD62P.

References

1 Watson, M.L. et al. (1990) J. Exp. Med. 172, 263–272.

2 Johnston, G.I. et al. (1990) J. Biol. Chem. 265, 21381–21385.

3 **McEver, R.P. et al. (1995) J. Biol. Chem. 270, 11025–11028.**

4 Ishiwata, N. et al. (1994) J. Biol. Chem. 269, 23708–23715.

5 Lasky, L.A. (1995) Annu. Rev. Biochem. 64, 113–139.

6 Johnston, G.I. et al. (1989) Cell 56, 1033–1044.

7 Ushiyama, S. et al. (1993) J. Biol. Chem. 268, 15229–15237.

8 Crovello, C.S. et al. (1995) Cell 82, 279–286.

9 Varki, A. (1994) Proc. Natl Acad. Sci. USA 91, 7390–7397.

10 **Rosen, S.D. and Bertozzi, C.R. (1996) Curr. Biol. 6, 261–264.**

11 Sammar, M. et al. (1994) Int. Immunol. 6, 1027–1036.

12 Tedder, T.F. et al. (1995) FASEB J. 9, 866–873.

13 Diacovo, T.G. et al. (1996) Science 273, 252–255.

14 Frenette, P.S. et al. (1996) Cell 84, 563–574.

15 Weller, A. et al. (1992) J. Biol. Chem. 267, 15176–15183.

16 Auchampach, J.A. et al. (1994) Gene 145, 251–255.

CD63 | ME491, MLA1, PTLGP40, granulophysin

Molecular weights
Polypeptide 25 505

SDS-PAGE
unreduced 53 kDa

Carbohydrate
N-linked sites 3
O-linked nil

Human gene location and size
12q12–q13; 4 kb [1]

Tissue distribution

CD63 is widely distributed on the surface and interior on both haematopoietic and non-haematopoietic cells. Expression is high on monocytes, macrophages and activated platelets, and low on lymphocytes and granulocytes [2].

Structure

CD63 is a member of the TM4 superfamily and is predicted to have four transmembrane regions, short cytoplasmic N- and C-termini, and two extracellular regions (reviewed in ref. 3).

Ligands and associated molecules

CD63 associates non-covalently with the TM4SF molecules CD9 and CD81, and with the integrins CD29/CD49c (VLA-3), CD29/CD49d (VLA-4) and CD29/CD49f (VLA-6) [4,5]. In human neutrophils, CD63 associates with the integrin CD11/CD18 and the Src family protein tyrosine kinases Lyn and Hck [6]. In rat lymph node cells, CD63 is associated with a protein tyrosine phosphatase [7]. No extracellular ligand has been identified for CD63.

Function

CD63 may play a role as a tumour suppressor gene since expression of CD63 in human melanoma cells reduces tumour spread and metastasis [8].

Database accession numbers

	PIR	SWISSPROT	EMBL/GENBANK	REFERENCE
Human	S01418	P08962	X07982	9
Rat	S16776	P28648	X61654	10
Mouse		P41731	D16432	11

Amino acid sequence of human CD63

```
AVEGGMKCVK FLLYVLLLAF CACAVGLIAV GVGAQLVLSQ TIIQGATPGS      50
LLPVVIIAVG VFLFLVAFVG CCGACKENYC LMITFAIFLS LIMLVEVAAA     100
IAGYVFRDKV MSEFNNNFRQ QMENYPKNNH TASILDRMQA DFKCCGAANY     150
TDWEKIPSMS KNRVPDSCCI NVTVGCGINF NEKAIHKEGC VEKIGGWLRK     200
NVLVVAAAAL GIAFVEVLGI VFACCLVKSI RSGYEVM                   223
```

References

[1] Hotta, H. et al. (1992) Biochem. Biophys. Res. Commun. 185, 436–442.

[2] Azorsa, D.O. and Hildreth, J.E.K. (1995) Leucocyte Typing V, 1352–1353.

[3] **Wright, M.D. and Tomlinson, M.G. (1994) Immunol. Today 15, 588–594.**

[4] Berditchevski, F. et al. (1996) Mol. Biol. Cell 7, 193–207.

[5] Mannion, B.A. et al. (1996) J. Immunol. 157, 2039–2047.

[6] Skubitz, K.M. et al. (1996) J. Immunol. 157, 3617–3626.

[7] Carmo, A.M. and Wright, M.D. (1995) Eur. J. Immunol. 25, 2090–2095.

[8] Radford, K.J. et al. (1995) Int. J. Cancer 62, 631–635.

[9] Hotta, H. et al. (1988) Cancer Res. 48, 2955–2962.

[10] Nishikata, H. et al. (1992) J. Immunol. 149, 862–870.

[11] Miyamoto, H. et al. (1994) Biochim. Biophys. Acta 1217, 312–316.

Molecular weights
Polypeptide | A form | 40 833
| B2 form | 30 434

SDS-PAGE
reduced | A form | 72 kDa

Carbohydrate
N-linked sites | 7
O-linked sites | unknown

Human gene location and size
Three genes, A, B and C are located on 1q21.1;
~ 9.4 kb each [1].

COOH

Domains

Exon boundaries

CEV YRC CHA YHC CET YWC

| S | C2 | C2 | C2 | TM | CY |

WVP VDT   RWG   KEL   LGL

KGL (B2 isoform)

Tissue distribution

CD64 is constitutively expressed on monocytes and macrophages; expression on monocytes can be strongly upregulated by treatment with interferon γ. Expression of CD64 can be induced by interferon γ on neutrophils and eosinophils [2-4]. CD64 is also expressed on dendritic cells [5]. B and C gene transcripts have been identified in monocytic cells. B2 transcripts are detected in all cells that express the A form of CD64, but a B2 protein has not been detected at the protein level [4,5].

Structure

The A gene encodes the high-affinity Fcγ receptor, a type I membrane protein with three IgSF extracellular domains [6]. A cDNA clone has been identified which encodes a variant of the A form (A') with a different cytoplasmic domain [6], but this alternative sequence is not present in the gene sequence reported in ref. 1. The B and C genes are very similar to the A gene except both contain stop codons in the third IgSF domain, suggesting that they encode soluble proteins with two IgSF domains (see B1 and C sequences below) [1]. B and C gene transcripts have been identified in monocytic cells. An alternatively spliced form of the B gene (B2) is similar to the A form but lacks the third IgSF domain [1,7]. A third alternatively spliced form of the B gene has also been identified but with a cryptic leader sequence [7].

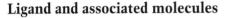
Ligand and associated molecules

CD64 is the high-affinity Fcγ receptor and binds monomeric (as well as aggregated) IgG [1-3]. CD64 associates with the γ chain homodimer of Fc receptors [8,9], possibly through the interaction between the His in CD64 and the Asp in the γ chain in their respective transmembrane regions [10]. The kinases Hck and Lyn can also be co-immunoprecipitated with CD64 from cell lysates [11].

Function

CD64 plays a role in antibody-dependent cytotoxicity, clearance of immune complexes, and phagocytosis of IgG opsonized targets. It also mediates release of cytokines including IL-1, IL-6, and TNFα [2-4]. The association of CD64 with the Fc receptor γ chain homodimer is required for its signal transduction activity. It has been shown that ligation of CD64 results in an increase in the Hck and Lyn kinase activities [11]. Although a B2 form has not been identified at the protein level, transfection of the B2 cDNA into COS cells showed binding to aggregated IgG but not monomeric IgG [7]. A nonsense mutation in the CD64 A gene has been indentified [12]. Because individuals homozygous for this mutation are apparently healthy, and the level of the B2 transcript is consistently high in their blood monocytes, it was speculated that the B2 form of CD64 may be functional [12].

Database accession numbers

	PIR	SWISSPROT	EMBL/GENBANK	REFERENCE
Human A	S03018	P12314	X14356	6
Human A'	S03019	P12315	X14355	6
Human A			M91645	5
Human B			M91646	5
Human C			M91647	5
Mouse	A46480	P26151	M31314	13,14

Amino acid sequence of human CD64

```
A   MWFLTTLLLW VPVDG                                            -1
A' ---------- -----                                            -1
B2 ---------- -----                                            -1
B1 ---------- -----                                            -1
C  ---------- -----                                            -1

A   QVDTTKAVIT LQPPWVSVFQ EETVTLHCEV LHLPGSSSTQ WFLNGTATQT     50
A' ---------S ---------- ---------- ---------- ----------     50
B2 ---------- ---------- ---------- ---------- ----------     50
B1 ---------- ---------- ---------- ---------- ----------     50
C  ---------- ---------- ---------- ---------- ----------     50

A   STPSYRITSA SVNDSGEYRC QRGLSGRSDP IQLEIHRGWL LLQVSSRVFT    100
A' ---------- ---------- ---------- ---------- ----------    100
B2 ---------- ---------- ---------- ---------- --------M    100
B1 ---------- ---------- ---------- ---------- --------M    100
C  ---------- ---------- ---------- ---------- -P--------    100
```

```
A   EGEPLALRCH AWKDKLVYNV LYYRNGKAFK FFHWNSNLTI LKTNISHNGT   150
A'  ---------- ---------- ---------- ---------- ----------   150
B2  ---------- ---------- ---------- ---------- ----------   150
B1  ---------- ---------- ---------- ---------- ----------   150
C   ---------- ---------- ---------- ---------- ----------   150

A   YHCSGMGKHR YTSAGISV.TV KELFPAPVLN ASVTSPLLEG NLVTLSCETK  200
A'  ---------- -------.-- ---------- ---------- ----------   201
B2  ---------- -------QY-- -.......... .......... ..........  172
B1  ---------- -------QY-- ---------- ---------- ----------   201
C   ---------- -------QY-- ---------- --------G- IWSP         195

A   LLLQRPGLQL YFSFYMGSKT LRGRNTSSEY QILTARREDS GLYWCEAATE   250
A'  ---------- ---------- ---------- ---------- ----------   250
B2  .......... .......... .......... .......... ..........   172
B1  --------                                                 259

A   DGNVLKRSPE LELQVLGLQL PTPVWFHVLF YLAVGIMFLV NTVLWVTIRK   300
A'  ---------- ---------- ---------- ---------- ----------   300
B2  .......... ......---- ---------- ---------- ----------   206

A   ELKRKKKWDL EISLDSGHEK KVTISLQEDR HLEEELKCQE QKEEQLQEGV   350
A'  ---------- -------GQA LEAPTQGCA                          329
B2  --------N- ---------- ---------- ---------- ----------   256

A   HRKEPQGAT                                                359
B2  ---------                                                265
```

The sequence of the A form is from ref. 1, and that of the A' from ref. 6. Amino acids identical to the top sequence are indicated by dashes. Gaps in the alignment are indicated by dots.

References
1 Ernst, L.K. et al. (1992) J. Biol. Chem. 267, 15692–15700.
2 Unkeless, J.C. et al. (1988) Annu. Rev. Immunol. 6, 251–281.
3 Ravetch, J.V. and Kinet, J.P. (1991) Annu. Rev. Immunol. 9, 457–492.
4 van de Winkel, J.G.J. and Capel, P.J.A. (1994) Immunol. Today 14, 215–221.
5 Fanger, N.A. et al. (1996) J. Immunol. 157, 541–548.
6 Allen, J.M. and Seed, B. (1989) Science 243, 378–381.
7 Porges, A.J. et al. (1992) J. Clin. Invest. 90, 2102–2109.
8 Scholl, P.R. and Geha, R.S. (1993) Proc. Natl Acad. Sci. USA 90, 8847–8850.
9 Ernst, L.K. et al. (1993) Proc. Natl Acad. Sci. USA 90, 6023–6027
10 Morton, H.C. et al. (1995) J. Biol. Chem. 270, 29781–29787.
11 Wang, A.V.T. et al. (1994) J. Exp. Med. 180, 1165–1170.
12 van de Winkel, J.G.J. et al. (1995) J. Immunol. 2896–2903.
13 Sears, D.W. et al. (1989) J. Immunol. 144, 371–378.
14 Osman, N. et al. (1992) J. Immunol. 148, 1570–1575.

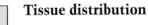

CD65　Ceramide dodecasaccharide 4c

Tissue distribution

CD65 is restricted to the myeloid lineage, with expression on most granulocytes and a proportion of monocytic cells. T cells, B cells, thymocytes, platelets and non-haematopoietic cells do not express CD65 [1,2].

Structure

CD65 mAbs were originally shown to bind to a ceramide dodecasaccharide [3]. The antigen consists of the oligosaccharide sequence:

NeuAcα2 → 3Galβ1 → 4GlcNAcβ1 → 3Galβ1
$$\qquad\qquad\qquad\qquad → 4GlcNAc(Fucα1 → 3)β1 → 3Galβ →$$

Recently, CD65 mAbs have been shown to recognize distinct epitopes of this carbohydrate [2]. The mAbs VIM-8 and VIM-11 recognize the following asialylated epitope that is expressed on granulocytes only:

Galβ1 → 4GlcNAcβ1 → 3Galβ1 → 4GlcNAc(Fucα1 → 3) →　　(CD65 epitope)

In contrast, mAb VIM-2 binds to the following sialylated epitope, which is expressed on both granulocytes and monocytes:

NeuAcα2 → 3Galβ1 → 4GlcNAcβ1 → 3Galβ1 → 4GlcNAc(Fucα1 → 3) →
$$\qquad\qquad\qquad\qquad\qquad\qquad\qquad\qquad\qquad (CD65s\ epitope)$$

Function

Unknown.

Comments

CD65 was retained as a provisional CDw antigen at the Fifth Leucocyte Typing Workshop because of the heterogeneity of the CD65 mAbs in terms of cellular and antigenic reactivity [1]. Since the CD65 mAbs have now been separated into two groups and their precise epitopes determined (see above), the VIM-2 mAb has been placed in a new cluster named CD65s [2].

References
[1]　Knapp, W. et al. (1995) Leucocyte Typing V, 876–882.
[2]　**Kniep, B. et al. (1996) J. Biochem. 119, 456–462.**
[3]　Macher, B.A. et al. (1988) J. Biol. Chem. 253, 10186–10191.

CD66 Carcinoembryonic antigen (CEA) family

Members

CD66a	BGP, biliary glycoprotein, NCA-160
CD66b	CGM6, W272, NCA-95 (previously CD67)
CD66c	NCA, NCA-90
CD66d	CGM1
CD66e	CEA

Molecular weights

Polypeptide	CD66a (BGPa)	53 796
	CD66b	31 493
	CD66c	31 247
	CD66d (CGM1a)	23 391

SDS-PAGE		
reduced	CD66a	160–180 kDa
	CD66b	95–100 kDa
	CD66c	90–95 kDa
	CD66d	~30 kDa (predicted)

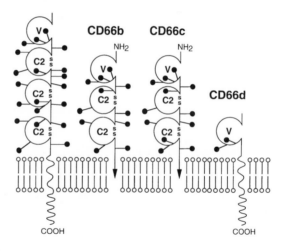

Carbohydrate

N-linked sites	CD66a	20
	CD66b	11
	CD66c	12
	CD66d	2
O-linked		unknown

Gene location
19q13.1–2

Domains

CD66a

		VHN		CEP		CYA		CST			
			YTL		YEC		YTC		YWC		
S	V		C2		C2		C2			TM	CY

The CEA family in humans and other mammals

The human CEA molecules are a family of closely related, IgSF domain-containing glycoproteins encoded by a dense cluster of at least 18 genes (within ~1.2 Mb) with 65–75% sequence identity. Based on sequence similarity and gene proximity this family can be divided into two subgroups, with 80–95% sequence identity within each subgroup[1]. The CEA subgroup (≥7 genes) encodes predominantly cell surface molecules, whereas the pregnancy-specific glycoprotein (PSG) subgroup (≥11 genes) encodes secreted molecules[1,2]. CEA and PSG subgroups have also been identified in the mouse and the rat. However molecules within the subgroups show greater intraspecies (>80%) than interspecies (~60%) identity, making it impossible to identify species homologues. Indeed homologues may not exist since sequence analysis suggests that there has been independent and parallel evolution of the CEA and PSG subgroups following the divergence of rodents and humans[1].

Tissue distribution

Products of four of the seven functional CEA family genes (CD66a–d) are known to be expressed by haematopoietic cells[1-3]. CD66e (CEA) has not been detected on haematopoietic cells and so is not considered further here[3]. Expression of these molecules on haematopoietic cells is generally restricted to the myeloid lineage, particularly in the case of CD66b[3]. These molecules are present at low levels on resting mature granulocytes but expression increases rapidly following activation with inflammatory agonists[2], probably as a result of exocytosis from storage granules[2]. CD66a, c and d are detected on some macrophages in tissue sections and CD66a has been reported on T cells and a subpopulation of activated NK cells[4]. CD66a, c and d are also expressed on a variety of epithelia and CD66a had been detected on some endothelia[3,5]. Soluble forms of CD66b and CD66c are present in plasma[6].

Structure

The extracellular portions of all CD66 molecules possess an N-terminal V-set IgSF domain which, like members of the CD2 family, lacks the canonical inter-β-sheet disulfide, followed by a variable number of C2-set IgSF domains[1]. CD66a, b and c are heavily glycosylated, with more than 60% of the mass contributed by N-linked glycans, and they bear sialylated Le^x (sLe^x, CD15s) structures[2]. CD66b and CD66c have GPI lipid anchors, whereas CD66a and CD66d have conventional transmembrane anchors as well as cytoplasmic domains. The CD66a and CD66d cytoplasmic domains each contain two YxxL/M motifs. In CD66d they resemble conventional ITAM-like motifs (YxxLx$_7$YxxM) whereas in CD66a they are spaced further apart (VxYxxLx$_{21}$IxYxxV) and resemble motifs which bind tyrosine phosphatases such as SHP-1 and -2. Activation of neutrophils leads to phosphorylation of tyrosine residues in the CD66a cytoplasmic domain[7]. Multiple splice variants have been identified for CD66a/BGP (at least 11) and CD66d/GCM1 (at least 3), the largest of which (termed BGPa and GCM1a) are shown below [1,2].

Ligands and associated molecules

CD66 molecules can mediate cell–cell adhesion by homotypic interactions and/or by heterotypic interactions with other CD66 molecules. CD66a, c and e exhibit both heterotypic and homotypic interactions whereas CD66b binds only heterotypically to CD66c and CD66e [8,9]. The binding sites for these interactions lie within their N-terminal V-set IgSF domains [8,9]. Unlike most IgSF adhesion molecules, homotypic adhesion involving CD66a is reportedly both cation and temperature dependent [8]. Carbohydrate structures on CD66c mediate binding to *E. coli* type 1 fimbriae [10], and may be important in presenting sLe^x-related ligands to the endothelial cell adhesion molecule CD66e [2]. CD66a associates with the cytoplasmic tyrosine kinases Src, Lyn and Hck [7,11]. Phosphorylated YxxL motifs in the cytoplasmic domain of CD66a bind to the SH2 domain of Src and activate the enzyme. MAbs specific for the GPI-anchored molecules CD66b and CD66c co-precipitate Lyn and Hck [7].

Function

The ability of CD66 molecules to mediate cell–cell adhesion and their rapid upregulation following activation suggests that they may contribute to the interactions of activated granulocytes with each other or with endothelia or epithelia. However, direct functional evidence for such a role is lacking. Crosslinking of CD66 molecules with antibodies can stimulate integrin-mediated neutrophil adhesion to endothelial cells, suggesting a possible signalling role [12].

Database accession numbers

	PIR	SWISSPROT	EMBL/GENBANK	REFERENCE
Human CD66a (BGPa)	A32164	P13688	X16354	1
Human CD66b	S13524	P31997	X52378	1
Human CD66c		P40199	M29541	1
Human CD66d (CGM1a)	S33323	P40198	L00692	1

Amino acid sequence of CD66a (BGPa)

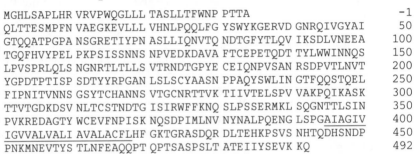

```
MGHLSAPLHR VRVPWQGLLL TASLLTFWNP PTTA                    -1
QLTTESMPFN VAEGKEVLLL VHNLPQQLFG YSWYKGERVD GNRQIVGYAI    50
GTQQATPGPA NSGRETIYPN ASLLIQNVTQ NDTGFYTLQV IKSDLVNEEA   100
TGQFHVYPEL PKPSISSNNS NPVEDKDAVA FTCEPETQDT TYLWWINNQS   150
LPVSPRLQLS NGNRTLTLLS VTRNDTGPYE CEIQNPVSAN RSDPVTLNVT   200
YGPDTPTISP SDTYYRPGAN LSLSCYAASN PPAQYSWLIN GTFQQSTQEL   250
FIPNITVNNS GSYTCHANNS VTGCNRTTVK TIIVTELSPV VAKPQIKASK   300
TTVTGDKDSV NLTCSTNDTG ISIRWFFKNQ SLPSSERMKL SQGNTTLSIN   350
PVKREDAGTY WCEVFNPISK NQSDPIMLNV NYNALPQENG LSPGAIAGIV   400
IGVVALVALI AVALACFLHF GKTGRASDQR DLTEHKPSVS NHTQDHSNDP   450
PNKMNEVTYS TLNFEAQQPT QPTSASPSLT ATEIIYSEVK KQ           492
```

Amino acid sequence of CD66b

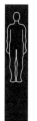

```
MGPISAPSCR WRIPWQGLLL TASLFTFWNP PTTA              -1
QLTIEAVPSN AAEGKEVLLL VHNLPQDPRG YNWYKGETVD ANRRIIGYVI   50
SNQQITPGPA YSNRETIYPN ASLLMRNVTR NDTGSYTLQV IKLNLMSEEV  100
TGQFSVHPET PKPSISSNNS NPVEDKDAVA FTCEPETQNT TYLWWVNGQS  150
LPVSPRLQLS NGNRTLTLLS VTRNDVGPYE CEIQNPASAN FSDPVTLNVL  200
YGPDAPTISP SDTYYHAGVN LNLSCHAASN PPSQYSWSVN GTFQQYTQKL  250
FIPNITTKNS GSYACHTTNS ATGRNRTTVR MITVSD              286
AVVQGSSPGL SARATVSIMI GVLARVALI                      +29
```

Amino acid sequence of CD66c

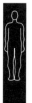

```
MGPPSAPPCR LHVPWKEVLL TASLLTFWNP PTTA              -1
KLTIESTPFN VAEGKEVLLL AHNLPQNRIG YSWYKGERVD GNSLIVGYVI   50
GTQQATPGPA YSGRETIYPN ASLLIQNVTQ NDTGFYTLQV IKSDLVNEEA  100
TGQLHVYPEL PKPSISSNNS NPVEDKDAVA FTCEPEVQNT TYLWWVNGQS  150
LPVSPRLQLS NGNMTLTLLS VKRNDAGSYE CEIQNPASAN RSDPVTLNVL  200
YGPDGPTISP SKANYRPGEN LNLSCHAASN PPAQYSWFIN GTFQQSTQEL  250
FIPNITVNNS GSYMCQAHNS ATGLNRTTVT MITVSG              286
SAPVLSAVAT VGITIGVLAR VALI                          +24
```

Amino acid sequence of CD66d (CGM1a)

```
MGPPSASPHR ECIPWQGLLL TASLLNFWNP PTTA              -1
KLTIESMPLS VAEGKEVLLL VHNLPQHLFG YSWYKGERVD GNSLIVGYVI   50
GTQQATPGAA YSGRETIYTN ASLLIQNVTQ NDIGFYTLQV IKSDLVNEEA  100
TGQFHVYQEN APGLPVGAVA GIVTGVLVGV ALVAALVCFL LLAKTGRTSI  150
QRDLKEQQPQ ALAPGRGPSH SSAFSMSPLS SAQAPLPNPR TAASIYEELL  200
KHDTNIYCRM DHKAEVAS                                 218
```

References
1 **Thompson, J.A. et al. (1991) J. Clin. Lab. Anal. 5, 344–366.**
2 Nagel, G. and Grunert, F. (1995) Tumor Biology 16, 17–22.
3 Schlossman, S.F. et al. (eds) (1995) Leucocyte Typing V: white cell differentiation antigens. Oxford University Press, Oxford.
4 Möller, M.J. et al. (1996) Int. J. Cancer 65, 740–745.
5 Prall, F. et al. (1996) J. Histochem. Cytochem. 44, 35–41.
6 Grunert, F. et al. (1995) Int. J. Cancer 63, 349–355.
7 **Skubitz, K.M. et al. (1995) J. Immunol. 155, 5382–5390.**
8 Teixeira, A.M. et al. (1994) Blood 84, 211–219.
9 Yamanaka, T. et al. (1996) Biochem. Biophys. Res. Commun. 219, 842–847.
10 Sauter, S.L. et al. (1993) J. Biol. Chem. 268, 15510–15516.
11 Brümmer, J. et al. (1995) Oncogene 11, 1649–1655.
12 Skubitz, K.M. et al. (1996) J. Leukocyte Biol. 60, 106–117.

CD68 Macrosialin (mouse)

Molecular weights
Polypeptide   35 367

SDS-PAGE
   reduced   110 kDa

Carbohydrate
N-linked sites   9
O-linked   ++

Human gene location and size
17p13; ~2 kb [1]

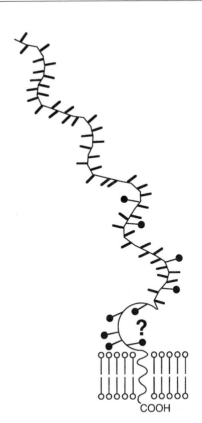

Tissue distribution

Present in the lysosomes, endosomes and, to a lesser extent, on the surface of macrophages, monocytes, neutrophils, basophils and large lymphocytes [2,3]. The antigen is also expressed in the cytoplasm of a number of cells in non-haematopoietic tissues, notably in the liver and in renal tubules and glomeruli [2]. Not all anti-CD68 antibodies give the same staining patterns, possibly as a result of tissue-specific glycosylation [2].

Structure

CD68 belongs to a family of acidic, highly glycosylated lysosomal-associated membrane proteins (lamps) that includes lamp-1 (CD107a) and lamp-2 (CD107b) [4,5]. The extracellular domains of lamps are partitioned into two related subdomains by a short linker rich in proline, threonine and serine residues [5]. In CD68 there is only one domain that is related to the lamps, and this is adjacent to the membrane [4]. The N-terminal region, which is very rich in Thr and Ser residues, shares no homology with the lamps [4] and is likely to be heavily O-glycosylated on the basis of comparison with the CD43 antigen. Expression cloning of the CD68 cDNA has produced two sequences that differ with respect to the length of the N-terminal domain and which might arise by alternative splicing [4]. The cytoplasmic domain contains a tyrosine residue which might direct the protein to the lysosomes [4,5]. Soluble forms of CD68 have been detected in serum and urine [2].

Ligands and associated moleules

Macrosialin from lysates of mouse peritoneal macrophages and a macrophage cell line has been shown to bind oxidized low-density lipoprotein [6]. Whether macrosialin participates in the uptake of oxidized-LDL or binds following its internalization remains to be determined.

Function

While the function of CD68 is unknown, lamps are the major components of lysosomal membranes and may protect the membranes from attack by acid hydrolases [5]. It is not clear whether the surface expression of CD68 is functionally significant or due to leakage from the lysosomes, as could be the case for the lamps [5]. Inflammatory agents upregulate macrosialin expression and this is accompanied by changes in the pattern of its glycosylation [7].

Comments

Expression cloning has identified macrosialin as the mouse homologue of CD68 [4,8]. Macrosialin is known to be O-glycosylated and its expression is restricted to macrophages and, at lower levels, dendritic cells (ref. 7 and references therein).

Database accession numbers

	PIR	SWISSPROT	EMBL/GENBANK	REFERENCE
Human	A48931	P34810	S57235	4
Mouse	S28587	P31996	X68273	8

Amino acid sequence of human CD68

```
MRLAVLFSGA LLGLLAAQGT G                                          -1
NDCPHKKSAT LLPSFTVTPT VTESTGTTSH RTTKSHKTTT HRTTTTGTTS          50
HGPTTATHNP TTTSHGNVTV HPTSNSTATS QGPSTATHSP ATTSHGNATV          100
HPTSNSTATS PGFTSSAHPE PPPPSPSPSP TSKETIGDYT WTNGSQPCVH          150
LQAQIQIRVM YTTQGGGEAW GISVLNPNKT KVQGSCEGAH PHLLLSFPYG          200
HLSFGFMQDL QQKVVYLSYM AVEYNVSFPH AAKWTFSAQN ASLRDLQAPL          250
GQSFSCSNSS IILSPAVHLD LLSLRLQAAQ LPHTGVFGQS FSCPSDRSIL          300
LPLIIGLILL GLLALVLIAF CIIRRRPSAY QAL                            333
```

References
1 Greaves, D.R. et al. Manuscript in preparation.
2 Pulford, K.A.F. et al. (1990) Int. Immunol. 2, 973–980.
3 Stockinger, H. (1989) Leucocyte Typing IV, 841–843.
4 Holness, C.L. and Simmons, D.L. (1993) Blood 81, 1607–1613.
5 **Fukuda, M. (1991) J. Biol. Chem. 266, 21327–21330.**
6 **Ramprasad, M.P. et al. (1995) Proc. Natl Acad. Sci. USA 92, 9580–9584.**
7 Rabinowitz, S.S. and Gordon, S. (1991) J. Exp. Med. 174, 827–836.
8 Holness, C.L. et al. (1993) J. Biol. Chem. 268, 9661–9666.

CD69

AIM, EA 1, MLR-3, Leu-23

Molecular weights
Polypeptide   22 559

SDS-PAGE
  reduced   ~28 and ~32 kDa
  unreduced   55–65 kDa

Carbohydrate
N-linked sites   1
O-linked   unknown

Human gene location and size
12p12.3–p13.2; ~15 kb [1,2]

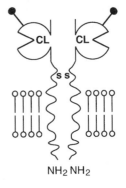

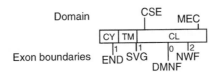

Tissue distribution

CD69 is widely expressed on hematopoietic cells including lymphocytes, neutrophils, eosinophils, platelets and epidermal Langerhans cells. It is not expressed on resting lymphocytes but is rapidly (within 2 h) induced upon activation of B, T and NK cells. CD69 is expressed on CD4+ or CD8+ thymocytes, germinal centre T cells, and T cells in regions of inflammation, consistent with it being a marker of T cell activation [3–5].

Structure

The human and mouse genes for CD69 are encoded within the NK gene complex on chromosomes 12 and 6, respectively [1,6]. Like other proteins encoded within the NK gene complex (CD95, CD161, NKG2, and Ly-49) [7], CD69 is a type II membrane glycoprotein expressed as a disulfide-linked homodimer [3–5]. The extracellular region has a C-type lectin domain. The cytoplasmic domain contain phosphorylation sites for serine/threonine kinases and is constitutively phosphorylated [3–5].

Function

CD69 is not expressed on resting peripheral blood lymphocytes but is amongst the earliest antigens to appear upon activation of lymphocytes, appearing within 2 h after stimulation. Expression requires mRNA synthesis, and is very transient, as the result of rapid degradation of the mRNA (which has a functional AU-rich motif in the 3′ untranslated region) [8]. Anti-CD69 mAbs can activate T and B cells, NK cells, platelets and neutrophils, suggesting that it may function as a signalling molecule [3–5].

Database accession numbers

	PIR	*SWISSPROT*	*EMBL/GENBANK*	*REFERENCE*
Human	JH0822	Q07108	L07555	3,4
Mouse		P37217	L23638	5

Amino acid sequence of human CD69

```
MSSENCFVAE NSSLHPESGQ ENDATSPHFS TRHEGSFQVP VLCAVMNVVF      50
ITILIIALIA LSVGQYNCPG QYTFSMPSDS HVSSCSEDWV GYQRKCYFIS     100
TVKRSWTSAQ NACSEHGATL AVIDSEKDMN FLKRYAGREE HWVGLKKEPG     150
HPWKWSNGKE FNNWFNVTGS DKCVFLKNTE VSSMECEKNL YWICNKPYK      199
```

References

1 Schnittger, S. et al. (1993) Eur. J. Immunol. 23, 2711–2713.
2 Santis, A.G. et al. (1994) Eur. J. Immunol. 24, 1692–1697.
3 Hamann, J. et al. (1993) J. Immunol. 150, 4920–4927.
4 López-Cabrera, M. et al. (1993) J. Exp. Med. 178, 537–547.
5 Ziegler, S.F. et al. (1993) Eur. J. Immunol. 23, 1643–1648.
6 Ziegler, S.F. et al. (1994) J. Immunol. 152, 1228–1236.
7 Gumperz, J.E. and Parham, P. (1995) Nature 378, 245–248.
8 **Santis, A.G. et al. (1995) Eur. J. Immunol. 25, 2142–2146.**

CD70

CD27L

Molecular weights
Polypeptide   21 147

Carbohydrate
N-linked sites   2
O-linked   unknown

Human gene location
19p13.3 [1,2]

Domains

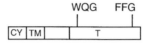

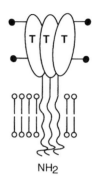

Tissue distribution

CD70 is expressed on most activated B cells and some activated T cells but is absent from resting lymphocytes, red blood cells, thymocytes, platelets, monocytes, neutrophils or dendritic cells [2].

Structure

CD70 is a member of the TNF superfamily [1-4]. Like other members of this superfamily, it is a type II membrane protein and is probably expressed as a trimer. The sequence similarity to TNF is in the C-terminal extracellular region [1-4].

Ligands and associated molecules

CD70 binds CD27, a member of the TNFR superfamily [1].

Function

Cells expressing CD70 can co-stimulate T cell proliferation, and enhance the generation of cytotoxic T cells and cytokine production [1,5]. CD70 binding to CD27 on B cells co-stimulates B cell proliferation and immunoglobulin production [6].

Database accession numbers

	PIR	SWISSPROT	EMBL/GENBANK	REFERENCE
Human	A40738	P32970	L08096	1

Amino acid sequence of human CD27

```
MPEEGSGCSV RRRPYGCVLR AALVPLVAGL VICLVVCIQR FAQAQQQLPL     50
ESLGWDVAEL QLNHTGPQQD PRLYWQGGPA LGRSFLHGPE LDKGQLRIHR    100
DGIYMVHIQV TLAICSSTTA SRHHPTTLAV GICSPASRSI SLLRLSFHQG    150
CTIVSQRLTP LARGDTLCTN LTGTLLPSRN TDETFFGVQW VRP           193
```

References
1 Goodwin, R.G. et al. (1993) Cell 73, 447–456.
2 Gruss, H.-J. and Dower, S.K. (1995) Blood 85, 3378–3404.

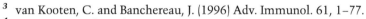

[3] van Kooten, C. and Banchereau, J. (1996) Adv. Immunol. 61, 1–77.

[4] Armitage, R.J. (1994) Curr. Opin. Immunol. 6, 407–413.

[5] **Hintzen, R.Q. et al. (1994) Immunol. Today 15, 307–311.**

[6] Kobata, T. et al. (1995) Proc. Natl Acad. Sci. USA 92, 11249–11253.

CD71 — Transferrin receptor, T9

Molecular weights
Polypeptide   84 901

SDS-PAGE
  reduced   90–95 kDa
  unreduced   180–190 kDa

Carbohydrate
N-linked sites   3
O-linked   +

Human gene location
3q26.2–qter; 31 kb [1]

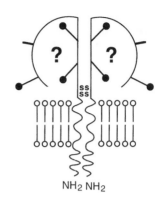

Tissue distribution

CD71 expression is very low on resting leucocytes but is upregulated upon activation, presumably reflecting the iron dependence of proliferation. In other tissues CD71 is expressed on most dividing cells and also on brain endothelium [1].

Structure

CD71 is a type II membrane glycoprotein that exists as a homodimer with interchain disulfide bonds at Cys89 and Cys98. It is acylated at Cys62 and phosphorylated at Ser24 by protein kinase C (reviewed in ref. 1). The CD71 internalization signal is the tetrapeptide sequence YTRF (amino acids 20–23), which structurally appears to be a tight turn [2]. CD71 can be cleaved by an unidentified protease, between Arg100 and Leu101, to yield a soluble truncated form. O-linked glycosylation at Thr104 decreases the susceptibility of the molecule to cleavage [3].

Ligands and associated molecules

The ligand for CD71 is transferrin, the serum iron-transport protein (reviewed in ref. 1). CD71 associates non-covalently with the TCR ζ chain in T cells, where it may play a role in signal transduction [4]. CD71 monomers have been reported to form a complex with the integrin CD29/CD49c (VLA-3) in some cell lines, via a disulfide bond interaction between CD71 and CD49c [5].

Function

CD71 plays a critical role in cell proliferation by controlling the supply of iron, which is essential for many metabolic pathways, through the binding and endocytosis of transferrin, the major iron-carrying protein [1]. The expression of CD71 is regulated at the post-transcriptional level through the control of mRNA stability and is closely linked to intracellular iron levels (reviewed in ref. 6). Upon iron deprivation, a cytoplasmic protein, known as the iron-response element binding protein (IRE-BP), stabilizes CD71 mRNA by binding to specific sequences, known as iron-response elements (IREs), within the 3' untranslated region of the CD71 mRNA. When iron levels are high, the IRE-BP affinity for IREs is lower and CD71 mRNA more susceptible to degradation. Nitric oxide can affect CD71 expression independently of intracellular iron concentration by activating IRE-BP binding to IREs and thus stabilizing CD71 mRNA[6].

Comment

Proteins that share sequence homology with CD71 have not previously been described. However we have noted that a 55 amino acid sequence (residues Phe237–Ile290) shares 43.6% identity with a region of streptococcal C5a peptidase (residues Tyr371–Ile425[7]). The ALIGN score for this comparison is 9.33 standard deviations, making the similarity highly significant.

Database accession numbers

	PIR	SWISSPROT	EMBL/GENBANK	REFERENCE
Human	A03259	P02786	X01060	8
Rat	A34549		M58040	9
Mouse	S29548		X57349	10

Amino acid sequence of human CD71

```
MMDQARSAFS NLFGGEPLSY TRFSLARQVD GDNSHVEMKL AVDEEENADN    50
NTKANVTKPK RCSGSICYGT IAVIVFFLIG FMIGYLGYCK GVEPKTECER   100
LAGTESPVRE EPGEDFPAAR RLYWDDLKRK LSEKLDSTDF TSTIKLLNEN   150
SYVPREAGSQ KDENLALYVE NQFREFKLSK VWRDQHFVKI QVKDSAQNSV   200
IIVDKNGRLV YLVENPGGYV AYSKAATVTG KLVHANFGTK KDFEDLYTPV   250
NGSIVIVRAG KITFAEKVAN AESLNAIGVL IYMDQTKFPI VNAELSFFGH   300
AHLGTGDPYT PGFPSFNHTQ FPPSRSSGLP NIPVQTISRA AAEKLFGNME   350
GDCPSDWKTD STCRMVTSES KNVKLTVSNV LKEIKILNIF GVIKGFVEPD   400
HYVVVGAQRD AWGPGAAKSG VGTALLLKLA QMFSDMVLKD GFQPSRSIIF   450
ASWSAGDFGS VGATEWLEGY LSSLHLKAFT YINLDKAVLG TSNFKVSASP   500
LLYTLIEKTM QNVKHPVTGQ FLYQDSNWAS KVEKLTLDNA AFPFLAYSGI   550
PAVSFCFCED TDYPYLGTTM DTYKELIERI PELNKVARAA AEVAGQFVIK   600
LTHDVELNLD YERYNSQLLS FVRDLNQYRA DIKEMGLSLQ WLYSARGDFF   650
RATSRLTTDF GNAEKTDRFV MKKLNDRVMR VEYHFLSPYV SPKESPFRHV   700
FWGSGSHTLP ALLENLKLRK QNNGAFNETL FRNQLALATW TIQGAANALS   750
GDVVWDIDNEF                                             760
```

References

1. Testa, U. et al. (1993) Crit. Rev. Oncog. 4, 241–276.
2. Trowbridge, I.S. et al. (1993) Annu. Rev. Cell Biol. 9, 129–161.
3. Rutledge, E.A. et al. (1994) J. Biol. Chem. 269, 31864–31868.
4. Salmeron, A. et al. (1995) J. Immunol. 154, 1675–1683.
5. Coppolino, M. et al. (1995) Biochem. J. 306, 129–134.
6. Hentze, M.W. and Kühn, L.C. (1996) Proc. Natl Acad. Sci. USA 93, 8175–8182.
7. Chen, C.C. and Cleary, P.P. (1990) J. Biol. Chem. 265, 3161–3167.

[8] Schneider, C. et al. (1984) Nature 311, 675–678.

[9] Roberts, K.P. and Griswold, M.D. (1990) Mol. Cell. Endocrinol. 14, 531–542.

[10] Trowbridge, I.S. et al. Unpublished.

CD72

Lyb-2, Ly-32.2, Ly-19.2 (mouse)

Molecular weights
Polypeptide   40 224

SDS-PAGE
  reduced   39 and 43 (major) kDa
  unreduced   86 (major) and 90 kDa

Carbohydrate
N-linked sites 1
O-linked   unknown

Gene location
9p [1]

Domain boundaries

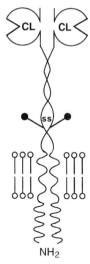

Tissue distribution

CD72 is expressed on all cells of the B cell lineage except plasma cells [2]. Anti-CD72 antibodies also label human tissue macrophages weakly.

Structure

CD72 is a member of a group of related cell surface molecules which includes the asialoglycoprotein receptors, CD23, and the Kupffer cell receptor [3]. These molecules are type II integral membrane glycoprotein with membrane-proximal stalk regions, which are predicted to form α helical coiled coils [4], and membrane-distal C-type lectin (CL) domains [3]. CD72 is expressed as a disulfide-linked homodimer [5]. The mouse alloantigens Ly-32.2, Ly-19.2 and Lyb-2 have been shown to be identical to mouse CD72 [6], for which multiple allelic [7] and splice [8] variants have been identified. The CD72 CL domain has a lower level of identity to other CL domains than is usually the case for this superfamily, and is missing key residues implicated in Ca^{2+} and carbohydrate binding [3], but the assignment of the CL domain is not in doubt.

Ligands and associated molecules

Purified CD5 has been reported to bind CD72 on cells [9] but this is controversial (see **CD5**). Lectin-like activity has not been demonstrated.

Function

Unknown. Exposure of B cells to CD72 antibodies activates a variety of signalling pathways and can induce MHC Class II expression and B cell proliferation [2]. However, the significance of these observations is not clear.

Database accession numbers

	PIR	SWISSPROT	EMBL/GENBANK	REFERENCE
Human	A43532	P21854	M54992	5
Mouse	A32331	P21855	J04170	10

Amino acid sequence of human CD72

```
MAEAITYADL RFVKAPLKKS ISSRLGQDPG ADDDGEITYE NVQVPAVLGV    50
PSSLASSVLG DKAAVKSEQP TASWRAVTSP AVGRILPCRT TCLRYLLLGL   100
LLTCLLLGVT AICLGVRYLQ VSQQLQQTNR VLEVTNSSLR QQLRLKITQL   150
GQSAEDLQGS RRELAQSQEA LQVEQRAHQA AEGQLQACQA DRQKTKETLQ   200
SEEQQRRALE QKLSNMENRL KPFFTCGSAD TCCPSGWIMH QKSCFYISLT   250
SKNWQESQKQ CETLSSKLAT FSEIYPQSHS YYFLNSLLPN GGSGNSYWTG   300
LSSNKDWKLT DDTQRTRTYA QSSKCNKVHK TWSWWTLESE SCRSSLPYIC   350
EMTAFRFPD                                               359
```

References

[1] von Hoegen, I. et al. (1991) Eur. J. Immunol. 21, 1425–1431.

[2] **Gordon, J. (1994) Immunol. Today 15, 411–417.**

[3] Day, A.J. (1994) Biochem. Soc. Trans. 22, 83–88.

[4] Beavil, A.J. et al. (1992) Proc. Natl Acad. Sci. USA 89, 753–757.

[5] von Hoegen, I. et al. (1990) J. Immunol. 144, 4870–4877.

[6] Robinson, W.H. et al. (1993) J. Immunol. 151, 4764–4772.

[7] Robinson, W.H. et al. (1992) J. Immunol. 149, 880–886.

[8] Ying, H. et al. (1995) J. Immunol. 154, 2743–2752.

[9] Van de Velde, H. et al. (1991) Nature 351, 662–665.

[10] Nakayama, E. et al. (1989) Proc. Natl Acad. Sci. USA 86, 1352–1356.

Molecular weights
Polypeptide   60 824

SDS-PAGE
  unreduced   70 kDa
  reduced   70 kDa

Carbohydrate
N-linked sites   4
O-linked   unknown

Human gene location
6q14–q21

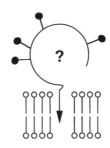

Tissue distribution

CD73 is expressed differentially on subsets of mature lymphocytes (10% of $CD4^+$ cells, 50% of $CD8^+$ cells and 70% of B cells)[1]. CD73 is also expressed on certain endothelial and epithelial cells[1]. Enzyme activity in peripheral T cells is 10-fold higher than in thymocytes, and in peripheral B cells enzyme activity is 5-fold higher than in umbilical cord B cells[1,2].

Structure

CD73 is GPI-linked. The site of GPI attachment has been confirmed by peptide analysis[3].

Function

CD73 catalyses the 5′ dephosphorylation of purine and pyrimidine ribo- and deoxyribonucleoside monophosphates to nucleosides that can be taken up by transport systems[2,4]. Co-stimulatory effects of CD73 mAb on human T lymphocytes do not require enzyme activity of CD73[5]. Inhibition of ecto-5′-nucleotidase activity by biochemical inhibitors or a polyclonal antiserum suppressed the generation and cytotoxicity of alloreactive cytotoxic T lymphocytes[2]. CD73 mediates binding of lymphocytes to cultured endothelial cells[6].

Comments

Ecto-5′-nucleotidase activity is abnormally low on lymphocytes of patients with various immunodeficiency diseases, including severe combined immunodeficiency, X-linked agammaglobulinaemia, common variable immunodeficiency, selective IgA deficiency, Wiskott–Aldrich syndrome and AIDS[1].

Database accession numbers

	PIR	SWISSPROT	EMBL/GENBANK	REFERENCE
Human	S11032	P21589	X55740	3
Mouse			L12059	7
Rat				8

Amino acid sequence of human CD73

```
MCPRAARAPA TLLLALGAVL WPAAGA                                  -1
WELTILHTND VHSRLEQTSE DSSKCVNASR CMGGVARLFT KVQQIRRAEP         50
NVLLLDAGDQ YQGTIWFTVY KGAEVAHFMN ALRYDAMALG NHEFDNGVEG        100
LIEPLLKEAK FPILSANIKA KGPLASQISG LYLPYKVLPV GDEVVGIVGY        150
TSKETPFLSN PGTNLVFEDE ITALQPEVDK LKTLNVNKII ALGHSGFEMD        200
KLIAQKVRGV DVVVGGHSNT FLYTGNPPSK EVPAGKYPFI VTSDDGRKVP        250
VVQAYAFGKY LGYLKIEFDE RGNVISSHGN PILLNSSIPE DPSIKADINK        300
WRIKLDNYST QELGKTIVYL DGSSQSCRFR ECNMGNLICD AMINNNLRHT        350
DEMFWNHVSM CILNGGGIRS PIDERNNGTI TWENLAAVLP FGGTFDLVQL        400
KGSTLKKAFE HSVHRYGQST GEFLQVGGIH VVYDLSRKPG DRVVKLDVLC        450
TKCRVPSYDP LKMDEVYKVI LPNFLANGGD GFQMIKDELL RHDSGDQDIN        500
VVSTYISKMK VIYPAVEGRI KFS                                     523
TGSHCHGSFS LIFLSLWAVI FVLYQ                                  +25
```

References
1 Thomson, L.F. et al. (1990) Tissue Antigens 55, 9–19.
2 **Shipp, M.A. and Look, A.T. (1993) Blood 82, 1052–1070.**
3 Misumi, Y. et al. (1990) Eur. J. Biochem. 191, 563–569.
4 Zimmermann, H. (1992) Biochem. J. 285, 345–365.
5 Gutensohn, W. et al. (1995) Cell. Immunol. 161, 213–217.
6 Airas, L. et al. (1995) J. Exp. Med. 182, 1603–1608.
7 Resta, R. et al. (1993) Gene 133, 171–177.
8 Misumi, Y. et al. (1990) J. Biol. Chem. 265, 2178–2183.

CD74

MHC Class II-associated invariant chain (Ii or Iγ)

Molecular weights
Polypeptides   26 399 / 24 376 / 33 388 / 31 365

SDS-PAGE
  reduced   33 / 35 / 41 / 43 kDa

Carbohydrate
N-linked sites   2 or 4
O-linked   +

Human gene location and size
5q32; 12 kb [1]

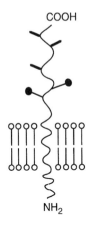

Tissue distribution

CD74 is mostly expressed intracellularly in MHC Class II-positive cells. There is moderate surface expression on B cells and weak surface expression on monocytes. CD74 is also expressed by a subset of activated T cells and some epithelial cells.

Structure

CD74 is a type II integral membrane glycoprotein [2]. It consists of four distinct forms which are generated by usage of two in-phase initiation codons (yielding products which differ in apparent M_r by 2 kDa) and by alternative splicing of exon 6b (yielding products which differ in apparent M_r by 8 kDa) [3,4]. The latter exon encodes a sequence of 64 amino acids, containing six cysteines, which has sequence similarity to thyroglobulin type I repeats centred around the Cys-Trp-Cys-Val motif. The shorter form of CD74 is illustrated above. CD74 contains N-linked and O-linked carbohydrates and minor forms are acylated, sulfated, phosphorylated or contain glycosaminoglycans.

Function

CD74 homotrimers associate in the endoplasmic reticulum (ER) with three MHC Class II $\alpha\beta$ dimers and this prevents the binding of endogenous peptides to Class II molecules [5-8]. The N-terminal cytoplasmic domain of CD74 contains targeting motifs which leads to its retention in the ER, or to targeting of Class II $\alpha\beta$ dimers into the endosomal–lysosomal pathway via the Golgi [5,6]. Subsequent proteolytic degradation of CD74 leaves a small fragment (Class II-associated invariant chain peptide (CLIP)) bound to Class II $\alpha\beta$ dimers in the peptide-binding groove. The interaction of Class II $\alpha\beta$/CLIP complexes with HLA-DM (a Class II-related $\alpha\beta$ dimer) in a specialized compartment releases the CLIP and allows the Class II molecules to bind peptides derived from exogenous proteins [8]. CD74-deficient mice have reduced levels of MHC Class II at the cell surface and these molecules lack the compact conformation indicative of bound peptide[9]. Consequently these mice have reduced numbers of peripheral CD4[+] T cells and their antigen-presenting cells present protein antigens very poorly.

Comments

Expression of CD74 and the MHC Class II α and β chains is co-regulated and induced by IFNγ [10]. Coordinate expression of these three genes may be directed by a segment of sequence homology at the 5' region of each gene[1].

Database accession numbers

	PIR	SWISSPROT	EMBL/GENBANK	REFERENCE
Human	A30060	P04233	X03339, X03340	1–3
Mouse	A02244	P04441	X00496	11
Rat	S02182	P10247	X14254	12

Amino acid sequence of human CD74

```
MHRRRSRSCR EDQKPV**M**DDQ RDLISNNEQL PMLGRRPGAP ESKCSRGALY     50
TGFSILVTLL LAGQATTAYF LYQQQGRLDK LTVTSQNLQL ENLRMKLPKP    100
PKPVSKMRMA TPLLMQALPM GALPQGPMQN ATKYGNMTED HVMHLLQNAD    150
PLKVYPPLKG SFPENLRHLK NTMETIDWKV FESWMHHWLL FEMSRHSLEQ    200
KPTDAPP**K**ES LELEDPSSGL GVTKQDLGPV PM                     232
```

Notes

1 The alternative N-terminal Met residue is bold and underlined.

2 Usage of exon 6b generates the following in-frame sequence inserted after Lys208 which is indicated bold and underlined above:

```
VLTKCQEEVS HIPAVHPGSF RPKCDENGNY LPLQCYGSIG YCWCVFPNGT    258
EVPNTRSRGH HNCS                                           272
```

References

1 O'Sullivan, D.M. et al. (1986) Proc. Natl Acad. Sci. USA 83, 4484–4488.

2 Claesson, L. et al. (1983) Proc. Natl Acad. Sci. USA 80, 7395–7399.

3 Strubin, M. et al. (1986) EMBO J. 5, 3483–3488.

4 O'Sullivan, D.M. et al. (1987) J. Exp. Med. 166, 444–460.

5 Lotteau, V. et al. (1990) Nature 348, 600–605.

6 **Lamb, C.A. et al. (1991) Proc. Natl Acad. Sci. USA 88, 5998–6002.**

7 Marks, M.S. et al. (1990) J. Cell Biol. 111, 839–855.

8 Cresswell, P. (1996) Cell 84, 505–507.

9 **Viville, S. et al. (1993) Cell 72, 635–648.**

10 Paulnock–King, D. et al. (1985) J. Immunol. 135, 632–636.

11 Koch, N. et al. (1987) EMBO J. 6, 1677–1683.

12 McKnight, A.J. et al. (1989) Nucleic Acids Res. 17, 3983–3984.

CDw75

Tissue distribution

CDw75 is expressed on sIg$^+$ mature B cells but not on plasma cells[1,2]. Expression is particularly high in germinal centres. The level of expression increases on activation of B cells. It is also expressed weakly on a fraction of T cells, on erythrocyte precursors in the bone marrow and on a broad range of epithelial cell types.

Structure

CDw75 is an ill-defined carbohydrate structure present on *N*-glycans which contains α2,6-linked sialic acid[1,2]. Some (but not all) cells lacking CDw75 express the antigen when transfected with the Golgi enzyme β-galactoside α2,6-sialyltransferase (EC 2.4.99.1)[1,2].

Ligands and associated molecules

No ligand has been identified. CDw75 is not a ligand for the lectin CD22, which binds the sialoglycoconjugate NeuAcα2 → 6Galβ1 → 4GlcNAc[3].

References
1 **Bast, B.J.E.G. et al. (1992) J. Cell Biol. 116, 423–435.**
2 Schlossman, S.F. et al. (1995) Leucocyte Typing V: white cell differentiation antigens. Oxford University Press, Oxford.
3 Engel, P. et al. (1993) J. Immunol. 150, 4719–4732.

CDw76

CDw76

Molecular weights

SDS-PAGE
   reduced   85, 67 kDa

Tissue distribution

CDw76 is a provisional CD cluster that represents two closely related but distinct carbohydrate epitopes, designated CD76.1 and CD76.2, recognized by the mAbs CRIS-4 and HD66, respectively[1]. It is likely that CDw76 will be subdivided in future to distinguish the CD76.1 and CD76.2 epitopes[1]. Both epitopes are strongly expressed on mature peripheral blood B cells and mantle zone B cells, but expression is weak or absent on germinal centre B cells and plasma cells. CD76.1 is expressed on resting T cells and some granulocytes but CD76.2 is absent on these cells. On activated T cells, expression of both CD76.1 and CD76.2 is upregulated. Amongst non-haematopoietic cells, CDw76 epitopes are expressed on various epithelial and some endothelial cells[1,2].

Structure

The CDw76 epitope is present on α2,6-sialylated polylactosamine structures and is thus not restricted to one particular glycoprotein or glycolipid. Both CDw76 mAbs have been shown to react with α2,6-sialylated type 2 chain oligosaccharide moieties of glycosphingolipids. The CD76.1 mAb detects sialylated glycosphingolipids with higher charge than does CD76.2. The CD76.1 and CD76.2 epitopes may be present on polylactosamine sequences of N-linked carbohydrate structures, but only CD76.1 may be present on O-linked structures[2]. The CD76.2 mAb immunoprecipitates two uncharacterized glycoproteins of 85 kDa and 67 kDa[2].

Function

Unknown.

References
[1] Engel, P. and Tedder, T.F. (1995) Leucocyte Typing V, 577–580.
[2] Schwartz-Albiez, R. et al. (1995) Leucocyte Typing V, 580–586.

CD77

Other names
Globotriaocylceramide (Gb$_3$)
Ceramide trihexoside
P^k blood group antigen
Burkitt's lymphoma-associated antigen (BLA)

Tissue distribution

Expressed on a subset of germinal centre tonsillar B cells [1,2]. CD77 is a useful marker for Burkitt's lymphoma [1,3] and it has been postulated that B cells expressing this antigen are the normal counterparts of Burkitt's lymphoma tumour cells. Lymphoblastoid cell lines, obtained by transformation of normal B cells with Epstein–Barr virus, do not express CD77 but the antigen is expressed on endothelium and some epithelial cells, as well as follicular dendritic cells and macrophages in lymphoid tissue [4].

Structure

CD77 mAbs react with Galα1 → 4Galβ1 → 4Glc-ceramide (Gb$_3$), which belongs to the globo-series of neutral glycosphingolipids [5].

Ligands and associated molecules

Co-capping experiments suggest that CD77 is associated with CD19 on the surface of Daudi B cells, while CD77-deficient cells show concomitant decreased expression of CD19, suggesting that CD77 influences the surface expression of CD19 [6].

Function

The function of CD77 is unknown. However, CD77 is a receptor for lectins on the pili of a certain strain of *Escherichia coli*. The vero toxin of *E. coli* and the Shiga toxin of *Shigella dysenteriae* specifically bind to Gb$_3$ [7]. Germinal centre B cells which express CD77 have been shown to be engaged in programmed cell death (apoptosis) [2], but it is not known whether the glycolipid is involved in this process.

References
1 Gregory, C.D. et al. (1987) J. Immunol. 139, 313–318.
2 **Mangeney, M. et al. (1991) Eur. J. Immunol. 21, 1131–1140.**
3 Wiels, J. et al. (1981) Proc. Natl Acad. Sci. USA 78, 6485–6488.
4 Möller, P. and Mielke, B. (1989) Leucocyte Typing IV, 175–177.
5 Nudelman, E. et al. (1983) Science 220, 509–511.
6 **Maloney, M.D. and Lingwood, C.A. (1994) J. Exp. Med. 180, 191–201.**
7 Karlsson, K.-A. (1989) Annu. Rev. Biochem. 58, 309–350.

CD79/BCR

Other names
CD79a (mb-1, Igα)
CD79b (B29, Igβ)
–B cell antigen receptor (mIg) complex

Molecular weights
Polypeptide   CD79a   21 841
               CD79b   23 083

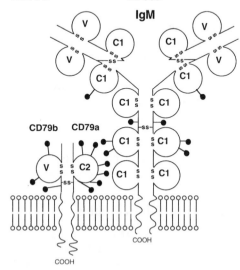

SDS-PAGE
reduced   mIgM heavy chain   73 kDa
           mIgD heavy chain   67 kDa
           Ig light chain   28 kDa
           CD79a   32–33 kDa
           CD79b   37–39 kDa

Carbohydrates
N-linked sites   CD79a   6
                  CD79b   3
O-linked   unknown

Human gene location and size
Ig heavy chain: 14q32.33
Ig κ light chain: 2p12
Ig λ light chain: 22q11.1–q11.2
CD79a: 19q13.2; 4.8 kb [1]
CD79b: 17q23; 3.9 kb [2]

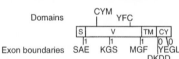

The structure and function of immunoglobulins are well reviewed and will not be considered in detail here.

Tissue distribution

CD79a and CD79b are restricted to B lymphocytes, first appearing on the surface at the pre-B cell stage and remaining through all stages of B cell differentiation prior to plasma cells [3]. The surrogate λ chain and a truncated heavy chain Dμ are expressed on pre-B cells [4,5].

Structure

CD79a and CD79b exist at the surface as a disulfide-linked heterodimer non-covalently associated with membrane Ig. It is proposed that each BCR complex contains two heterodimers of CD79a and CD79b [3]. Both CD79a and CD79b are composed of single IgSF domains [3]. All classes of heavy chains can associate with CD79a and CD79b [3]. The disulfide bond between CD79a and CD79b is likely to be between Cys residues that are found in identical sequences of Ser-Cys-Gly-Thr in both molecules. In each case this sequence is predicted to be part of β strand G of the Ig fold, and thus this disulfide bond probably stabilizes a domain:domain interaction rather than being between two hinge regions, as for example in CD8. The cytoplasmic domains of CD79a and CD79b contain ITAM motifs. In pre-B cells, CD79a and CD79b form a complex with a "surrogate" light chain built up from VpreB (V-like) and λ_5 (C-like) which associate non-covalently and either a heavy chain or a truncated Dμ chain [4,5].

Ligands and associated molecules

Membrane Ig binds antigen. Different pairs of BAP (BCR-associated proteins) molecules have been identified which specifically associate with IgM or IgD [6]. As with CD3/TCR, phosphorylated ITAM motifs of CD79a and CD79b bind to SH2 domains of B cell intracellular signalling molecules [7,8].

Function

Antigen binding leads to internalization and presentation of antigen to T cells via MHC molecules, or can signal the B cell directly, in the case of multivalent antigens which crosslink several mIg molecules [9]. Crosslinking of BCR leads to activation of B cells. This is dependent on CD79a and CD79b for signal transduction. Transmembrane signalling through surface Ig leads to rapid activation of a phospholipase C and tyrosine kinases [6-8]. CD79b and CD79a are both phosphorylated on tyrosine as a result of B cell activation [6-8].

Database accession numbers

	PIR	SWISSPROT	EMBL/GENBANK	REFERENCE
Human CD79a	A46477	P11912	L32754	[1]
Human CD79b	A46527	P40259	L27587	[2]
Mouse CD79a	A43540	P11911	X13450	[10]
Mouse CD79b	A31403	P15530	J03857	[11]

Amino acid sequence of human CD79a

```
MPGGPGVLQA LPATIFLLFL LSAVYLGPGC QA                    -1
LWMHKVPASL MVSLGEDAHF QCPHNSSNNA NVTWWRVLHG NYTWPPEFLG  50
PGEDPNGTLI IQNVNKSHGG IYVCRVQEGN ESYQQSCGTY LRVRQPPPRP  100
FLDMGEGTKN RIITAEGIIL LFCAVVPGTL LLFRKRWQNE KLGLDAGDEY  150
EDENLYEGLN LDDCSMYEDI SRGLQGTYQD VGSLNIGDVQ LEKP        194
```

Amino acid sequence of human CD79b

```
MARLALSPVP SHWMVALLLL LSAEPVPA                          -1
ARSEDRYRNP KGSACSRIWQ SPRFIARKRG FTVKMHCYMN SASGNVSWLW  50
KQEMDENPQQ LKLEKGRMEE SQNESLATLT IQGIRFEDNG IYFCQQKCNN  100
TSEVYQGCGT ELRVMGFSTL AQLKQRNTLK DGIIMIQTLL IILFIIVPIF  150
LLLDKDDSKA GMEEDHTYEG LDIDQTATYE DIVTLRTGEV KWSVGEHPGQ  200
E                                                      201
```

References

1 Hashimoto, S. et al. (1994) Immunogenetics 40, 287–295.
2 Hashimoto, S. et al. (1994) Immunogenetics 40, 145–149.
3 Reth, M. (1992) Annu. Rev. Immunol. 10, 97–121.
4 Melchers, F. et al. (1993) Immunol. Today 14, 60–68.
5 Horne, M.C. et al. (1996) Immunity 4, 145–158.
6 Reth, M. (1995) Immunol. Today 16, 310–313.
7 Cambier, J.C. et al. (1994) Annu. Rev. Immunol. 12, 457–486.
8 **DeFranco, A.L. (1995) Curr. Opin. Cell Biol. 7, 163–175.**
9 DeFranco, A.L. (1996) Curr. Biol. 6, 548–550.
10 Kashiwamura, S-I. et al. (1990) J. Immunol. 145, 337.
11 Hermanson, G.G. et al. (1988) J. Immunol. 85, 6890–6894.

CD80   B7, B7-1, B1

Molecular weights
Polypeptides   30 048

SDS-PAGE
   reduced   60 kDa
   unreduced   60 kDa

Carbohydrate
N-linked sites   8
O-linked   unknown

Human gene location and size
3q21; 32 kb [1,2]

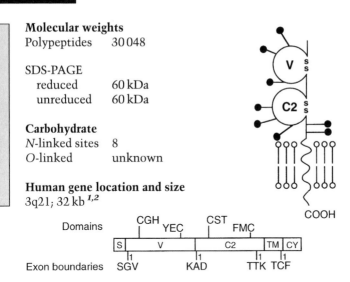

Domains

	CGH	YEC		CST	FMC		
S	V			C2		TM	CY

Exon boundaries   SGV [1]   KAD [1]   TTK [1]   TCF [1]

Tissue distribution [3]

CD80 is expressed at low levels on resting peripheral blood monocytes and dendritic cells. Expression is increased upon activation of B cells, T cells, and peripheral blood monocytes, and with culture of Langerhans cells. Signalling through the MHC Class II cytoplasmic domain may induce CD80 expression on B cells [4].

Structure

CD80 is structurally related to CD86 (25% identity). The extracellular portion contains two IgSF domains which are highly glycosylated [5]. In mice a splice variant has been identified which lacks the C2-set domain [6]. The sequence of the transmembrane domain is unusual in containing three cysteine residues, two of which are also present in CD86. The short cytoplasmic domain, which bears no similarity to the CD86 cytoplasmic domain, has a preponderance (9/19) of arginine residues and contains a potential site for calmodulin-dependent phosphorylation (RRES).

Ligands and associated molecules

CD80 binds to CD28 and CD152 (CTLA-4) using the same site on the GFCC'C'' β sheet of the V-set domain, though the C2-set domain may also contribute to binding [7-9]. CD80 binds CD152 with a slightly higher affinity than CD28 (K_d 0.4 and 4 μM, respectively) with both interactions having fast dissociation rate constants ($k_{off} \geq 0.4$ and $\geq 1.6 \, s^{-1}$, respectively) [10,11].

Function

The interaction of CD80 or CD86 with CD28 provides a potent co-stimulatory signal for T cells activated through the CD3 complex [3,12]. CD80 is expressed later than CD86 and appears to be less important in the primary immune response[3]. Mice deficient in CD80[13] are less severely affected than CD86-deficient mice and have nearly normal T_H1 and T_H2 responses[3]. Early reports that CD80 and CD86 ligation promote T_H1 and T_H2 responses, respectively, remain controversial[3].

Database accession numbers

	PIR	SWISSPROT	EMBL/GENBANK	REFERENCE
Human	A45803	P33681	M27533	5
Mouse	S17291	Q00609	X60958	14
Rat			U05593	15

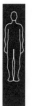

Amino acid sequence of human CD80

```
MGHTRRQGTS PSKCPYLNFF QLLVLAGLSH FCSG                    -1
VIHVTKEVKE VATLSCGHNV SVEELAQTRI YWQKEKKMVL TMMSGDMNIW    50
PEYKNRTIFD ITNNLSIVIL ALRPSDEGTY ECVVLKYEKD AFKREHLAEV   100
TLSVKADFPT PSISDFEIPT SNIRRIICST SGGFPEPHLS WLKREHLAEV   150
INTTVSQDPE TELYAVSSKL DFNMTTNHSF MCLIKYGHLR VNQTFNWNTT   200
KQEHFPDNLL PSWAITLISV NGIFVICCLT YCFAPRCRER RRNERLRRES   250
VRPV                                                    254
```

References

1 Freeman, G.J. et al. (1992) Blood 79, 489–494.
2 Selvakumar, A. et al. (1992) Immunogenetics 36, 175–181.
3 **Lenschow, D.J. et al. (1996) Annu. Rev. Immunol. 14, 233–258.**
4 Nabavi, N. et al. (1992) Nature 360, 266–268.
5 Freeman, G.J. et al. (1989) J. Immunol. 143, 2714–2722.
6 Inobe, M. et al. (1994) Biochem. Biophys. Res. Commun. 200, 443–449.
7 Peach, R.J. et al. (1995) J. Biol. Chem. 270, 21181–21187.
8 Linsley, P.S. et al. (1991) J. Exp. Med. 174, 561–569.
9 Linsley, P.S. et al. (1991) J. Exp. Med. 173, 721–730.
10 Greene, J.L. et al. (1996) J. Biol. Chem. 271, 26762–26771.
11 van der Merwe, P.A. et al., (1997) J. Exp. Med. (in press).
12 Linsley, P.S. and Ledbetter, J.A. (1993) Annu. Rev. Immunol. 11, 191–211.
13 Freeman, G.J. et al. (1993) Science 262, 907–909.
14 Freeman, G.J. et al. (1991) J. Exp. Med. 174, 625–631.
15 Judge, T.A. et al. (1995) Int. Immunol. 7, 171–178.

CD81   TAPA-1

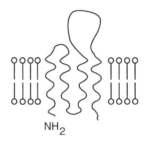

Molecular weights
Polypeptide   25 810

SDS-PAGE
  reduced   26 kDa

Carbohydrate
N-linked sites   0
O-linked   nil

Human gene location
11p15.5

NH₂

Tissue distribution

CD81 is expressed by most cell types[1] and consistent with this the CD81 gene has a housekeeping type promoter[2]. Amongst haematopoietic cells, CD81 is expressed by B and T cells, macrophages, dendritic cells, NK cells and eosinophils, but not by neutrophils, platelets and erythrocytes[3].

Structure

CD81 is a member of the TM4 superfamily and is predicted to have four trans-membrane regions, short cytoplasmic N- and C-termini, and two extracellular regions. Proteolysis studies of the CD81 protein, translated *in vitro* in microsomes, are consistent with the predicted topology of TM4SF molecules (reviewed in ref. 4).

Ligands and associated molecules

Co-immunoprecipitation and flow cytometric energy transfer studies have shown that CD81 associates non-covalently with a number of other molecules: CD19, CD21 and leu-13[5], MHC Class I and II, CD20, CD37, CD53 and CD82 in B cells[6]; CD4, CD8 and CD82 in T cells[7]; and CD9, CD63, and the integrins CD29/CD49c (VLA-3), CD29/CD49d (VLA-4) and CD29/CD49f (VLA-6) in several cell types[8,9]. No extracellular ligand has been identified for CD81.

Function

Mouse CD81 appears to play a role in early T cell development[10]. Engagement of CD81 with the mAb TAPA-1 induces B cell adhesion via the integrin CD29/CD49d (VLA-4)[11].

Database accession numbers

	PIR	SWISSPROT	EMBL/GENBANK	REFERENCE
Human	A35649	P18582	M33680	1
Mouse	A46472	P35762	S45012	2

Amino acid sequence of human CD81

```
MGVEGCTKCI KYLLFVFNFV FWLAGGVILG VALWLRHDPQ TTNLLYLELG    50
DKPAPNTFYV GIYILIAVGA VMMFVGFLGC YGAIQESQCL LGTFFTCLVI   100
LFACEVAAGI WGFVNKDQIA KDVKQFYDQA LQQAVVDDDA NNAKAVVKTF   150
HETLDCCGSS TLTALTTSVL KNNLCPSGSN IISNLFKEDC HQKIDDLFSG   200
KLYLIGIAAI VVAVIMIFEM ILSMVLCCGI RNSSVY                  236
```

References
1 Oren, R. et al. (1990) Mol. Cell. Biol. 10, 4007–4015.
2 Andria, M.L. et al. (1991) J. Immunol. 147, 1030–1036.
3 Tedder, T.F. et al. (1995) Leucocyte Typing V, 684–688.
4 **Wright, M.D. and Tomlinson, M.G. (1994) Immunol. Today 15, 588–594.**
5 **Fearon, D.T. and Carter, R.H. (1995) Annu. Rev. Immunol. 13, 127–149.**
6 Szöllosi, J. et al. (1996) J. Immunol. 157, 2939–2946.
7 Imai, T. et al. (1995) J. Immunol. 155, 1229–1239.
8 Berditchevski, F. et al. (1996) Mol. Biol. Cell 7, 193–207.
9 Mannion, B.A. et al. (1996) J. Immunol. 157, 2039–2047.
10 **Boismenu, R. et al. (1996) Science 271, 198–200.**
11 **Behr, S. and Schriever, F. (1995) J. Exp. Med. 182, 1191–1199.**

CD82   R2, C33, IA4, 4F9, KAI1

Molecular weight
Polypeptide   29 626

SDS-PAGE
    reduced   50–53 kDa

Carbohydrate
N-linked sites   3
O-linked   nil

Human gene location
11p11.2

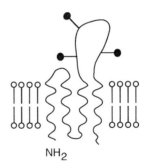

NH$_2$

Tissue distribution

CD82 is expressed by most cell types. Amongst haematopoietic cells, CD82 is expressed by B and T cells, NK cells, monocytes, granulocytes and platelets, but not by erythrocytes. CD82 is strongly upregulated on lymphocyte activation [1].

Structure

CD82 is a member of the TM4 superfamily and is predicted to have four transmembrane regions, short cytoplasmic N- and C-termini, and two extracellular regions (reviewed in ref. 2).

Ligands and associated molecules

Co-immunoprecipitation and flow cytometric energy transfer studies have shown that CD82 associates non-covalently with a number of other molecules: MHC Class I and II, CD20, CD37, CD53 and CD81 in B cells [3]; CD4, CD8 and CD81 in T cells [4]; and integrins including CD29/CD49d (VLA-4) in some cell lines [5]. No extracellular ligand has been identified for CD82.

Function

Expression of CD82 suppresses metastasis in tumour cells [6]. *In vitro* experiments have shown that CD82 can transduce signals in B cells, T cells and monocytes [7,8].

Database accession numbers

	PIR	SWISSPROT	EMBL/GENBANK	REFERENCE
Human	S16156	P27701	X53795	9
Mouse		P40237	D14883	10

Amino acid sequence of human CD82

```
MGSACIKVTK YFLFLFNLIF FILGAVILGF GVWILADKSS FISVLQTSSS    50
SLRMGAYVFI GVGAVTMLMG FLGCIGAVNE VRCLLGLYFA FLLLILIAQV   100
TAGALFYFNM GKLKQEMGGI VTELIRDYNS SREDSLQDAW DYVQAQVKCC   150
GWVSFYNWTD NAELMNRPEV TYPCSCEVKG EEDNSLSVRK GFCEAPGNRT   200
QSGNHPEDWP VYQEGCMEKV QAWLQENLGI ILGVGVGVAI IELLGMVLSI   250
CLCRHVHSED YSKVPKY                                       267
```

References
[1] Engel, P. et al. (1995) Leucocyte Typing V, 691–693.
[2] **Wright, M.D. and Tomlinson, M.G. (1994) Immunol. Today 15, 588–594.**
[3] Szöllosi, J. et al. (1996) J. Immunol. 157, 2939–2946.
[4] Imai, T. et al. (1995) J. Immunol. 155, 1229–1239.
[5] Mannion, B.A. et al. (1996) J. Immunol. 157, 2039–2047.
[6] Dong, J.-T. et al. (1995) Science 268, 884–886.
[7] Lebel-Binay, S. et al. (1995) J. Leukocyte Biol. 57, 956–963.
[8] Lebel-Binay, S. et al. (1995) J. Immunol. 155, 101–110.
[9] Gaugitsch, H.W. et al. (1991) Eur. J. Immunol. 21, 377–383.
[10] Nagira, M. et al. (1994) Cell. Immunol. 157, 144–157.

CD83 HB15

Molecular weights
Polypeptide   23 041

SDS-PAGE
  reduced   45 kDa
  unreduced   45 kDa

Carbohydrate
N-linked sites   3
O-linked   unknown

Human gene location
6p23–p21.3

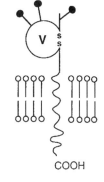

COOH

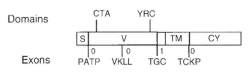

Domains

| S | V | | TM | CY |

Exons PATP VKLL TGC TCKP

CTA   YRC

Tissue distribution

CD83 is a marker for a subset of dendritic cells which include Langerhans cells in the skin, peripheral blood dendritic cells, and interdigitating reticulum cells within the T cell zones of lymphoid organs[1]. Expression is not restricted to dendritic cells since CD83 is also expressed on some germinal centre B cells and weakly on activated peripheral lymphocytes[2].

Structure

CD83 comprises a single V-set IgSF domain, a transmembrane region and a 39 amino acid C-terminal cytoplasmic tail[2]. The gene for CD83 has an unusual structure, with respect to most other IgSF molecules, in that the intron/exon boundaries encompassing the IgSF domain are of phase 0 and phase 1 rather than both being of phase 1[2]. There is also an intron within the coding sequence for the IgSF domain, but this is relatively common.

Function

Unknown.

Database accession numbers

	PIR	SWISSPROT	EMBL/GENBANK	REFERENCE
Human	S23066	Q01151	Z11697	2

Amino acid sequence of human CD83

```
MSRGLQLLLL SCAYSLAPA                                           -1
TPEVKVACSE DVDLPCTAPW DPQVPYTVSW VKLLEGGEER METPQEDHLR         50
GQHYHQKGQN GSFDAPNERP YSLKIRNTTS CNSGTYRCTL QDPDGQRNLS         100
GKVILRVTGC PAQRKEETFK KYRAEIVLLL ALVIFYLTLI IFTCKFARLQ         150
SIFPDFSKAG MERAFLPVTS PNKHLGLVTP HKTELV                        186
```

341

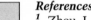

References

[1] Zhou, L.-J. and T.F. Tedder (1995) J. Immunol. 154, 3821–3835.
[2] Zhou, L.-J. et al. (1992) J. Immunol. 149, 735–742.

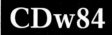

CDw84

Tissue distribution

CDw84 is highly expressed on macrophages and platelets. Expression is lower on T and B lymphocytes and absent from plasma cells [1].

Structure

Unknown.

Function

Unknown.

Reference
[1] Engel, P. et al. (1995) Leucocyte Typing V, 699–700.

CD85

Molecular weights

SDS-PAGE
    reduced   83 kDa
    unreduced   72 kDa

Tissue distribution

CD85 is highly expressed on plasma cells and monocytes. Expression is lower on mature B cells and not detectable on early lineage B cells, T cells, NK cells and non-haematopoietic cells. On tumour cells, CD85 is a marker for all acute lymphoblastic leukaemia (ALL) cells and hairy cell leukaemias, most B cell chronic lymphocytic leukaemia (B-CLL) and B cell non-Hodgkin's lymphoma (B-NHL), and some acute myeloid leukaemias [1,2].

Structure

Unknown.

Function

Unknown.

Comments

The molecular weight of the CD85 antigen on SDS-PAGE is controversial. The original value of 83 kDa under reducing conditions [2] was not confirmed by the Leucocyte Typing V Workshop, in which one laboratory reported a weight of 120 kDa and another laboratory reported weights of 90 kDa and 18 kDa [1]. A possible susceptibility of the protein to proteolysis was suggested as an explanation for this discrepancy [1].

References
[1] Engel, P. et al. (1995) Leucocyte Typing V, 701–702.
[2] Pulford, K. et al. (1991) Clin. Exp. Immunol. 85, 429–435.

CD86 B7-2, B70

Molecular weights
Polypeptide   35 254

SDS-PAGE
  reduced   70 kDa
  unreduced   70 kDa

Carbohydrate
N-linked sites 8
O-linked   unknown

Human gene location and size
3q13–q23 [1]; >22 kb [2]

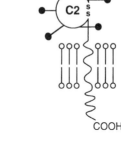

COOH

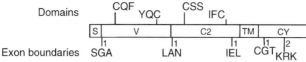

Tissue distribution

CD86 is expressed at high levels on resting peripheral blood monocytes and dendritic cells and at very low levels on resting B and T cells [3]. Activation of B cells, T cells, and monocytes and culture of Langerhans cells leads to increased expression of CD86. CD86 expression is induced more rapidly than CD80 expression (peaks at ~20 h versus ~60 h) and reaches higher levels. Expression is increased by IL-4 (B cells) and IFNγ (peripheral blood monocytes) and decreased by IL-10 (peripheral blood dendritic cells).

Structure

CD86 is an IgSF molecule structurally related to CD80 (25% amino acid identity). The extracellular domain contains two IgSF domains and is highly glycosylated [4,5]. The transmembrane domain contains two of the three cysteines seen in CD80. The cytoplasmic domain is completely unrelated to the CD80 cytoplasmic domain and contains three potential protein kinase C phosphorylation sites.

Ligands and associated molecules

Like CD80, the extracellular portion of CD86 binds to CD28 and CD152 (CTLA-4). Like CD80, CD86 binds CD28 with a lower avidity than CD152 [6], and binding involves residues in the V-domain [7]. CD86 binds CD152 with a lower avidity than CD80 [8].

Function

The interactions of CD80 and CD86 with CD28 provide important co-stimulatory signals for T cells activated through the CD3/TCR. CD86 is expressed earlier than CD80 and appears to dominate in the primary immune response[3]. Mice deficient in CD86 have more profound defects in T cell function (including T cell-dependent antibody responses) than CD80-deficient mice[3]. Early reports that CD86 and CD80 ligation favour T_H2 and T_H1 responses, respectively, remain controversial[3].

Database accession numbers

	PIR	SWISSPROT	EMBL/GENBANK	REFERENCE
Human	A48754	P42081	U404343	4,5
Mouse		P42082	L25606	9

Amino acid sequence of human CD86

```
MDPQCTMGLS NILFVMAFLL SGA                                -1
APLKIQAYFN ETADLPCQFA NSQNQSLSEL VVFWQDQENL VLNEVYLGKE   50
KFDSVHSKYM GRTSFDSDSW TLRLHNLQIK DKGLYQCIIH HKKPTGMIRI  100
HQMNSELSVL ANFSQPEIVP ISNITENVYI NLTCSSIHGY PEPKKMSVLL  150
RTKNSTIEYD GIMQKSQDNV TELYDVSISL SVSFPDVTSN MTIFCILETD  200
KTRLLSSPFS IELEDPQPPP DHIPWITAVL PTVIICVMVF CLILWKWKKK  250
KRPRNSYKCG TNTMEREESE QTKKREKIHI PERSDEAQRV FKSSKTSSCD  300
KSDTCF                                                 306
```

References

1 Fernandez-Ruiz, E. et al. (1995) Eur. J. Immunol. 25, 1453–1456.
2 Jellis, C.L. et al. (1995) Immunogenetics 42, 85–89.
3 **Lenschow, D.J. et al. (1996) Annu. Rev. Immunol. 14, 233–258.**
4 Azumo, M. et al. (1993) Nature 366, 76–79.
5 Freeman, G.J. et al. (1993) Science 262, 909–911.
6 Linsley, P.S. et al. (1994) Immunity 1, 793–801.
7 Peach, R.J. et al. (1995) J. Biol. Chem. 270, 21181–21187.
8 Greene, J.L. et al. (1996) J. Biol. Chem. 271, 26762–26771.
9 Freeman, G.J. et al. (1993) J. Exp. Med. 178, 2185–2192.

Molecular weights
Polypeptide   31 460

SDS-PAGE
  reduced   55–60 kDa

Carbohydrate
  N-linked sites 5
  O-linked sites unknown

Human gene location and size
19q13; ~23 kb [1].

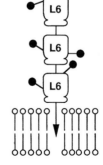

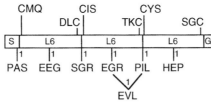

Tissue distribution

CD87 is expressed on monocytes and granulocytes and the level of expression is generally upregulated following activation of the cells [2]. It is also found on the activated subset of NK cells characterized as large granular lymphocytes [3]. Only 0–5% of resting T lymphocytes from normal donors are CD87+ but expression can be upregulated following treatment with phorbol esters, mitogens, anti-CD3 antibodies and certain combinations of cytokines [3]. Upregulation of CD87 is correlated with the expression of CD25 on T cells [4]. T cells from patients with viral infections are found to express high levels of CD87 [4].

Structure

CD87 is a heavily glycosylated, GPI-linked protein [5,6]. The extracelluar region consists of three Ly-6 domains [5-8]. A cDNA lacking exon 5 has been reported [1]. The N-terminal sequence has been determined [6].

Ligands and associated molecules

The ligand for CD87 is the urokinase plasminogen activator (uPA) [2,7]. CD87 has been shown to associate in monocytes with CD11a/CD18, CD11b/CD18 and Src-related kinases [9]. Its association with CD11b/CD18 has also been demonstrated on resting neutrophils [9,10].

Function

CD87 is the receptor for uPA, a serine protease that converts plasminogen to plasmin. The major function of CD87 is to retain and concentrate uPA at the cell surface for the local conversion of plasminogen to plasmin. This process is important for the pericellular proteolysis during extravasation of leucocytes and cancer cells[4,11,12]. The CD87–CD11b/CD18 complex on resting neutrophils dissociates when the cells become polarized following stimulation. CD87 accumulates at the lamellipodium and CD11b/CD18 at the uropod. This reversible interaction may be important in directing polarized uPA proteolytic activity during cell extravasation and migration[10,13].

Database accession numbers

	PIR	SWISSPROT	EMBL/GENBANK	REFERENCE
Human	A39743	Q03405	M83246	5
			X51675	7
Mouse	A55356	P35456	X62700	14
			U12235	15

Amino acid sequence of human CD87

```
MGHPPLLPLL LLLHTCVPAS WG                                  -1
LRCMQCKTNG DCRVEECALG QDLCRTTIVR LWEEGEELEL VEKSCTHSEK    50
TNRTLSYRTG LKITSLTEVV CGLDLCNQGN SGRAVTYSRS RYLECISCGS   100
SDMSCERGRH QSLQCRSPEE QCLDVVTHWI QEGEEGRPKD DRHLRGCGYL   150
PGCPGSNGFH NNDTFHFLKC CNTTKCNEGP ILELENLPQN GRQCYSCKGN   200
STHGCSSEET FLIDCRGPMN QCLVATGTHE PKNQSYMVRG CATASMCQHA   250
HLGDAFSMNH IDVSCCTKSG CNHPDLDVQY RSG                     283
AAPQPGPAHL SLTITLLMTA RLWGGTLLWT                         +30
```

References

1   Casey, J.R. et al. (1994) Blood 84, 1151–1156.
2   Miles, L.A. et al. (1987) Thromb. Haemost. 58, 936–942.
3   Nykjær, A. et al. (1992) FEBS Lett. 300, 13–17
4   **Nykjær, A. et al. (1994) J. Immunol. 152, 505–516.**
5   **Min, H.Y. et al. (1992) J. Immunol. 148, 3636–3642.**
6   Behrendt, N. et al. (1990) J. Biol. Chem. 6453–6460.
7   Roldan, A.L. et al. (1990) EMBO J. 9, 467–474.
8   Ploug, M. et al. (1993) J. Biol. Chem. 268, 17539–17546.
9   Bohuslav, J. et al. (1995) J. Exp. Med. 181, 1381–1390.
10 Xue, W. et al. (1994) J. Immunol. 152, 4630–4640.
11 Ellis, V. et al. (1991) J. Biol. Chem. 266, 12752–12758.
12 Bianchi, E. et al. (1994) Cancer Res. 54, 861–866.
13 **Kindzelskii, A.L. et al. (1996) J. Immunol. 156, 297–309.**
14 Kristensen, P. et al. (1991) J. Cell Biol. 115, 1763–1771.
15 Suh, T.T. et al. (1994) J. Biol. Chem. 269, 25992–25998.

CD88 C5a receptor

Molecular weights
Polypeptide   39 321

SDS-PAGE
  reduced   40 kDa

Carbohydrate
N-linked sites   1
O-linked sites   unknown

Human gene location and size
19q13.3–13.4; ~10 kb [1].

COOH

Tissue distribution

CD88 is expressed on cells of the myeloid lineage and smooth muscles [2,3]. It is also expressed on hepatocytes and on many cell types in the lung, including bronchial and alveolar epithelial cells, alveolar macrophages and vascular endothelial cells [3]. CD88 mRNA has also been detected in the heart, spleen, kidney and intestine but the cell types expressing CD88 have not been identified [3].

Structure

CD88 is a typical G protein-coupled receptor with seven transmembrane domains [4-6].

Ligands and associated molecules

CD88 binds C5a which is the N-terminal fragment (74 residues in the human) of the α chain of the complement component C5. This fragment is proteolytically cleaved from C5 during complement activation. CD88 is coupled to heterotrimeric G proteins inside the cell. In neutrophils, CD88 appears to couple exclusively to the G proteins Giα2 and Giα3, which are pertussis toxin sensitive [7].

Function

The binding of C5a to CD88 on neutrophils leads to a number of effects including (with increasing C5a concentrations) cytoskeletal remodelling, shedding of selectins, upregulation of adhesion molecules, chemotaxis, granule exocytosis and activation of NADPH oxidase [7]. A role in mucosal defense to infection is indicated by the failure of CD88 knockout mice to clear *Pseudomonas aeruginosa* introduced directly into the trachea [8]. Curiously, neutrophil migration into the lung was elevated. In contrast migration into the peritoneum in response to glycogen-induced inflammation was decreased [8].

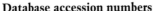

Database accession numbers

	PIR	SWISSPROT	EMBL/GENBANK	REFERENCE
Human	A37963	P21730	X57250	4
			M62505	5
Mouse		P30993	S46665	9

Amino acid sequence of human CD88

```
MNSFNYTTPD YGHYDDKDTL DLNTPVDKTS NTLRVPDILA LVIFAVVFLV    50
GVLGNALVVW VTAFEAKRTI NAIWFLNLAV ADFLSCLALP ILFTSIVQHH   100
HWPFGGAACS ILPSLILLNM YASILLLATI SADRFLLVFK PIWCQNFRGA   150
GLAWIACAVA WGLALLLTIP SFLYRVVREE YFPPKVLCGV DYSHDKRRER   200
AVAIVRLVLG FLWPLLTLTI CYTFILLRTW SRRATRSTKT LKVVVAVVAS   250
FFIFWLPYQV TGIMMSFLEP SSPTFLLLNK LDSLCVSFAY INCCINPIIY   300
VVAGQGFQGR LRKSLPSLLR NVLTEESVVR ESKSFTRSTV DTMAQKTQAV   350
```

References

1. Gerard, N.P. et al. (1993) Biochemistry 32, 1243–1250.
2. Hugli, T.E. and Müller-Eberhard, H.J. (1978) Adv. Immunol. 26, 1–53.
3. Haviland, D.L. et al. (1995) J. Immunol. 154, 1861–1869.
4. **Gerard, N.P. and Gerard, C. (1990) Nature 349, 614–617.**
5. Boulay, F. et al. (1991) Biochemistry 30, 2993–2999.
6. Rollins, T.E. et al. (1991) Proc. Natl Acad. Sci. USA 88, 971–975.
7. **Gerard, C. and Gerard, N.P. (1994) Annu. Rev. Immunol. 12, 758–808.**
8. **Höpken, U.E. et al. (1996) Nature 383, 86–89.**
9. Gerard, C. et al. (1992) J. Immunol. 149, 2600–2606.

Molecular weights

Polypeptide	a1	29 938
	a2	27 356
	a3	19 367

a1 isoform

SDS-PAGE
reduced   50–75 kDa

Carbohydrate

N-linked sites	a1	6
	a2	5
	a3	2
O-linked sites		unknown

Human gene location and size
19q13.4; ~12 kb [1].

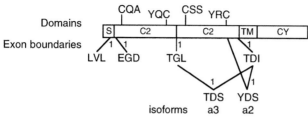

Tissue distribution

CD89 is expressed on most phagocytic cells in blood and mucosal tissues. It is also found on subpopulations of T and B lymphocytes [2-4]. The a1 and a2 products are differentially expressed. Whereas the a1 form is found on monocytes and neutrophils, the a2 form is expressed by alveolar macrophages [5]. Only the a1 and a2 forms have been detected at the protein level [5].

Structure

CD89 is a type I membrane protein with two IgSF domains [2]. However, at least six cDNA species have been identified. The a1, a2 and a3 clones encode transmembrane proteins and are generated by alternative splicing of exons [1,5]. An a' form, also derived from alternative splicing, has been found to have a cryptic leader sequence [6]. Two other forms have alternative sequences to the transmembrane segment and may code for soluble products. Genomic analysis suggests that CD89 is most closely related to the two Fcγ receptors CD16 and CD64 [1]. CD89 has an Arg within the transmembrane region; it is notable that there is a His residue at the equivalent position in CD64.

Ligands and associated molecules

CD89 binds both IgA1 and IgA2 via their Fc regions [7,8]. CD89 associates with the γ chain homodimer of Fc receptors [9]. This interaction involves the transmembrane segment of CD89 as shown by mutation of Arg209, which presumably forms a salt bridge with the Asp residue in the transmembrane segment of the γ chain [10].

Function

CD89 binds serum and secretory IgA1 and IgA2 with an affinity of about $5 \times 10^7 \text{M}^{-1}$ (see refs 3 and 4). Binding can trigger a number of cellular responses including phagocytosis, superoxide production, release of inflammatory mediators and antibody-dependent cellular cytotoxicity [7,8]. These responses require the interaction of CD89 with the FcR γ chain homodimer, possibly through tyrosine phosphorylation [9,10]. The differential expression of the a1 and a2 isoforms in blood leucocytes and alveolar macrophages may suggest their different roles in blood and mucosal defense [5].

Database accession numbers

	PIR	SWISSPROT	EMBL/GENBANK	REFERENCE
Human a1	JH0332	P24071	X54150	1,5
Human a2			U43774	5
Human a3			U43677	5

Amino acid sequence of human CD89 (a1 isoform)

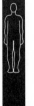

```
MDPKQTTLLC LVLCLGQRIQ A                                    -1
QEGDFPMPFI SAKSSPVIPL DGSVKIQCQA IREAYLTQLM IIKNSTYREI     50
GRRLKFWNET DPEFVIDHMD ANKAGRYQCQ YRIGHYRFRY SDTLELVVTG    100
LYGKPFLSAD RGLVLMPGEN ISLTCSSAHI PFDRFSLAKE GELSLPQHQS    150
GEHPANFSLG PVDLNVSGIY RCYGWYNRSP YLWSFPSNAL ELVVTDISHQ    200
DYTTQNLIRM AVAGLVLVAL LAILVENWHS HTALNKEASA DVAEPSWSQQ    245
MCQPGLTFAR TPSVCK                                         266
```

The a2 and a3 isoforms differ from the a1 isoform by lacking residues 154–195 and residues 100–195, respectively, through alternative splicing.

References
[1] de Wit, T.P.M. et al. (1995) J. Immunol. 155, 1203–1209.
[2] **Maliszewski, D.R. et al. (1990) J. Exp. Med. 172, 1665–1672.**
[3] Monteiro, R.C. et al. (1990) J. Exp. Med. 171, 597–613.
[4] Mazengera, R.L. et al. (1990) Biochem. J. 272, 159–165.
[5] **Patry, C. et al. (1996) J. Immunol. 156, 4442–4448.**
[6] Morton, H.C. et al. (1996) Immunogenetics 43, 246–247.
[7] **Mestecky, J. and McGhee, J.R. (1987) Adv. Immunol. 40, 153–245.**
[8] Kerr, M.A. (1990) Biochem. J. 271, 285–296.
[9] Pfefferkorn, L.C. and Yeaman, G.R. (1994) J. Immunol. 153, 3228–3236.
[10] Morton, H.C. et al. (1995) J. Biol. Chem. 270, 29781–29787.

CD90

Thy-1, theta

Molecular weights
Polypeptide   12 576

SDS-PAGE
  reduced   18 kDa
  unreduced   18 kDa

Carbohydrate
N-linked sites   3
O-linked   nil

Human gene location and size
11q23.3; ~8 kb [1]

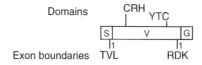

Tissue distribution

CD90 expression varies considerably among different species [2,3]. It is expressed on the prothymocyte subpopulation of human leucocytes, on all mouse and rat thymocytes, and on mouse but not rat T cells. Rat bone marrow cells also express CD90. In all three species the antigen is expressed abundantly in the brain and at varying levels in other non-lymphoid tissues [2,3].

Structure

CD90 is a GPI-anchored molecule consisting of a single IgSF V-set domain [2,3]. The N-terminus and site of addition of the GPI anchor of rat CD90 have been confirmed [3,4]. Although the protein sequence of rat CD90 is invariant, the brain and thymocyte forms of the protein have tissue- and site-specific glycosylation patterns [5]. The *Thy-1* gene maps to a region that also encodes the CD3 antigens and CD56 (NCAM) [1]. The mouse Thy-1 alloantigens Thy-1.1 and Thy-1.2 differ by a single amino acid at residue 89, namely Arg in Thy-1.1 and Gln in Thy-1.2 [3].

Ligands and associated molecules

CD90 associates non-covalently with the Src family tyrosine kinase Fyn [6].

Function

The function of CD90 is unknown. CD90 mAbs can activate T cells *in vitro*, which is a feature of other GPI-anchored proteins. The tyrosine kinase Fyn, that associates with Thy-1, is selectively required for activation through Thy-1 [6]. Thy-1 mAbs can also induce *bcl*-2-resistant thymocyte apoptosis

353

and a ligand for Thy-1 on thymic epithelial cells has been proposed[7]. Thy-1 expression on a neural cell line selectively inhibits neurite outgrowth on mature astrocytes *in vitro* and a Thy-1 ligand on astrocytes is suggested[8]. Thy-1 knockout mice have provided few clues concerning Thy-1 function. Such mice appear normal apart from having a slight defect in brain function: an impairment of long-term potentiation in the hippocampus is accompanied by normal spatial learning[9].

Database accession numbers

	PIR	SWISSPROT	EMBL/GENBANK	REFERENCE
Human	A02106	P04216	M11749	10
Rat	A02107	P01830	X03152	11
Mouse	A02108	P01831	X03151	12

Amino acid sequence of human CD90

```
MNLAISIALL LTVLQVSRG                                    -1
QKVTSLTACL VDQSLRLDCR HENTSSSPIQ YEFSLTRETK KHVLFGTVGV  50
PEHTYRSRTN FTSKYHMKVL YLSAFTSKDE GTYTCALHHS GHSPPISSQN  100
VTVLRDKLVK C                                            111
EGISLLAQNT SWLLLLLLSL SLLQATDFMS L                      +31
```

References

1. Silver, J. (1989) In Cell Surface Antigen Thy-1 (Reif, A.E. and Schlesinger, M., eds). Marcel Dekker, New York, pp. 241–269.
2. Williams, A.F. (1989) In Cell Surface Antigen Thy-1 (Reif, A.E. and Schlesinger, M., eds). Marcel Dekker, New York, pp. 49–69.
3. **Williams, A.F. and Gagnon, J. (1982) Science 216, 696–703.**
4. Tse, A.G. et al. (1985) Science 230, 1003–1008.
5. Williams, A.F. et al. (1993) Glycobiology 3, 339–348.
6. Lancki, D.W. et al. (1995) J. Immunol. 154, 4363–4370.
7. Hueber, A.O. et al. (1994) J. Exp. Med. 179, 785–796.
8. Tiveron, M.C. et al. (1992) Nature 355, 745–748.
9. Nosten-Bertrand, M. et al. (1996) Nature 379, 826–829.
10. Seki, T. et al. (1985) Proc. Natl Acad. Sci. USA 82, 6657–6661.
11. Seki, T. et al. (1985) Fedn. Proc. 44, 2865–2869.
12. Seki, T. et al. (1985) Science 227, 649–651.

Molecular weights
Polypeptide   502 671

SDS-PAGE
   reduced   ~500 + 85 kDa
   unreduced   ~500 + 85 kDa

Carbohydrate
N-linked sites   53
O-linked sites   unknown

Human gene location
12q13.1–q13.3

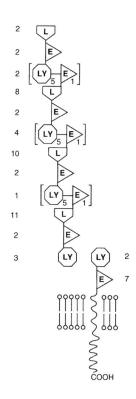

Tissue distribution

CD91 is expressed on the phagocytes of liver, lung and lymphoid tissues, but not on antigen-presenting cells. It is also expressed on neurons and astrocytes in the central nervous system, epithelial cells of the gastrointestinal tract, smooth muscle cells, fibroblasts, Leydig cells in the testis, granulosa cells in the ovary and dendritic cells of the kidney[1].

Structure

CD91 is a type I membrane protein. Its single chain precursor is cleaved to yield an N-terminal fragment of ~500 kDa and a C-terminal 85 kDa transmembrane fragment. The two fragments remain non-covalently associated with each other. The extracellular region is composed of 31 LDLR type A domains, 16 EGF type B1 domains, 40 LY domains containing the YWTD sequence and 6 EGF type B2 domains, arranged as shown[2,3]. The N-termini of both fragments have been determined by protein sequencing[2]. The cleavage site is shown indented in the sequence below. Highly homologous molecules are found in the mouse[4] (97% homology to human) and chicken[5] (83% homology to human). CD91 is a member of the LDLR supergene family, the other members are the LDLR, VLDLR and a glycoprotein of 330 kDa (gp330)[6]. In the figure, the domains of CD91 are not drawn out in full. The numbers appearing on either side indicate the number of repeats of that

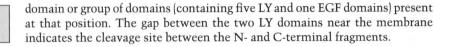

domain or group of domains (containing five LY and one EGF domains) present at that position. The gap between the two LY domains near the membrane indicates the cleavage site between the N- and C-terminal fragments.

Ligands and associated molecules

CD91 binds protease–inhibitor complexes such as protease/α_2-macroglobulin complexes and complexes between the tissue-type and urinary-type plasminogen activators and plasminogen activator inhibitor type 1. It also binds a variety of other molecules including lipoproteins, toxins, viruses and lactoferrin[6]. Several of its ligands do not cross-compete for binding, suggesting that there are multiple binding sites on CD91[7]. CD91 associates at a ratio of 1:2 with receptor-associated protein (RAP), a soluble 39 kDa protein which is localized to the rough endoplasmic reticulum[2,6,7].

Function

CD91 appears to be involved in the regulation of proteolytic activity and lipoprotein metabolism, amongst other things. The presence of the two NPXY motifs in its cytoplasmic segment suggests that it may bind to and remove its many ligands from the circulation by receptor-mediated endocytosis. RAP interferes with CD91 binding to its ligands, suggesting its role in preventing CD91 binding to intracellular proteins in the endoplasmic reticulum while en route to the cell surface[7].

Database accession numbers

	PIR	SWISSPROT	EMBL/GENBANK	REFERENCE
Human		Q07954	X13916	3
Mouse			X67469	4
Chicken		P98157	X74904	5

Amino acid sequence of human CD91

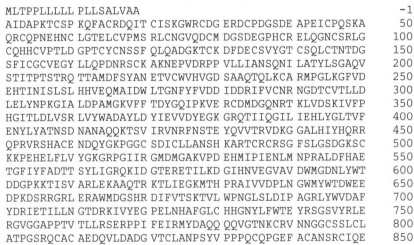

```
MLTPPLLLLL PLLSALVAA                                            -1
AIDAPKTCSP KQFACRDQIT CISKGWRCDG ERDCPDGSDE APEICPQSKA          50
QRCQPNEHNC LGTELCVPMS RLCNGVQDCM DGSDEGPHCR ELQGNCSRLG          100
CQHHCVPTLD GPTCYCNSSF QLQADGKTCK DFDECSVYGT CSQLCTNTDG          150
SFICGCVEGY LLQPDNRSCK AKNEPVDRPP VLLIANSQNI LATYLSGAQV          200
STITPTSTRQ TTAMDFSYAN ETVCWVHVGD SAAQTQLKCA RMPGLKGFVD          250
EHTINISLSL HHVEQMAIDW LTGNFYFVDD IDDRIFVCNR NGDTCVTLLD          300
LELYNPKGIA LDPAMGKVFF TDYGQIPKVE RCDMDGQNRT KLVDSKIVFP          350
HGITLDLVSR LVYWADAYLD YIEVVDYEGK GRQTIIQGIL IEHLYGLTVF          400
ENYLYATNSD NANAQQKTSV IRVNRFNSTE YQVVTRVDKG GALHIYHQRR          450
QPRVRSHACE NDQYGKPGGC SDICLLANSH KARTCRCRSG FSLGSDGKSC          500
KKPEHELFLV YGKGRPGIIR GMDMGAKVPD EHMIPIENLM NPRALDFHAE          550
TGFIYFADTT SYLIGRQKID GTERETILKD GIHNVEGVAV DWMGDNLYWT          600
DDGPKKTISV ARLEKAAQTR KTLIEGKMTH PRAIVVDPLN GWMYWTDWEE          650
DPKDSRRGRL ERAWMDGSHR DIFVTSKTVL WPNGLSLDIP AGRLYWVDAF          700
YDRIETILLN GTDRKIVYEG PELNHAFGLC HHGNYLFWTE YRSGSVYRLE          750
RGVGGAPPTV TLLRSERPPI FEIRMYDAQQ QQVGTNKCRV NNGGCSSLCL          800
ATPGSRQCAC AEDQVLDADG VTCLANPSYV PPPQCQPGEF ACANSRCIQE          850
```

```
RWKCDGDNDC LDNSDEAPAL CHQHTCPSDR FKCENNRCIP NRWLCDGDND    900
CGNSEDESNA TCSARTCPPN QFSCASGRCI PISWTCDLDD DCGDRSDESA    950
SCAYPTCFPL TQFTCNNGRC ININWRCDND NDCGDNSDEA GCSHSCSSTQ   1000
FKCNSGRCIP EHWTCDGDND CGDYSDETHA NCTNQATRPP GGCHTDEFQC   1050
RLDGLCIPLR WRCDGDTDCM DSSDEKSCEG VTHVCDPSVK FGCKDSARCI   1100
SKAWVCDGDN DCEDNSDEEN CESLACRPPS HPCANNTSVC LPPDKLCDGN   1150
DDCGDGSDEG ELCDQCSLNN GGCSHNCSVA PGEGIVCSCP LGMELGPDNH   1200
TCQIQSYCAK HLKCSQKCDQ NKFSVKCSCY EGWVLEPDGE SCRSLDPFKP   1250
FIIFSNRHEI RRIDLHKGDY SVLVPGLRNT IALDFHLSQS ALYWTDVVED   1300
KIYRGKLLDN GALTSFEVVI QYGLATPEGL AVDWIAGNIY WVESNLDQIE   1350
VAKLDGTLRT TLLAGDIEHP RAIALDPRDG ILFWTDWDAS LPRIEAASMS   1400
GAGRRTVHRE TGSGGWPNGL TVDYLEKRIL WIDARSDAIY SARYDGSGHM   1450
EVLRGHEFLS HPFAVTLYGG EVYWTDWRTN TLAKANKWTG HNVTVVQRTN   1500
TQPFDLQVYH PSRQPMAPNP CEANGGQGPC SHLCLINYNR TVSCACPHLM   1550
KLHKDNTTCY EFKKFLLYAR QMEIRGVDLD APYYNYIISF TVPDIDNVTV   1600
LDYDAREQRV YWSDVRTQAI KRAFINGTGV ETVVSADLPN AHGLAVDWVS   1650
RNLFWTSYDT NKKQINVARL DGSFKNAVVQ GLEQPHGLVV HPLRGKLYWT   1700
DGDNISMANM DGSNRTLLFS GQKGPVGLAI DFPESKLYWI SSGNHTINRC   1750
NLDGSGLEVI DAMRSQLGKA TALAIMGDKL WWADQVSEKM GTCSKADGSG   1800
SVVLRNSTTL VMHMKVYDES IQLDHKGTNP CSVNNGDCSQ LCLPTSETTR   1850
SCMCTAGYSL RSGQQACEGV GSFLLYSVHE GIRGIPLDPN DKSDALVPVS   1900
GTSLAVGIDF HAENDTIYWV DMGLSTISRA KRDQTWREDV VTNGIGRVEG   1950
IAVDWIAGNI YWTDQGFDVI EVARLNGSFR YVVISQGLDK PRAITVHPEK   2000
GYLFWTEWGQ YPRIERSRLD GTERVVLVNV SISWPNGISV DYQDGKLYWC   2050
DARTDKIERI DLETGENREV VLSSNNMDMF SVSVFEDFIY WSDRTHANGS   2100
IKRGSKDNAT DSVPLRTGIG VQLKDIKVFN RDRQKGTNVC AVANGGCQQL   2150
CLYRGRGQRA CACAHGMLAE DGASCREYAG YLLYSERTIL KSIHLSDERN   2200
LNAPVQPFED PEHMKNVIAL AFDYRAGTSP GTPNRIFFSD IHFGNIQQIN   2250
DDGSRRITIV ENVGSVEGLA YHRGWDTLYW TSYTTSTITR HTVDQTRPGA   2300
FERETVITMS GDDHPRAFVL DECQNLMFWT NWNEQHPSIM RAALSGANVL   2350
TLIEKDIRTP NGLAIDHRAE KLYFSDATLD KIERCEYDGS HRYVILKSEP   2400
VHPFGLAVYG EHIFWTDWVR RAVQRANKHV GSNMKLLRVD IPQQPMGIIA   2450
VANDTNSCEL SPCRINNGGC QDLCLLTHQG HVNCSCRGGR ILQDDLTCRA   2500
VNSSCRAQDE FECANGECIN FSLTCDGVPH CKDKSDEKPS YCNSRRCKKT   2550
FRQCSNGRCV SNMLWCNGAD DCGDGSDEIP CNKTACGVGE FRCRDGTCIG   2600
NSSRCNQFVD CEDASDEMNC SATDCSSYFR LGVKGVLFQP CERTSLCYAP   2650
SWVCDGANDC GDYSDERDCP GVKRPRCPLN YFACPSGRCI PMSWTCDKED   2700
DCEHGEDETH CNKFCSEAQF ECQNHRCISK QWLCDGSDDC GDGSDEAAHC   2750
EGKTCGPSSF SCPGTHVCVP ERWLCDGDKD CADGADESIA AGCLYNSTCD   2800
DREFMCQNRQ CIPKHFVCDH DRDCADGSDE SPECEYPTCG PSEFRCANGR   2850
CLSSRQWECD GENDCHDQSD EAPKNPHCTS PEHKCNASSQ FLCSSGRCVA   2900
EALLCNGQDD CGDSSDERGC HINECLSRKL SGCSQDCEDL KIGFKCRCRP   2950
GFRLKDDGRT CADVDECSTT FPCSQRCINT HGSYKCLCVE GYAPRGGDPH   3000
SCKAVTDEEP FLIFANRYYL RKLNLDGSNY TLLKQGLNNA VALDFDYREQ   3050
MIYWTDVTTQ GSMIRRMHLN GSNVQVLHRT GLSNPDGLAV DWVGGNLYWC   3100
DKGRDTIEVS KLNGAYRTVL VSSGLREPRA LVVDVQNGYL YWTDWGDHSL   3150
IGRIGMDGSS RSVIVDTKIT WPNGLTLDYV TERIYWADAR EDYIEFASLD   3200
GSNRHVVLSQ DIPHIFALTL FEDYVYWTDW ETKSINRAHK TTGTNKTLLI   3250
STLHRPMDLH VFHALRQPDV PNHPCKVNNG GCSNLCLLSP GGGHKCACPT   3300
NFYLGSDGRT CVSNCTASQF VCKNDKCIPF WWKCDTEDDC GDHSDEPPDC   3350
PEFKCRPGQF QCSTGICTNP AFICDGDNDC QDNSDEANCD IHVCLPSQFK   3400
CTNTNRCIPG IFRCNGQDNC GDGEDERDCP EVTCAPNQFQ CSITKRCIPR   3450
VWVCDRDNDC VDGSDEPANC TQMTCGVDEF RCKDSGRCIP ARWKCDGEDD   3500
CGDGSDEPKE ECDERTCEPY QFRCKNNRCV PGRWQCDYDN DCGDNSDEES   3550
```

```
CTPRPCSESE FSCANGRCIA GRWKCDGDHD CADGSDEKDC TPRCDMDQFQ    3600
CKSGHCIPLR WRCDADADCM DGSDEEACGT GVRTCPLDEF QCNNTLCKPL    3650
AWKCDGEDDC GDNSDENPEE CARFVCPPNR PFRCKNDRVC LWIGRQCDGT    3700
DNCGDGTDEE DCEPPTAHTT HCKDKKEFLC RNQRCLSSSL RCNMFDDCGD    3750
GSDEEDCSID PKLTSCATNA SICGDEARCV RTEKAAYCAC RSGFHTVPGQ    3800
PGCQDINECL RFGTCSQLCN NTKGGHLCSC ARNFMKTHNT CKAEGSEYQV    3850
LYIADDNEIR SLFPGHPHSA YEQAFQGDES VRIDAMDVHV KAGRVYWTNW    3900
HTGTISYRSL PPAAPPTTSN RHRR
                          QIDRGV THLNISGLKM PRGIAIDWVA    3950
GNVYWTDSGR DVIEVAQMKG ENRKTLISGM IDEPHAIVVD PLRGTMYWSD    4000
WGNHPKIETA AMDGTLRETL VQDNIQWPTG LAVDYHNERL YWADAKLSVI    4050
GSIRLNGTDP IVAADSKRGL SHPFSIDVFE DYIYGVTYIN NRVFKIHKFG    4100
HSPLVNLTGG LSHASDVVLY HQHKQPEVTN PCDRKKCEWL CLLSPSGPVC    4150
TCPNGKRLDN GTCVPVPSPT PPPDAPRPGT CNLQCFNGGS CFLNARRQPK    4200
CRCQPRYTGD KCELDQCWEH CRNGGTCAAS PSGMPTCRCP TGFTGPKCTQ    4250
QVCAGYCANN STCTVNQGNQ PQCRCLPGFL GDRCQYRQCS GYCENFGTCQ    4300
MAADGSRQCR CTAYFEGSRC EVNKCSRCLE GACVVNKQSG DVTCNCTDGR    4350
VAPSCLTCVG HCSNGGSCTM NSKMMPECQC PPHMTGPRCE EHVFSQQQPG    4400
HIASILIPLL LLLLLVLVAG VVFWYKRRVQ GAKGFQHQRM TNGAMNVEIG    4450
NPTYKMYEGG EPDDVGGLLD ADFALDPDKP TNFTNPVYAT LYMGGHGSRH    4500
SLASTDEKRE LLGRGPEDEI GDPLA                              4525
```

References

[1] **Moestrup, S.K. et al. (1992) Cell Tissue Res. 269, 375–382.**

[2] Kristensen, T. et al. (1990) FEBS Lett. 276, 151–155.

[3] Herz, J. et al. (1988) EMBO J. 7, 4119–4127.

[4] van Leuven, F. et al. (1993) Biochim. Biophys. Acta 1173, 71–74.

[5] Nimpf, P. et al. (1994) J. Biol. Chem. 269, 212–219.

[6] **Williams, S.E. et al. (1994) Ann. N.Y. Acad. Sci. 737, 1–13.**

[7] **Williams, S.E. et al. (1992) J. Biol. Chem. 267, 9035–9040.**

CDw92

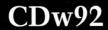

Molecular weights

SDS-PAGE
  reduced   70 kDa
  unreduced   70 kDa

Tissue distribution

CDw92 is expressed primarily by myeloid cells. Expression is stronger on monocytes than on granulocytes. Lymphocytes, endothelial cells, epithelial cells and fibroblasts are weakly positive for CDw92 [1].

Structure

Unknown.

Function

Unknown.

Reference
[1] Majdic, O. et al. (1995) Leucocyte Typing V, 984–985.

CD93

Molecular weights

SDS-PAGE
   reduced   120 kDa
   unreduced   110 kDa

Tissue distribution

CD93 is expressed on granulocytes, monocytes and endothelial cells, but absent from lymphocytes, red blood cells and platelets [1].

Structure

The structure of CD93 is unknown. However, treatment of KG1a cells (CD93⁺) with O-sialoglycoprotease, which selectively cleaves O-sialylated peptides, reduces the binding of all four anti-CD93 mAbs by greater than 90%. This suggests that CD93 is an O-sialoglycoprotein [1]. The anti-CD93 mAbs are not dependent on sialic acid for their reactivity, since neuraminidase treatment of KG1a cells does not abolish their binding.

Ligands and associated molecules

Unknown.

Function

Unknown.

Reference
[1] Mai, I. et al. (1995) Leucocyte Typing V, 986–988.

CD94 Kp43

Molecular weights
Polypeptide   20 497

SDS-PAGE [1]
    non-reduced   70 kDa (CD94/NKG2 heterodimer)
    reduced   30 kDa (plus ~40–43 kDa NKG2 subunit)

Carbohydrate
N-linked sites 2
O-linked   none

Human gene location
12p12.3–p13.1

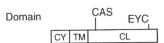

Tissue distribution

Expressed on most freshly-isolated NK cells but with wide variation in levels of expression [2,3]. Also present on a subset of $\gamma\delta$ and $\alpha\beta$ T cells [4].

Structure

CD94 is a type II transmembrane glycoprotein with a C-type lectin domain in its extracellular portion and a very short cytoplasmic domain. CD94 is structurally related to several other molecules with C-type lectin domains (Ly-49, CD161, NKG2 and CD69) which are encoded within the NK gene complex (human chromosome 12/mouse chromosome 6) and which all contribute to NK cell function [5]. Indeed, CD94 is expressed as a disulfide-linked heterodimer with a 40–43 kDa NKG2 subunit [1,6]. Based on transfection studies CD94 may also be expressed as a disulfide-linked homodimer [7].

Ligands and associated molecules

Functional studies suggest that CD94/NKG2 heterodimers may be involved in recognition of HLA-A, -B, and -C ligands, but there is currently no evidence for direct binding [1,6].

Function

CD94/NKG2 receptors play a role in recognition of MHC Class I molecules by NK cells and some cytotoxic T cells [1,6,8]. The ligation of CD94 on NK cells inhibits killing of target cells which express suitable MHC Class I molecule ligands. However, CD94 ligation appears to activate some NK cells, suggesting that there may be stimulatory and inhibitory forms of CD94 [8], probably due to the association of CD94 with different NKG2 subunits [6].

Database accession numbers

	PIR	SWISSPROT	EMBL/GENBANK	REFERENCE
Human			U30610	7

Amino acid sequence of human CD94

```
MAVFKTTLWR LISGTLGIIC LSLMATLGIL LKNSFTKLSI EPAFTPGPNI    50
ELQKDSDCCS CQEKWVGYRC NCYFISSEQK TWNESRHLCA SQKSSLLQLQ   100
NTDELDFMSS SQQFYWIGLS YSEEHTAWLW ENGSALSQYL FPSFETFNTK   150
NCIAYNPNGN ALDESCEDKN RYICKQQLI                          179
```

References

1 Phillips, J.H. et al. (1996) Immunity 5, 163–172.
2 Aramburu, J. et al. (1990) J. Immunol. 144, 3238–3247.
3 Moretta, A. et al. (1996) Annu. Rev. Immunol. 14, 619–648.
4 Mingari, M.C. et al. (1995) Int. Immunol. 7, 697–703.
5 Gumperz, J.E. and Parham, P. (1995) Nature 378, 245–248.
6 **Lazetic, S. et al. (1996) J. Immunol. 157, 4741–4745.**
7 Chang, C. et al. (1995) Eur. J. Immunol. 25, 2433–2437.
8 Pérez-Villar, J.J. et al. (1995) J. Immunol. 154, 5779–5788.

CD95

Fas, Apo-1

Molecular weights
Polypeptide   36 023

SDS-PAGE
   reduced   43 kDa

Carbohydrate
N-linked sites   2
O-linked   unknown

Human gene location
10q24.1

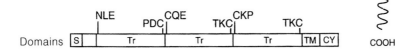

Domains

Tissue distribution

CD95 is expressed by activated lymphocytes, monocytes, neutrophils, fibroblasts and cell lines [1,2]. Mouse CD95 mRNA is also found in liver, heart, lung and ovary [1].

Structure

Fas is a member of the TNFR superfamily and contains three cysteine-rich repeats [1,2]. The cytoplasmic sequence contains a "death domain" motif which has similarity to the cytoplasmic domain of tumour necrosis factor receptor I [2,3].

Ligands and associated molecules

The extracellular region of CD95 binds to FasL. Intracellular molecules isolated by the yeast two hybrid technique as interacting with the CD95 cytoplasmic domain contain a "death domain" and include MORT/FADD [2–4]. FasL binding to CD95 recruits an ICE (interleukin-converting enzyme)-related protease via its association with MORT [5]. The C-terminal 15 amino acids of CD95 associate with a protein tyrosine phosphatase [2–4].

Function

FasL binding to CD95 induces apoptosis in activated mature lymphocytes, thus has a role in maintaining peripheral tolerance but does not appear critical in development [4,6]. Autoimmune disease in *lpr* mouse and in humans is associated with mutations in CD95 [3,4,6]. The mechanism of killing by CD95 is thought to involve ICE and ICE-like proteases [4]. FasL on cytotoxic T cells can induce cytolysis of target cells expressing CD95 [2,6,7].

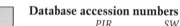

Database accession numbers

	PIR	SWISSPROT	EMBL/GENBANK	REFERENCE
Human	A40036	P25445	M67454	8
Mouse	A46484	P25446	M83649	9

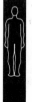

Amino acid sequence of human CD95

```
MLGIWTLLPL VLTSVA                                            -1
RLSSKSVNAQ VTDINSKGLE LRKTVTTVET QNLEGLHHDG QFCHKPCPPG       50
ERKARDCTVN GDEPDCVPCQ EGKEYTDKAH FSSKCRRCRL CDEGHGLEVE      100
INCTRTQNTK CRCKPNFFCN STVCEHCDPC TKCEHGIIKE CTLTSNTKCK      150
EEGSRSNLGW LCLLLLPIPL IVWVKRKEVQ KTCRKHRKEN QGSHESPTLN      200
PETVAINLSD VDLSKYITTI AGVMTLSQVK GFVRKNGVNE AKIDEIKNDN      250
VQDTAEQKVQ LLRNWHQLHG KKEAYDTLIK DLKKANLCTL AEKIQTIILK      300
DITSDSENSN FRNEIQSLV                                        319
```

References

1 Gruss, H.-J. and Dower, S.K. (1995) Blood 85, 3378–3404.

2 **Nagata, S. and Golstein, P. (1995) Science 267, 1449–1456.**

3 Cleveland, J.L. and Ihle, J.N. (1995) Cell 81, 479–482.

4 **van Parijs, L. and Abbas, A.K. (1996) Curr. Opin. Immunol. 8, 355–361.**

5 Fraser, A. and Evan, G. (1996) Cell 85, 781–784.

6 Lynch, D.H. et al. (1995) Immunol. Today 16, 569–574.

7 Takayama, H. et al. (1995) Adv. Immunol. 60, 289–321.

8 Itoh, N. et al. (1991) Cell 66, 233–243.

9 Watanabe-Fukunaga, R. et al. (1992) J. Immunol. 148, 1274–1279.

CD96　Tactile

Molecular weights
Polypeptide　61 258

SDS-PAGE
　reduced　　160 kDa
　unreduced　160, 180, 240 kDa

Carbohydrate
N-linked sites　15
O-linked probable　++++

Domains

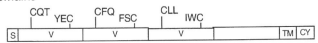

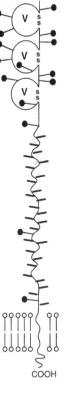

COOH

Tissue distribution

CD96 is expressed at low levels on peripheral T cells and NK cells and expression on both is increased on activation and reaches a maximum at 6–9 days [1,2]. CD96 is not expressed on B cells or monocytes [1,2]. CD96 is expressed on T cell lines [1,2].

Structure

The extracellular domain is made up of three IgSF domains followed by a membrane-proximal serine/threonine/proline-rich stalk region which is probably *O*-glycosylated. The N-terminal IgSF domain contains three Cys residues in addition to the pair predicted to form the intersheet disulfide. The cytoplasmic domain has a basic/proline-rich region. Some CD96 may exist as a homodimer [1,2].

Function

Unknown.

Database accession numbers

	PIR	SWISSPROT	EMBL/GENBANK	REFERENCE
Human	A46462	P40200	M88282	1

Amino acid sequence of human CD96

```
MEKKWKYCAV YYIIQIHFVK G                                    -1
VWEKTVNTEE NVYATLGSDV NLTCQTQTVG FFVQMQWSKV TNKIDLIAVY      50
HPQYGFYCAY GRPCESLVTF TETPENGSKW TLHLRNMSCS VSGRYECMLV     100
LYPEGIQTKI YNLLIQTHVT ADEWNSNHTI EIEINQTLEI PCFQNSSSKI     150
SSEFTYAWSV EDNGTQETLI SQNHLISNST LLKDRVKLGT DYRLHLSPVQ     200
IFDDGRKFSC HIRVGPNKIL RSSTTVKVFA KPEIPVIVEN NSTDVLVERR     250
FTCLLKNVFP KANITWFIDG SFLHDEKEGI YITNEERKGK DGFLELKSVL     300
TRVHSNKPAQ SDNLTIWCMA LSPVPGNKVW NISSEKITFL LGSEISSTDP     350
PLSVTESTLD TQPSPASSVS PARYPATSSV TLVDVSALRP NTTPQPSNSS     400
MTTRGFNYPW TSSGTDTKKS VSRIPSETYS SSPSGAGSTL HDNVFTSTAR     450
AFSEVPTTAN GSTKTNHVHI TGIVVNKPKD G̲M̲S̲W̲P̲V̲I̲V̲A̲A̲ ̲L̲L̲F̲C̲C̲M̲I̲L̲F̲G̲     500
L̲G̲V̲R̲K̲W̲C̲Q̲Y̲Q̲ KEIMERPPPF KPPPPPIKYT CIQEPNESDL PYHEMETL     548
```

References
1. Wang, P.L. et al. (1992) J. Immunol. 148, 2600–2608.
2. **Wang, P.L. and Krensky, A.M. (1995) In Leucocyte Typing V (Schlossman, S.F. et al., ed.) Oxford University Press, Oxford, pp. 1149–1150.**

CD97

Molecular weights
Polypeptide   79 665

SDS-PAGE
  reduced   78–85 kDa
  unreduced   78–85 kDa

Carbohydrate
N-linked sites   8
O-linked   unknown

Human gene location and size
19p13.12–p13.2; 12 kb [1]

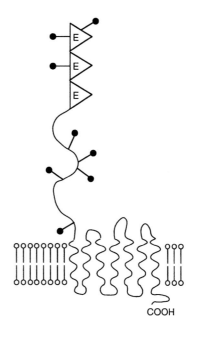

COOH

Tissue distribution

CD97 is constitutively expressed on granulocytes, monocytes and at low levels on resting T cells and B cells [2,3]. Expression is rapidly upregulated following activation of T cells and B cells [2,3].

Structure

CD97 has seven potential membrane spanning domains and three extracellular EGF domains [4]. There is a single RGD sequence. CD97 shows sequence similarity to EMR1 and F4/80 and is a member of the EGF-TM7 family [5]. The seven-span transmembrane region also shows approximately 25% sequence identity to members of the recently described glucagon/vasoactive intestinal peptide/calcitonin receptor family [6].

Ligands and associated molecules

COS cells expressing CD97 adhere to lymphocytes and erythrocytes. This interaction is blocked by mAbs specific for CD55, a proposed cellular ligand for CD97 [7]. Immunoprecipitation studies have identified a 58 kDa protein non-covalently associated with CD97 on the cell surface [2].

Function

Unknown.

Database accession numbers

	PIR	SWISSPROT	EMBL/GENBANK	REFERENCE
Human	S54875	P48960	X84700	4

Amino acid sequence of human CD97

```
MGGRVFLAFC VWLTLPGAET                               -1
QDSRGCARWC PQNSSCVNAT ACRCNPGFSS FSEIITTPTE TCDDINECAT 50
PSKVSCGKFS DCWNTEGSYD CVCSPGYEPV SGAKTFKNES ENTCQDVDEC 100
SSGQHQCDSS TVCFNTVGSY SCRCRPGWKP RHGIPNNQKD TVCEDMTFST 150
WTPPPGVHSQ TLSRFFDKVQ DLGRDSKTSS AEVTIQNVIK LVDELMEAPG 200
DVEALAPPVR HLIATQLLSN LEDIMRILAK SLPKGPFTYI SPSNTELTLM 250
IQERGDKNVT MGQSSARMKL NWAVAAGAED PGPAVAGILS IQNMTTLLAN 300
ASLNLHSKKQ AELEEIYESS IRGVQLRRLS AVNSIFLSHN NTKELNSPIL 350
FAFSHLESSD GEAGRDPPAK DVMPGPRQEL LCAFWKSDSD RGGHWATEVC 400
QVLGSKNGST TCQCSHLSSF TILMAHYDVE DWKLTLITRV GLALSLFCLL 450
LCILTFLLVR PIQGSRTTIH LHLCICLFVG STIFLAGIEN EGGQVGLRCR 500
LVAGLLHYCF LAAFCWMSLE GLELYFLVVR VFQGQGLSTR WLCLIGYGVP 550
LLIVGVSAAI YSKGYGRPRY CWLDFEQGFL WSFLGPVTFI ILCNAVIFVT 600
TVWKLTQKFS EINPDMKKLK KARALTITAI AQLFLLGCTW VFGLFIFDDR 650
SLVLTYVFTI LNCLQGAFLY LLHCLLNKKV REEYRKWACL VAGGSKYSEF 700
TSTTSGTGHN QTRALRASES GI                            722
```

References

1. Hamann, J. et al. (1996) Genomics 32, 144–147.
2. Eichler, W. et al. (1994) Scand. J. Immunol. 39, 111–115.
3. Pickl, W.F. et al. (1995) Leucocyte Typing V, 1151–1153.
4. **Hamann, J. et al. (1995) J. Immunol. 155, 1942–1950.**
5. McKnight, A.J. and Gordon, S. (1996) Immunol. Today 17, 283–287.
6. Segre, G.V. and Goldring, S.R. (1993) Trends Endocrinol. Metab. 4, 309–314.
7. **Hamann, J. et al. (1996) J. Exp. Med. 184, 1185–1189.**

Note added in proof

The isolation of further human CD97 cDNA clones indicates that there are five extracellular EGF domains (GENBANK accession number U76764), which may be alternatively spliced to generate the form of the molecule shown here (Gray, J.X. et al. (1996) J. Immunol. 157, 5438–5447). Further, the CD97 antigen is shown to be processed into two non-covalently associated subunits (CD97 α and β) prior to expression on the cell surface.

CD98 4F2, FRP-1, RL-388 (mouse)

Molecular weights
Polypeptides   57 039

SDS-PAGE
  reduced   80 kDa, 40 kDa
  unreduced   120 kDa

Carbohydrate
80 kDa chain: N-linked sites 4
              O-linked   unknown
40 kDa chain: non-glycosylated

Human gene location and size
11q; 8 kb [1]

? s — S-light chain (40 kD)

NH₂

Tissue distribution

CD98 is expressed at high levels on monocytes but very low levels on peripheral blood T and B cells, splenocytes, NK cells and granulocytes [2]. Con A and alloantigen-activated lymphocytes and activated NK cells express high levels of this antigen [2]. It is also expressed on some non-haematopoietic cells [2]. All human cell lines studied express CD98 [2]. Studies in mouse show CD98 is expressed at the beginning of haematopoiesis [3].

Structure

CD98 is a heterodimer consisting of a disulfide-linked glycosylated heavy chain (80–90 kDa) and a non-glycosylated light chain (40 kDa). The heavy chain is a type II integral membrane protein containing a 73 amino acid N-terminal cytoplasmic domain, a single transmembrane sequence and a large extracellular domain [4]. The N-terminus has been determined by amino acid sequencing [5].

Ligands and associated molecules

Unknown.

Function

A role in cell growth and death for CD98 is suggested by studies with mAbs [3]. CD98 mAb inhibits lectin-induced mitogenesis of human T cells by 50%, but does not inhibit the mixed lymphocyte reaction (MLR), antibody-dependent cellular cytotoxicity, T cell-mediated cytotoxicity or NK cell activity [2,3]. CD98 mAb had inhibitory effects on early haematopoietic progenitors [3]. CD98 mAbs induce cell fusion [5], homotypic aggregation and tyrosine phosphorylation [3]. Experiments in *Xenopus* oocytes suggesting CD98 is an amino acid transporter are controversial [3,7].

Database accession numbers

	PIR	SWISSPROT	EMBL/GENBANK	REFERENCE
Human	A28455	P08195	J02939	4
Mouse	S03600	P10852	X14309	6
Rat			X89225	7

Amino acid sequence of human CD98 heavy chain

```
MKEVELNELE PEKQPMNAAS GAAMSLAGAE KNGLVKIKVA EDEAEAAAAA    50
KFTGLSKEEL LKVAGSPGWV RTRWALLLLF WLGWLGMLAG AVVIIVRAPR   100
CRELPAQKWW HTGALYRIGD LQAFQGHGAG NLAGLKGRLD YLSSLKVKGL   150
VLGPIHKNQK DDVAQTDLLQ IDPNFGSKED FDSLLQSAKK KSIRVILDLT   200
PNYRGENSWF STQVDTVATK VKDALEFWLQ AGVDGFQVRD IENLKDASSF   250
LAEWQNITKG FSEDRLLIAG TNSSDLQQIL SLLESNKDLL LTSSYLSDSG   300
STGEHTKSLV TQYLNATGNR WCSWSLSQAR LLTSFLPAQL LRLYQLMLFT   350
LPGTPVFSYG DEIGLDAAAL PGQPMEAPVM LWDESSFPDI PGAVSANMTV   400
KGQSEDPGSL LSLFRRLSDQ RSKERSLLHG DFHAFSAGPG LFSYIRHWDQ   450
 NERFLVVLNF GDVGLSAGLQ ASDLPASASL PAKADLLLST QPGREEGSPL   500
ELERLKLEPH EGLLLRFPYA A                                 521
```

References
1 Gottesdiener, K.M. et al. (1988) Mol. Cell. Biol. 8, 3809–3819.
2 Haynes, B.F. et al. (1981) J. Immunol. 126, 1409–1414.
3 **Warren, A.P. et al. (1996) Blood 87, 3676–3687.**
4 Quackenbush, E. et al. (1987) Proc. Natl Acad. Sci. USA 84, 6526–6530.
5 Ohgimoto, S. et al. (1995) J. Immunol. 155, 3585–3592.
6 Parmacek, M.S. et al. (1989) Nucleic Acids Res. 17, 1915–1931.
7 Broer, S. et al. (1995) Biochem. J. 312, 863–870.

CD99　MIC2, E2, 12E7, HuLy-m6, FMC29

Molecular weights
Polypeptide　　16 728

SDS-PAGE
　reduced　　　32 kDa
　unreduced　　32 kDa

Carbohydrate
N-linked sites　nil
O-linked　　　+ abundant

Human gene location and size
MIC2X: Xp22.32–pter
MIC2Y: Yp11.2–pter; 52 kb [1]

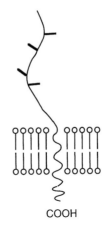

COOH

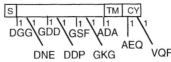

Exon boundaries

Tissue distribution

CD99 is expressed on all leucocyte lineages[2]. Expression is highest on thymocytes and falls on maturation[2]. Expression on CD4+ and CD8+ T cells is bimodal and within the CD4+ population, expression is higher on the CD45RA− subset[2]. NK cells and monocytes express high levels of CD99[2]. Expression of CD99 and Xga appears to be linked[3]. CD99 is highly expressed at the surface of Xg(a+) red blood cells and shows low expression on Xg(a−) red blood cells[3]. CD99 expression is high on Ewing's tumours[2].

Structure

The extracellular domain of CD99 contains five Gly-X-Y repeats, such as found in collagen and collagen-like proteins[5] and also contains three repeats of 16 amino acids[4]. CD99 contains a high content of Pro[4,5] and is highly glycosylated with O-linked sugars[6]. The N-terminus has been established by protein sequencing[6]. CD99 shares 48% amino acid identity (including conservative changes) to Xga antigen, originally defined as a blood group polymorphism[3]. The CD99 gene locus is in the pairing region of the human X and Y chromosomes and was the first pseudoautosomal gene to be described in man[1,3]. CD99X escapes X inactivation[1,3]. The CD99 gene is closely linked (within 10 kb) to the Xga gene[3].

Function

CD99 on thymocytes and T cells is involved in rosette formation with sheep or human erythrocytes[5,7]. CD99 mAbs induce homotypic adhesion of CD4+CD8+ thymocytes[7].

Database accession numbers

	PIR	SWISSPROT	EMBL/GENBANK	REFERENCE
Human	SO6786	P14209	X16996	5

Amino acid sequence of human CD99

```
MARGAALALL LFGLLGVLVA AP                               -1
DGGFDLSDAL PDNENKKPTA IPKKPSAGDD FDLGDAVVDG ENDDPRPPNP  50
PKPMPNPNPN HPSSSGSFSD ADLADGVSGG EGKGGSDGGG SHRKEGEEAD 100
APGVIPGIVG AVVVAVAGAI SSFIAYQKKK LCFKENAEQG EVDMESHRNA 150
NAEPAVQRTL LEK                                        163
```

References

1 Smith, M.J. et al. (1993) Hum. Mol. Genet. 2, 417–422.
2 **Tippett, P. (1995) Immunol. Invest. 24, 173–186.**
3 Ellis, N.A. et al. (1994) Nature Genet. 8, 285–289.
4 Sandrin, M.S. et al. (1992) Immunogenetics 35, 283–285.
5 Gelin, C. et al. (1989) EMBO J. 11, 3253–3259.
6 Aubrit, F. et al. (1989) Eur. J. Immunol. 19, 1431–1436.
7 Bernard, G. et al. (1995) J. Immunol. 154, 26–32.

CD100

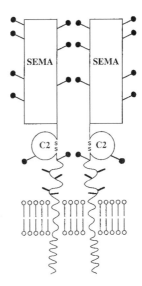

Molecular weights
Polypeptide   93 996

SDS-PAGE
   reduced   150 kDa
   unreduced   300 kDa

Carbohydrate
N-linked sites   9
O-linked   + probable

Tissue distribution

CD100 is expressed by B, T and NK cells, most myeloid cells, but is absent from bone marrow, erythrocytes, eosinophils and endothelial cells. The level of expression is low on resting cells but increased following activation [1,2]. CD100 mRNA is expressed in most tissues [1].

Structure

The CD100 molecule is a type I membrane glycoprotein that is a member of the semaphorin (sema) superfamily. CD100 consists of an N-terminal sema domain, followed by a C2-set IgSF domain, a 104 amino acid stalk, a hydrophobic transmembrane region and a 110 amino acid C-terminal cytoplasmic tail. The cytoplasmic region has potential sites for tyrosine and serine phosphorylation [1]. CD100 exists at the cell surface as a disulfide-linked homodimer. The cysteine residues involved in dimerization are not known [2].

Function

CD100 is thought to play a role in lymphocyte activation. Cells transfected with CD100 modify B cell signalling through CD40 by downregulating CD23 expression and by augmenting B cell aggregation and survival [1]. Antibody crosslinking of CD100 on T cells increases both CD2- and CD3-induced T cell proliferation [3]. The identification of CD100 as a semaphorin suggests a possible role in neuronal guidance [1].

Database accession numbers

	PIR	SWISSPROT	EMBL/GENBANK	REFERENCE
Human			U60800	1

Amino acid sequence of human CD100

```
MRMCTPIRGL LMALAVMFGT A                                        -1
MAFAPIPRIT WEHREVHLVQ FHEPDIYNYS ALLLSEDKDT LYIGAREAVF         50
AVNALNISEK QHEVYWKVSE DKKAKCAEKG KSKQTECLNY IRVLQPLSAT        100
SLYVCGTNAF QPACDHLNLT SFKFLGKNED GKGRCPFDPA HSYTSVMVDG        150
ELYSGTSYNF LGSEPIISRN SSHSPLRTEY AIPWLNEPSF VFADVIRKSP       200
DSPDGEDDRV YFFFTEVSVE YEFVFRVLIP RIARVCKGDQ GGLRTLQKKW       250
TSFLKARLIC SRPDSGLVFN VLRDVFVLRS PGLKVPVFYA LFTPQLNNVG       300
LSAVCAYNLS TAEEVFSHGK YMQSTTVEQS HTKWVRYNGP VPKPRPGACI       350
DSEARAANYT SSLNLPDKTL QFVKDHPLMD DSVTPIDNRP RLIKKDVNYT       400
QIVVDRTQAL DGTVYDVMFV STDRGALHKA ISLEHAVHII EETQLFQDFE       450
PVQTLLLSSK KGNRFVYAGS NSGVVQAPLA FCGKHGTCED CVLARDPYCA       500
WSPPTATCVA LHQTESPSRG LIQEMSGDAS VCPDKSKGSY RQHFFKHGGT       550
AELKCSQKSN LARVFWKFQN GVLKAESPKY GLMGRKNLLI FNLSEGDSGV       600
YQCLSEERVK NKTVFQVVAK HVLEVKVVPK PVVAPTLSVV QTEGSRIATK       650
VLVASTQGSS PPTPAVQATS SGAITLPPKP APTGTSCEPK IVINTVPQLH       700
SEKTMYLKSS DNRLLMSLFL FFFVLFLCLF FYNCYKGYLP RQCLKFRSAL       750
LIGKKKPKSD FCDREQSLKE TLVEPGSFSQ QNGEHPKPAL DTGYETEQDT       800
ITSKVPTDRE DSQRIDDLSA RDKPFDVKCE LKFADSDADG DI              842
```

References

[1] **Hall, K.T. et al. (1996) Proc. Natl Acad. Sci. USA 93, 11780–11785.**
[2] Herold, C. et al. (1995) Leucocyte Typing V, 288–289.
[3] Herold, C. et al. (1995) Int. Immunol. 7, 1–8.

Molecular weights
Polypeptide   115 042

SDS-PAGE
  reduced   126 kDa
  unreduced   200 kDa

Carbohydrate
N-linked sites   7
O-linked   nil

Human gene location
1p13

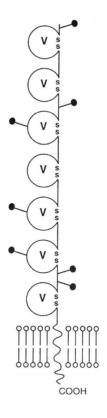

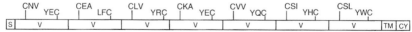

Domains

Tissue distribution

CD101 is expressed on monocytes, granulocytes, mucosal T cells, and on activated peripheral blood T cells. Expression is weak on resting T, B and NK cells, absent from platelets and weak or absent from most haematopoietic cell lines [1-3]. Northern blot analyses show CD101 mRNA to be present in PBLs, thymus, spleen, lung and small intestine, but not in other tissues [4].

Structure

The extracellular portion of the molecule contains seven V-set IgSF domains. The C-terminal cytoplasmic region is relatively short [4]. CD101 exists at the cell surface as a disulfide-linked homodimer. The cysteine residues involved are not known [1, 3].

Function

CD101 is thought to play a co-stimulatory role in TCR/CD3-mediated T cell activation [1-3]. The anti-CD101 mAb V7.1 inhibits the proliferative response of CD4⁺ and CD8⁺ T cells *in vitro* to alloantigens and immobilized CD3 mAbs, but not to mitogenic lectins[2]. Other CD101 mAbs are co-stimulatory for intraepithelial T lymphocytes when administered *in vitro* with suboptimal doses of CD3 mAb[3].

Database accession numbers

	PIR	SWISSPROT	EMBL/GENBANK	REFERENCE
Human			Z33642	4

Amino acid sequence of human CD101

```
MAGISYVASF FLLLTKLSIG                                 -1
QREVTVQKGP LFRAEGYPVS IGCNVTGHQG PSEQHFQWSV YLPTNPTQEV  50
QIISTKDAAF SYAVYTQRVR GGDVYVERVQ GNSVLLHISK LQMKDAGEYE 100
CHTPNTDENY YGSYRAKTNL IVIPDTLSAT MSSQTLGKEE GEPLALTCEA 150
SKATAQHTHL SVTWYLTQDG GGSQATEIIS LSKDFILVPG PLYTERFAAS 200
DVQLNKLGPT TFRLSIERLQ SSDQGQLFCE ATEWIQDPDE TWMFITKKQT 250
DQTTLRIQPA VKDFQVNITA DSLFAEGKPL ELVCLVVSSG RDPQLQGIWF 300
FNGTEIAHID AGGVLGLKND YKERASQGEL QLSKLGPKAF SLKIFSLGPE 350
DEGAYRCVVA EVMKTRTGSW QVLQRKQSPD SHVHLRKPAA RSVVVSTKNK 400
QQVVWEGETL AFLCKAGGAE SPLSVSWWHI PRDQTQPEFV AGMGQDGIVQ 450
LGALLWGTSY HGNTRLEKMD WATFQLEITF TAITDSGTYE CRVSEKSRNQ 500
ARDLSWTQKI SVTVKSLESS LQVSLMSRQP QVMLTNTFDL SCVVRAGYSD 550
LKVPLTVTWQ FQPASSHIFH QLIRITHNGT IEWGNFLSRF QKKTKVSQSL 600
FRSQLLVHDA TEQETGVYQC EVEVYDRNSL YNNPPPRASA ISHPLRIAVT 650
LPESKLKVNS RSQGQELSIN SNTDIECSIL SRSNGNLQLA IIWYFSPVST 700
NASWLKILEM DQTNVIKTGD EFHTPQRKQK FHTEKVSQDL FQLHILNVED 750
 SDRGKYHCAV EEWLLSTNGT WHKLGEKKSG LTELKLKPTG SKVRVSKVYW 800
TENVTEHREV AIRCSLESVG SSATLYSVMW YWNRENSGSK LLVHLQHDGL 850
LEYGEEGLRG HLHCYRSSST DFVLKLHQVE MEDAGMYWCR VAEWQLHGHP 900
SKWINKHPMS HSGWCSPCCL QSPRFLPGSA PRPPLLYFLF ICPFVLLLLL 950
LISLLCLYWK ARKLSTLRSN TRKEKALWVD LKEAGGVTTN RREDEEEDEG 1000
N                                                    1001
```

References
1. Gouttefangeas, C. et al. (1994) Int. Immunol. 6, 423–430.
2. Rivas, A. et al. (1995) J. Immunol. 154, 4423–4433.
3. **Russell, G.J. et al. (1996) J. Immunol. 157, 3366–3374.**
4. Ruegg, C.L. et al. (1995) J. Immunol. 154, 4434–4443.

CD102   ICAM-2

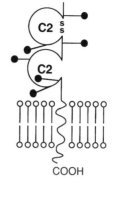

Molecular weights
Polypeptide   28 393

SDS-PAGE
  reduced   55–65 kDa
  unreduced   54–68 kDa

Carbohydrate
N-linked sites   6
O-linked   unknown

Human gene location
17q23–q25 [1]

COOH

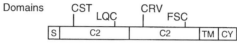

Domains

	CST	LQC	CRV	FSC		
S	C2		C2		TM	CY

Tissue distribution

CD102 is broadly expressed on leucocytes (with the exception of neutrophils) and is expressed constitutively and at high levels on vascular endothelium [2]. Expression is more restricted than CD54 (ICAM-1) and, unlike CD54, there is little or no induction of CD102 on lymphocytes and endothelial cells by inflammatory mediators [2].

Structure

CD102 is a highly glycosylated cell surface protein. The extracellular portion contains two IgSF C2-set domains and shares ~36% sequence identity with the two membrane-distal IgSF domains of CD54 (ICAM-1) and CD50 (ICAM-3).

Ligands and associated molecules

CD102 is a ligand for the leucocyte integrin CD11a/CD18 (LFA-1) [3], like the related proteins CD54 (ICAM-1) and CD50 (ICAM-3). CD102 has also been reported to bind CD11b/CD18 (Mac-1) [4].

Function

CD102 is the major LFA-1 ligand on endothelial cells that have not been activated by inflammatory stimuli, suggesting a possible role in lymphocyte recirculation [2]. Recombinant CD102 can co-stimulate T cell *in vitro*, suggesting a role in T cell activation [5].

Database accession numbers

	PIR	SWISSPROT	EMBL/GENBANK	REFERENCE
Human	S03967	P13598	X15606	3
Mouse	A46510	P35330	X65493	6

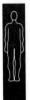

Amino acid sequence of human CD102

```
MSSFGYRTLT VALFTLICCP G                                    -1
SDEKVFEVHV RPKKLAVEPK GSLEVNCSTT CNQPEVGGLE TSLNKILLDE     50
QAQWKHYLVS NISHDTVLQC HFTCSGKQES MNSNVSVYQP PRQVILTLQP     100
TLVAVGKSFT IECRVPTVEP LDSLTLFLFR GNETLHYETF GKAAPAPQEA     150
TATFNSTADR EDGHRNFSCL AVLDLMSRGG NIFHKHSAPK MLEIYEPVSD     200
SQMVIIVTVV SVLLSLFVTS VLLCFIFGQH LRQQRMGTYG VRAAWRRLPQ     250
AFRP                                                      254
```

References
[1] Sansom, D. et al. (1991) Genomics 11, 462–464.
[2] **de Fougerolles, A.R. et al. (1991) J. Exp. Med. 174, 253–267.**
[3] Staunton, D.E. et al. (1989) Nature 339, 61–64.
[4] Xie, J. et al. (1995) J. Immunol. 155, 3619–3628.
[5] Damle, N.K. et al. (1992) J. Immunol. 148, 665–671.
[6] Xu, H. et al. (1992) J. Immunol. 149, 2650–2655.

Molecular weights
Polypeptide   127 746

SDS-PAGE
   reduced   150 + 25 kDa
   unreduced   175 kDa

Carbohydrate
N-linked sites   11
O-linked sites   unknown

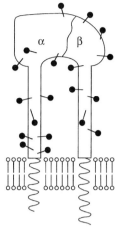

CD103(αE)/β7

Tissue distribution

αEβ7 is expressed primarily on intraepithelial lymphocytes and on 1–2% of peripheral blood lymphocytes[1]. Its level of expression can be upregulated by lymphocyte mitogens[2]. CD103 mRNA is found in the thymus and spleen as well as tissues such as lung, small intestine, and colon, which contain large populations of intraepithelial lymphocytes. It is also expressed in the prostate and ovary and in tissues such as the pancreas and testis, where β7 mRNA transcripts are not detectable[3].

Structure

CD103 is the integrin αE subunit (E for epithelial-associated), which usually forms a heterodimer with the integrin β7 subunit. It belongs to the subgroup of integrin α subunits with an I-domain. Unlike the other members of this group, it is cleaved into two chains, an N-terminal chain of 25 kDa and a C-terminal chain of 150 kDa, which remain linked by disulfide bonds. An extra segment of 55 residues (X-domain) is found immediately N-terminal to the I-domain. This segment (shown in bold below) contains the intrachain cleavage site (shown on new line) and a continuous stretch of 18 charged residues, 16 of which are acidic. The N-terminal sequences of both cleaved chains were determined at the protein level[3].

Ligands and associated molecules

The integrin αEβ7 binds E-cadherin[1,4].

Function

αEβ7 binds to E-cadherin on epithelial cells. This interaction may be of importance in the homing and retention of αEβ7-expressing lymphocytes in the intestinal epithelium[4–6].

Database accession numbers

	PIR	SWISSPROT	EMBL/GENBANK	REFERENCE
Human		P38570	L25851	3

Amino acid sequence of human CD103

```
MWLFHTLLCI ASLALLAA                                              -1
FNVDVARPWL TPKGGAPFVL SSLLHQDPST NQTWLLVTSP RTKRTPGPLH           50
RCSLVQDEIL CHPVEHVPIQ GEAPGSDRCP EPPRCFDMHS SAGPAPHSLS          100
SELTGTCSLL GPDLRPQAQA NFFDLENLLD PDARVDTGDC YSNKEGGGED          150
DVNTARQRR
          A LEKEEEEDKE EEEDEEEEEA GTEIAIILDG SGSIDPPDFQ          200
RAKDFISNMM RNFYEKCFEC NFALVQYGGV IQTEFDLRDS QDVMASLARV          250
QNITQVGSVT KTASAMQHVL DSIFTSSHGS RRKASKVMVV LTDGGIFEDP          300
LNLTTVINSP KMQGVERFAI GVGEEFKSAR TARELNLIAS DPDETHAFKV          350
TNYMALDGLL SKLRYNIISM EGTVGDALHY QLAQIGFSAQ ILDERQVLLG          400
AVGAFDWSGG ALLYDTRSRR GRFLNQTAAA AADAEAAQYS YLGYAVAVLH          450
KTCSLSYVAG APQYKHHGAV FELQKEGREA SFLPVLEGEQ MGSYFGSELC          500
PVDIDMDGST DFLLVAAPFY HVHGEEGRVY VYRLSEQDGS FSLARILSGH          550
PGFTNARFGF AMAAMGDLSQ DKLTDVAIGA PLEGFGADDG ASFGSVYIYN          600
GHWDGLSASP SQRIRASTVA PGLQYFGMSM AGGFDISGDG LADITVGTLG          650
QAVVFRSRPV VRLKVSMAFT PSALPIGFNG VVNVRLCFEI SSVTTASESG          700
LREALLNFTL DVDVGKQRRR LQCSDVRSCL GCLREWSSGS QLCEDLLLMP          750
TEGELCEEDC FSNASVKVSY QLQTPEGQTD HPQPILDRYT EPFAIFQLPY          800
EKACKNKLFC VAELQLATTV SQQELVVGLT KELTLNINLT NSGEDSYMTS          850
MALNYPRNLQ LKRMQKPPSP NIQCDDPQPV ASVLIMNCRI GHPVLKRSSA          900
HVSVVWQLEE NAFPNRTADI TVTVTNSNER RSLANETHTL QFRHGFVAVL          950
SKPSIMYVNT GQGLSHHKEF LFHVHGENLF GAEYQLQICV PTKLRGLQVA         1000
AVKKLTRTQA STVCTWSQER ACAYSSVQHV EEWHSVSCVI ASDKENVTVA         1050
AEISWDHSEE LLKDVTELQI LGEISFNKSL YEGLNAENHR TKITVVFLKD         1100
EKYHSLPIII KGSVGGLLVL IVILVILFKC GFFKRKYQQL NLESIRKAQL         1150
KSENLLEEEN                                                     1160
```

References
1. Parker, C. M. et al. (1992) Proc. Natl Acad. Sci. USA 89, 1924–1928.
2. Schieferdecker, H.L. et al. (1990) J. Immunol. 144, 2541–2549.
3. **Shaw, S. K. et al. (1994) J. Biol. Chem. 269, 6016–6025.**
4. Cepek, K. L. et al. (1994) Nature 372, 190–193.
5. Cepek, K. L. et al. (1993) J. Immunol. 150, 3459–3470.
6. **Shaw, S. K. and Brenner, M. B. (1995) Semin. Immunol. 7, 335–342.**

Molecular weights

Polypeptide	(no insert)	192 267
	(insert-1)	197 979
	(insert-2)	199 599

SDS-PAGE
reduced	220 kDa
unreduced	210 kDa

Carbohydrates
N-linked sites	5
O-linked sites	unknown

Human gene location
17q11–qter

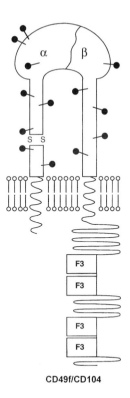

CD49f/CD104

Tissue distribution

CD104 is expressed in conjunction with CD49f as the α6β4 integrin on the hemidesmosomes of stratified epithelia [1]. It is also expressed on cells which do not have hemidesmosomes including simple epithelia and Schwann cells [2,3], and a subset of endothelial cells in the mouse [4].

Structure

CD104 is the integrin β4 subunit, which forms a heterodimer with the integrin α6 subunit (CD49f). It has only 48 out of the 56 cysteine residues normally conserved in the extracellular portion of integrin β subunits. It also has an unusually large cytoplasmic domain of about 1000 residues which includes four fibronectin type III domains. Three alternative forms have been identified by cDNA analysis; they contain either no inserts, or insert-1 at position 1343, or insert-2 at position 1413 (refs 5–7). Both inserts are between the second and third fibronectin type III domains and are shown in bold indented lines in the sequence below. cDNA isolated from the placenta contains a mixture of the short form (no inserts) and the one having only insert-2, whereas carcinoma cell lines appear to express only the form with insert-1 [6]. Immunoprecipitation studies suggest that free β4 subunit, i.e. not in association with any α subunit, may be present on carcinoma cell lines [2]. The N-terminus of CD104 has been determined [8].

Ligands and associated molecules

CD104 combines with CD49f to form the $\alpha6\beta4$ integrin, which is an integral component of hemidesmosomes in stratified epithelia [1,9].

Function

Hemidesmosomal CD49f/CD104 ($\alpha6\beta4$) plays an important role in the adhesion of epithelia to basement membranes, via interactions with laminin and/or kalinin anchoring filaments [1,9,10]. Unlike other integrins, CD49f/CD104 interacts with intracellular keratin filaments rather than the actin cytoskeleton. Frameshift and deletion mutations have been identified in a patient with junctional epidermolysis bullosa and pyloric atresia [11].

Database accession numbers

	PIR	SWISSPROT	EMBL/GENBANK	REFERENCE
Human	S08465	P16144	X51841	5
	A36429		X53587	6
	S12380		X52186	7
Mouse			L04678	12

Amino acid sequence of human CD104

```
MAGPRPSPWA RLLLAALISV SLSGTLA                                  -1
NRCKKAPVKS CTECVRVDKD CAYCTDEMFR DRRCNTQAEL LAAGCQRESI          50
VVMESSFQIT EETQIDTTLR RSQMSPQGLR VRLRPGEERH FELEVFEPLE         100
SPVDLYILMD FSNSMSDDLD NLKKMGQNLA RVLSQLTSDY TIGFGKFVDK         150
VSVPQTDMRP EKLKEPWPNS DPPFSFKNVI SLTEDVDEFR NKLQGERISG         200
NLDAPEGGFD AILQTAVCTR DIGWRPDSTH LLVFSTESAF HYEADGANVL         250
AGIMSRNDER CHLDTTGTYT QYRTQDYPSV PTLVRLLAKH NIIPIFAVTN         300
YSYSYYEKLH TYFPVSSLGV LQEDSSNIVE LLEEAFNRIR SNLDIRALDS         350
PRGLRTEVTS KMFQKTRTGS FHIRRGEVGI YQVQLRALEH VDGTHVCQLP         400
EDQKGNIHLK PSFSDGLKMD AGIICDVCTC ELQKEVRSAR CSFNGDFVCG         450
QCVCSEGWSG QTCNCSTGSL SDIQPCLREG EDKPCSGRGE CQCGHCVCYG         500
EGRYEGQFCE YDNFQCPRTS GFLCNDRGRC SMGQCVCEPG WTGPSCDCPL         550
SNATCIDSNG GICNGRGHCE CGRCHCHQQS LYTDTICEIN YSAIHPGLCE         600
DLRSCVQCQA WGTGEKKGRT CEECNFKVKM VDELKRAEEV VVRCSFRDED         650
DDCTYSYTME GDGAPGPNST VLVHKKKDCP PGSFWWLIPL LLLLLPLLAL         700
LLLLCWKYCA CCKACLALLP CCNRGHMVGF KEDHYMLREN LMASDHLDTP         750
MLRSGNLKGR DVVRWKVTNN MQRPGFATHA ASINPTELVP YGLSLRLARL         800
CTENLLKPDT RECAQLRQEV EENLNEVYRQ ISGVHKLQQT KFRQQPNAGK         850
KQDHTIVDTV LMAPRSAKPA LLKLTEKQVE QRAFHDLKVA PGYYTLTADQ         900
DARGMVEFQE GVELVDVRVP LFIRPEDDDE KQLLVEAIDV PAGTATLGRR         950
LVNITIIKEQ ARDVVSFEQP EFSVSRGDQV ARIPVIRRVL DGGKSQVSYR        1000
TQDGTAQGNR DYIPVEGELL FQPGEAWKEL QVKLLELQEV DSLLRGRQVR        1050
RFHVQLSNPK FGAHLGQPHS TTIIIRDPDE LDRSFTSQML SSQPPPHGDL        1100
GAPQNPNAKA AGSRKIHFNW LPPSGKPMGY RVKYWIQGDS ESEAHLLDSK        1150
VPSVELTNLY PYCDYEMKVC AYGAQGEGPY SSLVSCRTHQ EVPSEPGRLA        1200
FNVVSSTVTQ LSWAEPAETN GEITAYEVCY GLVNDDNRPI GPMKKVLVDN        1250
PKNRMLLIEN LRESQPYRYT VKARNGAGWG PEREAIINLA TQPKRPMSIP        1300
IIPDIPIVDA QSGEDYDSFL MYSDDVLRSP SGSQRPSVSD DT               
                                          GCGWKFEP           1350
LLGEELDLRR VTWRLPPELI PRLSASSGRS SDAEAPTAPR TTAARAGRAA        1400
```

AVPRSATPGP PG

```
        EHLVNGRM DFAFPGSTNS LHRMTTTSAA AYGTHLSPHV   1450
PHRVLSTSST LTRDYNSLTR SEHSHSTTLP RDYSTLTSVS SH
                                        GLPPIWEH   1500
GRSRLPLSWA LGSRSRAQMK GFPPSRGPRD SIILAGRPAA PSWGP
                                           DSRLT   1550
AGVPDTPTRL VFSALGPTSL RVSWQEPRCE RPLQGYSVEY QLLNGGELHR   1600
LNIPNPAQTS VVVEDLLPNH SYVFRVRAQS QEGWGREREG VITIESQVHP   1650
QSPLCPLPGS AFTLSTPSAP GPLVFTALSP DSLQLSWERP RRPNGDIVGY   1700
LVTCEMAQGG GPATAFRVDG DSPESRLTVP GLSENVPYKF KVQARTTEGF   1750
GPEREGIITI ESQDGGPFPQ LGSRAGLFQH PLQSEYSSIT TTHTSATEPF   1800
LVDGPTLGAQ HLEAGGSLTR HVTQEFVSRT LTTSGTLSTH MDQQFFQT   1848
```

References

1. Garrod, D.R. (1993) Curr. Opin. Cell Biol. 5, 30–40.
2. Sonnenberg, A. et al. (1990) J. Cell Sci. 96, 207–217.
3. Natali, P.G. et al. (1992) J. Cell Sci. 103, 1243–1247.
4. Kennel, S.J. et al. (1992) J. Cell Sci. 101, 145–150.
5. Suzuki, S. and Naitoh, Y. (1990) EMBO J. 39, 757–763.
6. **Tamura, R.N. et al. (1990) J. Cell Biol. 111, 1593–1604.**
7. Hogervorst, F. et al. (1990) EMBO J. 9, 765–770.
8. Kajiji, S. (1989) EMBO J. 8, 673–680.
9. **Dowling, J. et al. (1996) J. Cell Biol. 134, 559–572.**
10. Niessen, C.M. et al. (1994) Exp. Cell Res. 211, 360–367.
11. Vidal, F. et al. (1995) Nature Genet. 10, 229–234.
12. Kennel, S.J. et al. (1993) Gene 130, 209–216.

CD105 Endoglin

Molecular weights
Polypeptide   68 095

SDS-PAGE
   reduced   95 kDa
   unreduced   170 kDa

Carbohydrate
N-linked sites   5
O-linked   +

Human gene location
9q34.1

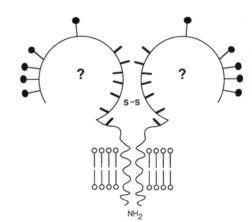

Tissue distribution

CD105 is present on endothelial cells. It is absent from most normal B and T cells, but is present on some leukaemic cells of B lymphoid and myeloid origin and on a subset of bone marrow cells[1,2]. CD105 expression can be induced on the surface of *in vitro* activated macrophages and macrophage cell lines[3,4].

Structure

CD105 is present at the cell surface as a disulfide-linked homodimer. O-glycosylation of CD105 has been demonstrated by digestion with O-glycanase. The O-glycosylation is likely to be on the membrane-proximal region that contains a high proportion of Thr, Ser and Pro residues[1]. The N-terminus has been established by protein sequencing. The sequence shows some patches of similarity with another receptor for TGFβ namely TGFβ receptor type III (β-glycan). The highest similarity is between the cytoplasmic domains at 70%, with an overall sequence identity of 30%[5].

Ligands and associated molecules

CD105 is a receptor for transforming growth factor β (TGFβ). CD105 binds with high affinity both the β1 isoform ($K_d = 50$ pM) and β3 isoform but not the β2 isoform of TGFβ[5]. CD105 exist in two forms (L and S isoforms) derived from alternative splicing in the cytoplasmic domain and both these isoforms bind TGFβ[6].

Function

CD105 is one of several receptors for the various isoforms of TGFβ, which in turn is one of a family of proteins involved in regulation of cell differentiation, migration of cells and control of the immune response. The level of CD105 increases in response to TGFβ. Cell lines transfected with CD105 show modulation of some of the effects of TGFβ although the mechanism is unclear[4].

Comments

Mutations in the gene for CD105 have been found in the disease hereditary haemorrhagic telangiectasia which is characterized by multisystemic vascular dysplasia and recurrent haemorrhage[7,8].

Database accession numbers

	PIR	SWISSPROT	EMBL/GENBANK	REFERENCE
Human	S37628	P17813*	X72012	1
Mouse	S42844		X77952	9

* Partial sequence (see EMBL entry for full length).

Amino acid sequence of human CD105 (L-endoglin isoform)

```
MDRGTLPLAV ALLLASCSLS PTSLA                         -1
ETVHCDLQPV GPERGEVTYT TSQVSKGCVA QAPNAILEVH VLFLEFPTGP  50
SQLELTLQAS KQNGTWPREV LLVLSVNSSV FLHLQALGIP LHLAYNSSLV 100
TFQEPPGVNT TELPSFPKTQ ILEWAAERGP ITSAAELNDP QSILLRLGQA 150
QGSLSFCMLE ASQDMGRTLE WRPRTPALVR GCHLEGVAGH KEAHILRVLP 200
GHSAGPRTVT VKVELSCAPG DLDAVLILQG PPYVSWLIDA NHNMQIWTTG 250
EYSFKIFPEK NIRGFKLPDT PQGLLGEARM LNASIVASFV ELPLASIVSL 300
HASSCGGRLQ TSPAPIQTTP PKDTCSPELL MSLIQTKCAD DAMTLVLKKE 350
LVAHLKCTIT GLTFWDPSCE AEDRGDKFVL RSAYSSCGMQ VSASMISNEA 400
VVNILSSSSP QRKKVHCLNM DSLSFQLGLY LSPHFLQASN TIEPGQQSFV 450
QVRVSPSVSE FLLQLDSCHL DLGPEGGTVE LIQGRAAKGN CVSLLSPSPE 500
GDPRFSFLLH FYTVPIPKTG TLSCTVALRP KTGSQDQEVH RTVFMRLNII 550
SPDLSGCTSK GLVLPAVLGI TGGAFLIGAL LTAALWYIYS HTRSPSKREP 600
VVAVAAPASS ESSSTNHSIG STQSTPCSTS SMA                 633
```

The C-terminal amino acid sequence of the human S-endoglin isoform[6] is as follows:

```
SPDLSGCTSK GLVLPAVLGI TGGAFLIGAL LTAALWYIYS HTREYPRPPQ 600
```

References
1. Gougos, A. and Letarte, M. (1990) J. Biol. Chem. 265, 8361–8364.
2. Rokhlin, O.W. et al. (1995) J. Immunol. 154, 4456–4465.
3. Lastres, P. et al. (1992) Eur. J. Immunol. 22, 393–397.
4. **Lastres, P. et al. (1996) J. Cell Biol. 133, 1109–1121.**
5. Cheifetz, S. et al. (1992) J. Biol. Chem. 267, 19027–19030.
6. Bellon, T. et al. (1993) Eur. J. Immunol. 23, 2340–2345.
7. **McAllister, K.A. et al. (1994) Nature Genet. 8, 345–351.**
8. http://www3.ncbi.nlm.nih.gov:80/htbin-post/Omim/dispmim?131195.
9. Ge, A.Z. and Butcher, E.C. (1994) Gene 138, 201–206.

CD106

VCAM-1, INCAM-110

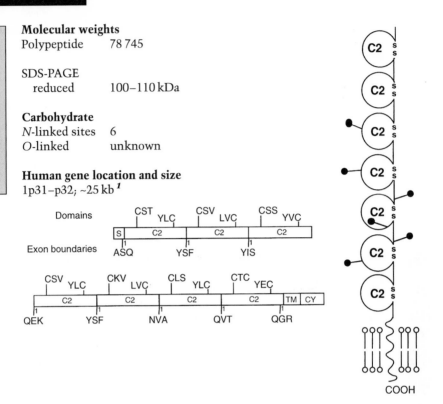

Molecular weights
Polypeptide   78 745

SDS-PAGE
  reduced   100–110 kDa

Carbohydrate
N-linked sites   6
O-linked   unknown

Human gene location and size
1p31–p32; ~25 kb [1]

Tissue distribution

CD106 is expressed predominantly on vascular endothelium but has also been identified on follicular and interfollicular dendritic cells, some macrophages, bone marrow stromal cells, and non-vascular cell populations within joints, kidney, muscle, heart, placenta and brain [2,3]. Expression on endothelial cells as well as many other cells is induced by inflammatory stimuli and cytokines [2,4]. Activated endothelial cells can release soluble forms of CD106 which can be detected in the blood [5].

Structure

CD106 has seven IgSF C2-set domains in its extracellular portion. Domains 1–3 show substantial sequence similarity to domains 4–5, consistant with an internal duplication event during CD106 evolution. Alternative splicing can produce a six IgSF domain form lacking domain 4 or, in the mouse, a GPI-anchored form of CD106 comprising domains 1–3 [2,3]. The structures of domains 1 and 2 have been determined by X-ray crystallography; as a result domain 1 was classified as an I-type IgSF domain on structural grounds [6,7]. The domains 1+2 and 4+5 fragments are closely related to the two IgSF domains of MAdCAM-1, which also binds the integrin α4β7 [7,8]. These portions of CD106 and MAdCAM-1 are also related to domains 1+2 of the β2 (CD18) integrin binding molecules CD50, CD54 and CD102. The membrane-distal domains of all these molecules have atypical disulfides between the B–C and F–G loops as well as an (I/L)(D/E)(S/T)xL motif in the C–D loop, which forms part of the integrin binding site[7]. CD106 is highly conserved between humans and rodents (~76% overall, 100% within cytoplasmic domain).

Ligands and associated molecules

CD106 binds the integrins $\alpha4\beta1$ (CD49d/CD29, VLA-4) and $\alpha4\beta7$[9]. VLA-4 is the dominant ligand in cells expressing both integrins[9]. CD106 has two independent binding sites for VLA-4 in domains 1 and 4, respectively[3]. Both sites lie on the GFC β-sheets of these domains and include the conserved C–D loop motif IDSPL[3].

Function

Endothelial CD106 contributes to the extravasation of lymphocytes, monocytes, basophils and eosinophils (but not neutrophils) from blood vessels, particularly at sites of inflammation[2-4]. Unlike the $\beta2$ integrins, the CD106/VLA-4 interaction can mediate both the initial tethering and rolling of lymphocytes on endothelium as well as their subsequent arrest and firm adhesion[10]. CD106 expressed in non-vascular tissues has been implicated in the interaction of haematopoietic progenitors with bone marrow stromal cells, B cell binding to follicular dendritic cells, co-stimulation of T cells, and embryonic development[2-4]. Mice deficient in CD106 have defects in the development of the placenta and heart and die during embryogenesis[11].

Database accession numbers (full-length form)

	PIR	SWISSPROT	EMBL/GENBANK	REFERENCE
Human	A41288	P19320	M73255	1
Mouse	JN0581	P29533	M84487	12
Rat	JS0675	P29534	M84488	12

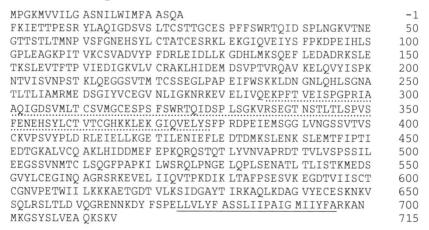

Amino acid sequence of human CD106

```
MPGKMVVILG ASNILWIMFA ASQA                              -1
FKIETTPESR YLAQIGDSVS LTCSTTGCES PFFSWRTQID SPLNGKVTNE   50
GTTSTLTMNP VSFGNEHSYL CTATCESRKL EKGIQVEIYS FPKDPEIHLS  100
GPLEAGKPIT VKCSVADVYP FDRLEIDLLK GDHLMKSQEF LEDADRKSLE  150
TKSLEVTFTP VIEDIGKVLV CRAKLHIDEM DSVPTVRQAV KELQVYISPK  200
NTVISVNPST KLQEGGSVTM TCSSEGLPAP EIFWSKKLDN GNLQHLSGNA  250
TLTLIAMRME DSGIYVCEGV NLIGKNRKEV ELIVQEKPFT VEISPGPRIA  300
AQIGDSVMLT CSVMGCESPS FSWRTQIDSP LSGKVRSEGT NSTLTLSPVS  350
FENEHSYLCT VTCGHKKLEK GIQVELYSFP RDPEIEMSGG LVNGSSVTVS  400
CKVPSVYPLD RLEIELLKGE TILENIEFLE DTDMKSLENK SLEMTFIPTI  450
EDTGKALVCQ AKLHIDDMEF EPKQRQSTQT LYVNVAPRDT TVLVSPSSIL  500
EEGSSVNMTC LSQGFPAPKI LWSRQLPNGE LQPLSENATL TLISTKMEDS  550
GVYLCEGINQ AGRSRKEVEL IIQVTPKDIK LTAFPSESVK EGDTVIISCT  600
CGNVPETWII LKKKAETGDT VLKSIDGAYT IRKAQLKDAG VYECESKNKV  650
SQLRSLTLD VQGRENNKDY FSPELLVLYF ASSLIIPAIG MIIYFARKAN  700
MKGSYSLVEA QKSKV                                       715
```

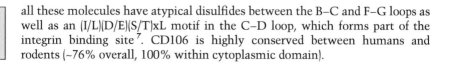

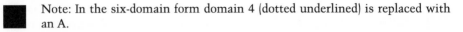

Note: In the six-domain form domain 4 (dotted underlined) is replaced with an A.

References

1. Cybulsky, M.I. et al. (1991) Proc. Natl Acad. Sci. USA 88, 7859–7863.
2. Bevilacqua, M.P. (1993) Annu. Rev. Immunol. 11, 767–804.
3. Vonderheide, R.H. et al. (1994) J. Cell. Biol. 125, 215–222.
4. **Carlos, T.M. and Harlan, J.M. (1994) Blood 84, 2068–2101.**
5. Gearing, A.J.H. and Newman, W. (1993) Immunol. Today 14, 506–512.
6. Harpaz, Y. and Chothia, C. (1994) J. Mol. Biol. 238, 528–539.
7. **Jones, E.Y. et al. (1995) Nature 373, 539–544.**
8. Shyjan, A.M. et al. (1996) J. Immunol. 156, 2851–2857.
9. Berlin, C. et al. (1993) Cell 74, 185–195.
10. Butcher, E.C. and Picker, L.J. (1996) Science 272, 60–66.
11. Kwee, L. et al. (1995) Development 121, 489–503.
12. Hession, C. et al. (1992) Biochem. Biophys. Res. Commun. 183, 163–169.

CD107a, CD107b

Other names
CD107a: lysosome-associated membrane protein-1 (lamp-1), lgp-120 (rat)
CD107b: lamp-2, lgp-110 (rat)

Molecular weights

Polypeptide	CD107a	41955
	CD107b	42012

SDS-PAGE

reduced	CD107a	120 kDa
	CD107b	120 kDa
unreduced	CD107a	120 kDa
	CD107b	120 kDa

Carbohydrate

N-linked sites	CD107a	19
	CD107b	17
O-linked	CD107a	+
	CD107b	+

Human gene location and size
CD107a: 13q34
CD107b: Xq24; >40 kb [1]

CD107a   CD107b

Tissue distribution

CD107a is expressed by granulocytes, T cells, macrophages, dendritic cells, activated platelets, endothelial cells, tonsillar epithelium and melanoma cells [2,3]. CD107b is expressed by granulocytes, activated platelets, TNFα-activated endothelial cells, tonsillar epithelium and melanoma cells [2,3].

Structure

CD107a and CD107b are both type I membrane glycoproteins, with 39% amino acid sequence identity, and constitute the major sialoglycoproteins on lysosomal membranes [3,4]. A smaller proportion of CD107a and CD107b can be detected on the plasma membrane. Both molecules are heavily glycosylated, containing 19 (CD107a) or 17 (CD107b) N-glycans, some of which are composed of very complex poly-N-acetyllactosamines [5]. Carbohydrates constitute 55–65% of the total mass in both CD107a and CD107b. The major portion of each molecule is located on the luminal side of lysosomes, anchored by a transmembrane region with a short cytoplasmic tail [3,4]. In both molecules the intraluminal portion comprises two internally related domains, separated by a hinge region rich in Pro and Ser residues (CD107a), or Pro and Thr residues (CD107b), which is O-glycosylated [6]. Both CD107a and CD107b contain the sequence GYXX in their cytoplasmic tail. This motif is also present in the cytoplasmic tail of CD63 and lysosomal acid phosphatase (LAP), both of which are transported to lysosomes [3]. The N-termini of CD107a and CD107b mature proteins have been determined by amino acid sequence analysis [4].

Ligands and associated molecules

Both CD107a and CD107b have been identified as ligands for galaptin, an S-type lectin (galectin) present in extracellular matrix, through its recognition of N-acetyllactosamine oligosaccharide chains[7]. In addition, CD62E binds to the sialyl-Lewis x structures displayed by poly-N-acetyllactosamines on CD107a[8,9].

Function

It has been suggested that CD107a and CD107b protect the inner surface of the lysosomal membrane by forming a barrier to soluble lysosomal hydrolases[3]. The upregulated expression of CD107a and CD107b on the surface of several tumour cell lines has been associated with their enhanced metastatic potential, where they may increase adhesion to extracellular matrix and endothelium[7-9].

Comments

Alternatively spliced forms of the CD107b gene are expressed in a tissue-specific manner[10].

Database accession numbers

	PIR	SWISSPROT	EMBL/GENBANK	REFERENCE
Human CD107a	A23656	P11279	J04182	4
Human CD107b	B23656	P13473	J04183	4
Mouse CD107a	A28067	P11438	J03881, M32015	11
Mouse CD107b	A35560	P17047	J05287	13
Rat CD107a	A30200	P14562	M34959	12
Rat CD107b	A36288	P17046	D90211	14

Amino acid sequence of human CD107a

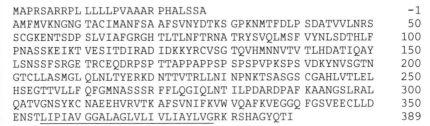

```
MAPRSARRPL LLLLPVAAAR PHALSSA                            -1
AMFMVKNGNG TACIMANFSA AFSVNYDTKS GPKNMTFDLP SDATVVLNRS    50
SCGKENTSDP SLVIAFGRGH TLTLNFTRNA TRYSVQLMSF VYNLSDTHLF   100
PNASSKEIKT VESITDIRAD IDKKYRCVSG TQVHMNNVTV TLHDATIQAY   150
LSNSSFSRGE TRCEQDRPSP TTAPPAPPSP SPSPVPKSPS VDKYNVSGTN   200
GTCLLASMGL QLNLTYERKD NTTVTRLLNI NPNKTSASGS CGAHLVTLEL   250
HSEGTTVLLF QFGMNASSSR FFLQGIQLNT ILPDARDPAF KAANGSLRAL   300
QATVGNSYKC NAEEHVRVTK AFSVNIFKVW VQAFKVEGGQ FGSVEECLLD   350
ENSTLIPIAV GGALAGLVLI VLIAYLVGRK RSHAGYQTI               389
```

Amino acid sequence of human CD107b

```
MVCFRLFPVP GSGLVLVCLV LGAVRSYA                           -1
LELNLTDSEN ATCLYAKWQM NFTVRYETTN KTYKTVTISD HGTVTYNGSI    50
CGDDQNGPKI AVQFGPGFSW IANFTKAAST YSNDSVSFSY NTGDNTTFPD   100
AEDKGILTVD ELLAIRIPLN DLFRCNSLST LEKNDVVQHY WDVLVQAFVQ   150
NGTVSTNEFL CDKDKTSTVA PTIHTTVPSP TTTPTPKEKP EAGTYSVNNG   200
NDTCLLATMG LQLNITQDKV ASVININPNT THSTGSCRSH TALLRLNSST   250
IKYLDFVFAV KNENRFYLKE VNISMYLVNG SVFSIANNNL SYWDAPLGSS   300
YMCNKEQTVS VSGAFQINTF DLRVQPFNVT QGKYSTAQDC SADDDNFLVP   350
IAVGAALAGV LILVLLAYFI GLKHHHAGYE QF                      382
```

References
1   Sawada, R. et al. (1993) J. Biol. Chem. 268, 9014–9022 (erratum: J. Biol. Chem. 268, 13010).
2   Azorsa, D.O. et al. (1995) Leucocyte Typing V, 1351.
3   **Fukuda, M. (1991) J. Biol. Chem. 266, 21327–21330.**
4   Fukuda, M. et al. (1988) J. Biol. Chem. 263, 18920–18928.
5   Carlsson, S.R. et al. (1988) J. Biol. Chem. 263, 18911–18919.
6   Carlsson, S.R. et al. (1993) Arch. Biochem. Biophys. 304, 65–73.
7   Woynarowska, B. et al. (1994) J. Biol. Chem. 269, 22797–22803.
8   Sawada, R. et al. (1993) J. Biol. Chem. 268, 12675–12681.
9   Sawada, R. et al. (1994) J. Biol. Chem. 269, 1425–1431.
10 Konecki, D.S. et al. (1995) Biochem. Biophys. Res. Commun. 215, 757–767.
11 Chen, J.W. et al. (1988) J. Biol. Chem. 263, 8754–8758.
12 Howe, C.L. et al. (1988) Proc. Natl Acad. Sci. USA 85, 7577–7581.
13 Cha, Y. et al. (1990) J. Biol. Chem. 265, 5008–5013.
14 Noguchi, Y. et al. (1989) Biochem. Biophys. Res. Commun. 164, 1113–1120.

CDw108

Molecular weights

SDS-PAGE
   reduced   80 kDa
   unreduced   75 kDa

Tissue distribution

CDw108 is expressed weakly on some lymphoid, myeloid and stromal cells, and highly expressed on the leukaemic T cell line HPB-ALL [1].

Structure

CDw108 is a GPI-linked glycoprotein that contains 20% of *N*-linked carbohydrate by mass [1].

Function

Unknown.

Comments

The CDw108 antigen is identical to the JMH erythrocyte blood group antigen [2].

References
[1] Klickstein, L.B. and Springer, T.A. (1995) Leucocyte Typing V, 1477–1478.
[2] Mudad, R. et al. (1995) Transfusion 35, 566–570.

CD109 Gov$^{a/b}$ alloantigen

Molecular weights

SDS-PAGE
reduced   175 kDa
unreduced   175 kDa

Carbohydrate
N-linked sites   yes
O-linked sites   no

Tissue distribution

CD109 carries the epitopes for the Gov$^{a/b}$ alloantigen on platelets [1]. It is also expressed on activated T cells, human umbilical vein endothelial cells and several tumor cell lines. It is not expressed on resting lymphocytes, neutrophils, or erythrocytes [1,2].

Structure

CD109 is a GPI-linked protein on T cells, tumour cells and endothelial cells [3]. However, only about 50% of the antigen can be released from platelets by phosphatidylinositol-specific phospholipase C [1]. Multiple chains are observed by immunoprecipitation but the lower bands are proteolytic products of the single chain at 175 kDa. Two N-linked sites have been found by peptide mapping [4]. No change in polypeptide chain size is observed with O-glycanase [1].

Function

Unknown. Alloantibodies against CD109 have been identified in patients following multiple platelet transfusions [5]. The alloantigenicity of CD109 has been implicated in post-transfusion purpura and alloimmune neonatal thrombocytopenia [1].

References
[1] **Smith, J.W. et al. (1995) Blood 86, 2807–2814.**
[2] Brashem-Stein, C. et al. (1988) J. Immunol. 140, 2330–2333.
[3] Haregewoin, A. et al. (1994) Cell. Immunol. 156, 357–370.
[4] Sutherland, D.R. et al. (1991) Blood 77, 84–93.
[5] Kelton, J.G. et al. (1990) Blood 75, 2172–2176.

Molecular weights
Polypeptide   107 350

SDS-PAGE
    reduced   145 kDa

Carbohydrate
N-linked sites   10
O-linked   unknown

Human gene location and size
4q11–q12; >70 kb [1]

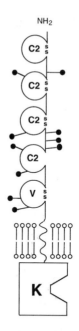

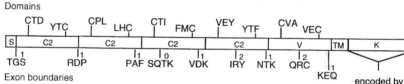

Domains

CTD   YTC   CPL   LHC   CTI   FMC   VEY   YTF   CVA   VEC

| S | C2 | C2 | C2 | C2 | V | TM | K |

Exon boundaries

TGS   RDP   PAF SQTK   VDK   IRY   NTK   QRC   KEQ

encoded by 12 exons

Tissue distribution

Human CD117 is expressed on 1–4% of bone marrow cells, the majority of which (50–70%) also express CD34 and comprise pluripotent haematopoietic progenitor cells [2]. CD117 is also expressed on human mast cells and acute myeloid leukaemic cells, while CD117 mRNA has been detected in melanocytes, primordial germ cells, small cell lung cancers and seminomas [2]. In the mouse, CD117 is expressed on almost all haematopoietic progenitor cells including colony-forming cells reactive to IL-3, GM-CSF and M-CSF, but not on B-lineage progenitors which form colonies in response to IL-7 [3]. It is also expressed on the surface of mouse mast cells, melanocytes, spermatogonia and oocytes [3].

Structure

CD117 belongs to subclass III within the family of growth factor receptors with tyrosine kinase activity, that also includes CD115 (M-CSFR) and the PDGF receptors type A and B (CD140a and CD140b) [4,5]. The extracellular domain of CD117 consists of five IgSF domains (four C2-set and one V-set), followed by a transmembrane sequence and a cytoplasmic region containing a tyrosine kinase domain, which is interrupted by an insertion sequence of 77 amino acids [4].

Ligands and associated molecules

The natural ligand for CD117 is c-kit ligand (also known as stem cell growth factor, steel factor and mast cell growth factor), a growth factor which is biologically active in both membrane-bound and soluble form (see **c-kitL**)[6]. CD117 transduces transmembrane signals by interaction with phosphatidylinositol 3-kinase, Raf1 and, to some extent, phospholipase C-γ[7].

Function

The interaction of c-kit ligand with CD117 is crucial for the development of haematopoietic, gonadal and pigment stem cells (reviewed in ref. 8). c-kit ligand also increases the sensitivity of human mucosal mast cells to crosslinking of the high-affinity IgE receptor[9]. In mice, mutations of the *W* and *Sl* loci, which encode CD117 and c-kit ligand respectively, lead to alterations of coat colour (white spotting), anaemia and defective gonad development[8]. In humans, naturally occurring mutations within the CD117 gene have been identified as the cause of piebaldism, an autosomal dominant disorder of pigmentation. These mutations are reviewed in OMIM entries 164920 and 172800 (see Chapter 1 for methods to access OMIM).

Comment

The feline v-kit oncogene has lost the extracellular and transmembrane domains as well as the proximal cytoplasmic and the C-terminal amino acids. The last 49 amino acids have been replaced by five amino acids due to fusion with the feline leukaemia polymerase gene[4].

Database accession numbers

	PIR	SWISSPROT	EMBL/GENBANK	REFERENCE
Human	S01426	P10721	X06182	4
Mouse	S00474	P05532	Y00864	10

Amino acid sequence of human CD117

```
MRGARGAWDF LCVLLLLLRV QT                                 -1
GSSQPSVSPG EPSPPSIHPG KSDLIVRVGD EIRLLCTDPG FVKWTFEILD    50
ETNENKQNEW ITEKAEATNT GKYTCTNKHG LSNSIYVFVR DPAKLFLVDR   100
SLYGKEDNDT LVRCPLTDPE VTNYSLKGCQ GKPLPKDLRF IPDPKAGIMI   150
KSVKRAYHRL CLHCSVDQEG KSVLSEKFIL KVRPAFKAVP VVSVSKASYL   200
LREGEEFTVT CTIKDVSSSV YSTWKRENSQ TKLQEKYNSW HHGDFNYERQ   250
ATLTISSARV NDSGVFMCYA NNTFGSANVT TTLEVVDKGF INIFPMINTT   300
VFVNDGENVD LIVEYEAFPK PEHQQWIYMN RTFTDKWEDY PKSENESNIR   350
YVSELHLTRL KGTEGGTYTF LVSNSDVNAA IAFNVYVNTK PEILTYDRLV   400
NGMLQCVAAG FPEPTIDWYF CPGTEQRCSA SVLPVDVQTL NSSGPPFGKL   450
VVQSSIDSSA FKHNGTVECK AYNDVGKTSA YFNFAFKGNN KEQIHPHTLF   500
TPLLIGFVIV AGMMCIIVMI LTYKYLQKPM YEVQWKVVEE INGNNYVYID   550
```

```
PTQLPYDHKW EFPRNRLSFG KTLGAGAFGK VVEATAYGLI KSDAAMTVAV   600
KMLKPSAHLT EREALMSELK VLSYLGNHMN IVNLLGACTI GGPTLVITEY   650
CCYGDLLNFL RRKRDSFICS KQEDHAEAAL YKNLLHSKES SCSDSTNEYM   700
DMKPGVSYVV PTKADKRRSV RIGSYIERDV TPAIMEDDEL ALDLEDLLSF   750
SYQVAKGMAF LASKNCIHRD LAARNILLTH GRITKICDFG LARDIKNDSN   800
YVVKGNARLP VKWMAPESIF NCVYTFESDV WSYGIFLWEL FSLGSSPYPG   850
MPVDSKFYKM IKEGFRMLSP EHAPAEMYDI MKTCWDADPL KRPTFKQIVQ   900
LIEKQISEST NHIYSNLANC SPNRQKPVVD HSVRINSVGS TASSSQPLLV   950
HDDV                                                    954
```

References

1 Vandenbark, G.R. et al. (1992) Oncogene 7, 1259–1266.
2 Bühring, H–J. et al. (1995) Leucocyte Typing V, 1882–1888.
3 Ogawa, M. et al. (1991) J. Exp. Med. 174, 63–71.
4 **Yarden, Y. et al. (1987) EMBO J. 6, 3341–3351.**
5 Ullrich, A. and Schlessinger, J. (1990) Cell 61, 203–212.
6 Callard, R.E. and Gearing, A.J.H. (1994) The Cytokine FactsBook. Academic Press, London.
7 Lev, S. et al. (1991) EMBO J. 10, 647–654.
8 **Witte, O.N. (1990) Cell 63, 5–6.**
9 Bischoff, S.C. et al. (1992) J. Exp. Med. 175, 237–244.
10 Qiu, F. et al. (1988) EMBO J. 7, 1003–1011.

CD120a, CD120b

Other names
TNFRI and TNFRII (tumour necrosis factor receptors I and II)
TNF-R55 and TNF-R75

Molecular weights
Polypeptide	CD120a	48 307
	CD120b	46 091

SDS-PAGE
reduced	CD120a	50–60 kDa
	CD120b	75–85 kDa

Carbohydrate
N-linked sites	CD120a	3
	CD120b	2
O-linked	CD120a	nil
	CD120b	probable +

Human gene locations and size
CD120a: 12p13.2
CD120b: 1p36.3–p36.2; 43 kb [1]

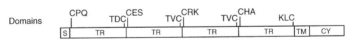

CD120a

Domains						
	CPQ	CES CRK CHA				
	TDC	TVC TVC			KLC	
S	TR	TR	TR	TR	TM	CY

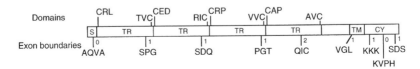

CD120b

Domains						
	CRL CED CRP CAP					
	TVC RIC VVC AVC					
S	TR	TR	TR	TR	TM	CY

Exon boundaries
|0| |1| |1| |1| |2| |1| |1| |0| |1|
| AQVA | SPG | SDQ | PGT | QIC | | VGL | KKK | SDS |
| | | | | | | | | KVPH |

Tissue distribution
Most cell types express both of the two receptors for TNF. CD120a is con-stitutively expressed at a low level and CD120b expression is inducible [2,3].

Structure
Both receptors are members of the TNFR superfamily, and contain four cysteine-rich repeats, but are <25% identical to each other, i.e. no more similar to each other than to the other members of this family of receptors [4–6]. The structure of a complex between the trimeric lymphotoxin α (LTα) and three molecules of the extracellular domain of CD120a has been determined by X-ray crystallography [7]. The structure of the extracellular domain of CD120a has also been determined in the absence of ligand, and it

forms a dimer but it is not known whether this occurs at the membrane[8]. CD120a contains a 'death domain' within the cytoplasmic region[9].

Ligands and associated molecules

Both receptors bind TNFα and LTα with relatively high affinity $(K_d < 10^{-9} \text{M}^{-1})$[10]. Membrane bound and soluble TNF and LTα bind to CD120a and CD120b[2]. A third TNF-like protein, lymphotoxin β (LTβ) forms heterocomplexes with LTα at the cell surface but these do not bind CD120a or CD120b but to a separate lymphotoxin-beta receptor[11]. Several different proteins can associate directly or indirectly with the cytoplasmic parts of CD120a and b, including TNF receptor-associated factors (TRAF), TNF receptor-associated proteins (TRAP), TNF receptor-associated kinase (TRAK) and TRADD (TNFR1-associated death domain protein)[3,12]. The 'death domain' within the cytoplasmic region of CD120a self-associates[10].

Function

CD120a and CD120b are receptors for both TNFα and TNFβ (LTα) which are cytokines produced primarily by macrophages/monocytes, activated T cells and NK cells in response to bacterial, viral and parasitic infections[13]. TNF mediates a wide variety of effects including tumour necrosis, anorexia, fever, induction of other cytokines, cell differentiation and apoptosis. The most effective cell killing occurs when membrane bound TNF crosslinks both CD120a and CD120b[2]. Crosslinking of the TNF receptors by soluble or membrane bound TNF leads to signalling which is mediated by a variety of associated molecules leading to different pathways[2,3,14]. Signalling is mainly mediated through CD120a[3].

Database accession numbers

	PIR	SWISSPROT	EMBL/GENBANK	REFERENCE
Human CD120a	A34899	P19438	M33294	5,6
Human CD120b	A35356	P20333	M35857	4
Rat CD120a	B36555	P22934	M63122, M75862	15
Mouse CD120a			M60468, X59238	16
Mouse CD120b			M60469	16

Amino acid sequence of human CD120a

```
MGLSTVPDLL LPLVLLELLV G                                    -1
IYPSGVIGLV PHLGDREKRD SVCPQGKYIH PQNNSICCTK CHKGTYLYND     50
CPGPGQDTDC RECESGSFTA SENHLRHCLS CSKCRKEMGQ VEISSCTVDR     100
DTVCGCRKNQ YRHYWSENLF QCFNCSLCLN GTVHLSCQEK QNTVCTCHAG     150
FFLRENECVS CSNCKKSLEC TKLCLPQIEN VKGTEDSGTT VLLPLVIFFG     200
LCLLSLLFIG LMYRYQRWKS KLYSIVCGKS TPEKEGELEG TTTKPLAPNP     250
SFSPTPGFTP TLGFSPVPSS TFTSSSTYTP GDCPNFAAPR REVAPPYQGA     300
DPILATALAS DPIPNPLQKW EDSAHKPQSL DTDDPATLYA VVENVPPLRW     350
KEFVRRLGLS DHEIDRLELQ NGRCLREAQY SMLATWRRRT PRREATLELL     400
GRVLRDMDLL GCLEDIEEAL CGPAALPPAP SLLR                      434
```

Amino acid sequence of human CD120b

```
MAPVAVWAAL AVGLELWAAA HA                                     -1
LPAQVAFTPY APEPGSTCRL REYYDQTAQM CCSKCSPGQH AKVFCTKTSD       50
TVCDSCEDST YTQLWNWVPE CLSCGSRCSS DQVETQACTR EQNRICTCRP      100
GWYCALSKQE GCRLCAPLRK CRPGFGVARP GTETSDVVCK PCAPGTFSNT      150
TSSTDICRPH QICNVVAIPG NASMDAVCTS TSPTRSMAPG AVHLPQPVST      200
RSQHTQPTPE PSTAPSTSFL LPMGPSPPAE GSTGDFALPV GLIVGVTALG      250
LLIIGVVNCV IMTQVKKKPL CLQREAKVPH LPADKARGTQ GPEQQHLLIT      300
APSSSSSSLE SSASALDRRA PTRNQPQAPG VEASGAGEAR ASTGSSDSSP      350
GGHGTQVNVT CIVNVCSSSD HSSQCSSQAS STMGDTDSSP SESPKDEQVP      400
FSKEECAFRS QLETPETLLG STEEKPLPLG VPDAGMKPS                  439
```

References

1 Santee, S. and Owen-Schaub, L. (1996) J. Biol. Chem. 271, 21151–21159.
2 Grell, M. et al. (1995) Cell 83, 793–802.
3 **Vandenabeele, P. et al. (1995) Trends Cell Biol. 5, 392–399.**
4 Smith, C.A. et al. (1990) Science 248, 1019–1023.
5 Schall, T.J. et al. (1990) Cell 61, 631–370.
6 Loetscher, H. et al. (1990) Cell 61, 351–359.
7 Banner, D.W. et al. (1993) Cell 73, 431–45.
8 Naismith, J. et al. (1995) J. Biol. Chem. 270, 13303–13307.
9 Boldin, M. et al. (1995) J. Biol. Chem. 270, 387–391.
10 Brockhaus, M. et al. (1990) Proc. Natl Acad. Sci. USA 87, 3127–3131.
11 Crowe, P. et al. (1994) Science 264, 707–710.
12 Darnay, B. et al. (1995) J. Biol. Chem. 270, 14867–14870.
13 Tracey, K. and Cerami, A. (1993) Annu. Rev. Cell Biol. 9, 317–343.
14 **Liu, Z.-g. et al. (1996) Cell 87, 565–576.**
15 Himmler, A. et al. (1990) DNA Cell Biol. 9, 705–715.
16 Lewis, M. et al. (1991) Proc. Natl Acad. Sci. USA 88, 2830–2834.

CD134   OX40, MRC OX40, ACT35 antigen

Molecular weights
Polypeptide   26 602

SDS-PAGE
   reduced   47–51 kDa
   unreduced   51–55 kDa

Carbohydrate
N-linked sites   2
O-linked   probable +

Human gene location
1p36 [1,2]

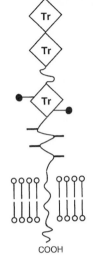

Domains

	CVG		CGP		CPP				
		TVC		TVC		AIC			
S	Tr		Tr		Tr			TM	CY

Tissue distribution

CD134 was originally named MRC OX40 after the first antibody. CD134 is specifically expressed on activated T cells with maximum expression at 24 h after stimulation [1-5]. In the rat, CD134 is only found on activated rat CD4[+] T cells with 32 000 sites per cell [3] and in human it is described as predominantly on CD4[+] cells [2]. In mouse, CD134 is expressed on both activated CD4[+] and CD4[+]CD8α[+] cells [4].

Structure

CD134 is a member of the TNFR superfamily, with three complete Cys-rich repeats [1,3,6]. The membrane-proximal hinge region contains possible sites for O-linked glycosylation [2,3].

Ligands and associated molecules

CD134 binds to OX40 ligand (OX40L) [7] and there is no evidence for another ligand [4]. The affinity of monomeric CD134 for OX40L is 190 nM and of trimeric OX40L for CD134 on the surface of activated T cells is 0.2 nM [8]. Three CD134 receptors bind one OX40L trimer [8].

Function

OX40L binding to CD134 on T cells co-stimulates proliferation [1]. Crosslinking OX40L on activated B cells stimulates proliferation and antibody production [5]. Similarly, blocking the OX40L–CD134 interaction reduced antibody production, suggesting a role in differentiation into plasma cells[5].

Database accession numbers

	PIR	SWISSPROT	EMBL/GENBANK	REFERENCE
Human		P43489	X75962	2
Rat	S12783	P15725	X17037	3
Mouse		P47741	Z21674	9

Amino acid sequence of human CD134

```
MCVGARRLGR GPCAALLLLG LGLSTVTG                               -1
LHCVGDTYPS NDRCCHECRP GNGMVSRCSR SQNTVCRPCG PGFYNDVVSS       50
KPCKPCTWCN LRSGSERKQL CTATQDTVCR CRAGTQPLDS YKPGVDCAPC       100
PPGHFSPGDN QACKPWTNCT LAGKHTLQPA SNSSDAICED RDPPATQPQE       150
TQGPPARPIT VQPTEAWPRT SQGPSTRPVE VPGGRAVAAI LGLGLVLGLL       200
GPLAILLALY LLRRDQRLPP DAHKPPGGGS FRTPIQEEQA DAHSTLAKI        249
```

References
1. Gruss, H.-J. and Dower, S.K. (1995) Blood 85, 3378–3404.
2. Latza, U. et al. (1994) Eur. J. Immunol. 24, 677–683.
3. Mallett, S. et al. (1990) EMBO J. 9, 1063–1068.
4. Al-Shamkhani, A. et al. (1996) Eur. J. Immunol. 26, 1695–1699.
5. **Stuber, E. and Strober, W. (1996) J. Exp. Med. 183, 979–989.**
6. van Kooten, C. and Banchereau, J. (1996) Adv. Immunol. 61, 1–77.
7. Baum, P.R. et al. (1994) EMBO J. 13, 3992–4001.
8. Al-Shamkhani, A. et al. (1997) J. Biol. Chem. 272, 5275–5282.
9. Calderhead, D.M. et al. (1993) J. Immunol. 151, 5261–5271.

CD135

STK-1, FLT3, flk-2

Molecular weights
Polypeptide   110 131

SDS-PAGE
  reduced (doublet)   130/160 kDa

Carbohydrate
N-linked sites   10
O-linked sites   unknown

Human gene location
13q12

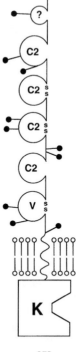

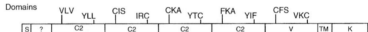

Tissue distribution

CD135 is expressed on CD34⁺ haematopoietic stem cells[1]. It has also been detected in mouse brain[2].

Structure

CD135 has five IgSF domains, a single transmembrane segment, and a cytoplasmic region containing a protein kinase domain with an internal kinase insert domain[1,2]. It is a member of the type III receptor tyrosine kinase family which includes c-kit, M-CSFR (CD115) and PDGFR (CD140)[3]. A short sequence that shows no similarity to other proteins precedes the first IgSF domain. The IgSF domains contain a number of cysteines in atypical positions and so the domain assignments are tentative. Domains 1 and 2 show substantial similarity to domains 4 and 5, suggesting an internal duplication event during evolution. Cell lines expressing CD135 show protein products of 130 and 160 kDa, probably due to differential glycosylation.

Ligands and associated molecules

CD135 binds FLT3 ligand[4].

Function

CD135 is likely to be involved in growth and differentiation of primitive haematopoietic cells. Antisense RNA of CD135 has been shown to inhibit colony-forming activity of long-term bone marrow culture cells [1].

Database accession numbers

	PIR	SWISSPROT	EMBL/GENBANK	REFERENCE
Human		P36888	U02687	1
Mouse	A39931	Q00342	M64689	2
			X59398	5

Amino acid sequence of human CD135

```
MPALARDAGT VPLLVVFSAM IFGTIT                                 -1
NQDLPVIKCV LINHKNNDSS VGKSSSYPMV SESPEDLGCA LRPQSSGTVY        50
EAAAVEVDVS ASITLQVLVD APGNISCLWV FKHSSLNCQP HFDLQNRGVV       100
SMVILKMTET QAGEYLLFIQ SEATNYTILF TVSIRNTLLY TLRRPYFRKM       150
ENQDALVCIS ESVPEPIVEW VLCDSQGESC KEESPAVVKK EEKVLHELFG       200
TDIRCCARNE LGRECTRLFT IDLNQTPQTT LPQLFLKVGE PLWIRCKAVH       250
VNHGFGLTWE LENKALEEGN YFEMSTYSTN RTMIRILFAF VSSVARNDTG       300
YYTCSSSKHP SQSALVTIVG KGFINATNSS EDYEIDQYEE FCFSVRFKAY       350
PQIRCTWTFS RKSFPCEQKG LDNGYSISKF CNHKHQPGEY IFHAENDDAQ       400
FTKMFTLNIR RKPQVLAEAS ASQASCFSDG YPLPSWTWKK CSDKSPNCTE       450
EITEGVWNRK ANRKVFGQWV SSSTLNMSEA IKGFLVKCCA YNSLGTSCET       500
ILLNSPGPFP FIQDNISFYA TIGVCLLFIV VLTLLICHKY KKQFRYESQL       550
QMVQVTGSSD NEYFYVDFRE YEYDLKWEFP RENLEFGKVL GSGAFGKVMN       600
ATAYGISKTG VSIQVAVKML KEKADSSERE ALMSELKMMT QLGSHENIVN       650
LLGACTLSGP IYLIFEYCCY GDLLNYLRSK REKFHRTWTE IFKEHNFSFY       700
PTFQSHPNSS MPGSREVQIH PDSDQISGLH GNSFHSEDEI EYENQKRLEE       750
EEDLNVLTFE DLLCFAYQVA KGMEFLEFKS CVHRDLAARN VLVTHGKVVK       800
ICDFGLARDI MSDSNYVVRG NARLPVKWMA PESLFEGIYT IKSDVWSYGI       850
LLWEIFSLGV NPYPGIPVDA NFYKLIQNGF KMDQPFYATE EIYIIMQSCW       900
AFDSRKRPSF PNLTSFLGCQ LADAEEAMYQ NVDGRVSECP HTYQNRRPFS       950
REMDLGLLSP QAQVEDS                                          967
```

References
[1] **Small, D. et al. (1994) Proc. Natl Acad. Sci. USA 91, 459–463.**
[2] Matthews, W. et al. (1991) Cell 65, 1143–1152.
[3] Ullrich, A. and Schlessinger, J. (1990) Cell 61, 203–212.
[4] Hannum, C. et al. (1994) Nature 368, 643–648.
[5] Rosnet, O. et al. (1991) Oncogene 6, 1641–1650.

CDw137 4-1BB ILA

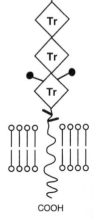

Molecular weight
Polypeptide   26 079

SDS-PAGE
    reduced   28–30 kDa
    unreduced   28–30, 55 (major form) and 110 kDa

Carbohydrate
N-linked sites   2
O-linked   probable +

Human gene location
1p36

COOH

Domains

CPP   CTP   CCF
    AEC   KGC   VVC
S | Tr | Tr | Tr | TM | CY

Tissue distribution

Human CDw137 mRNA is absent from resting T cells but on activation is induced in T and B cells and in monocytes [1]. It is also detected in activated non-lymphoid cells [1]. Expression on the surface of activated human T cells was indicated with peptide antibodies [1]. Peptide antibodies showed that mouse CDw137 is expressed on activated thymocytes and activated splenic T cells, CD4+ and CD8+ T cells [2,3]. Mouse CDw137 mRNA was not found in activated B cells [2].

Structure

CDw137 encodes for a transmembrane protein that contains three TNFR repeats [3-6]. The second and third Cys residues in the first repeat of CDw137 are not adjacent, as they are in the first repeats of other members of this superfamily, but are separated by two amino acids, as they are in a typical second repeat [3,5,6]. The cytoplasmic domain of mouse CDw137 contains a sequence, CSCRCP, which resembles the CXCP motif for the Lck recognition site found in CD4 and CD8 [5,7]. Human CDw137 has a slightly different sequence CSCRFP. The cytoplasmic domain contains a high proportion of consecutive acidic residues [5,7]. SDS-PAGE analysis revealed disulfide-linked forms of CDw137 but it is not clear from sequence analysis how these form or their physiological significance [2].

Ligands and associated molecules

CDw137 binds to 4-1BBL, a type II membrane protein of the TNF superfamily [3,4]. CDw137 has been reported to bind to extracellular matrix [3]. Lck is co-precipitated with mouse CDw137 and Cys20 and Cys23 of Lck are critical for the association [7].

Function

4-1BBL binding to CDw137 can co-stimulate T cell growth and this can be blocked by soluble CDw137 [8,9]. Reciprocally, CDw137 binding to 4-1BBL can co-stimulate B cells [1].

Database accession numbers

	PIR	SWISSPROT	EMBL/GENBANK	REFERENCE
Human		Q07011	U03397	4
Mouse	B32393	P20334	J04492	10

Amino acid sequence of human CDw137

```
MGNSCYNIVA TLLLVLN                                            -1
FERTRSLQDP CSNCPAGTFC DNNRNQICSP CPPNSFSSAG GQRTCDICRQ        50
CKGVFRTRKE CSSTSNAECD CTPGFHCLGA GCSMCEQDCK QGQELTKKGC       100
KDCCFGTFND QKRGICRPWT NCSLDGKSVL VNGTKERDVV CGPSPADLSP       150
GASSVTPPAP AREPGHSPQI ISFFLALTST ALLFLLFFLT LRFSVVKRGR       200
KKLLYIFKQP FMRPVQTTQE EDGCSCRFPE EEEGGCEL                    238
```

References

1 Schwartz, H. et al. (1995) Blood 85, 1043–1052.
2 Pollock, K.E. et al. (1993) J. Immunol. 150, 771–781.
3 Gruss, H.-J. and Dower, S.K. (1995) Blood 85, 3378–3404.
4 **Alderson, M.R. et al. (1994) Eur. J. Immunol. 24, 2219–2227.**
5 Armitage, R.J. (1994) Curr. Opin. Immunol. 6, 407–413.
6 van Kooten, C. and Banchereau, J. (1996) Adv. Immunol. 61, 1–77.
7 Kim, Y-J. et al. (1993) J. Immunol. 151, 1255–1262.
8 Hurtado, J.C. et al. (1995) J. Immunol. 155, 3360–3367.
9 DeBenedette, M.A. et al. (1995) J. Exp. Med. 181, 985–992.
10 Kwon, B.S. and Weissman, S.M. (1989) Proc. Natl Acad. Sci. USA 86, 1963–1967.

CD138

Syndecan-1

Molecular weights

Polypeptide		30 507
SDS-PAGE		
unreduced	(immature B cells)	92 kDa
	(plasma cells)	85 kDa

Carbohydrate

N-linked sites	1
O-linked sites	probably +
Glycosaminoglycans	5

Human gene location
2p23

COOH

Tissue distribution

CD138 is expressed on pre-B cells, immature B cells and plasma cells, but not on mature circulating B lymphocytes. It is also expressed on the basolateral surfaces of epithelial cells, embryonic mesenchymal cells, vascular smooth muscle cells, endothelium and neural cells [1-4].

Structure

CD138 has an extended backbone with five glycosaminoglycan (GAG) attachment sites [5,6]. Site utilization varies: in the mouse, the three distal sites (Ser20, Ser28 and Ser30) are usually modified by heparan sulfate, whereas the two sites close to the membrane (Ser190 and Ser200; equivalent to Ser189 and Ser199 in the human), are usually occupied by chondroitin sulfate [7]. In addition, the structure of the GAG chains may be cell type-specific [8]. CD138 is highly conserved (>90%) between the human and the mouse. The single N-glycosylation site may serve to regulate the glycanation of the distal cluster [5,9]. CD138 is closely related to syndecan-2 (fibroglycan), syndecan-3 (N-syndecan) and syndecan-4 (amphiglycan or ryudocan); although the extracellular protein cores are different they have very similar transmembrane and cytoplasmic domains [3]. Their expression patterns also vary, suggesting that they have tissue-specific functions.

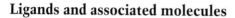

Ligands and associated molecules

CD138 has been shown to bind many extracellular matrix proteins through its heparan sulfate side-chains, including fibronectin, collagen types I, III and V, tenascin, thrombospondin and antithrombin III[2,3]. The cytoplasmic region of CD138 is known to interact with actin-rich microfilaments[10]. CD138 on the cell surface may be regulated to form oligomeric complexes, since antibody-induced clustering causes CD138 to become insoluble in non-ionic detergents[11]. This aggregation is mediated by the transmembrane segment[10]. CD138 has been shown to bind fibroblast growth factor 2 (FGF-2)[12].

Function

CD138 is an extracellular matrix receptor[2-4]. It may serve as a co-receptor for FGF and related molecules. FGF-2 appears to require an association with heparan sulfate-bearing molecules (such as CD138) to transduce signals via the FGF receptor[12,13].

Database accession numbers

	PIR	SWISSPROT	EMBL/GENBANK	REFERENCE
Human	A41176	P18827	J05392	5
			X60306	6
Mouse	S06619	P18828	X15487	9
			Z22532	14

Amino acid sequence of human CD138

```
MRRAALWLWL CALALSL                                             -1
QPALPQIVAT NLPPEDQDGS GDDSDNFSGS GAGALQDITL SQQTPSTWKD         50
TQLLTAIPTS PEPTGLEATA ASTSTLPAGE GPKEGEAVVL PEVEPGLTAR        100
EQEATPRPRE TTQLPTTHQA STTTATTAQE PATSHPHRDM QPGHHETSTP        150
AGPSQADLHT PHTEDGGPSA TERAAEDGAS SQLPAAEGSG EQDFTFETSG        200
ENTAVVAVEP DRRNQSPVDQ GATGASQGLL DRKEVLGGVI AGGLVGLIFA        250
VCLVGFMLYR MKKKDEGSYS LEEPKQANGG AYQKPTKQEE FYA              293
```

References

1   Sanderson, R.D. et al. (1989) Cell Regul. 1, 27–35.
2   **Bernfield, M. et al. (1992) Annu. Rev. Cell Biol. 8, 365–393.**
3   **Couchman, J.R. and Woods, A. (1996) J. Cell. Biochem. 61, 578–584.**
4   David, G. (1993) FASEB J. 7, 1023–1030.
5   Mali, M. et al. (1990) J. Biol. Chem. 265, 6884–6889.
6   Lories, V. et al. (1992) J. Biol. Chem. 267, 1116–1122.
7   Kokenyesi, R. and Bernfield, M. (1994) J. Biol. Chem. 269, 12304–12309.
8   Kato, M. et al. (1994) J. Biol. Chem. 269, 18881–18890.
9   Saunders, S. et al. (1989) J. Cell Biol. 108, 1547–1556.
10 Carey, D.J. et al. (1996) J. Biol. Chem. 271, 15253–15260.
11 Miettinen, H.M. et al. (1994) J. Cell Sci. 107, 1571–1581.
12 Yayon, A. et al. (1991) Cell 64, 841–848.
13 Aviezer, D. et al. (1994) Cell 79, 1005–1013.
14 Vihinen, T. et al. (1993) J. Biol. Chem. 268, 17261–17269.

CD147

Other names
EMMPRIN (human)
M6 (human)
OX-47 (rat)
CE9 (rat)
Basigin (mouse)
gp42 (mouse)
Neurothelin (chicken)
HT7 (chicken)
5A11 (chicken)

Molecular weights
Polypeptide   27 563

SDS-PAGE
  reduced   65 kDa
  unreduced   54 kDa

Carbohydrate
N-linked sites   3
O-linked   unknown

Human gene location
19p13.3

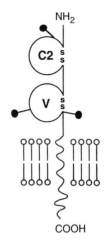

Domains

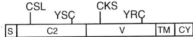

Tissue distribution

The CD147 antigen has a broad expression pattern in both haematopoietic and non-haematopoietic tissues in all four species and is upregulated upon cell activation. CD147 is expressed weakly on resting leucocytes but is strongly upregulated on activated lymphocytes and monocytes[1]. CD147 is expressed on various epithelial cells with some differences between species, e.g. rat[2,3], mouse[4] and chicken[5].

Structure

The CD147 antigen consists of two IgSF domains, a transmembrane sequence containing a charged residue (Glu) and a cytoplasmic domain of 40 residues. The N-terminal IgSF domain belongs to the C2-set and the membrane proximal domain belongs to the V-set. This is unusual since most members of the IgSF that contain V- and C2-set domains have the opposite arrangement[2]. In the chicken, the second domain belongs to the C2-set[5]. The extent of CD147 glycosylation is tissue-specific and is responsible for a variation in the apparent molecular mass from 40 kDa to 68 kDa[3]. Within the transmembrane region, the charged residue (Glu) is noteworthy because charged residues are rarely found in transmembrane segments of proteins

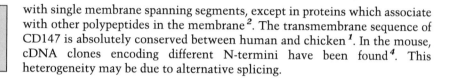

with single membrane spanning segments, except in proteins which associate with other polypeptides in the membrane[2]. The transmembrane sequence of CD147 is absolutely conserved between human and chicken[1]. In the mouse, cDNA clones encoding different N-termini have been found[4]. This heterogeneity may be due to alternative splicing.

Function

Human CD147 (EMMPRIN – extracellular matrix metalloproteinase inducer) on tumour cells is thought to bind an unknown ligand on fibroblasts, which stimulates their production of collagenase and other extracellular matrix metalloproteinases, thus enhancing tumour cell invasion and metastasis[6]. CD147 knockout mice are abnormal in their response to odour and their lymphocytes show an increased mitogenic response upon mixed lymphocyte reaction[7]. An adhesion role for chicken CD147 has been proposed, since the 5A11 mAb inhibits neural extensions of retinal glial cells and reduces retinal cell re-aggregation *in vitro*[8].

Database accession numbers

	PIR	SWISSPROT	EMBL/GENBANK	REFERENCE
Human M6	A46506	P35613	X64364	1
Rat CD147	A45444	P26453	X54640	2
Mouse Basigin	JX0107	P18572	D00611	9
Chicken HT7	S10147	P17790	X52751	5

Amino acid sequence of human CD147

```
MAAALFVLLG FALLGTHGAS G                                        -1
AAGTVFTTVE DLGSKILLTC SLNDSATEVT GHRWLKGGVV LKEDALPGQK         50
TEFKVDSDDQ WGEYSCVFLP EPMGTANIQL HGPPRVKAVK SSEHINEGET         100
AMLVCKSESV PPVTDWAWYK ITDSEDKALM NGSESRFFVS SSQGRSELHI         150
ENLNMEADPG QYRCNGTSSK GSDQAIITLR VRSHLAALWP FLGIVAEVLV         200
LVTIIFIYEK RRKPEDVLDD DDAGSAPLKS SGQHQNDKGK NVRQRNSS           248
```

References
1 Kasinrerk, W. et al. (1992) J. Immunol. 149, 847–854.
2 Fossum, S. et al. (1991) Eur. J. Immunol. 21, 671–679.
3 Nehme, C.L. et al. (1995) Blood 310, 693–698.
4 Kanekura, T. et al. (1991) Cell Struct. Funct. 16, 23–30.
5 Seulberger, H. et al. (1990) EMBO J. 9, 2151–2158.
6 **Biswas, C. et al. (1995) Cancer Res. 55, 434–439.**
7 **Igakura, T. et al. (1996) Biochem. Biophys. Res. Commun. 224, 33–36.**
8 Fadool, J.M. and Linser, P.J. (1993) Dev. Dynamics 196, 252–262.
9 Altruda, F. et al. (1989) Gene 85, 445–451.

CD148

HTPTη, DEP-1

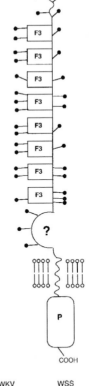

Molecular weights
Polypeptide   141 815

SDS-PAGE
  reduced   220–250 kDa

Carbohydrate
N-linked sites   34
O-linked   unknown

Human gene location
11p11.2

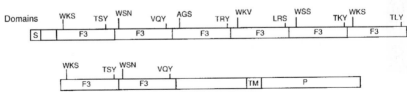

Domains

	WKS		TSY	WSN		VQY		AGS		TRY		WKV		LRS		WSS		TKY		WKS		TLY
S	F3				F3				F3				F3				F3				F3	

	WKS		TSY	WSN		VQY					
	F3				F3				TM		P

Tissue distribution

Messenger RNA analysis indicates that CD148 is expressed on a variety of cell types. Protein expression has been demonstrated in haematopoietic, particularly myeloid, cell lines by immunoblotting [1-3].

Structure

CD148 is a type I membrane glycoprotein with eight fibronectin type III (Fn3) domains and a single cytoplasmic phosphotyrosine phosphatase domain [4]. A further two Fn3 domains have been proposed in the membrane-proximal region but the alignments are not typical of Fn3 domains [1]. CD148 contains a particularly high content of N-linked glycosylation sites.

Function

The levels of expression of CD148 increase on contact between epithelial cell lines suggesting a role in contact inhibition of cell growth [2,5].

Database accession numbers

	PIR	SWISSPROT	EMBL/GENBANK	REFERENCE
Human			D37781	2
Mouse			D45212	3

Amino acid sequence of human CD148

```
MKPAAREARL PPRSPGLRWA LPLLLLLLRL GQILCA                          -1
GGTPSPIPDP SVATVATGEN GITQISSTAE SFHKQNGTGT PQVETNTSED           50
GESSGANDSL RTPEQGSNGT DGASQKTPSS TGPSPVFDIK AVSISPTNVI          100
LTWKSNDTAA SEYKYVVKHK MENEKTITVV HQPWCNITGL RPATSYVFSI          150
TPGIGNETWG DPRVIKVITE PIPVSDLRVA LTGVRKAALS WSNGNGTASC          200
RVLLESIGSH EELTQDSRLQ VNISGLKPGV QYNINPYLLQ SNKTKGDPLG          250
TEGGLDASNT ERSRAGSPTA PVHDESLVGP VDPSSGQQSR DTEVLLVGLE          300
PGTRYNATVY SQAANGTEGQ PQAIEFRTNA IQVFDVTAVN ISATSLTLIW          350
KVSDNESSSN YTYKIHVAGE TDSSNLNVSE PRAVIPGLRS STFYNITVCP          400
VLGDIEGTPG FLQVHTPPVP VSDFRVTVVS TTEIGLAWSS HDAESFQMHI          450
TQEGAGNSRV EITTNQSIII GGLFPGTKYC FEIVPKGPNG TEGASRTVCN          500
RTVPSAVFDI HVVYVTTTEM WLDWKSPDGA SEYVYHLVIE SKHGSNHTST          550
YDKAITLQGL IPGTLYNITI SPEVDHVWGD PNSTAQYTRP SNVSNIDVST          600
NTTAATLSWQ NFDDASPTYS YCLLIEKAGN SSNATQVVTD IGITDATVTE          650
LIPGSSYTVE IFAQVGDGIK SLEPGRKSFC TDPASMASFD CEVVPKEPAL          700
VLKWTCPPGA NAGFELEVSS GAWNNATHLE SCSSENGTEY RTEVTYLNFS          750
TSYNISITTV SCGKMAAPTR NTCTTGITDP PPPDGSPNIT SVSHNSVKVK          800
FSGFEASHGP IKAYAVILTT GEAGHPSADV LKYTYDDFKK GASDTYVTYL          850
IRTEEKGRSQ SLSEVLKYEI DVGNESTTLG YLQWEAGTSG LLPACVAGFT          900
NITFHPQNKG LIDGAESYVS FSRYSDAVSL PQDPGVICGA VFGCIFGALV          950
IVTVGGFIFW RKKRKDAKNN EVSFSQIKPK KSKLIRVENF EAYFKKQQAD         1000
SNCGFAEEYE DLKLVGISQP KYAAELAENR GKNRYNNVLP YDISRVKLSV         1050
QTHSTDDYIN ANYMPGYHSK KDFIATQGPL PNTLKDFWRM VWEKNVYAII         1100
MLTKCVEQGR TKCEEYWPSK QAQDYGDITV AMTSEIVLPE WTIRDFTVKN         1150
IQTSESHPLR QFHFTSWPDH GVPDTTDLLI NFRYLVRDYM KQSPPESPIL         1200
VHCSAGVGRT GTFIAIDRLI YQIENENTVD VYGIVYDLRM HRPLMVQTED         1250
QYVFLNQCVL DIVRSQKDSK VDLIYQNTTA MTIYENLAPV TTFGKTNGYI         1300
A                                                             1301
```

References

1 Honda, H. et al. (1994) Blood 84, 4186–4194.
2 Ostman, A. et al. (1994) Proc. Natl Acad. Sci. USA 91, 9680–9684.
3 Kuramochi, S. et al. (1996) FEBS Lett. 378, 7–14.
4 Fauman, E.B. and Saper, M.A. (1996) Trends Biochem. Sci. 21, 413–417.
5 **Keane, M.M. et al. (1996) Cancer Res. 56, 4236–4243.**

CDw150 SLAM

Molecular weights
Polypeptide   34 486

SDS-PAGE
   reduced   70 kDa

Carbohydrate
N-linked sites   8
O-linked   unknown

Domains

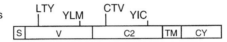

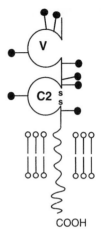

Tissue distribution

Constitutively expressed on immature thymocytes, some CD45RO^{high} memory T cells, and a proportion of B cells. Rapidly induced on all T and B cells following activation[1].

Structure

CDw150 contains two highly glycosylated IgSF domains and has structural features placing it within the CD2 family, which includes CD48, CD58, 2B4 and Ly-9[1,2]. Two variant cDNAs have been identified which correspond to alternatively spliced mRNA transcripts[1]. One encodes a soluble protein lacking the transmembrane region (207–236). The second one encodes a truncated molecule in which residue 261 is followed by the sequence DTHHQTSDLF. The cytoplasmic motif contains three Tyr-containing motifs (Y/hydrophobic/X/hydrophobic) suggestive of SH2-binding sites.

Function

The CDw150 mAb A12 enhances Ag-induced proliferation of CD4$^+$ T cells and can directly stimulate proliferation of previously activated T cells even as an Fab fragment[1]. This mAb increases IFNγ, but not IL-4, production on Ag-activated T$_H$0, T$_H$1 and T$_H$2 clones.

Database accession numbers

	PIR	SWISSPROT	EMBL/GENBANK	REFERENCE
Human			U33017	1

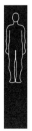

Amino acid sequence of human CDw150

```
MDPKGLLSLT FVLFLSLAFG ASYGTGG                               -1
RMMNCPKILR QLGSKVLLPL TYERINKSMN KSIHIVVTMA KSLENSVENK       50
IVSLDPSEAG PPRYLGDRYK FYLENLTLGI RESRKEDEGW YLMTLEKNVS      100
VQRFCLQLRL YEQVSTPEIK VLNKTQENGT CTLILGCTVE KGDHVAYSWS      150
EKAGTHPLNP ANSSHLLSLT LGPQHADNIY ICTVSNPISN NSQTFSPWPG      200
CRTDPSETKP WAVYAGLLGG VIMILIMVVI LQLRRRGKTN HYQTTVEKKS      250
LTIYAQVQKP GPLQKKLDSF PAQDPCTTIY VAATEPVPES VQETNSITVY      300
ASVTLPES                                                    308
```

References

1 **Cocks, B.G. et al. (1995) Nature 376, 260–263.**
2 Davis, S.J. and van der Merwe, P.A. (1996) Immunol. Today 17, 177–187.

CD151 PETA-3

Molecular weight
Polypeptide   28 295

SDS-PAGE
   reduced   27 kDa

Carbohydrate
N-linked sites   1
O-linked   nil

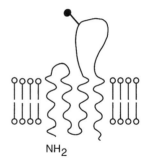

NH$_2$

Tissue distribution

CD151 is expressed by platelets, megakaryocytes and monocytes, but not by lymphocytes, granulocytes or haematopoietic progenitor cells. The expression of this antigen is not confined to haematopoietic cells, since epithelial and endothelial cells express CD151 [1].

Structure

CD151 is a member of the TM4 superfamily and is predicted to have four transmembrane regions, short cytoplasmic N- and C-termini, and two extracellular regions (reviewed in ref. 2).

Function

The CD151 mAb, 14A2.H1, activates platelets *in vitro* [3].

Database accession numbers

	PIR	SWISSPROT	EMBL/GENBANK	REFERENCE
Human		P48509	U14650	[4]

Amino acid sequence of human CD151

```
MGEFNEKKTT CGTVCLKYLL FTYNCCFWLA GLAVMAVGIW TLALKSDYIS    50
LLASGTYLAT AYILVVAGTV VMVTGVLGCC ATFKERRNLL RLYFILLLII   100
FLLEIIAGIL AYAYYQQLNT ELKENLKDTM TKRYHQPGHE AVTSAVDQLQ   150
QEFHCCGSNN SQDWRDSEWI RSQEAGGRVV PDSCCKTVVA LCGQRDHASN   200
IYKVEGGCIT KLETFIQEHL RVIGAVGIGI ACVQVFGMIF TCCLYRSLKL   250
EHY                                                     253
```

References
[1] Ashman, L.K. et al. (1991) Br. J. Haematol. 79, 263–270.
[2] **Wright, M.D. and Tomlinson, M.G. (1994) Immunol. Today 15, 588–594.**
[3] Roberts, J.J. et al. (1995) Br. J. Haematol. 89, 853–860.
[4] **Fitter, S. et al. (1995) Blood 86, 1348–1355.**

CD152   CTLA-4

Molecular weights
Polypeptide   20 343

SDS-PAGE
  reduced   33 kDa
  unreduced   50 kDa

Carbohydrate
N-linked sites   1
O-linked   unknown

Human gene location and size
2 q33; 6 kb [1,2]

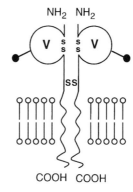

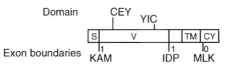

Tissue distribution

CD152 is expressed on activated but not resting T lymphocytes. Expression peaks at ~24 h and then subsides by 72 h [3], but is always 30–50-fold lower than CD28 [4]. CD28 ligation is particularly effective in inducing CD152 expression [3]. CD152 mRNA is frequently present in the absence of cell surface CD152 protein, suggesting post-transcriptional regulation of cell surface expression [3].

Structure

CD152 is structurally similar to CD28 (31% identity), binds the same ligands (see below), and the two genes are less than 150 kb apart [5], suggesting that they share a common ancestor in evolution. CD152 has been particularly highly conserved during evolution; the cytoplasmic domains of human and mouse CD152 are identical [2]. CD152 exists primarily as a disulfide-linked dimer [6] but non-disulfide-linked forms have been reported [3].

Ligands and associated molecules

Like CD28, CD152 binds both CD80 and CD86. The binding site for CD80 includes a highly conserved motif (MYPPPY) in the CDR3-like loop [7]. CD80 and CD86 bind CD152 with K_ds of 0.4 and 2.2 μM, respectively and dissociate rapidly ($k_{off} \geq 0.4\,s^{-1}$) [8,9]. The CD152 cytoplasmic domain has been reported to interact with the SH2 domain of the tyrosine phosphatase SHP-2 (PTP1D, SYP) through the phosphotyrosine motif pYVKM [10]. An association with phosphatidylinositol 3-kinase has also been reported, apparently through the same motif [11].

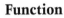

Function

Unlike CD28, CD152 negatively regulates T cell activation. Anti-CD152 monoclonal antibodies enhance T cell responses *in vitro* and *in vivo*[12,13] and CD152-deficient mice develop a fatal lymphoproliferative disorder[14,15]. Although the mechanism of this effect is not known, CD152 may inhibit tyrosine kinase signalling through the TCR through its association with tyrosine phosphatases such as SHP-2[10].

Database accession numbers

	PIR	SWISSPROT	EMBL/GENBANK	REFERENCE
Human	S08614	P16410	M74363	2
Mouse	A29063	P09793	X05719	16

Amino acid sequence of human CD152

```
MACLGFQRHK AQLNLATRTW PCTLLFFLLF IPVFCKA              -1
MHVAQPAVVL ASSRGIASFV CEYASPGKAT EVRVTVLRQA DSQVTEVCAA  50
TYMMGNELTF LDDSICTGTS SGNQVNLTIQ GLRAMDTGLY ICKVELMYPP 100
PYYLGIGNGA QIYVIDPEPC PDSDFLLWIL AAVSSGLFFY SFLLTAVSLS 150
KMLKKRSPLT TGVYVKMPPT EPECEKQFQP YFIPIN               186
```

References

1 Dariavach, P. et al. (1988) Eur. J. Immunol. 18, 1901–1905.
2 Harper, K. et al. (1991) J. Immunol. 147, 1037–1044.
3 Lenschow, D.J. et al. (1996) Annu. Rev. Immunol. 14, 233–258.
4 **Linsley, P.S. and Ledbetter, J.A. (1993) Annu. Rev. Immunol. 11, 191–211.**
5 Buonavista, N. et al. (1992) Genomics 13, 856–861.
6 Linsley, P.S. et al. (1995) J. Biol. Chem. 270, 15417–15424.
7 Peach, R.J. et al. (1994) J. Exp. Med. 180, 2049–2058.
8 Greene, J.L. et al. (1996) J. Biol. Chem. 271, 26762–26771.
9 van der Merwe, P.A. et al., (1997) J. Exp. Med. 185, 393–403.
10 Marengére, L.E.M. et al. (1996) Science 272, 1170–1173.
11 Schneider, H. et al. (1995) J. Exp. Med. 181, 351–355.
12 Kearney, E.R. et al. (1995) J. Immunol. 155, 1032–1036.
13 **Leach, D.R. et al. (1996) Science 271, 1734–1736.**
14 Tivol, E.A. et al. (1995) Immunity 3, 541–547.
15 Waterhouse, P. et al. (1995) Science 270, 985–988.
16 Brunet, J.F. et al. (1987) Nature 328, 267–270.

CD153 CD30L

Molecular weights
Polypeptide   26 017

SDS-PAGE
  reduced   40 kDa
  unreduced   40 kDa plus dimers and with
                     mouse CD153 higher oligomers

Carbohydrate
N-linked sites   5
O-linked   unknown

Human gene location
9q33 [1]

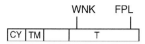

or oligomers

NH2

Domain

WNK   FPL

| CY | TM | | T |

Tissue distribution

CD153 is mainly expressed on activated peripheral blood T cells and macrophages [1,2]. Messenger RNA for human CD153 is restricted to T cells and monocyte/macrophages activated in a particular way and was not found in activated B cells [1]. Unlike CD30, CD153 is not expressed on Hodgkin's lymphoma-derived cell lines [2].

Structure

CD153 is a member of the TNF superfamily [1-4]. Like other members of this superfamily, it is a type II membrane protein with the C-terminal extracellular region showing similarity to TNF [1-4]. CD153 has two cysteines which do not align with other members of the family which may form disulfide-linked multimers [1]. It is not clear whether the protein is normally a dimer, trimer or higher oligomer [1].

Ligands and associated molecules

CD153 binds to CD30, a member of the TNFR superfamily.

Function

The CD153–CD30 interaction co-stimulates T cell proliferation [1,2], upregulates expression of adhesion molecules and stimulates cytokine release [2]. A role for the CD153–CD30 interaction in deletion of thymocytes in the thymus is suggested from studies with CD30-deficient mice [5]. CD30+ T cell clones produce T_H2-type cytokines. A role for the CD153–CD30 interaction in T_H2-type autoimmune disease has been suggested [2,6].

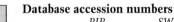

Database accession numbers

	PIR	SWISSPROT	EMBL/GENBANK	REFERENCE
Human	A40710	P32971	L09753	*1*
Mouse	B40710	P32972	L09754	*1*

Amino acid sequence of human CD153

```
MDPGLQQALN GMAPPGDTAM HVPAGSVASH LGTTSRSYFY LTTATLALCL      50
VFTVATIMVL VVQRTDSIPN SPDNVPLKGG NCSEDLLCIL KRAPFKKSWA     100
YLQVAKHLNK TKLSWNKDGI LHGVRYQDGN LVIQFPGLYF IICQLQFLVQ     150
CPNNSVDLKL ELLINKHIKK QALVTVCESG MQTKHVYQNL SQFLLDYLQV     200
NTTISVNVDT FQYIDTSTFP LENVLSIFLY SNSD                      234
```

References

1. Smith, C.A. et al. (1993) Cell 73, 1349–1360.
2. **Gruss, H.-J. and Dower, S.K. (1995) Blood 85, 3378–3404.**
3. Armitage, R.J. (1994) Curr. Opin. Immunol. (1994) 6, 407–413.
4. van Kooten, C. and Banchereau, J. (1996) Adv. Immunol. 61, 1–77.
5. Amakawa, R. et al. (1996) Cell, 84, 551–562.
6. Del Prete, G. et al. (1995) Immunol. Today 16, 76–80.

CD154   CD40L

Molecular weights
Polypeptide   29 274

SDS-PAGE
    reduced   33 kDa

Carbohydrate
N-linked sites   1
O-linked   unknown

Human gene location
Xq26.3–27.1; 13 kb [1]

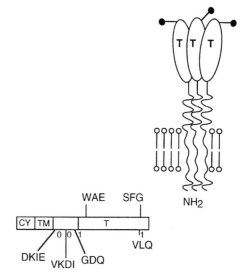

Domain

Exon boundaries

WAE SFG NH2

CY TM   T

DKIE VKDI GDQ VLQ

Tissue distribution

CD154 is absent from resting lymphocytes but is rapidly expressed on activation. It is present mostly on CD4⁺ cells but also a small population of CD8⁺ cells and γδ T cells [1-3]. It is also expressed on activated basophils and mast cells [1-3].

Structure

CD154 is a member of the TNF superfamily [1-3]. Like other members of this superfamily, it is a type II membrane protein expressed as a trimer with the similarity to TNF being in the C-terminal extracellular region [1-3]. The crystal structure of the extracellular region has confirmed the similarity to TNF with differences in loop regions predicted to be involved in CD40 binding [4]. Trimeric CD154 is predicted to bind three CD40 molecules [3].

Ligands and associated molecules

CD154 binds to CD40, a member of the TNFR superfamily.

Function

CD154 binding to CD40 on B cells is required for secondary immune responses and germinal centre formation [1-3]. Mutations in CD154 which abolish binding to CD40 cause the immunodeficiency disease, hyper-IgM syndrome which is characterized by lack of isotype switching in Ig production and lack of germinal centres [1-3]. There is evidence for a role for the CD154–CD40 interaction in negative selection and peripheral tolerance [1-3]. Mice deficient in CD40 or CD154 have increased susceptibility to parasite infection, pointing to a role in cell-mediated immunity as well as the humoral response [5].

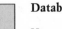

Database accession numbers

	PIR	SWISSPROT	EMBL/GENBANK	REFERENCE
Human	S28017	P29965	Z15017	6
Mouse	S21738	P27548	X65453	7

Amino acid sequence of human CD154

```
MIETYNQTSP RSAATGLPIS MKIFMYLLTV FLITQMIGSA LFAVYLHRRL       50
DKIEDERNLH EDFVFMKTIQ RCNTGERSLS LLNCEEIKSQ FEGFVKDIML      100
NKEETKKENS FEMQKGDQNP QIAAHVISEA SSKTTSVLQW AEKGYYTMSN      150
NLVTLENGKQ LTVKRQGLYY IYAQVTFCSN REASSQAPFI ASLCLKSPGR      200
FERILLRAAN THSSAKPCGQ QSIHLGGVFE LQPGASVFVN VTDPSQVSHG      250
TGFTSFGLLK L                                                261
```

References

1 van Kooten, C. and Banchereau, J. (1996) Adv. Immunol. 61, 1–77.

2 Gruss, H.-J. and Dower, S.K. (1995) Blood 85, 3378–3404.

3 Foy, T.M. et al. (1996) Annu. Rev. Immunol. 14, 591–617.

4 Karpusas, M. et al. (1995) Structure 3, 1031–1039.

5 Noelle, R.J. (1996) Immunity 4, 415–419.

6 Hollenbaugh D. et al. (1992). EMBO J. 11, 4313–4321

7 Armitage, R.J. et al. (1992) Nature 357, 80–82.

Members [1]
NKR-P1A (CD161, NKR-P1 gene 2, mNKR-P1.7 (mouse); 3.2.3, NKR-P1 (rat))
NKR-P1B (NKR-P1 gene 34 (mouse))
NKR-P1C (NK1.1, NKR-P1 gene 40, mNKR-P1.9 (mouse))

Molecular weights (human CD161)
Polypeptide   25 415

SDS-PAGE
   reduced   ~40–44 kDa
   unreduced   ~80–85 kDa

Carbohydrate (human CD161)
N-linked sites   4
O-linked   none

Human gene location
12p12.3–p13.1

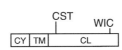

Tissue distribution

These molecules are found on most natural killer (NK) cells and a subset of T cells. In humans the only NKR-P1 molecule identified (CD161, NKR-P1A) is present on ~90% of NK cells, ~25% of T cells (both CD4 and CD8 cells) [4], and a subset of very immature thymocytes [5]. In the rat, NKR-P1A is found on all NK cells at high levels and at low levels on most neutrophils and a subset of T cells [6,7]. In the mouse NKR-P1C (NK1.1) is expressed on all NK cells as well as subsets of thymocytes and peripheral T cells. Transcripts of all three mouse genes have been detected in a single cell, suggesting that multiple NKR-P1 molecules can be expressed simultaneously by NK cells [1]. T lineage cells expressing NK1.1 form a functionally distinct group (termed 'natural T' or NT cells) characterized by expression of a TCR with an invariant α chain (Vα14–Jα281), restriction by CD1, and rapid expression of cytokines (including IL-4, -5 and -10) upon activation [8]. Several common laboratory strains of mice (e.g. BALB/c) appear not to express NKR-P1 molecules [3].

Structure

The NKR-P1 family members are structurally related to several other proteins encoded within the NK gene complex, including Ly-49 proteins, CD69, CD94 and NKG2 [9]. The NKR-P1 locus lies 0.41 cM distal to the Ly-49 locus on mouse chromosome 6 [1,2]. These molecules are all type II transmembrane glycoproteins with a C-type lectin domain in their extracellular portion and are expressed as disulfide-linked homodimers on the cell surface (human NKR-P1A may have a monomeric form as well [5]). Three distinct genes have been cloned in the mouse and there are preliminary reports of at least four distinct genes existing in the rat [1] but only one gene has been identified thus far in humans. The three mouse proteins show 73–87% amino acid identity with each other, 61–74% identity with rat NKR-P1A, and 46–47% identity with human NKR-P1A [4,10]. Rat NKR-P1A is most closely related to mouse NKR-P1A [1], but it is not clear which mouse gene is the homologue of human NKR-P1A [4]. There is evidence for alternatively spliced mouse NKR-P1A transcripts [1]. The cytoplasmic domains contains conserved potential Tyr- (YXXL) and Ser- (SPXSLXXDXC) phosphorylation sites [4].

Ligands and associated molecules

The C-type lectin domain of rat NKR-P1A has been reported to bind to a variety of carbohydrate structures [11] but the biological relevance of these interactions is under re-evaluation [12].

Function

Studies in the rat suggest that the NKR-P1A molecule functions as a specific receptor for certain NK cell targets, with ligation of NKR-P1A activating NK cell killing [1,13]. T cells expressing NKR-P1A are capable of cytotoxicity following culture in IL-2 [7]. In the mouse antibodies to NKR-P1C can (1) activate NK cells and (2) block NK cell killing of target cells [14]. However, certain common mouse strains appear to not express NKR-P1 gene products and yet exhibit normal NK cell function [1,3]. NKR-P1A has also been implicated in NK cell function in humans but studies with antibodies indicate that receptor ligation may activate or inhibit lytic function in different NK cell clones [4]. NKR-P1 is not essential for the development of natural T cells since this cell population is unchanged in mice lacking NKR-P1 [8].

Database accession numbers

	PIR	SWISSPROT	EMBL/GENBANK	REFERENCE
Human NKR-P1A (CD161)	I38700		U11276	4
Mouse NKR-P1A	A46467	P27811	M77676	10
Mouse NKR-P1B	B46467	P27812	M77677	10
Mouse NKR-P1C	C46467	P27814	M77678	10
Rat NKR-P1A	A35917	P27471	M62891	15

Amino acid sequence of human NKR-P1A (CD161)

```
MDQQAIYAEL NLPTDSGPES SSPSSLPRDV CQGSPWHQFA LKLSCAGIIL    50
LVLVVTGLSV SVTSLIQKSS IEKCSVDIQQ SRNKTTERPG LLNCPIYWQQ   100
LREKCLLFSH TVNPWNNSLA DCSTKESSLL LIRDKDELIH TQNLIRDKAI   150
LFWIGLNFSL SEKNWKWING SFLNSNDLEI RGDAKENSCI SISQTSVYSE   200
YCSTEIRWIC QKELTPVRNK VYPDS                             225
```

References

1 Yokoyama, W.M. and Seaman, W.E. (1993) Annu. Rev. Immunol. 11, 613–635.

[2] Yokoyama, W.M. et al. (1991) J. Immunol. 147, 3229–3236.
[3] Giorda, R. et al. (1992) J. Immunol. 149, 1957–1963.
[4] Lanier, L.L. et al. (1994) J. Immunol. 153, 2417–2427.
[5] Poggi, A. et al. (1996) Eur. J. Immunol. 26, 1266–1272.
[6] Chambers, W.H. et al. (1989) J. Exp. Med. 169, 1373–1389.
[7] Brissette-Storkus, C. et al. (1994) J. Immunol. 152, 388–396.
[8] Bix, M. and Locksley, R.M. (1995) J. Immunol. 155, 1020–1022.
[9] Gumperz, J.E. and Parham, P. (1995) Nature 378, 245–248.
[10] Giorda, R. and Trucco, M. (1991) J. Immunol. 147, 1701–1708.
[11] Bezouska, K. et al. (1994) Nature 372, 150–157.
[12] Feizi, T. (1996) Nature 380, 559.
[13] Ryan, J.C. et al. (1995) J. Exp. Med. 181, 1911–1915.
[14] Kung, S.K.P. and Miller, R.G. (1995) J. Immunol. 154, 1624–1633.
[15] Giorda, R. et al. (1990) Science 249, 1298–1300.

Molecular weights
Polypeptide   41 301
                  38 608 (without propeptide)

SDS-PAGE
  reduced   ~120 kDa
  unreduced   ~220 kDa

Carbohydrate
N-linked sites   3
O-linked   +++

Human gene location
12q24; ~11 kb [1]

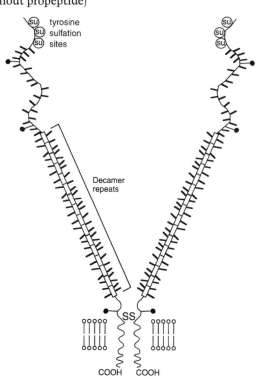

Tissue distribution

CD162 is expressed on neutrophils, monocytes and most lymphocytes [2,3]. On neutrophils CD162 in concentrated on the tips of microvilli [2]. In the mouse CD162 mRNA is detected in most tissues [4].

Structure

CD162 is a highly extended (~50 nm long [5]) mucin-like type I transmembrane glycoprotein which is expressed as a disulfide-linked homodimer [2]. A 23 residue propeptide is cleaved off at a consensus cleavage site (RxRR) for paired basic amino acid-converting enzyme (PACE) [5]. The region immediately following the propeptide contains many negatively charged residues as well as three tyrosines, within a tyrosine-sulfation consensus site [6]. This sulfotyrosine region is poorly conserved in the mouse but retains a negative charge and two tyrosine residues [4]. It is followed by a heavily O-glycosylated, mucin-like segment which includes 16 repeats of the decamer A(T/M)EAQTTX(P/L)(A/T) [1,7]. A human CD162 variant has been identified in cell lines which lacks one of the decameric repeats [1,7]. This is not due to alternative splicing as the CD162 protein is encoded by a single exon [1]. Only 10 decamer repeats are present in mouse CD162 [4].

Ligands and associated molecules

CD162 binds to CD62P (P-selectin) [2,8], CD62E (E-selectin) [2], and CD62L (L-selectin) [9,10]. CD62P binds with a relatively high affinity, apparently utilizing both carbohydrate (fucosylated, sialylated O-glycans) and protein determinants, with the latter including sulfotyrosine-containing N-terminal region [2,6,8]. CD62L binding also requires this sulfotyrosine-containing region [10]. In contrast, CD62E binds with a ~50-fold lower avidity than CD62P and does not require the sulfotyrosine-containing region [2,6,8]. CD62P does not bind all cells which express CD162, presumably because of differences in glycosylation and/or tyrosine sulfation [3]. For example, CD62P will bind activated but not resting T cells, despite no change in the CD162 expression level [3].

Function

CD162 is the major CD62P ligand on neutrophils [2] and T lymphocytes [3]. This interaction mediates the tethering and rolling of these cells on endothelial cells under physiological flow [2,11,12], an important initial step in leucocyte extravasation [2]. Interactions between CD162 and CD62L can mediate neutrophil–neutrophil interactions, which may amplify neutrophil extravasation [9].

Database accession numbers

	PIR	SWISSPROT	EMBL/GENBANK	REFERENCE
Human	A57468		U02297	7
			U25956	1
Mouse			X91144	4

Amino acid sequence of human CD162 [1]

```
MPLQLLLLLI LLGPGNSL                                           -1
QLWDTWADEA EKALGPLLAR DRRQATEYEY LDYDFLPETE PPEMLRNSTD        50
TTPLTGPGTP ESTTVEPAAR RSTGLDAGGA VTELTTELAN MGNLSTDSAA       100
MEIQTTQPAA TEAQTTQPVP TEAQTTPLAA TEAQTTRLTA TEAQTTPLAA       150
TEAQTTPPAA TEAQTTQPTG LEAQTTAPAA MEAQTTAPAA MEAQTTPPAA       200
MEAQTTQTTA MEAQTTAPEA TEAQTTQPTA TEAQTTPLAA MEALSTEPSA       250
TEALSMEPTT KRGLFIPFSV SSVTHKGIPM AASNLSVNYP VGAPDHISVK       300
QCLLAILILA LVATIFFVCT VVLAVRLSRK GHMYPVRNYS PTEMVCISSL       350
LPDGGEGPSA TANGGLSKAK SPGLTPEPRE DREGDDLTLH SFLP             394
```

The propeptide cleaved by PACE is in bold; the decamer repeat absent in one CD162 variant is dotted underlined [1].

References
1. Veldman, G.M. et al. (1995) J. Biol. Chem. 270, 16470–16475.
2. McEver, R.P. et al. (1995) J. Biol. Chem. 270, 11025–11028.
3. Vachino, G. et al. (1995) J. Biol. Chem. 270, 21966–21974.

4 Yang, J. et al. (1996) Blood 87, 4176–4186.

5 **Li, F. et al. (1996) J. Biol. Chem. 271, 6342–6348.**

6 Li, F. et al. (1996) J. Biol. Chem. 271, 3255–3265.

7 Sako, D. et al. (1993) Cell 75, 1179–1186.

8 **Rosen, S.D. and Bertozzi, C.R. (1996) Curr. Biol. 6, 261–264.**

9 Walcheck, B. et al. (1996) J. Clin. Invest. 98, 1081–1087.

10 Spertini, O. et al. (1996) J. Cell Biol. 135, 523–531.

11 Alon, R. et al. (1994) J. Cell Biol. 127, 1485–1495.

12 Norman, K.E. et al. (1995) Blood 86, 4417–4421.

Molecular weights

Polypeptide	116 654
variant 1	120 495
variant 2	121 027

SDS-PAGE

reduced	130 kDa
unreduced	110 kDa

Carbohydrate

N-linked sites	11
O-linked sites	unknown

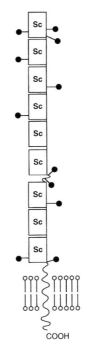

COOH

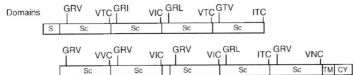

Tissue distribution

CD163 is restricted to the monocyte/macrophage lineage. It is present on all circulating monocytes and most tissue macrophages[1], with the exceptions of tingible body macrophages, macrophages in the mantle zone and germinal centers of lymphoid follicles, interdigitating reticulum cells, and Langerhans cells[2]. Multinucleated cells within inflammatory lesions *in vivo* do not express CD163[3].

Structure

CD163 is a type I membrane protein[4]. The extracellular domain consists of nine SRCR domains. Domains 5–9 show similarity to a long-range repeat of domains 2–6 and 7–11 of the WC1 antigen[5] with a characteristic insertion (31 amino acids in CD163) between domains 6 and 7. Three membrane bound forms of CD163 identified at the cDNA level are generated by alternative splicing within the cytoplasmic region; the predominant form is the short form[4]. The N-terminus has been determined by protein sequencing[4].

Function

Unknown.

Database accession numbers

	PIR	SWISSPROT	EMBL/GENBANK	REFERENCE
Human	S36077		Z22968	4
Human variant 1	S36078		Z22969	4
Human variant 2	S36079		Z22970	4

Amino acid sequence of human CD163

```
MVLLEDSGSA DFRRHFVNLS PFTITVVLLL SACFVTSSLG             -1
GTDKELRLVD GENKCSGRVE VKVQEEWGTV CNNGWSMEAV SVICNQLGCP   50
TAIKAPGWAN SSAGSGRIWM DHVSCRGNES ALWDCKHDGW GKHSNCTHQQ  100
DAGVTCSDGS NLEMRLTRGG NMCSGRIEIK FQGRWGTVCD DNFNIDHASV  150
ICRQLECGSA VSFSGSSNFG EGSGPIWFDD LICNGNESAL WNCKHQGWGK  200
HNCDHAEDAG VICSKGADLS LRLVDGVTEC SGRLEVRFQG EWGTICDDGW  250
DSYDAAVACK QLGCPTAVTA IGRVNASKGF GHIWLDSVSC QGHEPAVWQC  300
KHHEWGKHYC NHNEDAGVTC SDGSDLELRL RGGGSRCAGT VEVEIQRLLG  350
KVCDRGWGLK EADVVCRQLG CGSALKTSYQ VYSKIQATNT WLFLSSCNGN  400
ETSLWDCKNW QWGGLTCDHY EEAKITCSAH REPRLVGGDI PCSGRVEVKH  450
GDTWGSICDS DFSLEAASVL CRELQCGTVV SILGGAHFGE GNGQIWAEEF  500
QCEGHESHLS LCPVAPRPEG TCSHSRDVGV VCSRYTEIRL VNGKTPCEGR  550
VELKTLGAWG SLCNSHWDIE DAHVLCQQLK CGVALSTPGG ARFGKGNGQI  600
WRHMFHCTGT EQHMGDCPVT ALGASLCPSE QVASVICSGN QSQTLSSCNS  650
SSLGPTRPTI PEESAVACIE SGQLRLVNGG GRCAGRVEIY HEGSWGTICD  700
DSWDLSDAHV VCRQLGCGEA INATGSAHFG EGTGPIWLDE MKCNGKESRI  750
WQCHSHKEDAG QNCRHKEDAG VICSEFMSLR LTSEASREAC AGRLEVFYNG  800
AWGTVGKSSM SETTVGVVCR QLGCADKGKI NPASLDKAMS IPMWVDNVQC  850
PKGPDTLWQC PSSPWEKRLA SPSEETWITC DNKIRLQEGP TSCSGRVEIW  900
HGGSWGTVCD DSWDLDDAQV VCQQLGCGPA LKAFKEAEFG QGTGPIWLNE  950
VKCKGNESSL WDCPARRWGH SECGHKEDAA VNCTDISVQK TPQKATTGRS 1000
SRQSSFIAVG ILGVVLLAIF VALFFLTKKR RQRQRLAVSS RGENLVHQIQ 1050
```

```
   YREMNSCLNA DDLDLMNSSG GHSEPH                          1076
v1 YREMNSCLNA DDLDLMNSSE NSHESADFSA AELISVSKFL PISGMEKEAI 1100
v2 YREMNSCLNA DDLDLMNSSG LWVLGGSIAQ GFRSVAAVEA QTFYFDKQLK 1100
```

```
v1 LSHTEKENGN L                                         1111
v2 KSKNVIGSLD AYNGQE                                    1116
```

Note: v1 and v2 indicate the cytoplasmic sequences of the variants 1 and 2, respectively.

References

1. Radzun, H.J. et al. (1987) Blood 69, 1320–1327.
2. Pulford, K. et al. (1992) Immunology 75, 588–595.
3. Backe, E. et al. (1991) J. Clin. Pathol. 44, 936-945.
4. **Law, S.K.A. et al. (1993) Eur. J. Immunol. 23, 2320–2325.**
5. Wijngaard, P.L.J. et al. (1992) J. Immunol. 149, 3273-3277.

CD166

ALCAM, CD6L, BEN, SC-1, DM-GRASP, neurolin, KG-CAM

Molecular weights
Polypeptide   62 293

SDS-PAGE
   reduced   105 kDa
   unreduced   105 kDa

Carbohydrate
N-linked sites 8
O-linked   unknown

Human gene location
3q13.1–q13.2 [1]

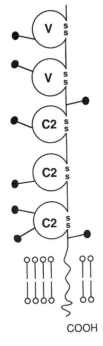

COOH

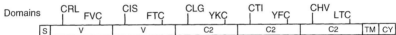

Domains	CRL	FVC	CIS	FTC	CLG	YKC	CTI	YFC	CHV	LTC		
S	V		V		C2		C2		C2		TM	CY

Tissue distribution

CD166 has a broad tissue distribution including cortical and medullary thymic epithelial cells[2] and activated T cells[1]. The avian equivalent, BEN[3] is expressed on epithelial cells of the Bursa. In the nervous system, CD166 is expressed on neurons and the distribution of BEN is well-characterized on developing sensory and motor neurons[3,4].

Structure

CD166 is a member of the IgSF with the Ig domains arranged as V-V-C2-C2-C2 as in MUC18[1,3,4]. The IgSF domains are followed by a transmembrane region and short (32 amino acid) cytoplasmic domain[1].

Ligands and associated molecules

CD166 on thymic epithelial cells, via its N-terminal IgSF V-set domain, mediates binding to the membrane proximal scavenger receptor domain of CD6 on thymocytes[1,5]. A homophilic interaction has been described for the chicken homologue[6].

Function

Through its interaction with CD166 in the thymus, CD6 may have a role in T cell development. A role in axonal guidance is postulated based on inhibitory effects with mAbs [4,7].

Database accession numbers

	PIR	SWISSPROT	EMBL/GENBANK	REFERENCE
Human			L38608	1
Mouse			L25274	4
Chicken		P42292	X64301	3

Amino acid sequence of human CD166

```
MESKGASSCR LLFCLLISAT VFRPGLG                          -1
WYTVNSAYGD TIIIPCRLDV PQNLMFGKWK YEKPDGSPVF IAFRSSTKKS  50
VQYDDVPEYK DRLNLSENYT LSISNARISD EKRFVCMLVT EDNVFEAPTI 100
VKVFKQPSKP EIVSKALFLE TEQLKKLGDC ISEDSYPDGN ITWYRNGKVL 150
HPLEGAVVII FKKEMDPVTQ LYTMTSTLEY KTTKADIQMP FTCSVTYYGP 200
SGQKTIHSEQ AVFDIYYPTE QVTIQVLPPK NAIKEGDNIT LKCLGNGNPP 250
PEEFLFYLPG QPEGIRSSNT YTLMDVRRNA TGDYKCSLID KKSMIASTAI 300
TVHYLDLSLN PSGEVTRQIG DALPVSCTIS ASRNATVVWM KDNIRLRSSP 350
SFSSLHYQDA GNYVCETALQ EVEGLKKRES LTLIVEGKPQ IKMTKKTDPS 400
GLSKTIICHV EGFPKPAIQW TITGSGSVIN QTEESPYING RYYSKIIISP 450
EENVTLTCTA ENQLERTVNS LNVSAISIPE HDEADEISDE NREKVNDQAK 500
LIVGIVVGLL LAALVAGVVY WLYMKKSKTA SKHVNKDLGN MEENKKLEEN 550
NHKTEA                                                556
```

References
1 **Bowen, M.A. et al. (1995) J. Exp. Med. 181, 2213–2220.**
2 Patel, D.D. et al. (1995) J. Exp. Med. 181, 1563–1568.
3 Pourquie, O. et al. (1992) Proc. Natl Acad. Sci. USA 89, 5261–5265.
4 Kanki, J.P. et al. (1994) J. Neurobiol. 25, 831–845.
5 Bajorath, J. et al. (1995) Protein Sci. 4, 1644–1647.
6 Tanaka, H. et al. (1991) Neuron 7, 535–545.
7 Burns, F.R. et al. (1991) Neuron 7, 209–220.

114/A10

Molecular weights
Polypeptide   56915

SDS-PAGE
  reduced   150 kDa (mean)
                 100–300 kDa (cell type variation)

Carbohydrate
N-linked sites   3
O-linked   probable +++

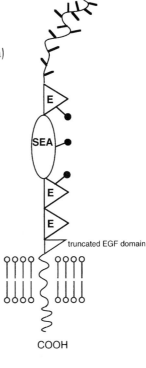

truncated EGF domain

COOH

Domains

		CNP		CDH		CSQ	RKC			
			SSC		PLC					
S		E		SEA	E		E		TM	CY

Tissue distribution

The 114/A10 antigen is expressed on mouse haematopoietic cells and cell lines that are responsive to IL-3, including primary erythroid, myeloid and multipotent progenitors [1].

Structure

The extracellular N-terminus consists of eight highly conserved Ser/Thr-rich repeats of about 27 residues each, followed by three complete EGF domains and one truncated EGF domain. Between EGF domains 1 and 3 there is a region of 120 residues with similarity to the recently defined SEA module which is commonly found in proteins with O-glycosylation [2]. Each Ser/Thr-rich repeat contains one Ser–Gly motif which could potentially serve as an attachment site of glycosaminoglycan side-chains [1]. However, digestions with glycosidases fail to demonstrate the presence of glycosaminoglycans. Instead it is suggested that the size heterogeneity of the 114/A10 molecule is the result of differential post-translational modification with sialylated *O*-linked carbohydrates, which are probably present in the repeats [3].

Function

The tissue distribution has prompted speculation that 114/A10 might play a regulatory role in the cellular response to IL-3. Further speculation has concerned the group of Arg residues, between the first and second EGF domains, that may be a site for cleavage by proteases. This would release a soluble product, containing the Ser/Thr repeats and a single EGF domain, which might function as a cytokine [1].

Database accession numbers

	PIR	SWISSPROT	EMBL/GENBANK	REFERENCE
Mouse	A33533	P19467	J04634	1

Amino acid sequence of mouse 114/A10

```
MKGFLLLSLS LLLVTVG                                              -1
SSSQASSTTS SSGGTSPPTT VQSQSPGSSS QASTTTSSSG GASPPTTVQS          50
QSPGSSSQAS TTTSSSGGAS PPTTVQSQSP GSSSQASTTT SSSGGASPPT         100
TVQSQSPGSS SQASTTTSSS GGASPPTTVQ SQSPGSSSQA STTTSSSGGA         150
SPPTTVQSQS PGSSSQVSTT TSSSGGASPP TTVQSQSPGS SSQPGPTQPS         200
GGASSSTVPS GGSTGPSDLC NPNPCKGTAS CVKLHSKHFC LCLEGYYYNS         250
SLSSCVKGTT FPGDISMSVS ETANLEDENS VGYQELYNSV TDFFETTFNK         300
TDYGQTVIIK VSTAPSRSAR SAMRDATKDV SVSVVNIFGA DTKETEKSVS         350
SAIETAIKTS GNVKDYVSIN LCDHYGCVGN DSSKCQDILQ CTCKPGLDRL         400
NPQVPFCVAV TCSQPCNAEE KEQCLKMDNG VMDCVCMPGY QRANGNRKCE         450
ECPFGYSGMN CKDQFQLILT IVGTIAGALI LILLIAFIVS ARSKNKKKDG         500
EEQRLIEDDF HNLRLRQTGF SNLGADNSIF PKVRTGVPSQ TPNPYANQRS         550
MPRPDY                                                         556
```

References
[1] Dougherty, G.J. et al. (1989) J. Biol. Chem. 264, 6509–6514.
[2] Bork, P. and Patthy, L. (1995) Protein Sci. 4, 1421–1425.
[3] Kay, R. et al. (1990) J. Biol. Chem. 265, 4962–4968.

2B4

Molecular weights
Polypeptide   43 091

SDS-PAGE
  reduced   66 kDa
  unreduced   66 kDa

Carbohydrate
N-linked sites 7
O-linked   nil

Domains

| PSN | YLL | CLV | YTC |

| S | V | C2 | TM | CY |

COOH

Tissue distribution

Expressed in mice on all NK cells and T cells capable of non-MHC-restricted cytotoxicity [1,2]. The latter include dendritic epidermal (γδ) T cells and a subset of T cells cultured in IL-2 [1,2].

Structure

The extracellular portion of this IgSF domain-containing glycoprotein exhibits several structural features that place it within the CD2 family of the IgSF (see **CD2**), which probably arose from a series of gene duplication events [3,4]. In addition to CD2 and 2B4 this family includes CD48, CD58, Ly-9, and CD150. The mouse 2B4 gene is situated on mouse chromosome 1 near the gene for Ly-17 (mouse CD32) [5], placing it close to the Ly-9 and CD48 loci [3,6]. The membrane-proximal IgSF domain is particularly highly glycosylated.

Function

The expression of 2B4 on all NK cells as well as T cells capable of non-MHC-restricted cytotoxicity suggests that it may contribute to the latter process. Treatment with a 2B4 mAb activates these cells and augments non-MHC-restricted cytotoxicity [1,2,5,7].

Database accession numbers

	PIR	SWISSPROT	EMBL/GENBANK	REFERENCE
Mouse			L19057	5

Amino acid sequence of mouse 2B4

```
MLGQAVLFTT FLLLRAHQ                                           -1
GQDCPDSSEE VVGVSGKPVQ LRPSNIQTKD VSVQWKKTEQ GSHRKIEILN        50
WYNDGPSWSN VSFSDIYGFD YGDFALSIKS AKLQDSGHYL LEITNTGGKV       100
CNKNFQLLIL DHVETPNLKA QWKPWTNGTC QLFLSCLVTK DDNVSYAFWY       150
RGSTLISNQR NSTHWENQID ASSLHTYTCN VSNRASWANH TLNFTHGCQS       200
VPSNFRFLPF GVIIVILVTL FLGAIICFCV WTKKRKQLQF SPKEPLTIYE       250
YVKDSRASRD QQGCSRASGS PSAVQEDGRG QRELDRRVSE VLEQLPQQTF       300
PGDRGTMYSM IQCKPSDSTS QEKCTVYSVV QPSRKSGSKK RNQNYSLSCT       350
VYEEVGNPWL KAHNPARLSR RELENFDVYS                             380
```

References

1. Garni-Wagner, B.A. et al. (1993) J. Immunol. 151, 60–70.
2. **Schuhmachers, G. et al. (1995) J. Invest. Dermatol. 105, 592–596.**
3. Wong, Y.W. et al. (1990) J. Exp. Med. 171, 2115–2130.
4. Davis, S.J. and van der Merwe, P.A. (1996) Immunol. Today 17, 177–187.
5. Mathew, P.A. et al. (1993) J. Immunol. 151, 5328–5337.
6. Kingsmore, S.F. et al. (1995) Immunogenetics 42, 59–62.
7. Schuhmachers, G. et al. (1995) Eur. J. Immunol. 25, 1117–1120.

4-1BBL CDw137L

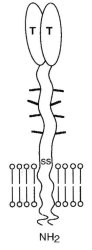

Molecular weights
Polypeptide   26 625

SDS-PAGE
  reduced   50 kDa
  nonreduced   97 kDa

Carbohydrate
N-linked sites   0
O-linked   probable

Human gene location
19p13.3 [1]

Domain

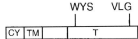

WYS   VLG

| CY | TM | T |

Tissue distribution

4-1BBL is expressed on activated T and B lymphocytes [2,3]. On cell lines, highest expression was found on IgG⁺ B cell lymphomas with an estimated site number of 3680 and on macrophage lines [3]. Messenger RNA for 4-1BBL is widespread [1].

Structure

4-1BBL is a member of the TNF superfamily [3,5,6]. Like other members of this superfamily, it is a type II membrane protein with the similarity to TNF being in the C-terminal extracellular region. Unusually, 4-1BBL is expressed as a disulfide-linked homodimer not a trimer [1]. Dimerization probably occurs through the cysteine in the serine/proline-rich membrane-proximal stalk [1]. Mouse 4-1BBL has three potential N-linked glycosylation sites [4].

Ligands and associated molecules

4-1BBL binds to CDw137, a member of the TNFR superfamily.

Function

Cells expressing 4-1BBL can co-stimulate T cell growth and this can be inhibited by soluble 4-1BBL [4,7,8]. Reciprocally, cells expressing recombinant CDw137 can co-stimulate proliferation by B cells [2]. These experiments suggest a role for the 4-1BBL/CDw137 interaction in T and B cell growth [2,7,8].

Database accession numbers

	PIR	SWISSPROT	EMBL/GENBANK	REFERENCE
Human		P41273	U03398	1
Mouse		P41274	L15435	4

Amino acid sequence of human 4-1BBL

```
MEYASDASLD PEAPWPPAPR ARACRVLPWA LVAGLLLLLL LAAACAVFLA      50
CPWAVSGARA SPGSAASPRL REGPELSPDD PAGLLDLRQG MFAQLVAQNV     100
LLIDGPLSWY SDPGLAGVSL TGGLSYKEDT KELVVAKAGV YYVFFQLELR     150
RVVAGEGSGS VSLALHLQPL RSAAGAAALA LTVDLPPASS EARNSAFGFQ     200
GRLLHLSAGQ RLGVHLHTEA RARHAWQLTQ GATVLGLFRV TPEIPAGLPS     250
PRSE                                                      254
```

References

[1] **Alderson, M.R. et al. (1994) Eur. J. Immunol. 24, 2219–2227.**

[2] Pollock, K. et al. (1994) Eur. J. Immunol. 24, 367–374.

[3] Gruss, H.-J. and Dower, S.K. (1995) Blood 85, 3378–3404.

[4] Goodwin, R.G. et al. (1993) Eur. J. Immunol. 23, 2631–2641.

[5] Armitage, R.J. (1994) Curr. Opin. Immunol. 6, 407–413.

[6] van Kooten, C. and Banchereau, J. (1996) Adv. Immunol. 61, 1–77.

[7] DeBenedette, M.A. et al. (1995) J. Exp. Med. 181, 985–992.

[8] Hurtado, J.C. et al. (1995) J. Immunol. 155, 3360–3367.

Aminopeptidase A

APA

Other names
Glutamyl aminopeptidase (EC 3.4.11.7)
BP-1/6C3 (mouse)
gp160

Molecular weights
Polypeptide   109 245

SDS-PAGE
  reduced   160 kDa
  unreduced   280–500 kDa

Carbohydrate
N-linked sites   13
O-linked   unknown

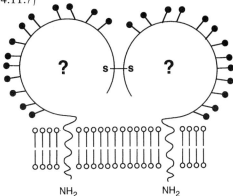

Tissue distribution

Aminopeptidase A (APA) is expressed in mice on early B lineage cells and on a population of thymic cortical epithelial cells, but not on mature lymphocytes (reviewed in refs 1 and 2). IL-7 has been shown to selectively induce APA expression on pre-B cells coincident with their growth[3]. Expression on bone marrow stromal cell lines correlates with their ability to support growth of B lineage cells[4]. The molecule is widely expressed on other tissues including vascular endothelium, kidney glomeruli and tubules, and the brush border of small intestine[1,2,5]. Northern blot analysis indicates a similar expression pattern in humans[6].

Structure

APA is a disulfide-linked homodimer of a type II integral membrane protein[2,6,7]. The extracellular region contains a typical zinc binding motif (shown below). Human APA shows sequence similarity to human CD13 (aminopeptidase N or APN). The molecule can be phosphorylated[8].

Ligands and associated molecules

APA binds to a wide range of oligopeptides[9].

Function

APA is a zinc-dependent metallopeptidase that cleaves N-terminal Glu or Asp residues from peptides[6,9,10]. For example, in the kidney APA removes the N-terminal Asp residues of angiotensins I and II, rendering them less potent as vasoconstrictors. In mice the BP-1 mAb blocks APA enzymatic activity and inhibits IL-7-driven proliferation of pre-B cells in the context of the bone marrow microenvironment, but does not inhibit the growth of purified pre-B cells in response to IL-7[11]. This suggests that APA cleaves, and inactivates, a peptide which serves as a natural inhibitor of B cell precursor proliferation.

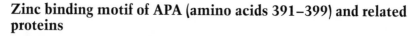

Zinc binding motif of APA (amino acids 391–399) and related proteins

APA	VA**HEL**V**H**Q̲W
Human CD13 (APN)	IA**HELAH**Q̲W
Rat APN	IA**HELAH**Q̲W
E. coli APN	IG**HE**YF**H**NW

Database accession numbers

	PIR	SWISSPROT	EMBL/GENBANK	REFERENCE
Human	A48287	Q07075	L14721	6
Mouse	S30398	P16406	M29961	1
Rat		P50123	S73583	12

Amino acid sequence of human aminopeptidase A

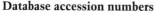

```
MNFAEREGSK RYCIQTKHVA ILCAVVVGVG LIVGLAVGLT RSCDSSGDGG    50
PGTAPAPSHL PSSTASPSGP PAQDQDICPA SEDESGQWKN FRLPDFVNPV   100
HYDLHVKPLL EEDTYTGTVS ISINLSAPTR YLWLHLRETR ITRLPELKRP   150
SGDQVQVRRC FEYKKQEYVV VEAEEELTPS SGDGLYLLTM EFAGWLNGSL   200
VGFYRTTYTE NGRVKSIAAT DHEPTDARKS FPCFDEPNKK ATYTISITHP   250
KEYGALSNMP VAKEESVDDK WTRTTFEKSV PMSTYLVCFA VHQFDSVKRI   300
SNSGKPLTIY VQPEQKHTAE YAANITKSVF DYFEEYFAMN YSLPKLDKIA   350
IPDFGTGAME NWGLITYRET NLLYDPKESA SSNQQRVATV VAHELVHQWF   400
GNIVTMDWWE DLWLNEGFAS FFEFLGVNHA ETDWQMRDQM LLEDVLPVQE   450
DDSLMSSHPI IVTVTTPDEI TSVFDGISYS KGSSILRMLE DWIKPENFQK   500
GCQMYLEKYQ FKNAKTSDFW AALEEASRLP VKEVMDTWTR QMGYPVLNVN   550
GVKNITQKRF LLDPRANPSQ PPSDLGYTWN IPVKWTEDNI TSSVLFNRSE   600
KEGITLNSSN PSGNAFLKIN PDHIGFYRVN YEVATWDSIA TALSLNHKTF   650
SSADRASLID DAFALARAQL LDYKVALNLT KYLKREENFL PWQRVISAVT   700
YIISMFEDDK ELYPMIEEYF QGQVKPIADS LGWNDAGDHV TKLLRSSVLG   750
FACKMGDREA LNNASSLFEQ WLNGTVSLPV NLRLLVYRYG MQNSGNEISW   800
NYTLEQYQKT SLAQEKEKLL YGLASVKNVT LLSRYLDLLK DTNLIKTQDV   850
FTVIRYISYN SYGKNMAWNW IQLNWDYLVN RYTLNNRNLG RIVTIAEPFN   900
TELQLWQMES FFAKYPQAGA GEKPREQVLE TVKNNIEWLK QHRNTIREWF   950
FNLLESG                                                 957
```

References

1 Wu, Q. et al. (1990) Proc. Natl Acad. Sci. USA 87, 993–997.
2 Adkins, B. et al. (1988) Immunogenetics 27, 180–186.
3 Welch, P.A. et al. (1990) Int. Immunol. 2, 697–705.
4 Whitlock, C.A. et al. (1987) Cell 48, 1009–1021.
5 Li, L. et al. (1993) Tissue Antigens 42, 488–496.
6 Li, L. et al. (1993) Genomics 17, 657–664.
7 Cooper, M.D. et al. (1986) Nature 321, 616–618.
8 Wu, Q. et al. (1989) J. Immunol. 143, 3303–3308.
9 Nanus, D.M. et al. (1993) Proc. Natl Acad. Sci. USA 90, 7069–7073.
10 **Wu, Q. et al. (1991) Proc. Natl Acad. Sci. USA 88, 676–680.**
11 **Welch, P.A. (1995) Int. Immunol. 7, 737–746.**
12 Song, L. et al. (1994) Am. J. Physiol. 267, F546–F557.

B-G

Molecular weights
Polypeptide (bg14/8)   41 576

SDS-PAGE
  reduced   35–55 kDa
  unreduced   90–160 kDa

Carbohydrate
N-linked sites   nil
O-linked   nil

Domain

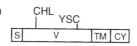

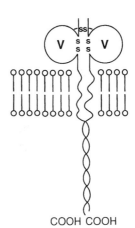

COOH COOH

Tissue distribution

Chicken B-G molecules are expressed on red blood cells, thrombocytes, B and T lymphocytes, bursal B cells, thymocytes and various non-haematopoietic cells [1,2].

Structure

The multigene family of chicken B-G molecules is encoded within the chicken MHC [1-3]. Structural information is given for erythrocyte B-G which is expressed mainly as a disulfide-linked dimer and contains no oligosaccharide [1,2]. On other cells B-G molecules may be monomeric or multimeric and be glycosylated [1,2]. The extracellular domain consists of a single IgSF V-set domain which shows polymorphism and similarity to myelin oligodendrodyte glycoprotein (MOG) [3,4]. A subfamily of the IgSF containing BT, MOG, B-G, CD80 and CD86 has been suggested [4]. The cytoplasmic domains contain different numbers of seven amino acid α helical repeats giving rise to size polymorphism [1,2]. B-G has been identified as a polymorphic family in another species of birds, namely the pheasant [5].

Function

The function of B-G molecules is unknown [2].

Database accession numbers

	PIR	SWISSPROT	EMBL/GENBANK	REFERENCE
Chicken bg14/8			M61860	6

Amino acid sequence of chicken B-G (bg14/8)

```
MAFTSGCNHP SFTLPWRTLL PYLVALHLLQ PGSA                  -1
QITVVAPSLR VTAIVGQDVV LRCHLSPCKD VRNSDIRWIQ QRSSRLVHHY  50
RNGVDLGQME EYKGRTELLR DGLSDGNLDL RITAVTSSDS GSYSCAVQDG 100
DAYAEAVVNL EVSDPFSMII LYWTVALAVI ITLLVGSFVV NVFLHRKKVA 150
QSRELKRKDA ELVEKAAALE RKDAELAEQA AQSKQRDAML DKHVLKLEEK 200
TDEVENWNSV LKKDSEEMGY GFGDLKKLAA ELEKHSEEMG TRDLKLERLA 250
AKLEHQTKEL EKQHSQFQRH FQNMYLSAGK QKKMVTKLEE HCEWMVRRNV 300
KLEIPAVKVG QQAKESEEQK SELKEHHEET GQQAKESEKQ KSELKERHEE 350
MAEQTEAVVV ETEE                                       364
```

References

1 **Kaufman, J. et al. (1991) CRC Crit. Rev. Immunol. 11, 113–143.**
2 Kaufman, J. and Salomonsen, J. (1992) Immunol. Today 13, 1–3.
3 Trowsdale, J. (1995) Immunogenetics 41, 1–17.
4 Linsley, P.S. et al. (1994) Protein Sci. 3, 1341–1343.
5 Jarvi, S.I. et al. (1996) Immunogenetics 43, 125–135.
6 Miller, M.M. et al. (1991) Proc. Natl Acad. Sci. USA 88, 4377–4381.

Chemokine receptors

The complex family of chemokine receptors has been extensively detailed in two other books in the FactsBook series [1,2] and recently reviewed in ref. 3. A separate entry is included for one well-characterized example for which antibodies are available, IL-8R (CXCR1/CDw128).

Nomenclature
An amended nomenclature was adopted for the chemokine receptors at the Gordon Conference on Chemotactic Cytokines (June 1996). The C-C chemokines (β chemokine family) share a group of five known receptors designated CCR1–CCR5. The C-X-C chemokines (α chemokine family) bind to the four receptors designated CXCR1–CXCR4. In addition, the Duffy antigen on erythrocytes acts as a receptor for a wide range of C-C and C-X-C chemokines.

Molecular weights
Apparent M_r of 46–52 kDa.

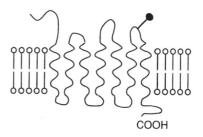

COOH

Tissue distribution

The tissue distribution of chemokine receptors has not yet been well defined, through the lack of specific monoclonal antibodies. However, mRNA analyses suggests that these receptors are widely distributed on leucocytes. The Duffy antigen is expressed on erythrocytes, T cells and endothelial cells in the spleen, lung, brain and kidney.

Structure

The chemokine receptors are seven transmembrane-spanning G protein-linked receptors. The CCR5 molecule is depicted in the figure.

Ligands and associated molecules

One feature of the chemokine receptors is that a number of receptors can bind several ligands and vice versa. The CCR1–CCR5 receptors bind to members of the C-C chemokine family, such as RANTES (CCR1, CCR3, CCR4 and CCR5), MIP-1α (CCR1, CCR4 and CCR5) and MCP-1 (CCR2) [3]. The CXCR1-CXCR4 receptors bind to members of the C-X-C chemokine family, either specifically such as IL-8 binding to CXCR1 (CDw128) and SDF-1 binding to CXCR4 (LESTR/fusin), or in a shared manner such as CXCR3 binding to both IP10 and Mig [3]. These interactions are usually of a high affinity, but are often within a range of affinities; for example MIP-1α binds to CCR5 with $K_d = 5$ nM whereas RANTES binds to CCR5 with $K_d = 470$ nM. The chemokine receptors are coupled to heterotrimeric G proteins (believed to be of the Giα class) located at the cytoplasmic face of the cell membrane.

Function

Chemokine–chemokine receptor interactions play an important role in the chemotactic recruitment of leucocytes to sites of infection and tissue damage. The signalling process involves G protein activation, leading to the generation of inositol trisphosphate with subsequent release of intracellular Ca^{2+}, opening of Ca^{2+} channels and activation of protein kinase C [4]. A recent development has been the finding that several chemokine receptors can function as cofactors (in concert with CD4) for HIV-1 infection of $CD4^+$ T cells and macrophages: CXCR4 (LESTR/fusin) acts as a cofactor for fusion and entry of T cell line-tropic strains of HIV-1, whereas CCR5 and, for some HIV-1 strains, CCR3 act as cofactors for macrophage-tropic isolates of HIV-1 [5–10]. Dual-tropic strains of HIV-1 may utilize CXCR4, CCR5 or CCR2 as cofactors for infection of target cells [10].

Comments

There are examples of viral gene products, such as US28 (cytomegalovirus) and ECRF3 (herpes saimiri virus), which have been shown to bind chemokines [3]. The Duffy antigen functions as a receptor for the malarial parasite *Plasmodium vivax*[11].

References
[1] Vaddi, K. et al. (1997) The Chemokine FactsBook. Academic Press, London.
[2] Callard, R.E. and Gearing, A.J.H. (1993) The Cytokine FactsBook. Academic Press, London.
[3] **Premack, B.A. and Schall, T.J. (1996) Nature Med. 2, 1174–1178.**
[4] Bokoch, G.M. (1995) Blood 86, 1649–1660.
[5] **Feng, Y. et al. (1996) Science 272, 872–877.**
[6] Deng, H.K. et al. (1996) Nature 381, 661–666.
[7] Dragic, T. et al. (1996) Nature 381, 667–673.
[8] Alkhatib, G. et al. (1996) Science 272, 1955–1958.
[9] **Choe, H. et al. (1996) Cell 85, 1135–1148.**
[10] Doranz, B.J. et al. (1996) Cell 85, 1149–1158.
[11] Horuk, R. et al. (1993) Science 261, 1182–1184.

c-kitL
c-kit ligand, mast/stem cell growth factor, steel factor

Molecular weights

Polypeptide 27 906 (longer membrane form)
18 458 or 18 529 (predominant soluble form)

SDS-PAGE
reduced 28–36 kDa (soluble form)
unreduced 28–36 kDa (soluble form)

Carbohydrate
N-linked sites 4 or 5
O-linked +

Human gene location
12q22

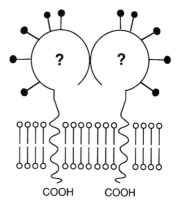

Tissue distribution

c-kitL is expressed by bone marrow stromal cells, fibroblasts, oocytes and in a range of tissues such as the liver, lung, kidney, testis and brain [1,2].

Structure

c-kitL is expressed both on the cell surface and, following proteolytic cleavage, in a soluble form [1,2]. Both membrane bound and secreted c-kitL are biologically active. The soluble form, and presumably also the membrane bound form, exists as a dimer [3]. Intramolecular disulfide bonds are formed between Cys4–89 and 43–138 (mature numbering) and the molecule contains considerable secondary structure including α helices and β sheets [1,3]. Together both *N*- and *O*-linked glycosylation accounts for approximately 30% of the total weight of c-kitL [3]. Alternative splicing gives rise to a second form of the molecule that lacks 28 amino acids (150–177; mature protein numbering), including one of the five potential *N*-linked glycosylation sites and the protease recognition site, which therefore yields soluble c-kitL less efficiently and is predominantly membrane bound [1].

Ligands and associated molecules

c-kitL binds to CD117 (c-kit), a cell surface receptor with Tyr kinase activity (see **CD117**).

Function

c-kitL is an early-acting haematopoietic growth factor, critical to the development of several distinct lineages from haematopoietic progenitors [1,2]. c-kitL also stimulates the proliferation of mast cells, as well as myeloid and lymphoid progenitors in bone marrow cultures, and functions as a survival factor for primordial germ cells [1,4].

Comment

c-kitL is analogous to PDGF and M-CSF, insofar as each growth factor is dimeric and their receptors (CD117 (c-kitL), PDGFRA/PDGFRB (CD140a/CD140b) and CD115 (c-fms)) constitute subclass III within the family of growth factor receptors with Tyr kinase activity[5]. Mutations at the *Sl* locus, which encodes mouse c-kitL, lead to alterations of coat colour (white coats), anaemia, defective mast cell development and defective gonad development[6,7].

Database accession numbers

	PIR	SWISSPROT	EMBL/GENBANK	REFERENCE
Human	A35974	P21583	M59964	8
Mouse	A35972	P20826	M38436	9
Rat	B35974	P21581	M59966	8

Amino acid sequence of human c-kitL

```
MKKTQTWILT CIYLQLLLFN PLVKT                             -1
EGICRNRVTN NVKDVTKLVA NLPKDYMITL KYVPGMDVLP SHCWISEMVV   50
QLSDSLTDLL DKFSNISEGL SNYSIIDKLV NIVDDLVECV KENSSKDLKK  100
SFKSPEPRLF TPEEFFRIFN RSIDAFKDFV VASETSDCVV SSTLSPEKDS  150
RVSVTKPFML PPVAASSLRN DSSSSNRKAK NPPGDSSLHW AAMALPALFS  200
LIIGFAFGAL YWKKRQPSLT RAVENIQINE EDNEISMLQE KEREFQEV    248
```

The longer membrane form of c-kitL (shown above) is cleaved following Ala164 or Ala165 (mature numbering) to yield soluble c-kitL.

References
1 **Galli, S.J. et al. (1994) Adv. Immunol. 55, 1–96.**
2 Callard, R.E. and Gearing, A.J.H. (1994) The Cytokine FactsBook. Academic Press, London.
3 Arakawa, T. et al. (1991) J. Biol. Chem. 266, 18942–18948.
4 Godin, I. et al. (1991) Nature 352, 807–809.
5 Ullrich, A. and Schlessinger, J. (1990) Cell 61, 203–212.
6 Witte, O.N. (1990) Cell 63, 5–6.
7 Copeland, N.G. et al. (1990) Cell 63, 175–183.
8 Martin, F.H. et al. (1990) Cell 63, 203–211.
9 Anderson, D.M. et al. (1990) Cell 63, 235–243.

CMRF35 antigen

Molecular weight
Polypeptide   22 606

SDS-PAGE
  unknown

Carbohydrate
N-linked sites   2
O-linked   probable +

Note
No protein data has thus far been obtained.

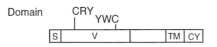

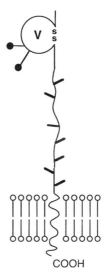

Tissue distribution

The CMRF35 antigen is expressed on human granulocytes, monocytes, neutrophils, NK cells, 25% of circulating T cells and 15% of circulating B cells [1].

Structure

The extracellular domain of the CMRF35 antigen contains a single IgSF V-set domain closely related to the first, third and fourth IgSF domains of the poly Ig receptor on epithelial cells [2]. This suggests that the two molecules evolved from a common precursor [2]. A Pro- and Ser-rich sequence that is likely to be O-glycosylated forms a hinge-like region linking the V-set domain to a transmembrane sequence that contains a charged residue (Glu) [2]. The presence of this charged residue suggests that the CMRF35 antigen may associate with other molecules in the membrane.

Function

Mitogenic stimulation of peripheral blood lymphocytes reduces both mRNA levels and cell surface expression of the CMRF35 antigen [1,2].

Amino acid sequence of human CMRF35

```
MTARAWASWR SSALLLLLVP                                          -1
GYFPLSHPMT VAGPVGGSLS VQCRYEKEHR TLNKFWCRPP QILRCDKIVE         50
TKGSAGKRNG RVSIRDSPAN LSFTVTLENL TEEDAGTYWC GVDTPWLRDF        100
HDPIVEVEVS VFPAGTTTAS SPQSSMGTSG PPTKLPVHTW PSVTRKDSPE        150
PSPHPGSLFS NVRFLLLVLL ELPLLLSMLG AVLWVNRPQR SSRSRQNWPK        200
GENQ                                                          204
```

References
[1] Daish, A. et al. (1993) Immunology 79, 55–63.
[2] Jackson, D.G. et al. (1992) Eur. J. Immunol. 22, 1157–1163.

DEC-205

Molecular weights
Polypeptide   194 529

SDS-PAGE
   reduced   205 kDa

Carbohydrate
N-linked sites   17
O-linked   nil

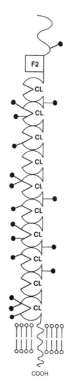

Domains

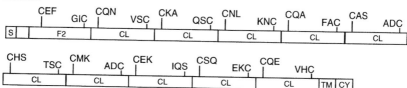

Tissue distribution

Mouse DEC-205 is recognized by the monoclonal antibody NLDC-145 [1]. Using this antibody the antigen was originally reported to be expressed on dendritic cells in the spleen, lymph nodes, Peyer's patches, thymic medulla and skin (Langerhans cells) and on epithelial cells in the thymic cortex and intestinal villi [1]. A rabbit polyclonal antibody raised against purified DEC-205 has subsequently detected low levels of expression on mature B cells, granulocytes, thioglycollate-elicited macrophages, thymocytes, mature T cells from spleen and lymph node, bone marrow stromal cells, the epithelia of the lung and on brain capillaries [2–4].

Structure

DEC-205 is a type I membrane glycoprotein comprising an N-terminus Cys-rich domain that shows sequence similarity to the B subunit of the plant protein ricin D, followed by a fibronectin type II domain, ten C-type lectin domains, transmembrane and cytoplasmic regions[5]. The molecule shows overall sequence similarity to the macrophage mannose receptor, the M-type receptor for secretory phospholipases A_2 and a fourth, widely expressed, member of this C-type lectin family[6]. The N-terminus of DEC-205 has been confirmed by protein sequencing[5].

Ligands and associated molecules

Unknown.

Function

Electron microscopy studies using gold-labelled monoclonal and polyclonal anti-DEC-205 antibodies have shown that dendritic cells rapidly internalize the antigen by means of coated pits and vesicles[5]. The molecule is delivered to a multivesicular compartment that resembles MHC Class II-containing vesicles. Dendritic cells treated with rabbit anti-DEC-205 antibodies were also found to induce activation of rabbit IgG-specific T cell clones more efficiently than cells treated with non-immune rabbit IgG[5]. Together these data suggest that DEC-205 contributes to antigen presentation.

Database accession numbers

	PIR	SWISSPROT	EMBL/GENBANK	REFERENCE
Mouse			U19271	5

Amino acid sequence of mouse DEC-205

```
MRTGRVTPGL AAGLLLLLLR SFGLVEP                            -1
SESSGNDPFT IVHENTGKCI QPLSDWVVAQ DCSGTNNMLW KWVSQHRLFH    50
LESQKCLGLD ITKATDNLRM FSCDSTVMLW WKCEHHSLYT AAQYRLALKD   100
GYAVANTNTS DVWKKGGSEE NLCAQPYHEI YTRDGNSYGR PCEFPFLIGE   150
TWYHDCIHDE DHSGPWCATT LSYEYDQKWG ICLLPESGCE GNWEKNEQIG   200
SCYQFNNQEI LSWKEAYVSC QNQGADLLSI HSAAELAYIT GKEDIARLVW   250
LGLNQLYSAR GWEWSDFRPL KFLNWDPGTP VAPVIGGSSC ARMDTESGLW   300
QSVSCESQQP YVCKKPLNNT LELPDVWTYT DTHCHVGWLP NNGFCYLLAN   350
ESSSWDAAHL KCKAFGADLI SMHSLADVEV VVTKLHNGDV KKEIWTGLKN   400
TNSPALFQWS DGTEVTLTYW NENEPSVPFN KTPNCVSYLG KLGQWKVQSC   450
EKKLRYVCKK KGEITKDAES DKLCPPDEGW KRHGETCYKI YEKEAPFGTN   500
CNLTITSRFE QEFLNYMMKN YDKSLRKYFW TGLRDPDSRG EYSWAVAQGV   550
KQAVTFSNWN FLEPASPGGC VAMSTGKTLG KWEVKNCRSF RALSICKKVS   600
EPQEPEEAAP KPDDPCPEGW HTFPSSLSCY KVFHIERIVR KRNWEEAERF   650
CQALGAHLPS FSRREEIKDF VHLLKDQFSG QRWLWIGLNK RSPDLQGSWQ   700
WSDRTPVSAV MMEPEFQQDF DIRDCAAIKV LDVPWRRVWH LYEDKDYAYW   750
KPFACDAKLE WVCQIPKGST PQMPDWYNPE RTGIHGPPVI IEGSEYWFVA   800
DPHLNYEEAV LYCASNHSFL ATITSFTGLK AIKNKLANIS GEEQKWWVKT   850
SENPIDRYFL GSRRRLWHHF PMTFGDECLH MSAKTWLVDL SKRADCNAKL   900
PFICERYNVS SLEKYSPDPA AKVQCTEKWI PFQNKCFLKV NSGPVTFSQA   950
SGICHSYGGT LPSVLSRGEQ DFIISLLPEM EASLWIGLRW TAYERINRWT  1000
DNRELTYSNF HPLLVGRRLS IPTNFFDDES HFHCALILNL KKSPLTGTWN  1050
FTSCSERHSL SLCQKYSETE DGQPWENTSK TVKYLNNLYK IISKPLTWHG  1100
ALKECMKEKM RLVSITDPYQ QAFLAVQATL RNSSFWIGLS SQDDELNFGW  1150
```

```
SDGKRLQFSN WAGSNEQLDD CVILDTDGFW KTADCDDNQP GAICYYPGNE    1200
TEEEVRALDT AKCPSPVQST PWIPFQNSCY NFMITNNRHK TVTPEEVQST    1250
CEKLHPKAHS LSIRNEEENT FVVEQLLYFN YIASWVMLGI TYENNSLMWF    1300
DKTALSYTHW RTGRPTVKNG KFLAGLSTDG FWDIQSFNVI EETLHFYQHS    1350
ISACKIEMVD YEDKHNGTLP QFIPYKDGVY SVIQKKVTWY EALNACSQSG    1400
GELASVHNPN GKLFLEDIVN RDGFPLWVGL SSHDGSESSF EWSDGRAFDY    1450
VPWQSLQSPG DCVVLYPKGI WRREKCLSVK DGAICYKPTK DKKLIFHVKS    1500
SKCPVAKRDG PQWVQYGGHC YASDQVLHSF SEAKQVCQEL DHSATVVTIA    1550
DENENKFVSR LMRENYNITM RVWLGLSQHS LDQSWSWLDG LDVTFVKWEN    1600
KTKDGDGKCS ILIASNETWR KVHCSRGYAR AVCKIPLSPD YTGIAILFAV    1650
LCLLGLISLA IWFLLQRSHI RWTGFSSVRY EHGTNEDEVM LPSFHD        1696
```

References

1 Kraal, G. et al. (1986) J. Exp. Med. 163, 981–997.
2 Swiggard, W.J. (1995) Cell. Immunol. 165, 302–311.
3 Inaba, K. et al. (1995) Cell. Immunol. 163, 148–156.
4 Witmer–Pack, M.D. et al. (1995) Cell. Immunol. 163, 157–162.
5 **Jiang, W. et al. (1995) Nature 375, 151–155.**
6 Wu, K. et al. (1996) J. Biol. Chem. 271, 21323–21330.

DNAM-1 DNAX accessory molecule 1

Molecular weights
Polypeptide   36 497

SDS-PAGE
  reduced   65 kDa
  unreduced   65 kDa

Carbohydrate
N-linked sites   8
O-linked   nil

Human gene location
18q22.3

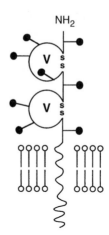

Tissue distribution

DNAM-1 is expressed on the majority of T cells, NK cells, monocytes, some B cells and some thymocytes. It is absent from erythrocytes and granulocytes[1].

Structure

The extracellular region consists of two IgSF domains which are unusually both V-set. The N-terminus has been established by protein sequencing[1].

Ligands and associated molecules

COS cells transfected with DNAM-1 bind to a variety of haematopoietic and non-haematopoietic cells indicating the presence of a widely distributed ligand[1].

Function

DNAM-1 mAb blocks NK and cytotoxic T cell killing[1]. Crosslinking of DNAM-1 causes phosphorylation of tyrosine residues in DNAM-1 indicating a possible role in signalling[1].

Database accession number

	PIR	SWISSPROT	EMBL/GENBANK	REFERENCE
Human			U56102	1

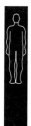

Amino acid sequence of human DNAM-1

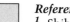

```
MDYPTLLLAL LHVYRALC                                              -1
EEVLWHTSVP FAENMSLECV YPSMGILTQV EWFKIGTQQD SIAIFSPTHG           50
MVIRKPYAER VYFLNSTMAS NNMTLFFRNA SEDDVGYYSC SLYTYPQGTW          100
QKVIQVVQSD SFEAAVPSNS HIVSEPGKNV TLTCQPQMTW PVQAVRWEKI          150
QPRQIDLLTY CNLVHGRNFT SKFPRQIVSN CSHGRWSVIV IPDVTVSDSG          200
LYRCYLQASA GENETFVMRL TVAEGKTDNQ YTLFVAGGTV LLLLFVISIT          250
TIIVIFLNRR RRRERRDLFT ESWDTQKAPN NYRSPISTGQ PTNQSMDDTR          300
EDIYVNYPTF SRRPKTRV                                             318
```

Reference
[1] Shibuya, A. (1996) Immunity 4, 573–581.

ESL-1
E-selectin ligand 1, MG-160, cysteine-rich FGF receptor

Molecular weights
Polypeptide   131 023

SDS-PAGE
  reduced   150 kDa
  unreduced   130 kDa

Carbohydrate
N-linked sites   5
O-linked   unknown

Human gene location
16q22–q23 [1]

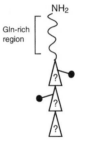

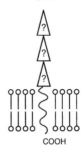

10 more cysteine-rich repeats

Tissue distribution

ESL-1 is expressed in virtually all cells [1–3]. However, the glycoform which binds to E-selectin has only been detected in cells of the myeloid lineage [3].

Structure

ESL-1 is a large cysteine-rich type I membrane glycoprotein with a short cytoplasmic domain and five potential N-linked glycosylation sites in the extracellular region. A glutamine-rich N-terminal segment (~70 amino acids) is followed by 16 repeats of a novel, 50–60 amino acid long, cysteine-rich motif [2]. Mouse ESL-1 is likely to be the homologue (98% identical) of the rat Golgi glycoprotein MG-160 [2]. ESL-1 may also be a splice variant of the cysteine-rich fibroblast growth factor (FGF) receptor, identified in the chicken [4] and the human (Genbank U28811). Apart from the glutamine-rich N-terminal segment, ESL-1 is >98% identical to the human cysteine-rich FGF receptor [3].

Ligands and associated proteins

E-selectin (CD62E) binds to a glycoform of ESL-1 expressed on myeloid cells (but not other cells) [3]. Binding requires N-linked carbohydrates on ESL-1 containing both sialic acid and fucose [3]. Proteins (MG-160, cysteine-rich FGF receptor) which may be species homologues of ESL-1 bind to fibroblast growth factor [1,4].

Function

Studies *in vitro* suggest that ESL-1 is a major E-selectin ligand on myeloid cells [3] but the functional significance of this interaction has not been tested *in vivo*. It is not known what role, if any, the protein has in Golgi function.

Database accession numbers

	PIR	SWISSPROT	EMBL/GENBANK	REFERENCE
Mouse			X84037	[3]
Rat MG-160			U08136	[2]

Amino acid sequence of mouse ESL-1

```
MAVCGRVRGM FRLSAALPLL LLAAAGA                                 -1
QNGHGQGQGP GTNFGPFPGQ GGGGSPAGQQ PPQQPQLSQQ QQQPPPQQQQ        50
QQQQQSLFAA GGLPARRGGA GPGGTGGGWK LAEEESCRED VTRVCPKHTW       100
SNNLAVLECL QDVREPENEI SSDCNHLLWN YKLNLTTDPK FESVAREVCK       150
STISEIKECA EEPVGKGYMV SCLVDHRGNI TEYQCHQYIT KMTAIIFSDY       200
RLICGFMDDC KNDINLLKCG SIRLGEKDAH SQGEVVSCLE KGLVKEAEEK       250
EPKIQVSELC KKAILRVAEL SSDDFHLDRH LYFACRDDRE RFCENTQAGE       300
GRVYKCLFNH KFEESMSEKC REALTTRQKL IAQDYKVSYS LAKSCKSDLK       350
KYRCNVENLP RSREARLSYL LMCLESAVHR GRQVSSECQG EMLDYRRMLM       400
EDFSLSPEII LSCRGEIEHH CSGLHRKGRT LHCLMKVVRG EKGNLGMNCQ       450
QALQTLIQET DPGADYRIDR ALNEACESVI QTACKHIRSG DPMILSCLME       500
HLYTEKMVED CEHRLLELQY FISRDWKLDP VLYRKCQGDA SRLCHTHGWN       550
ETSELMPPGA VFSCLYRHAY RTEEQGRRLS RECRAEVQRI LHQRAMDVKL       600
DPALQDKCLI DLGKWCSEKT ETGQELECLQ DHLDDLAVEC RDIVGNLTEL       650
ESEDIQIEAL LMRACEPIIQ NFCHDVADNQ IDSGDLMECL IQNKHQKDMN       700
EKCAIGVTHF QLVQMKDFRF SYKFKMACKE DVLKLCPNIK KKVDVVICLS       750
TTVRNDTLQE AKEHRVSLKC RKQLRVEELE MTEDIRLEPD LYEACKSDIK       800
NYCSTVQYGN AQIIECLKEN KKQLSTRCHQ KVFKLQETEM MDPELDYTLM       850
RVCKQMIKRF CPEADSKTML QCLKQNKNSE LMDPKCKQMI TKRQITQNTD       900
YRLNPVLRKA CKADIPKFCH GILTKAKDDS ELEGQVISCL KLRYADQRLS       950
SDCEDQIRII IQESALDYRL DPQLQLHCSD EIANLCAEEA AAQEQTGQVE      1000
ECLKVNLLKI KTELCKKEVL NMLKESKADI FVDPVLHTAC ALDIKHHCAA      1050
ITPGRGRQMS CLMEALEDKR VRLQPECKKR LNDRIEMWSY AAKVAPADGF      1100
SDLAMQVMTS PSKNYILSVI SGSICILFLI GLMCGRITKR VTRELKDR        1148
```

References

[1] Mourelatos, Z. et al. (1995) Genomics 28, 354–355.

[2] Gonatas, J.O. et al. (1995) J. Cell Sci. 108, 457–467.

[3] **Steegmaier, M. et al. (1995) Nature 373, 615–620.**

[4] Burrus, L.W. et al. (1992) Mol. Cell. Biol. 12, 5600–5609.

F4/80

EGF module-containing mucin-like hormone receptor 1 (EMR1) (human)

Molecular weights
Polypeptide   98 892

SDS-PAGE
  reduced   160 kDa
  unreduced   160 kDa

Carbohydrate
N-linked sites   10
O-linked   +
Glycosaminoglycan   1

Human gene location (EMR1)
19p13.3

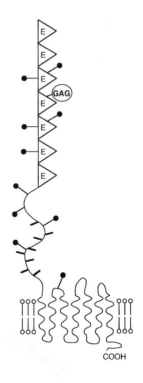

Tissue distribution

The F4/80 monoclonal antibody has been used to detect mouse macrophage populations in a wide range of tissues[1]. F4/80+ macrophages are located in the splenic red pulp, liver (Kupffer cells), medullary region of lymph nodes, brain (microglia), gut (lamina propria), bone marrow stroma, skin (Langerhans cells) and peritoneum[2]. Blood monocytes, thymic macrophages and macrophages in the lung express lower levels of the F4/80 molecule. The sequence of human EMR1 is available, however antibodies specific for EMR1 have not yet been developed. Limited RT-PCR analysis suggests that the human molecule is highly expressed on peripheral blood monocytes and a number of haematopoietic cell lines[3].

Structure

F4/80 is a member of the recently described EGF-TM7 family which also includes the CD97 molecule[4]. The deduced amino acid sequence of F4/80 comprises seven extracellular EGF domains, followed by a region of 277 amino acids and seven transmembrane-spanning regions with sequence similarities to the G protein-coupled transmembrane receptors[5]. F4/80 has also been shown to be extensively N-glycosylated, moderately O-glycosylated and contains a chondroitin sulfate glycosaminoglycan attachment[6].

Ligands and associated molecules

Unknown.

Function

Unknown.

Comments

The mouse F4/80 and human EMR1 polypeptide sequences share 68% overall amino acid identity, although mouse F4/80 contains seven extracellular EGF domains compared to the six in EMR1 [4,5]. F4/80 and EMR1 are either species homologues or are members of a closely related group of proteins.

Database accession numbers

	PIR	SWISSPROT	EMBL/GENBANK	REFERENCE
Human EMR1			X81479	3
Mouse			X93328	5

Amino acid sequence of mouse F4/80

```
MWGFWLLLFW GFSGMYRWGM TTLPTLG                             -1
QTLGGVNECQ DTTTCPAYAT CTDTTDSYYC TCKRGFLSSN GQTNFQGPGV    50
ECQDVNECLQ SDSPCGPNSV CTNILGRAKC SCLRGFSSST GKDWILGSLD   100
NFLCADVDEC LTIGICPKYS NCSNSVGSYS CTCQPGFVLN GSICEDEDEC   150
VTRDVCPEHA TCHNTLGSYY CTCNSGLESS GGGPMFQGLD ESCEDVDECS   200
RNSTLCGPTF ICINTLGSYS CSCPAGFSLP TFQILGHPAD GNCTDIDECD   250
DTCPLNSSCT NTIGSYFCTC HPGFASSNGQ LNFKDLEVTC EDIDECTQDP   300
LQCGLNSVCT NVPGSYICGC LPDFQMDPEG SQGYGNFNCK RILFKCKEDL   350
ILQSEQIQQC QAVQGRDLGY ASFCTLVNAT FTILDNTCEN KSAPVSLQSA   400
ATSVSLVLEQ ATTWFELSKE ETSTLGTILL ETVESTMLAA LLIPSGNASQ   450
MIQTEYLDIE SKVINEECKE NESINLAARG DKMNVGCFII KESVSTGAPG   500
VAFVSFAHME SVLNERFFED GQSFRKLRMN SRVVGGTVTG EKKEDFSKPI   550
IYTLQHIQPK QKSERPICVS WNTDVEDGRW TPSGCEIVEA SETHTVCSCN   600
RMANLAIIMA SGELTMEFSL YIISHVGTVI SLVCLALAIA TFLLCRAVQN   650
HNTYMHLHLC VCLFLAKILF LTGIDKTDNQ TACAIIAGFL HYLFLACFFW   700
MLVEAVMLFL MVRNLKVVNY FSSRNIKMLH LCAFGYGLPV LVVIISASVQ   750
PRGYGMHNRC WLNTETGFIW SFLGPVCMII TINSVLLAWT LWVLRQKLCS   800
VSSEVSKLKD TRLLTFKAIA QIFILGCSWV LGIFQIGPLA SIMAYLFTII   850
NSLQGAFIFL IHCLLNRQVR DEYKKLLTRK TDLSSHSQTS GILLSSMPST   900
SKMG                                                     904
```

References
1 Austyn, J.M. and Gordon, S. (1981) Eur. J. Immunol. 11, 805–815.
2 Gordon, S. et al. (1992) Curr. Top. Microbiol. Immunol. 181, 1–37.
3 Baud, V. et al. (1995) Genomics 26, 334–344.
4 McKnight, A.J. and Gordon, S. (1996) Immunol. Today 17, 283–287.
5 **McKnight, A.J. et al. (1996) J. Biol. Chem. 271, 486–489.**
6 Haidl, I.D. and Jefferies, W.A. (1996) Eur. J. Immunol. 26, 1139–1146.

FasL

Molecular weights
Polypeptide   31 485

SDS-PAGE
reduced   38–42 kDa

Carbohydrate
N-linked sites   3
O-linked   probable ++

Human gene location and size
1q23; 8 kb [1]

Domain

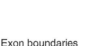

WED   FFG

| CY | TM | | T |

REST   TGK

Exon boundaries

IGH

NH₂

Tissue distribution

In contrast to Fas, FasL is mainly restricted to activated T lymphocytes and is induced rapidly [2]. FasL mRNA has been identified in rodent testis and eye and expression confirmed in the latter with a mAb [2].

Structure

FasL is a member of the TNF superfamily [2-5] and its amino acid sequence is highly conserved across species [1]. Like other members of this superfamily, it is a type II membrane protein expressed as a trimer with the similarity to TNF being in the C-terminal extracellular region [3,5]. The cytoplasmic domain is proline rich and contains a consensus SH3 binding motif [1]. The TNF-like extracellular region can be found in soluble form [3]. Other members of the TNF superfamily are clustered on chromosome 1 [1].

Ligands and associated molecules

The extracellular region of FasL binds to CD95 (Fas), a member of the TNFR superfamily.

Function

FasL binding to CD95 induces apoptosis in activated mature lymphocytes, thus has a role in maintaining peripheral tolerance but does not appear critical in development [2,7]. Autoimmune disease in gld⁻/⁻ mouse is due to mutations in FasL [2,7]. FasL on cytotoxic T cells can induce cytolysis of CD95-expressing target cells [7,8].

Database accession numbers

	PIR	SWISSPROT	EMBL/GENBANK	REFERENCE
Human		P48023	U11821	1
Mouse		P41047	S76752	6
Rat		P36940	U03470	5

Amino acid sequence of human FasL

```
MQQPFNYPYP QIYWVDSSAS SPWAPPGTVL PCPTSVPRRP GQRRPPPPPP     50
PPPLPPPPPP PPLPPLPLPP LKKRGNHSTG LCLLVMFFMV LVALVGLGLG    100
MFQLFHLQKE LAELRESTSQ MHTASSLEKQ IGHPSPPPEK KELRKVAHLT    150
GKSNSRSMPL EWEDTYGIVL LSGVKYKKGG LVINETGLYF VYSKVYFRGQ    200
SCNNLPLSHK VYMRNSKYPQ DLVMMEGKMM SYCTTGQMWA RSSYLGAVFN    250
LTSADHLYVN VSELSLVNFE ESQTFFGLYK L                        281
```

References

1 Takahashi T. et al. (1994) Int. Immunol. 6, 1567–1574.
2 **van Parijs, L. and Abbas, A.K. (1996) Curr. Opin. Immunol. 8, 355–361.**
3 Gruss, H.-J. and Dower, S.K. (1995) Blood 85, 3378–3404.
4 **Nagata, S. and Golstein, P. (1995) Science 267, 1449–1456.**
5 Suda, T. et al. (1993) Cell 75, 1169–1178.
6 Lynch, D.H. et al. (1994) Immunity 1, 131–136.
7 Lynch, D.H. et al. (1995) Immunol. Today 16. 569–574.
8 Takayama, H. et al. (1995) Adv. Immunol. 60, 289–321.

Molecular weights

Polypeptide		
	α	29 596
	β	26 533
	γ	9667

SDS-PAGE		
reduced	α	45–65 kDa
	β	27 kDa
	γ	7–10 kDa
unreduced	α	45–65 kDa
	β	27 kDa
	γ	20 kDa

Carbohydrate

N-linked sites	α	7
	β	0
	γ	0
O-linked	α	probable +
	β	unknown
	γ	nil

Human gene location and size

α chain: 1q23
β chain: 11q13; 10 kb [1]
γ chain: 1q23; 4 kb [2]

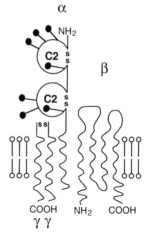

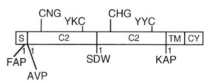

human FcεR1α

Tissue distribution

FcεRI was once thought to be expressed only on mast cells and basophils [3], but has recently been identified on eosinophils [4], monocytes [5], and Langerhans cells in the skin [6].

Structure

FcεRI is a multisubunit structure composed of an α chain, β chain and disulfide-linked γ homodimer [3]. In the human, but not the mouse, FcεRI is thought to exist as both $\alpha\beta\gamma_2$ and $\alpha\gamma_2$ complexes [7]. FcεRIα has an extracellular region composed of two IgSF domains followed by a highly conserved transmembrane region. Within the transmembrane region a sequence of nine amino acids is conserved in human, rat and mouse, of which eight residues are also identical in the CD16 transmembrane region [8]. FcεRIβ is a member of the CD20/FcεRIβ superfamily which includes CD20 and HTm4. These molecules are predicted to have four transmembrane regions, cytoplasmic N- and C-termini, and short extracellular loops [9]. FcεRIγ is identical to the γ subunit of CD16[8]. FcεRIγ has 86% amino acid identity between human, rat and mouse and is related to the ζ and η chains that are associated with the CD3/TCR complex[2]. The C-terminal cytoplasmic regions of FcεRIβ and FcεRIγ each contain an immunoreceptor tyrosine-based activation motif (ITAM)[10]. FcεRI shows no sequence similarity to the low-affinity IgE receptor CD23[8].

Ligands and associated molecules

FcεRIα binds to monomeric IgE with high affinity (K_a of $10^{10}\,\text{M}^{-1}$) and a stoichiometry of 1:1. The binding site involves the second IgSF domain of FcεRIα which interacts with the N-terminal segment of the Cε3 domain of IgE[3]. The cytoplasmic tails of FcεRIβ and FcεRIγ associate non-covalently with the non-receptor protein tyrosine kinases Lyn and Syk, respectively[7].

Function

As the high-affinity receptor for IgE, FcεRI on basophils and mast cells plays a central role in allergic reactions. When a multivalent allergen binds to FcεRI-bound IgE, FcεRI molecules are crosslinked and a signalling response is initiated. The result is cellular degranulation, a rapid release of histamine and other stored mediators, and the secretion of pro-inflammatory cytokines. These factors combine to induce the symptoms of immediate hypersensitivity[3]. The precise functions of the α, β and γ FcεRI subunits in this process are becoming clear. The α chain performs the ligand binding role by binding to IgE[3], whereas the β chain serves to amplify signals that are transduced through the γ homodimer[7]. The function of FcεRI on monocytes and Langerhans cells, in which the β chain is not expressed, is not clear, although FcεRI on these cells is upregulated in atopic individuals[5,6]. On eosinophils, FcεRI can mediate a cytotoxicity response against a metazoan parasite[4]. Indeed, the physiological role of FcεRI in a normal immune response is thought to be in protection against parasites.

Comments

1 The α and γ genes of FcεRI are linked to other Fc receptor genes on chromosome 1[8].
2 A common variant of FcεRIβ, Ile181Leu within the fourth transmembrane region, shows a strong association with atopic IgE responses[11].

Database accession numbers

	PIR	SWISSPROT	EMBL/GENBANK	REFERENCE
Human α	S00682	P12319	X06948	8
Human β	S21154	Q01362	D10583	1
Human γ	A35241	P30273	M33195	8
Rat α	A27116	P12371	M17153	8
Rat β	A31231	P13386	M22923	8
Rat γ	S02118	P20411		8
Mouse α	A34342	P20489	J05018	8
Mouse β	B34342	P20490	J05019	8
Mouse γ		P20491	J05020	8

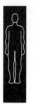

Amino acid sequence of human FcεRIα

```
MAPAMESPTL LCVALLFFAP DGVLA                                     -1
VPQKPKVSLN PPWNRIFKGE NVTLTCNGNN FFEVSSTKWF HNGSLSEETN          50
SSLNIVNAKF EDSGEYKCQH QQVNESEPVY LEVFSDWLLL QASAEVVMEG         100
QPLFLRCHGW RNWDVYKVIY YKDGEALKYW YENHNISITN ATVEDSGTYY         150
CTGKVWQLDY ESEPLNITVI KAPREKYWLQ FFIPLLVVIL FAVDTGLFIS         200
TQQQVTFLLK IKRTRKGFRL LNPHPKPNPK NN                            232
```

Amino acid sequence of human FcεRIβ

```
MDTESNRRAN LALPQEPSSV PAFEVLEISP QEVSSGRLLK SASSPPLHTW          50
LTVLKKEQEF LGVTQILTAM ICLCFGTVVC SVLDISHIEG DIFSSFKAGY         100
PFWGAIFFSI SGMLSIISER RNATYLVRGS LGANTASSIA GGTGITILII         150
NLKKSLAYIH IHSCQKFFET KCFMASFSTE IVVMMLFLTI LGLGSAVSLT         200
ICGAGEELKG NKVPEDRVYE ELNIYSATYS ELEDPGEMSP PIDL               244
```

Amino acid sequence of human FcεRIγ

```
MIPAVVLLLL LLVEQAAA                                             -1
LGEPQLCYIL DAILFLYGIV LTLLYCRLKI QVRKAAITSY EKSDGVYTGL          50
STRNQETYET LKHEKPPQ                                             68
```

References

1. Kuster, H. et al. (1992) J. Biol. Chem. 267, 12782–12787.
2. Kuster, H. et al. (1990) J. Biol. Chem. 265, 6448–6452.
3. Sutton, B.J. and Gould, H.J. (1993) Nature 366, 421–428.
4. Gounni, A.S. et al. (1994) Nature 367, 183–186.
5. Maurer, D. et al. (1994) J. Exp. Med. 179, 745–750.
6. Bieber, T. (1994) Immunol. Today 15, 52–53.
7. **Lin, S. et al. (1996) Cell 85, 985–995.**
8. Ravetch, J.V. and Kinet, J.-P. (1991) Annu. Rev. Immunol. 9, 457–492.
9. Adra, C.N. et al. (1994) Proc. Natl Acad. Sci. USA 91, 10178–10182.
10. Jouvin, M.-H. et al. (1995) Semin. Immunol. 7, 29–35.
11. Shirakawa, T. et al. (1994) Nature Genet. 7, 125–130.

FLT3 ligand   flk-2 (fetal liver kinase 2) ligand

Molecular weights
Polypeptide   23 716

SDS-PAGE
  soluble: reduced   30 kDa

Carbohydrate
N-linked   2
O-linked   unknown

Human gene location and size
19q13.3; 5.9 kb [1]

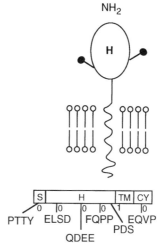

Exon boundaries

PTTY ELSD FQPP EQVP
              QDEE   PDS

Tissue distribution

mRNA for human and mouse FLT3 ligand is widespread in adult and fetal tissue with highest expression in spleen and lung [2]. Human FLT3 mRNA is high in peripheral blood mononuclear cells [1]. Surface expression has been demonstrated on cell lines by binding of recombinant FLT3 [3]. A mouse thymic stromal line secretes a soluble form of FLT3 ligand [2].

Structure

FLT3 ligand has an organization similar to c-kit ligand and macrophage colony-stimulating factor (M-CSF) and contains a four helix bundle, a single transmembrane and a short cytoplasmic domain [1,4]. Alternative splicing of exon 6 gives rise to a soluble form [2]. The native ligand has been reported to form a homodimer [2].

Ligands and associated molecules

FLT3 ligand binds to FLT3 (flk-2) receptor.

Function

FLT3 ligand binding to its receptor stimulates growth of primitive haematopoietic cells [5].

Database accession numbers

	PIR	SWISSPROT	EMBL/GENBANK	REFERENCE
Human		P49771	U04806	2
Mouse		P49772	U04807	2

Amino acid sequence of human FLT3 ligand

```
MTVLAPAWSP TTYLLLLLLL SSGLSG                                  -1
TQDCSFQHSP ISSDFAVKIR ELSDYLLQDY PVTVASNLQD EELCGGLWRL        50
VLAQRWMERL KTVAGSKMQG LLERVNTEIH FVTKCAFQPP PSCLRFVQTN       100
ISRLLQETSE QLVALKPWIT RQNFSRCLEL QCQPDSSTLP PPWSPRPLEA       150
TAPTAPQPPL LLLLLLPVGL LLLAAAWCLH WQRTRRRTPR PGEQVPPVPS       200
PQDLLLVEH                                                    209
```

References

1 Lyman, S.D. et al. (1995) Oncogene 11, 1165–1172.
2 Hannum, C. et al. (1994) Nature 368, 643–648.
3 Brasel, K. et al (1995) Leukemia 9, 1212–1218.
4 Mott, H. and Campbell, I.D. (1995) Curr. Opin. Struct. Biol. 5, 114–121.
5 **Lyman, S.D. et al. (1995) Curr. Opin. Hematol. 2, 177–181.**

Molecular weights
Polypeptide   38 402

SDS-PAGE
  reduced   55–70 kDa

Carbohydrate
N-linked sites   3
O-linked   unknown

Human gene location and size
19; 6 kb [1]

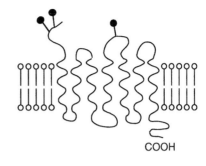

Tissue distribution

FPR is expressed by neutrophils, monocytes, macrophages and liver parenchymal cells [2-4].

Structure

FPR contains seven hydrophobic membrane spanning regions and is a member of the rhodopsin superfamily of G protein-coupled receptors [2,3,5]. It is closely related to the other chemoattractant receptors of the family, such as the IL-8, C5a and MIP-1α receptors. The third cytoplasmic loop contains a potential protein kinase A phosphorylation site and the C-terminal region is rich in Ser and Thr residues [2]. The cDNA clone originally reported to encode the rabbit FPR is actually the rabbit homologue of the IL-8 receptor (type A; CDw128) [6,7]. There are two human FPR isoforms that differ by two amino acids (Leu101 and Ala346 in the sequence shown below are replaced by Val and Glu, respectively) and by significant differences in the 5′ and 3′ untranslated regions. These probably represent allelic variants [2].

Ligands and associated molecules

FPR binds N-formyl peptides of bacterial and mitochondrial origin, such as the prototype fMLP (formyl-Met-Leu-Phe) ($K_d = 1$–2 nM). Putative natural ligands for FPR have also been described [8]. The reconstitution of a functional human FPR in *Xenopus* oocytes requires a complementary human factor [3].

Function

N-formyl peptides interact with FPR to induce neutrophil chemotaxis, phagocytosis, production of superoxide radicals and release of proteolytic enzymes from intracellular granules [2,3]. The binding of fMLP to FPR activates phospholipase C, via a pertussis toxin-sensitive G protein. The resulting production of diacylglycerol and phosphoinositides induces the activation of protein kinase C and mobilization of intracellular calcium. Other activation pathways of the receptor include the stimulation of phospholipases A2 and D [3].

Comments

The genes for two FPR-like receptors FPRL1 and FPRL2, which show 69% and 56% amino acid sequence identity to FPR, have also been mapped to human chromosome 19[9]. The FPRL1 molecule is a low-affinity receptor for fMLP ($K_d = 430$ nM), whereas FPRL2 does not bind fMLP and has no known ligand [10,11].

Database accession numbers

	PIR	SWISSPROT	EMBL/GENBANK	REFERENCE
Human	A35495	P21462	M60626, M60627	2
Mouse		P33766	L22181	10

Amino acid sequence of human FPR

```
METNSSLPTN ISGGTPAVSA GYLFLDIITY LVFAVTFVLG VLGNGLVIWV    50
AGFRMTHTVT TISYLNLAVA DFCFTSTLPF FMVRKAMGGH WPFGWFLCKF   100
LFTIVDINLF GSVFLIALIA LDRCVCVLHP VWTQNHRTVS LAKKVIIGPW   150
VMALLLTLPV IIRVTTVPGK TGTVACTFNF SPWTNDPKER INVAVAMLTV   200
RGIIRFIIGF SAPMSIVAVS YGLIATKIHK QGLIKSSRPL RVLSFVAAAF   250
FLCWSPYQVV ALIATVRIRE LLQGMYKEIG IAVDVTSALA FFNSCLNPML   300
YVFMGQDFRE RLIHALPASL ERALTEDSTQ TSDTATNSTL PSAEVALQAK   350
```

References
1   Murphy, P.M. et al. (1993) Gene 133, 285–290.
2   **Boulay, F. et al. (1990) Biochemistry 29, 11123–11133.**
3   Murphy, P.M. and McDermott, D. (1991) J. Biol. Chem. 266, 12560–12567.
4   McCoy, R. et al. (1995) J. Exp. Med. 182, 207–217.
5   Dohlman, H.G. et al. (1991) Annu. Rev. Biochem. 60, 653–688.
6   Thomas, K.M. et al. (1990) J. Biol. Chem. 265, 20061–20064.
7   Thomas, K.M. et al. (1991) J. Biol. Chem. 266, 14839–14841.
8   **Gao, J-L. et al. (1994) J. Exp. Med. 180, 2191–2197.**
9   Bao, L. et al. (1992) Genomics 13, 437–440.
10 Gao, J-L. and Murphy, P.M. (1993) J. Biol. Chem. 268, 25395–25401.
11 Durstin, M. et al. (1994) Biochem. Biophys. Res. Commun. 201, 174–179.

Galectin 3
Mac-2, εBP, IgEBP, CBP-35, CBP-30, RL29, L29, L31, L34, LBL etc.

Molecular weights
Polypeptide   27 482

SDS-PAGE
  reduced   35 kDa
  unreduced   35 kDa, 67 kDa, 80 kDa

Carbohydrate
N-linked sites   0
O-linked   unknown

Human gene location
1p13 [1]

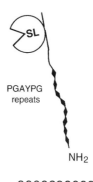

Domain

Tissue distribution

Tissue distribution

The highest levels of galectin 3 are found on thioglycollate-elicited macrophages $(1.7 \times 10^5$ sites/cell)[2], basophils, mast cells, some epithelial cells and some sensory neurons [1-3]. It is likely that cell surface expression is due to the carbohydrate recognition domain binding to cell surface glycoproteins as surface expression is reduced by inhibitory sugars [3].

Structure

Galectins, previously known as S-type lectins, contain carbohydrate binding domains which have sequence similarity in the carbohydrate binding sites and have affinity for β-galactoside sugars [1]. Galectin 3 consists of two distinct regions: the N-terminal region is rich in Pro and Gly residues and contains multiple repeats of the sequence PGAYPG or slight variations thereof, and the C-terminal region contains the carbohydrate binding domain [1,3,4]. The protein contains no hydrophobic sequences that may function as signal sequences or transmembrane domains and is secreted by unknown mechanisms [1,3]. Galectin 3 can form multimers through its N-terminal region and this is not dependent on disulfide formation [3,4].

Ligands and associated molecules

Galectin 3 binds IgE and FcεRI [4]. Another ligand is a secreted glycoprotein, Mac-2 binding protein, which contains a scavenger receptor cysteine-rich domain [3]. Binding activities can be inhibited by galactose [1,3].

Function

A role for galectin 3 in crosslinking IgE receptors is postulated [4]. Galectin 3 is the major non-integrin laminin binding protein of inflammatory macrophages and an antiadhesive role is suggested [3]. A recent study describes the activation of neutrophils by recombinant galectin 3 which is dependent on both its lectin binding activity and the N-terminal region[5]. An intracellular role for galectin 3 has been suggested based on localization of the protein in the nucleus[1]. There is evidence for galectin 3 as a factor in RNA splicing[6]. Activity was carbohydrate-dependent, in contrast to a report describing RNA binding by galectin 3[7].

Database accession numbers

	PIR	SWISSPROT	EMBL/GENBANK	REFERENCE
Human	A35820	P17931	J02921	[8]
Rat	A23148	P08699	J02962	[9]
Mouse	A28651	P16110	X16834	[10]

Amino acid sequence of human galectin 3

```
MADNFSLHDA LSGSGNPNPQ GWPGAWGNQP AGAGGYPGAS YPGAYPGQAP    50
PGAYPGQAPP GAYHGAPGAY PGAPAPGVYP GPPSGPGAYP SSGQPSAPGA   100
YPATGPYGAP AGPLIVPYNL PLPGGVVPRM LITILGTVKP NANRIALDFQ   150
RGNDVAFHFN PRFNENNRRV IVCNTKLDNN WGREERQSVF PFESGKPFKI   200
QVLVEPDHFK VAVNDAHLLQ YNHRVKKLNE ISKLGISGDI DLTSASYTMI   250
```

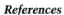

References
[1] Barondes, S.H. et al. (1994) J. Biol. Chem. 269, 20807–20810.
[2] Ho, M.-K. and Springer, T.A. (1982) J. Immunol. 128, 1221–1227.
[3] Hughes, R.C. (1994) Glycobiology 4, 5–12.
[4] Liu, F-T. (1993) Immunol. Today 14, 486–490.
[5] Yamaoka, A. et al. (1995) J. Immunol. 154, 3479–3487.
[6] Dagher, S.F. et al. (1995) Proc. Natl Acad. Sci. USA 92, 1213–1217.
[7] Wang, L. et al. (1995) Biochem. Biophys. Res. Commun. 217, 292–303.
[8] Cherayil, B.J. et al. (1990) Proc. Natl Acad. Sci. USA 87, 7324–7328.
[9] Albrandt, K. et al. (1987) Proc. Natl Acad. Sci. USA 84, 6859–6863.
[10] Cherayil, B.J. et al. (1989) J. Exp. Med. 170, 1959–1972.

Molecular weights
Polypeptide G-CSFR1   89 618

Carbohydrate
N-linked sites   9
O-linked   unknown

Human gene location and size
1p35–p34.3; ~16.5 kb [1]

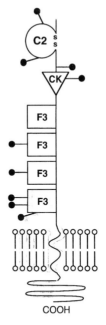

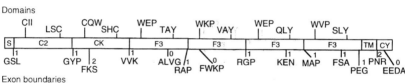

Domains

	CII		CQW		WEP		WKP		WEP		WVP		
		LSC		SHC		TAY		VAY		QLY		SLY	
S	C2		CK		F3		F3		F3		F3		TM	CY
1			1		1		0		1		1		1		2
GSL		GYP	2	VVK	ALVG	1		0	RGP	KEN	MAP	FSA	1 PNR	0
			FKS			RAP	FWKP						PEG	EEDA

Exon boundaries

Tissue distribution

CD114 is expressed on neutrophils and their bone marrow precursors, endothelial cells, platelets, myeloid leukaemias and carcinoma cell lines [2,3].

Structure

The extracellular region of CD114 consists of an IgSF C2-set domain, followed by a cytokine receptor domain and four fibronectin type III domains, the first of which contains the WSXWS motif characteristic of many Class I cytokine receptor family members [2]. Four forms of human CD114 (G-CSFR1, G-CSFR2, G-CSFR3 and G-CSFR4/D7) have been identified by cDNA cloning that differ at the C-terminal region of the molecule and are probably generated by alternative splicing [2,4]. The polypeptide encoded by G-CSFR2 appears to be a secreted form of CD114. The cytoplasmic domains of the remaining three forms have a high content of Ser and Pro residues. Based on crosslinking experiments, the estimated molecular weight of CD114 is 150 kDa [2].

Ligands and associated molecules

A single class of high-affinity binding sites for G-CSF (K_d = 100–500 pM) is detected on the cell surface[2]. The monomeric form of purified murine CD114 binds G-CSF with low affinity while its oligomeric forms show high-affinity binding, which suggests that the high-affinity receptor may be formed by a homodimer of the CD114 protein[3,5]. Following the binding of G-CSF to CD114, the Janus family Tyr kinases Jak1 and Jak2 and the transcriptional activator Stat3 are Tyr phosphorylated[6]. Mutational analysis has shown that the cytokine receptor domain and the WSXWS motif are necessary for G-CSF binding, and that a region of the cytoplasmic domain is essential for signal transduction[3].

Function

G-CSF stimulates the proliferation and differentiation of neutrophils from their bone marrow precursors, activates mature neutrophils and causes proliferation and migration of endothelial cells[7–9].

Database accession numbers

	PIR	SWISSPROT	EMBL/GENBANK	REFERENCE
Human	JH0330	Q99062	X55721	2
Mouse	A34898	P40223	M32699	10

The accession numbers for the alternatively spliced forms of human CD114 are M59819 (G-CSFR2), M59820 (G-CSFR3) and X5572 (G-CSFR4/D7).

Amino acid sequence of human CD114 (G-CSFR1)

```
MARLGNCSLT WAALIILLLP GSLE                                  -1
ECGHISVSAP IVHLGDPITA SCIIKQNCSH LDPEPQILWR LGAELQPGGR      50
QQRLSDGTQE SIITLPHLNH TQAFLSCCLN WGNSLQILDQ VELRAGYPPA     100
IPHNLSCLMN LTTSSLICQW EPGPETHLPT SFTLKSFKSR GNCQTQGDSI     150
LDCVPKDGQS HCCIPRKHLL LYQNMGIWVQ AENALGTSMS PQLCLDPMDV     200
VKLEPPMLRT MDPSPEAAPP QAGCLQLCWE PWQPGLHINQ KCELRHKPQR     250
GEASWALVGP LPLEALQYEL CGLLPATAYT LQIRCIRWPL PGHWSDWSPS     300
LELRTTERAP TVRLDTWWRQ RQLDPRTVQL FWKPVPLEED SGRIQGYVVS     350
WRPSGQAGAI LPLCNTTELS CTFHLPSEAQ EVALVAYNSA GTSRPTPVVF     400
SESRGPALTR LHAMARDPHS LWVGWEPPNP WPQGYVIEWG LGPPSASNSN     450
KTWRMEQNGR ATGFLLKENI RPFQLYEIIV TPLYQDTMGP SQHVYAYSQE     500
MAPSHAPELH LKHIGKTWAQ LEWVPEPPEL GKSPLTHYTI FWTNAQNQSF     550
SAILNASSRG FVLHGLEPAS LYHIHLMAAS QAGATNSTVL TLMTLTPEGS     600
ELHIILGLFG LLLLLTCLCG TAWLCCSPNR KNPLWPSVPD PAHSSLGSWV     650
PTIMEEDAFQ LPGLGTPPIT KLTVLEEDEK KPVPWESHNS SETCGLPTLV     700
QTYVLQGDPR AVSTQPQSQS GTSDQVLYGQ LLGSPTSPGP GHYLRCDSTQ     750
PLLAGLTPSP KSYENLWFQA SPLGTLVTPA PSQEDDCVFG PLLNFPLLQG     800
IRVHGMEALG SF                                             812
```

References

1 Seto, Y. et al. (1992) J. Immunol. 148, 259–266.
2 Larsen, A. et al. (1990) J. Exp. Med. 172, 1559–1570.
3 Fukunaga, R. et al. (1991) EMBO J. 10, 2855–2865.

[4] Fukunaga, R. et al. (1990) Proc. Natl Acad. Sci. USA 87, 8702–8706.

[5] Fukunaga, R. et al. (1990) J. Biol. Chem. 265, 14008–14015.

[6] Tian, S.S. et al. (1994) Blood 84, 1760–1764

[7] Nicola, N.A. (1989) Annu. Rev. Biochem. 58, 45–77.

[8] Arai, K. et al. (1990) Annu. Rev. Biochem. 59, 783–836.

[9] **Callard, R.E. and Gearing, A.J.H. (1994) The Cytokine FactsBook. Academic Press, London.**

[10] Fukunaga, R. et al. (1990) Cell 61, 341–350.

Subunits
CD116 (α chain)
CDw131 (βc chain)

Molecular weights

Polypeptide	CD116	43 777
	CDw131	95 707

Carbohydrate

N-linked sites	CD116	11
	CDw131	3
O-linked	CD116	unknown
	CDw131	unknown

Human gene location and size
CD116: Xp22.32, Yp11.3; ≥45 kb [1]
CDw131: 22q12.2–q13.1

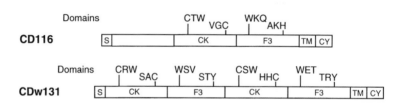

Tissue distribution

The GM-CSFR is expressed on monocytes, neutrophils, eosinophils, fibroblasts and endothelial cells. It is also present on myelocytic and promyelocytic cell lines, osteogenic sarcoma cell lines, osteoblast-like cells and breast and lung carcinoma cell lines [2].

Structure

The human GM-CSF receptor is formed by the association of CD116 and CDw131, which is the β chain common also to the IL-3R and IL-5R [3]. Crosslinking experiments show that the molecular weights of CD116 and CDw131 are 70–85 kDa and 120–140 kDa respectively [2,4]. The extracellular region of CD116 consists of an N-terminal region of about 100 amino acids with sequence similarities to that present in CDw123 (IL-3R α chain) and CDw125 (IL-5R α chain), followed by a cytokine receptor domain and a fibronectin type III domain that contains the WSXWS motif [2,3]. A soluble form of CD116 which binds GM-CSF with relatively low affinity ($K_d = 3$–4 nM) has been identified by PCR cloning [5-7]. In addition, an alternatively spliced form of CD116 with an altered cytoplasmic tail has been described [7]. The structure of CDw131 is described in the entry for the IL-3R.

Ligands and associated molecules

CD116 binds GM-CSF with low affinity $(K_d = 1-8 \text{ nM})$[2]. CDw131, which does not bind GM-CSF, associates with CD116 to generate a high-affinity receptor for GM-CSF $(K_d = 30-120 \text{ pM})$[4]. The GM-CSFR is believed to bind and mediate phosphorylation of the Janus family Tyr kinase, Jak2[8]. In the mouse it has been shown that CDw131 is essential for signal transduction[9].

Function

GM-CSF promotes the growth and differentiation of neutrophils, eosinophils and monocytes from multipotential bone marrow precursors. It is also a growth factor for erythroid progenitors, endothelial cells, megakaryocytes and T cells[10-12]. GM-CSF induces the tyrosine phosphorylation of a similar set of proteins as IL-3[13]. GM-CSF activates p21^{ras} and induces glucose transport, ion fluxes and the expression of a variety of genes[14,15].

Comment

The human CD116 gene has been mapped to the pseudoautosomal region of the X and Y chromosomes[16].

Database accession numbers

	PIR	SWISSPROT	EMBL/GENBANK	REFERENCE
Human CD116	S06945	P15509	X17648	2

Amino acid sequence of human CD116

```
MLLLVTSLLL CELPHPAFLL IP                                     -1
EKSDLRTVAP ASSLNVRFDS RTMNLSWDCQ ENTTFSKCFL TDKKNRVVEP        50
RLSNNECSCT FREICLHEGV TFEVHVNTSQ RGFQQKLLYP NSGREGTAAQ       100
NFSCFIYNAD LMNCTWARGP TAPRDVQYFL YIRNSKRRRE IRCPYYIQDS       150
GTHVGCHLDN LSGLTSRNYF LVNGTSREIG IQFFDSLLDT KKIERFNPPS       200
NVTVRCNTTH CLVRWKQPRT YQKLSYLDFQ YQLDVHRKNT QPGTENLLIN       250
VSGDLENRYN FPSSEPRAKH SVKIRAADVR ILNWSSWSEA IEFGSDDGNL       300
GSVYIYVLLI VGTLVCGIVL GFLFKRFLRI QRLFPPVPQI KDKLNDNHEV       350
EDEIIWEEFT PEEGKGYREE VLTVKEIT                               378
```

The accession numbers and amino acid sequence of CDw131, that is common to the IL-3R, IL-5R and GM-CSFR, are given in the **IL-3R** entry.

References

1. Rappold, G. et al. (1992) Genomics 14, 455–461.
2. Gearing, D.P. et al. (1989) EMBO J. 8, 3667–3676.
3. **Nicola, N.A. and Metcalf, D. (1991) Cell 67, 1–4.**
4. Hayashida, K. et al. (1990) Proc. Natl Acad. Sci. USA 87, 9655–9659.
5. Ashworth, A. and Kraft, A. (1990) Nucleic Acids Res. 18, 7178.
6. Raines, M.A. et al. (1991) Proc. Natl Acad. Sci. USA 88, 8203–8207.
7. Crosier, K.E. et al. (1991) Proc. Natl Acad. Sci. USA 88, 7744–7748.
8. Witthuhn, B.A. et al. (1993) Cell 74, 227–236.

9   Kitamura, T. et al. (1991) Proc. Natl Acad. Sci. USA 88, 5082–5086.

10 Nicola, N.A. et al. (1989) Annu. Rev. Biochem. 58, 45–77.

11 **Arai, K. et al. (1990) Annu. Rev. Biochem. 59, 783–836.**

12 Callard, R.E. and Gearing, A.J.H. (1994) The Cytokine FactsBook. Academic Press, London.

13 Isfort, R.J. and Ihle, J.N. (1990) Growth Factors 2, 213–220.

14 Satoh, T. et al. (1991) Proc. Natl Acad. Sci. USA 88, 3314–3318.

15 Vairo, G. and Hamilton , J.A. (1991) Immunol. Today 12, 362–369.

16 Gough, N.M. et al. (1990) Nature 345, 734–736.

GlyCAM-1 · Glycosylation-dependent cell adhesion molecule 1, Sgp50

Molecular weights
Polypeptide   14 154

SDS-PAGE
   reduced   50 kDa
   unreduced   50 kDa

Carbohydrate
N-linked sites   1
O-linked   +++

Mouse gene location and size
15; ~2.5 kb [1]

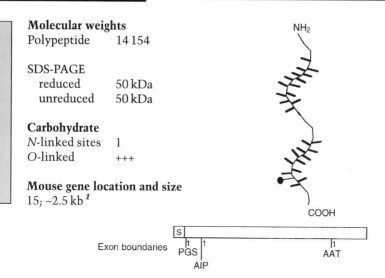

Tissue distribution

GlyCAM-1 is expressed by peripheral and mesenteric lymph node (LN) high endothelial venules (HEVs), the lactating mammary gland, and unknown cells in the lung [2,3]. Expression has also been reported by HEV-like vessels at sites of chronic inflammation [4]. GlyCAM-1 is a secreted molecule and is detectable in blood and milk [3].

Structure

GlyCAM-1 is a heavily *O*-glycosylated soluble secreted glycoprotein. Two segments within the extracellular region (residues 23–44 and 74–103) contain a high proportion (~50%) of serine and threonine residues and are likely to possess a mucin-like structure [2]. The N-terminus of the mature polypeptide has been established by protein sequencing [2].

Ligands and associated molecules

CD62L binds to carbohydrate structures present in some glycoforms of GlyCAM-1 expressed by HEVs. The exact ligand has yet to be identified but binding requires sialylation, sulfation and (probably) fucosylation of GlyCAM-1 carbohydrates. Notably, *O*-linked carbohydrates of GlyCAM-1 from LN HEV contain sulfated forms of sialylated Lewis x (sLe^x, Sia$\alpha2 \rightarrow 3$Gal$\beta1 \rightarrow 4$(Fuc$\alpha1 \rightarrow 3$)GlcNAc), which contain all three groups [5]. In contrast, milk GlyCAM-1, which does not bind CD62L, is not sulfated [3].

Function

As a ligand for CD62L, GlyCAM-1 was initially proposed to enhance lymphocyte adhesion to LN HEVs. However, the identification of GlyCAM-1 as a secreted molecule suggests that it may function instead to modulate CD62L-mediated adhesion[6]. Consistent with an inhibitory role, expression of GlyCAM-1 in the draining LN is dramatically decreased following antigen priming[7]. Soluble GlyCAM-1 can induce, via an interaction with cell surface CD62L, rapid activation of $\beta2$ (CD18) integrins on naive T cells[8].

Database accession numbers

	PIR	SWISSPROT	EMBL/GENBANK	REFERENCE
Mouse	A41908	Q02596	M93428	2
Rat	A47167	Q04807	L08100	9

Amino acid sequence of mouse GlyCAM-1

```
MKFFTVLLFV SLAATSLAL                                          -1
LPGSKDELQM KTQPTDAIPA AQSTPTSYTS EESTSSKDLS KEPSIFREEL        50
ISKDNVVIES TKPENQEAQD GLRSGSSQLE ETTRPTTSAA TTSEENLTKS       100
SQTVEEELGK IIEGFVTGAE DIISGASRIT KS                          132
```

References
[1] Dowbenko, D. et al. (1993) J. Biol. Chem. 268, 4525–4529.
[2] Lasky, L.A. et al. (1992) Cell 69, 927–938.
[3] **Lasky, L.A. (1995) Annu. Rev. Biochem. 64, 113–139.**
[4] Onrust, S.V. et al. (1996) J. Clin. Invest. 97, 54–64.
[5] Hemmerich, S. et al. (1995) J. Biol. Chem. 270, 12035–12047.
[6] Brustein, M. et al. (1992) J. Exp. Med. 176, 1415–1419.
[7] Hoke, D. et al. (1995) Curr. Biol. 5, 670–678.
[8] Hwang, S.T. et al. (1996) J. Exp. Med. 184, 1343–1348.
[9] Dowbenko, D. et al. (1993) J. Biol. Chem. 268, 14399–14403.

gp42

Molecular weights
Polypeptide   21 217

SDS-PAGE
    reduced   40–45 kDa
    unreduced   40–45 kDa

Carbohydrate
N-linked sites   3
O-linked   unknown

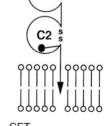

Tissue distribution

The antigen is not expressed on freshly isolated rat NK cells or T cells but its expression is selectively induced on NK cells in the presence of high concentrations of IL-2 *in vitro*[1].

Structure

gp42 is a GPI-anchored antigen consisting of two IgSF C2-set domains. The N-terminus and site of addition of the GPI anchor have not been determined but are predicted below.

Function

The function of gp42 is unknown. However, like other GPI-anchored molecules, gp42 may be capable of transmitting intracellular signals since anti-gp42 mAbs cross-linked with secondary antibodies induce increases in intracellular Ca^{2+} and inositol phosphates in a rat leukaemic cell line[2]. gp42 mAbs do not block the natural killer activity of NK cells[1].

Database accession numbers

	PIR	SWISSPROT	EMBL/GENBANK	REFERENCE
Rat	JH0372	P23505	X56448	2

Amino acid sequence of rat gp42

```
MLLWMVLLLC VSMTEA                                             -1
QELFQDPVLS RLNSSETSDL LLKCTTKVDP NKPASELFYS FYKDNHIIQN        50
RSHNPLFFIS EANEENSGLY QCVVDAKDGT IQKKSDYLDI DLCTSVSQPV       100
LTLQHEATNL AEGDKVKFLC ETQLGSLPIL YSFYMDGEIL GEPLAPSGRA       150
ASLLISVKAE WSGKNYSCQA ENKVSRDISE PKKFPLVVSG T                191
ASMKSTTV VIWLPVSCLV GWPWLLRF                                 +26
```

References
[1] Imboden, J.B. et al. (1989) J. Immunol. 143, 3100–3103.
[2] Seaman, W.E. et al. (1991) J. Exp. Med. 173, 251–260.

gp49

Molecular weights

Polypeptide	gp49B1	35 032
SDS-PAGE	gp49A	reduced 49 kDa
	gp49A	unreduced 49 kDa

gp49B1

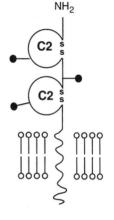

Carbohydrate

N-linked sites	2
O-linked	nil

Domains

gp49B1

Exon boundaries

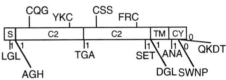

Tissue distribution

gp49 is present on mouse mast cells and their precursors [1].

Structure

The extracellular region consists of two IgSF domains, followed by a hydrophobic transmembrane domain and a cytoplasmic domain [2]. The N-terminus of gp49A has been determined by protein sequencing [2]. gp49A and gp49B1 differ in amino acid sequence by 9% except for an extra 32 residues at the C-terminal of gp49B1. The cytoplasmic domain of gp49B1 contains an ITIM motif. The 5.6 kb gene which encodes gp49B1 is alternatively spliced to produce gp49B2 which lacks a transmembrane region [3].

Function

The activation of bone marrow cultured mast cells by crosslinking of the FcεRI, or with a calcium ionophore or with PMA leads to phosphorylation of serine residues on gp49 [1].

Database accession numbers

	PIR	SWISSPROT	EMBL/GENBANK	REFERENCE
Mouse gp49B1	A5343		U05264	3

Amino acid sequence of mouse gp49B1

```
MIAMLTVLLY LGLILEPRTA VQA                                   -1
GHLPKPIIWA EPGSVIAAYT SVITWCQGSW EAQYYHLYKE KSVNPWDTQV      50
PLETRNKAKF NIPSMTTSYA GIYKCYYESA AGFSEHSDAM ELVMTGAYEN     100
PSLSVYPSSN VTSGVSISFS CSSSIVFGRF ILIQEGKHGL SWTLDSQHQA     150
NQPSYATFVL DAVTPNHNGT FRCYGYFRNE PQVWSKPSNS LDLMISETKD     200
QSSTPTEDGL ETYQKILIGV LVSFLLLFFL LLFLILIGYQ YGHKKKANAS     250
VKNTQSENNA ELNSWNPQNE DPQGIVYAQV KPSRLQKDTA CKETQDVTYA     300
QLCIRTQEQN NS                                             312
```

References

[1] Katz, H.R. et al. (1989) J. Immunol. 142, 919–926.

[2] Arm, J.P. et al. (1991) J. Biol. Chem. 266, 15966–15973.

[3] **Castells, M.C. et al. (1994) J. Biol. Chem. 266, 8393–8401.**

HTm4

Molecular weights
Polypeptide   22971

Carbohydrate
N-linked sites   nil
O-linked   unknown

Human gene location
11q12–q13.1

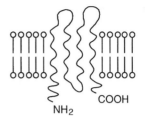

Tissue distribution

Northern blot and reverse transcriptase-PCR analyses suggest that HTm4 mRNA expression is restricted to cells of haematopoietic origin [1].

Structure

HTm4 is a member of the CD20/FcεRIβ superfamily of leucocyte surface antigens which includes CD20 and the β subunit of the high-affinity receptor for IgE (FcεRIβ). These molecules are predicted to have four transmembrane regions, cytoplasmic N- and C-termini, and short extracellular loops [1]. The gene for HTm4 maps to the same region of the genome as CD20 and FcεRIβ [1]. The CD20/FcεRIβ superfamily shares no sequence similarity with members of the TM4SF which also have four transmembrane regions.

Function

HTm4 cDNA was identified as a marker of haematopoietic cells by subtractive hybridization screening of cDNA libraries. The function of HTm4 is not known, although the sequence similarity to CD20 and FcεRIβ would suggest a role in signal transduction and/or as a subunit of receptor complexes [1].

Database accession numbers

	PIR	SWISSPROT	EMBL/GENBANK	REFERENCE
Human			L35848	[1]

Amino acid sequence of human HTm4

```
MASHEVDNAE LGSASAHGTP GSETGPEELN TSVYHPINGS PDYQKAKLQV   50
LGAIQILNAA MILALGVFLG SLQYPYHFQK HFFFFTFYTG YPIWGAVFFC  100
SSGTLSVVAG IKPTRTWIQN SFGMNIASAT IALVGTAFLS LNIAVNIQSL  150
RSCHSSSESP DLCNYMGSIS NGMVSLLLIL TLLELCVTIS TIAMWCNANC  200
CNSREEISSP PNSV                                        214
```

Reference
[1] Adra, C.N. et al. (1994) Proc. Natl Acad. Sci. USA 91, 10178–10182.

Subunits
CD119 (α chain)
IFNγ accessory factor 1 (IFNγ AF-1)

CD119   IFNγ AF-1

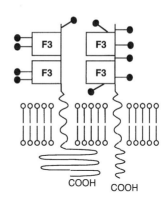

Molecular weights

Polypeptide	CD119	52 563
	IFNγ AF-1	35 034

SDS-PAGE		
reduced	CD119	90–100 kDa

Carbohydrate

N-linked sites	CD119	5
	IFNγ AF-1	6
O-linked	CD119	probable +
	IFNγ AF-1	probable +

Human gene location
CD119: 6q23–q24
IFNγ AF-1: 21q22.1–q22.2

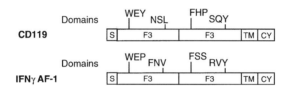

Tissue distribution

The IFNγR is expressed on monocytes, macrophages, T cells, B cells, NK cells, neutrophils, fibroblasts, epithelial cells, endothelium and a wide range of tumour cells [1,2].

Structure

The functional IFNγR consists of a complex formed between CD119 and IFNγ AF-1. Both CD119 and IFNγ AF-1 belong to the Class II cytokine receptor family, each consisting of two extracellular fibronectin type III domains, followed by a transmembrane region and a 222 amino acid (CD119) or 69 amino acid (IFNγ AF-1) cytoplasmic tail [1,3]. The WSXWS motif, characteristic of Class I cytokine receptors, is absent from both fibronectin type III domains in CD119 and IFNγ AF-1.

Ligands and associated molecules

The IFNγR binds IFNγ with high affinity (K_d = 1 nM–10 pM) [4]. Although CD119 alone can bind IFNγ with high affinity (K_d = 50 pM) the species-specific accessory factor (IFNγ AF-1), which interacts with the extracellular region of CD119, is required for signal transduction [1,3]. In Colo-205 cells, a human

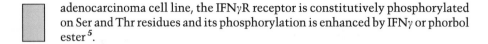

adenocarcinoma cell line, the IFNγR receptor is constitutively phosphorylated on Ser and Thr residues and its phosphorylation is enhanced by IFNγ or phorbol ester [5].

Function

IFNγ plays a key role in the initiation and effector phases of immune responses, including macrophage activation, B and T cell differentiation, activation of NK cells and upregulating the expression of MHC Class I and II antigens in several cell types [2,6].

Comments

The IFNγ AF-1 protein reconstitutes IFNγ-induced Class I MHC expression, but not viral resistance, when transfected into heterologous cells together with the human CD119 and HLA-B7 genes [3]. This suggests that other accessory factors are necessary for IFNγ-mediated activities such as antiviral responses. Despite normal T cell responses, CD119-deficient mice show increased susceptibility to infection by *Listeria monocytogenes* and vaccinia virus, but are resistant to endotoxic shock [7,8].

Database accession numbers

	PIR	SWISSPROT	EMBL/GENBANK	REFERENCE
Human CD119	A31555	P15260	J03143	1
Human IFNγ AF-1		P38484	U05875, U05877	3
Mouse CD119	A34368	P15261	M26711	9

Amino acid sequence of human CD119

```
MALLFLLPLV MQGVSRA                                              -1
EMGTADLGPS SVPTPTNVTI ESYNMNPIVY WEYQIMPQVP VFTVEVKNYG          50
VKNSEWIDAC INISHHYCNI SDHVGDPSNS LWVRVKARVG QKESAYAKSE         100
EFAVCRDGKI GPPKLDIRKE EKQIMIDIFH PSVFVNGDEQ EVDYDPETTC         150
YIRVYNVYVR MNGSEIQYKI LTQKEDDCDE IQCQLAIPVS SLNSQYCVSA         200
EGVLHVWGVT TEKSKEVCIT IFNSSIKGSL WIPVVAALLL FLVLSLVFIC         250
FYIKKINPLK EKSIILPKSL ISVVRSATLE TKPESKYVSL ITSYQPFSLE         300
KEVVCEEPLS PATVPGMHTE DNPGKVEHTE ELSSITEVVT TEENIPDVVP         350
GSHLTPIERE SSSPLSSNQS EPGSIALNSY HSRNCSESDH SRNGFDTDSS         400
CLESHSSLSD SEFPPNNKGE IKTEGQELIT VIKAPTSFGY DKPHVLVDLL         450
VDDSGKESLI GYRPTEDSKE FS                                       472
```

Amino acid sequence of human IFNγ AF-1

```
MRPTLLWSLL LLLGVFAAAA AAPPDPL                                   -1
SQLPAPQHPK IRLYNAEQVL SWEPVALSNS TRPVVYRVQF KYTDSKWFTA          50
DIMSIGVNCT QITATECDFT AASPSAGFPM DFNVTLRLRA ELGALHSAWV         100
TMPWFQHYRN VTVGPPENIE VTPGEGSLII RFSSPFDIAD TSTAFFCYVV         150
HYWEKGGIQQ VKGPFRSNSI SLDNLKPSRV YCLQVQAQLL WNKSNIFRVG         200
HLSNISCYET MADASTELQQ VILISVGTFS LLSVLAGACF FLVLKYRGLI         250
KYWFHTPPSI PLQIEEYLKD PTQPILEALD KDSSPKDDVW DSVSIISFPE         300
KEQEDVLQTL                                                     310
```

References

[1] Aguet, M. et al. (1988) Cell 55, 273–280.

[2] **Callard, R.E. and Gearing, A.J.H. (1994) The Cytokine FactsBook. Academic Press, London.**

[3] **Soh, J. et al. (1994) Cell 76, 793–802.**

[4] Langer, J.A. and Pestka, S. (1988) Immunol. Today 9, 393–400.

[5] Khurana Hershey, G.K. et al. (1990) J. Biol. Chem. 265, 17868–17875.

[6] Arai, K. et al. (1990) Annu. Rev. Biochem. 59, 783–836.

[7] Huang, S. et al. (1993) Science 259, 1742–1745.

[8] Car, B.D. et al. (1994) J. Exp. Med. 179, 1437–1444.

[9] Gray, P.W. et al. (1989) Proc. Natl Acad. Sci. USA 86, 8497–8501.

IL-1R Interleukin 1 receptor

Subunits
CD121a (IL-1R type I)
CDw121b (IL-1R type II)
IL-1R accessory protein (IL-1R AcP)

Molecular weights
Polypeptide	CD121a	63 487
	CDw121b	43 988
	IL-1R AcP	63 428

SDS-PAGE
reduced	CD121a	80 kDa
	CDw121b	60–70 kDa
unreduced	IL-1R AcP	70–90 kDa

Carbohydrate
N-linked sites	CD121a	6
	CDw121b	5
	IL-1R AcP	7
O-linked	CD121a	unknown
	CDw121b	unknown
	IL-1R AcP	unknown

Human gene location and size
CD121a: 2q12; ~75 kb [1]
CDw121b: 2q12–q22; ~38 kb [1]

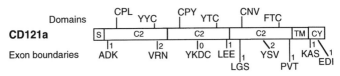

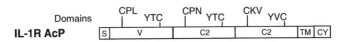

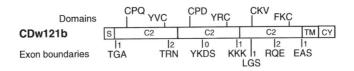

Tissue distribution
CD121a is expressed by T cells, thymocytes, fibroblasts, chondrocytes, synovial cells, hepatocytes, endothelial cells and keratinocytes [2]. CDw121b is predominantly expressed by B cells, monocytes, macrophages and neutrophils [3,4]. CDw121b mRNA is present in a number of cells, including T cells [4].

Structure

The extracellular region of both CD121a and CDw121b consists of three C2-set IgSF domains and the molecules have 28% amino acid sequence identity[2,4]. CD121a has a 213 amino acid cytoplasmic tail that is highly conserved across species (78% sequence identity between human and mouse) and is necessary for signal transduction[2,5]. In contrast, the cytoplasmic tail of CDw121b is only 29 amino acids long[4]. The N-terminal IgSF domains of CD121a and CDw121b are encoded by an exon flanked with the normal phase 1 intron/exon boundary at the N-terminus, but with an unusual phase 2 intron predicted between the F and G strands rather than after the G strand. Soluble forms of CD121a and CDw121b have been identified[6,7]. The IL-1R AcP also contains three extracellular IgSF domains[8].

Ligands and associated molecules

Both CD121a and CDw121b bind IL-1α and IL-1β, but with different affinities[2,4]. A second subunit of the IL-1R complex has been cloned from mouse 3T3-L1 cells, the widely expressed IL-1R AcP[8]. There is approximately 25% overall sequence homology between mouse IL-1R AcP and both CD121a and CDw121b from human, mouse and rat. A complex of CD121a and IL-1R AcP forms a high-affinity IL-1 binding site at the cell surface[8]. Alternative splicing of the IL-1R AcP gene may generate a soluble form of the molecule. There is an IL-1 receptor antagonist (IL-1ra) that inhibits the function of IL-1 in vivo and in vitro by binding to both CD121a and CDw121b[9,10]. The IL-1ra is unable to stimulate the kinase activity or the internalization of CD121a[11].

Function

IL-1 mediates thymocyte and T cell activation, fibroblast proliferation, induction of acute phase proteins and inflammatory reactions through binding to CD121a[12,13]. IL-1 bound to CD121a on fibroblasts induces phosphorylation of several proteins, including the EGF receptor and the heat shock protein p27[2,14]. CDw121b appears to be dispensable for IL-1 signalling and may act as a decoy receptor[15].

Comments

Vaccinia virus contains an open reading frame with strong resemblance to a soluble form of CDw121b[16]. The genes encoding human CD121a and CDw121b are linked on the same chromosome, together with the genes encoding IL-1α and IL-1β[4]. The ST2 antigen (also termed T1 or Fit-1) has approximately 25% amino acid sequence identity to CD121a and CDw121b[17]. The extracellular region of ST2 contains three C2-set IgSF domains and the molecule exists in both a soluble and membrane bound form[17,18]. ST2 does not appear to function as a receptor for either IL-1α, IL-1β or IL-1ra, but binds to a cell surface ligand expressed by a range of cell types[19].

Database accession numbers

	PIR	SWISSPROT	EMBL/GENBANK	REFERENCE
Human CD121a	A36187	P14778	M27492	[2]
Human CDw121b	S17428	P27930	X59770	[4]
Mouse CD121a	A32604	P13504	M20658	[20]
Mouse CDw121b		P27931	X59769	[4]
Mouse IL-1R AcP			X85999	[8]
Rat CD121a		Q02955	M95578	[21]
Rat CDw121b		P43303	Z22812	[22]

Amino acid sequence of human CD121a

```
MKVLLRLICF IALLISS                                         -1
LEADKCKERE EKIILVSSAN EIDVRPCPLN PNEHKGTITW YKDDSKTPVS      50
TEQASRIHQH KEKLWFVPAK VEDSGHYYCV VRNSSYCLRI KISAKFVENE     100
PNLCYNAQAI FKQKLPVAGD GGLVCPYMEF FKNENNELPK LQWYKDCKPL     150
LLDNIHFSGV KDRLIVMNVA EKHRGNYTCH ASYTYLGKQY PITRVIEFIT     200
LEENKPTRPV IVSPANETME VDLGSQIQLI CNVTGQLSDI AYWKWNGSVI     250
DEDDPVLGED YYSVENPANK RRSTLITVLN ISEIESRFYK HPFTCFAKNT     300
HGIDAAYIQL IYPVTNFQKH MIGICVTLTV IIVCSVFIYK IFKIDIVLWY     350
RDSCYDFLPI KASDGKTYDA YILYPKTVGE GSTSDCDIFV FKVLPEVLEK     400
QCGYKLFIYG RDDYVGEDIV EVINENVKKS RRLIIILVRE TSGFSWLGGS     450
SEEQIAMYNA LVQDGIKVVL LELEKIQDYE KMPESIKFIK QKHGAIRWSG     500
DFTQGPQSAK TRFWKNVRYH MPVQRRSPSS KHQLLSPATK EKLQREAHVP     550
LG                                                        552
```

Amino acid sequence of human CDw121b

```
MLRLYVLVMG VSA                                             -1
FTLQPAAHTG AARSCRFRGR HYKREFRLEG EPVALRCPQV PYWLWASVSP      50
RINLTWHKND SARTVPGEEE TRMWAQDGAL WLLPALQEDS GTYVCTTRNA     100
SYCDKMSIEL RVFENTDAFL PFISYPQILT LSTSGVLVCP DLSEFTRDKT     150
DVKIQWYKDS LLLDKDNEKF LSVRGTTHLL VHDVALEDAG YYRCVLTFAH     200
EGQQYNITRS IELRIKKKKE ETIPVIISPL KTISASLGSR LTIPCKVFLG     250
TGTPLTTMLW WTANDTHIES AYPGGRVTEG PRQEYSENNE NYIEVPLIFD     300
PVTREDLHMD FKCVVHNTLS FQTLRTTVKE ASSTFSWGIV LAPLSLAFLV     350
LGGIWMHRRC KHRTGKADGL TVLWPHHQDF QSYPK                     385
```

Amino acid sequence of mouse IL-1R AcP

```
MGLLWYLMSL SFYGILQSHA                                      -1
SERCDDWGLD TMRQIQVFED EPARIKCPLF EHFLKYNYST AHSSGLTLIW      50
YWTRQDRDLE EPINFRLPEN RISKEKDVLW FRPTLLNDTG NYTCMLRNTT     100
YCSKVAFPLE VVQKDSCFNS AMRFPVHKMY IEHGIHKITC PNVDGYFPSS     150
VKPSVTWYKG CTEIVDFHNV LPEGMNLSFF IPLVSNNGNY TCVVTYPENG     200
RLFHLTRTVT VKVVGSPKDA LPPQIYSPND RVVYEKEPGE ELVIPCKVYF     250
SFIMDSHNEV WWTIDGKKPD DVTVDITINE SVSYSSTEDE TRTQILSIKK     300
VTPEDLRRNY VCHARNTKGE AEQAAKVKQK VIPPRYTVEL ACGFGATVFL     350
VVVLIVVYHV YWLEMVLFYR AHFGTDETIL DGKEYDIYVS YARNVEEEEF     400
VLLTLRGVLE NEFGYKLCIF DRDSLPGGIV TDETLSFIQK SRRLLVVLSP     450
NYVLQGTQAL LELKAGLENM ASRGNINVIL VQYKAVKDMK VKELKRAKTV     500
LTVIKWKGEK SKYPQGRFWK QLQVAMPVKK SPRWSSNDKQ GLSYSSLKNV     550
```

References

1 Sims, J.E. et al. (1995) Cytokine 7, 483–490.

2 Sims, J.E. et al. (1989) Proc. Natl Acad. Sci. USA 86, 8946–8950.

3 Spriggs, M.K. et al. (1990) J. Biol. Chem. 265, 22499–22505.

4 McMahan, C.J. et al. (1991) EMBO J. 10, 2821–2832.

5 Curtis, B.M. et al. (1989) Proc. Natl Acad. Sci. USA 86, 3045–3049.

6 Svenson, M. et al. (1995) Eur. J. Immunol. 25, 2842–2850.

7 Symons, J.A. et al. (1995) Proc. Natl Acad. Sci. USA 92, 1714–1718.

8 **Greenfeder, S.A. et al. (1995) J. Biol. Chem. 270, 13757–13765.**

9 Eisenberg, S.P. et al. (1990) Nature 343, 341–346.

10 Dinarello, C.A. and Thompson, R.C. (1991) Immunol. Today 12, 404–410.

11 Dripps, D.J. et al. (1991) J. Biol. Chem. 266, 10331–10336.

12 Di Giovine, F.S. and Duff, G.W. (1990) Immunol. Today 11, 13–20.

13 **Callard, R.E. and Gearing, A.J.H. (1994) The Cytokine FactsBook. Academic Press, London.**

14 Kaur, P. et al. (1989) FEBS Lett. 258, 269–273.

15 **Colotta, F. et al. (1993) Science 261, 472–475.**

16 Alcamí, A. and Smith, G.L. (1995) Immunol. Today 16, 474–478.

17 Tominaga, S. (1989) FEBS Lett. 258, 301–304.

18 Bergers, G. et al. (1994) EMBO J. 13, 1176–1188.

19 Gayle, M.A. et al. (1996) J. Biol. Chem. 271, 5784–5789.

20 Sims, J.E. et al. (1988) Science 241, 585–589.

21 Hart, R.P. et al. (1993) J. Neuroimmunol. 44, 49–56.

22 Bristulf, J. et al. (1994) Eur. Cytokine Network 5, 319–330.

Subunits
CD25 (α chain)
CD122 (β chain)
CD132 (γc chain)

Other names
CD25: Tac antigen, p55
CD122: p75
CD132: cytokine receptor common
  γ chain, p64

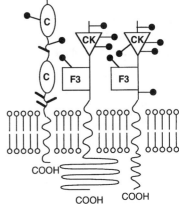

Molecular weights

Polypeptide	CD25	28 447
	CD122	58 359
	CD132	39 920

SDS-PAGE reduced	CD25	55 kDa
	CD122	70–75 kDa
	CD132	64 kDa

Carbohydrate

N-linked sites	CD25	2
	CD122	4
	CD132	6
O-linked	CD25	abundant +
	CD122	unknown
	CD132	unknown

Human gene location and size
CD25: 10p14–p15; >25 kb [1]
CD122: 22q11.2–q13; 24.3 kb [2]
CD132: Xq13; 4.2 kb [3]

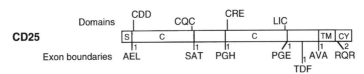

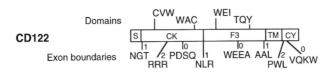

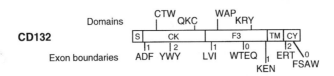

Tissue distribution

The IL-2R is expressed on activated cells including T cells, B cells and monocytes. The CD25 subunit of the human IL-2R is also present on a subset of thymocytes, HTLV-I transformed T and B cells, EBV transformed B cells, myeloid precursors and oligodendrocytes. Natural killer (NK) cells, certain B cell lines and a subpopulation of resting T cells constitutively express the CD122 subunit, which is upregulated 5- to 10-fold following T cell activation. IL-2 induces the expression of the CD25 subunit on NK cells [4,5].

Structure

The IL-2R exists in three alternative forms made up from the individual components of CD25, CD122 and CD132. CD25 contains two CCP domains, is rich in O-linked carbohydrates, and has a short cytoplasmic tail (13 amino acids) [6]. The extracellular region of CD122 consists of a cytokine receptor domain and a fibronectin type III domain that contains the WSXWS motif. Its cytoplasmic tail (286 amino acids) contains Ser-rich, acidic and Pro-rich regions [7]. Similarly, the extracellular region of CD132 also contains a cytokine receptor domain and a fibronectin type III domain containing the WSXWS sequence. Its cytoplasmic tail (86 amino acids) has a region of limited homology to SH2 subdomains 4 and 5 of Src-related kinases [8]. CD132 is also a component of the IL-4R, IL-7R, IL-9R and IL-15R.

Ligands and associated molecules

The functional high affinity IL-2R (K_d = 10 pM) is composed of a non-covalently associated CD25/CD122/CD132 heterotrimer. The isolated CD25 subunit constitutes a low-affinity IL-2R (K_d = 10 nM), while the CD122/CD132 heterodimer binds IL-2 with intermediate affinity (K_d = 1 nM). Both the high- and intermediate-affinity receptors are important for IL-2 signalling.

Function

IL-2 induces the activation and proliferation of T cells, thymocytes, NK cells, B cells and macrophages [4,9]. The WSXWS motif of CD122 is essential for IL-2 binding, while its cytoplasmic Ser-rich region is necessary for signal transduction [10,11]. CD122 associates with the Lck tyrosine kinase through its cytoplasmic acidic region [11]. The interaction of IL-2 with its high-affinity receptor induces Tyr phosphorylation of CD122 and several other proteins [11]. CD25 is phosphorylated on Ser and Thr residues [4].

Comments

Proteolytic cleavage of membrane-bound CD25 generates a soluble form present in human serum [5]. Mutations in the CD132 gene are responsible for X-linked severe combined immunodeficiency (SCID) in humans [12].

Database accession numbers

	PIR	SWISSPROT	EMBL/GENBANK	REFERENCE
Human CD25	A01856	P01589	X01057	[6]
Human CD122	A30342	P14784	M26062	[7]
Human CD132	A42565	P31785	D11086	[8]
Mouse CD25	A01857	P01590	K02891	[13]
Mouse CD122	A35052	P16297	M28052	[15]
Mouse CD132	JN0592	P34902	L20048	[16]
Rat CD25	A46535	P26897	M55049	[14]
Rat CD122		P26896	M55050	[14]

Amino acid sequence of human CD25

```
MDSYLLMWGL LTFIMVPGCQ A                                      -1
ELCDDDPPEI PHATFKAMAY KEGTMLNCEC KRGFRRIKSG SLYMLCTGNS       50
SHSSWDNQCQ CTSSATRNTT KQVTPQPEEQ KERKTTEMQS PMQPVDQASL      100
PGHCREPPPW ENEATERIYH FVVGQMVYYQ CVQGYRALHR GPAESVCKMT      150
HGKTRWTQPQ LICTGEMETS QFPGEEKPQA SPEGRPESET SCLVTTTDFQ      200
IQTEMAATME TSIFTTEYQV AVAGCVFLLI SVLLLSGLTW QRRQRKSRRT      250
I                                                          251
```

Amino acid sequence of human CD122

```
MAAPALSWRL PLLILLLPLA TSWASA                                 -1
AVNGTSQFTC FYNSRANISC VWSQDGALQD TSCQVHAWPD RRRWNQTCEL       50
LPVSQASWAC NLILGAPDSQ KLTTVDIVTL RVLCREGVRW RVMAIQDFKP      100
FENLRLMAPI SLQVVHVETH RCNISWEISQ ASHYFERHLE FEARTLSPGH      150
TWEEAPLLTL KQKQEWICLE TLTPDTQYEF QVRVKPLQGE FTTWSPWSQP      200
LAFRTKPAAL GKDTIPWLGH LLVGLSGAFG FIILVYLLIN CRNTGPWLKK      250
VLKCNTPDPS KFFSQLSSEH GGDVQKWLSS PFPSSSFSPG GLAPEISPLE      300
VLERDKVTQL LLQQDKVPEP ASLSSNHSLT SCFTNQGYFF FHLPDALEIE      350
ACQVYFTYDP YSEEDPDEGV AGAPTGSSPQ PLQPLSGEDD AYCTFPSRDD      400
LLLFSPSLLG GPSPPSTAPG GSGAGEERMP PSLQERVPRD WDPQPLGPPT      450
PGVPDLVDFQ PPPELVLREA GEEVPDAGPR EGVSFPWSRP PGQGEFRALN      500
ARLPLNTDAY LSLQELQGQD PTHLV                                 525
```

Amino acid sequence of human CD132

```
MLKPSLPFTS LLFLQLPLLG VG                                     -1
LNTTILTPNG NEDTTADFFL TTMPTDSLSV STLPLPEVQC FVFNVEYMNC       50
TWNSSSEPQP TNLTLHYWYK NSDNDKVQKC SHYLFSEEIT SGCQLQKKEI      100
HLYQTFVVQL QDPREPRRQA TQMLKLQNLV IPWAPENLTL HKLSESQLEL      150
NWNNRFLNHC LEHLVQYRTD WDHSWTEQSV DYRHKFSLPS VDGQKRYTFR      200
VRSRFNPLCG SAQHWSEWSH PIHWGSNTSK ENPFLFALEA VVISVGSMGL      250
IISLLCVYFW LERTMPRIPT LKNLEDLVTE YHGNFSAWSG VSKGLAESLQ      300
PDYSERLCLV SEIPPKGGAL GEGPGASPCN QHSPYWAPPC YTLKPET        347
```

References

[1] Leonard, W.J. et al. (1985) Science 230, 633–639.
[2] Shibuya, H. et al. (1990) Nucleic Acids Res. 18, 3697–3703.
[3] Noguchi, M. et al. (1993) J. Biol. Chem. 268, 13601–13608.
[4] Waldmann, T.A. (1989) Annu. Rev. Biochem. 58, 875–911.
[5] Waldmann, T.A. (1991) J. Biol. Chem. 266, 2681–2684.

6   Leonard, W.J. et al. (1984) Nature 311, 626–631.

7   **Hatakeyama, M. et al. (1989) Science 244, 551–556.**

8   Takeshita, T. et al. (1992) Science 257, 379–382.

9   **Callard, R.E. and Gearing, A.J.H (1994) The Cytokine FactsBook. Academic Press, London.**

10 Miyazaki, T. (1991) EMBO J. 10, 3191–3197.

11 Hatakeyama, M. et al. (1991) Science 252, 1523–1528.

12 **Noguchi, M. et al. (1993) Cell 73, 147–157.**

13 Miller, J. et al. (1985) J. Immunol. 134, 4212–4217.

14 Page, T.H. and Dallman, M.J. (1991) Eur. J. Immunol. 21, 2133–2138.

15 Kono, T. et al. (1990) Proc. Natl Acad. Sci. USA 87, 1806–1810.

16 Cao, X. et al. (1993) Proc. Natl Acad. Sci. USA 90, 8464–8468.

Subunits
CDw123 (α chain)
CDw131 (βc chain)

Molecular weights
Polypeptide	CDw123	41 282
	CDw131	95 707

Carbohydrate
N-linked sites	CDw123	6
	CDw131	3
O-linked	CDw123	unknown
	CDw131	unknown

Human gene location and size
CDw123: Xp22.3, Yp13.3; ~40 kb [1]
CDw131: 22q12.2–q13.1

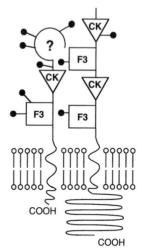

CDw123   CDw131

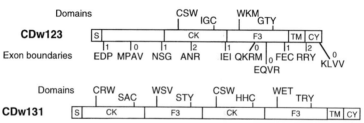

Tissue distribution

The IL-3R is expressed on bone marrow multipotential haematopoietic precursors, on neutrophil, basophil, eosinophil, monocyte and megakaryocyte committed precursors and on the erythroid lineage. It is also present on some myelocytic leukaemias and pre-B lymphomas and leukaemias [2].

Structure

The IL-3R is formed by the association of CDw123 and a common β chain (βc chain, CDw131) that is also a component of the receptors for GM-CSF and IL-5 [3,4]. CDw131 does not bind any of these cytokines in isolation [5]. Based on crosslinking experiments the estimated molecular weights of CDw123 and CDw131 are 70 kDa and 120–140 kDa respectively [3]. CDw123 consists of an N-terminal region of about 100 amino acids, similar in sequence to that present in CDw125 (IL-5R α chain) and CD116 (GM-CSFR α chain), followed by a cytokine receptor domain and a fibronectin type III domain [3,6,7]. The extracellular region of CDw131 can be divided into two homologous units, each one containing a cytokine receptor domain and a fibronectin type III domain [5,6]. The cytoplasmic tail of CDw131 contains Pro- and Ser-rich regions, similar to those found in other cytokine receptor subunits including CD122 (IL-2R β chain), CD124 (IL-4R α chain) and CD114 (G-CSFR)[8].

Ligands and associated molecules

CDw123 binds IL-3 with very low affinity (K_d = 80–90 nM), while its association with CDw131 generates a high affinity receptor for IL-3 (K_d = 110–180 pM)[3]. A 110 kDa Ser/Thr kinase that is activated following IL-3 stimulation was shown to be constitutively associated with the IL-3R[9].

Function

IL-3 promotes the growth and differentiation of multipotential haematopoietic precursors and of erythroid, neutrophil, basophil, monocyte, eosinophil and megakaryocyte committed precursors. In the mouse, IL-3 also activates mast cells and pre-B cells[10,11]. IL-3 induces the Tyr phosphorylation of several proteins and activates Ras[12,13]. The signalling mechanisms of the IL-3 receptor are reviewed in ref. 14.

Comments

In the mouse, two proteins with 91% amino acid sequence identity have been identified: the AIC2A and the AIC2B proteins[8,15]. Both AIC2A and AIC2B can associate with the murine CDw123 homologue to form distinct high-affinity IL-3Rs[16]. The AIC2B protein is a common component of the murine IL-3R, IL-5R and GM-CSFR[3,4]. The overall sequence of both proteins is similar to that of human CDw131[5,8,15]. The human CDw123 gene has been mapped to the pseudoautosomal region of the X and Y chromosomes[17].

Database accession numbers

	PIR	SWISSPROT	EMBL/GENBANK	REFERENCE
Human CDw123	A40266	P26951	M74782	3
Human CDw131	A39255	P32927	M59941	5
Mouse CDw123	S22909	P26952	X64534	16
Mouse AIC2A	A40091	P26954	M29855	8
Mouse AIC2B	A35782	P26955	M34397	15

Amino acid sequence of human CDw123

```
MVLLWLTLLL IALPCLLQ                                          -1
TKEDPNPPIT NLRMKAKAQQ LTWDLNRNVT DIECVKDADY SMPAVNNSYC       50
QFGAISLCEV TNYTVRVANP PFSTWILFPE NSGKPWAGAE NLTCWIHDVD       100
FLSCSWAVGP GAPADVQYDL YLNVANRRQQ YECLHYKTDA QGTRIGCRFD       150
DISRLSSGSQ SSHILVRGRS AAFGIPCTDK FVVFSQIEIL TPPNMTAKCN       200
KTHSFMHWKM RSHFNRKFRY ELQIQKRMQP VITEQVRDRT SFQLLNPGTY       250
TVQIRARERV YEFLSAWSTP QRFECDQEEG ANTRAWRTSL LIALGTLLAL       300
VCVFVICRRY LVMQRLFPRI PHMKDPIGDS FQNDKLVVWE AGKAGLEECL       350
VTEVQVVQKT                                                  360
```

Amino acid sequence of human CDw131

```
MVLAQGLLSM ALLALC                                                     -1
WERSLAGAEE TIPLQTLRCY NDYTSHITCR WADTQDAQRL VNVTLIRRVN               50
EDLLEPVSCD LSDDMPWSAC PHPRCVPRRC VIPCQSFVVT DVDYFSFQPD              100
RPLGTRLTVT LTQHVQPPEP RDLQISTDQD HFLLTWSVAL GSPQSHWLSP              150
GDLEFEVVYK RLQDSWEDAA ILLSNTSQAT LGPEHLMPSS TYVARVRTRL              200
APGSRLSGRP SKWSPEVCWD SQPGDEAQPQ NLECFFDGAA VLSCSWEVRK              250
EVASSVSFGL FYKPSPDAGE EECSPVLREG LGSLHTRHHC QIPVPDPATH              300
GQYIVSVQPR RAEKHIKSSV NIQMAPPSLN VTKDGDSYSL RWETMKMRYE              350
HIDHTFEIQY RKDTATWKDS KTETLQNAHS MALPALEPST RYWARVRVRT              400
SRTGYNGIWS EWSEARSWDT ESVLPMWVLA LIVIFLTTAV LLALRFCGIY              450
GYRLRRKWEE KIPNPSKSHL FQNGSAELWP PGSMSAFTSG SPPHQGPWGS              500
RFPELEGVFP VGFGDSEVSP LTIEDPKHVC DPPSGPDTTP AASDLPTEQP              550
PSPQPGPPAA SHTPEKQASS FDFNGPYLGP PHSRSLPDIL GQPEPPQEGG              600
SQKSPPPGSL EYLCLPAGGQ VQLVPLAQAM GPGQAVEVER RPSQGAAGSP              650
SLESGGGPAP PALGPRVGGQ DQKDSPVAIP MSSGDTEDPG VASGYVSSAD              700
LVFTPNSGAS SVSLVPSLGL PSDQTPSLCP GLASGPPGAP GPVKSGFEGY              750
VELPPIEGRS PRSPRNNPVP PEAKSPVLNP GERPADVSPT SPQPEGLLVL              800
QQVGDYCFLP GLGPGPLSLR SKPSSPGPGP EIKNLDQAFQ VKKPPGQAVP              850
QVPVIQLFKA LKQQDYLSLP PWEVNKPGEV C                                  881
```

References
1. Kosugi, H. et al. (1995) Biochem. Biophys. Res. Commun. 208, 360–367.
2. Park, L.S. et al. (1989) J. Biol. Chem. 264, 5420–5427.
3. Kitamura, T. et al. (1991) Cell 66, 1165–1174.
4. **Nicola, N.A. and Metcalf, D. (1991) Cell 67, 1–4.**
5. Hayashida, K. et al. (1990) Proc. Natl Acad. Sci. USA 87, 9655–9659.
6. Bazan, J.F. (1990) Proc. Natl Acad. Sci. USA 87, 6934–6938.
7. Patthy, L. (1990) Cell 61, 13–14.
8. Itoh, N. et al. (1990) Science 247, 324–327.
9. Liu, L. et al. (1995) J. Biol. Chem. 270, 22422–22427.
10. Arai, K. et al. (1990) Annu. Rev. Biochem. 59, 783–836.
11. **Callard, R.E. and Gearing, A.J.H. (1994) The Cytokine FactsBook. Academic Press, London.**
12. Isfort, R.J. and Ihle, J.N. (1990) Growth Factors 2, 213–220.
13. Satoh, T. et al. (1991) Proc. Natl Acad. Sci. USA 88, 3314–3318.
14. Vairo, G. and Hamilton, J.A. (1991) Immunol. Today 12, 362–369.
15. Gorman, D.M. et al. (1990) Proc. Natl Acad. Sci. USA 87, 5459–5463.
16. Hara, T. and Miyajima, A. (1992) EMBO J. 11, 1875–1884.
17. Kremer, E. et al. (1993) Blood 82, 22–28.

IL-4R Interleukin 4 receptor

Subunits
CD124 (α chain)
CD132 (γc chain)
IL-13R α chain

Molecular weights
Polypeptide	CD124	87 067
	CD132	39 920
	IL-13R α chain	41 457

Carbohydrate
N-linked sites	CD124	6
	CD132	6
	IL-13R α chain	4
O-linked	CD124	unknown
	CD132	unknown
	IL-13R α chain	unknown

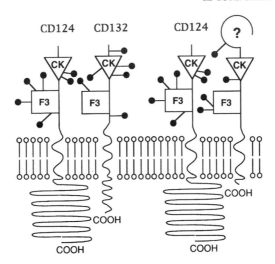

Human gene location and size
CD124: 16p11.2–p12.1
CD132: Xq13; 4.2 kb [1]

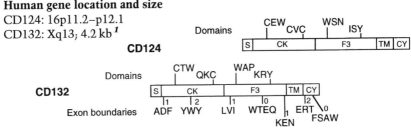

Tissue distribution

The IL-4R is expressed on mature B and T cells, haematopoietic precursors, fibroblasts, epithelial and endothelial cells [2].

Structure

CD124 is a member of the cytokine receptor superfamily. The extracellular domain consists of a cytokine receptor domain and a fibronectin type III domain containing the WSXWS motif [3,4]. The 596 amino acid cytoplasmic tail contains Pro- and Ser-rich regions, similar to those present in the IL-2R β chain (CD122), G-CSFR (CD114) and the GM-CSFR/IL-3R/IL-5R common β chain (CDw131) [4]. CD124 associates with CD132 (see **IL-2R**) to form a heterodimeric receptor complex at the cell surface [5,6]. In addition a second type of IL-4R is formed through the association of CD124 and the IL-13R α chain [7,8]. A soluble form of the mouse IL-4R is produced by alternative splicing of CD124 [9].

Ligands and associated molecules

High-affinity IL-4Rs ($K_d = 50-100$ pM) may be composed of CD124/CD132 or CD124/IL-13R α chain [4,7]. IL-4-induced signal transduction involves IL-4R binding and activation of two Janus family Tyr kinases (Jak1 and Jak3) [7]. These Tyr kinases activate signal transducers and activators of transcription (Stat) proteins; denoted IL-4 Stat(s) in the case of IL-4 [7,10]. IL-4 induces association of PI 3-kinase with the mouse IL-4R [11].

Function

IL-4 is a growth factor for pre-activated B cells and T cells. IL-4 enhances IgG1 and IgE production, differentiation of T_H2-type CD4+ T cells and the expression of MHC Class II molecules on B cells and macrophages. IL-4 also induces macrophage activation and synergizes with colony-stimulating factors in promoting the growth of haematopoietic cells [12,13]. IL-4, and IL-13, induces Tyr phosphorylation of CD124 [14].

Comments

The soluble form of mouse IL-4R binds IL-4 with high affinity, inhibits the biological activity of IL-4 and prevents the degradation of the cytokine [15]. A recombinant extracellular domain of the human IL-4R is a powerful antagonist of its specific ligand [16].

Database accession numbers

	PIR	SWISSPROT	EMBL/GENBANK	REFERENCE
Human CD124	A60386	P24394	X52425	3
Mouse CD124	A33380	P16382	M27959	9
Mouse CD124 (secreted form)			M27960	9
Rat CD124			X69903	17

The accession numbers and amino acid sequence of CD132, which is common to the IL-2R, IL-4R, IL-7R, IL-9R and IL-15R, are given in the **IL-2R** entry. The IL-13R α chain is detailed in the **IL-13R** entry.

Amino acid sequence of human CD124

```
MGWLCSGLLF PVSCLVLLQV ASSGN                              -1
MKVLQEPTCV SDYMSISTCE WKMNGPTNCS TELRLLYQLV FLLSEAHTCI    50
PENNGGAGCV CHLLMDDVVS ADNYTLDLWA GQQLLWKGSF KPSEHVKPRA   100
PGNLTVHTNV SDTLLLTWSN PYPPDNYLYN HLTYAVNIWS ENDPADFRIY   150
NVTYLEPSLR IAASTLKSGI SYRARVRAWA QCYNTTWSEW SPSTKWHNSY   200
REPFEQHLLL GVSVSCIVIL AVCLLCYVSI TKIKKEWWDQ IPNPARSRLV   250
AIIIQDAQGS QWEKRSRGQE PAKCPHWKNC LTKLLPCFLE HNMKRDEDPH   300
KAAKEMPFQG SGKSAWCPVE ISKTVLWPES ISVVRCVELF EAPVECEEEE   350
EVEEEKGSFC ASPESSRDDF QEGREGIVAR LTESLFLDLL GEENGGFCQQ   400
DMGESCLLPP SGSTSAHMPW DEFPSAGPKE APPWGKEQPL HLEPSPPASP   450
TQSPDNLTCT ETPLVIAGNP AYRSFSNSLS QSPCPRELGP DPLLARHLEE   500
VEPEMPCVPQ LSEPTTVPQP EPETWEQILR RNVLQHGAAA APVSAPTSGY   550
QEFVHAVEQG GTQASAVVGL GPPGEAGYKA FSSLLASSAV SPEKCGFGAS   600
SGEEGYKPFQ DLIPGCPGDP APVPVPLFTF GLDREPPRSP QSSHLPSSSP   650
EHLGLEPGEK VEDMPKPPLP QEQATDPLVD SLGSGIVYSA LTCHLCGHLK   700
QCHGQEDGGQ TPVMASPCCG CCCGDRSSPP TTPLRAPDPS PGGVPLEASL   750
CPASLAPSGI SEKSKSSSSF HPAPGNAQSS SQTPKIVNFV SVGPTYMRVS   800
```

References

[1] Noguchi, M. et al. (1993) J. Biol. Chem. 268, 13601–13608.

[2] Park, L.S. et al. (1987) J. Exp. Med. 166, 476–488.

[3] Idzerda, R.L. et al. (1990) J. Exp. Med. 171, 861–873.

[4] Galizzi, J-P. et al. (1990) Int. Immunol. 2, 669–675.

[5] Kondo, M. et al. (1993) Science 262, 1874–1877.

[6] Russell, S.M. et al. (1993) Science 262, 1880–1883.

[7] Lin, J-X. et al. (1995) Immunity 2, 331–339.

[8] **Hilton, D.J. et al. (1996) Proc. Natl Acad. Sci. USA 93, 497–501.**

[9] Mosley, B. et al. (1989) Cell 59, 335–348.

[10] Hou, J. et al. (1994) Science 265, 1701–1706.

[11] Izuhara, K. and Harada, N. (1993) J. Biol. Chem. 268, 13097–13102.

[12] Arai, K. et al. (1990) Annu. Rev. Biochem. 59, 783–836.

[13] **Callard, R.E. and Gearing, A.J.H. (1994) The Cytokine FactsBook. Academic Press, London.**

[14] Smerz-Bertling, C. and Duschl, A. (1995) J. Biol. Chem. 270, 966–970.

[15] Fernandez-Botran, R. and Vitetta, E.S. (1991) J. Exp. Med. 174, 673–681.

[16] Garrone, P. et al. (1991) Eur. J. Immunol. 21, 1365–1369.

[17] Richter, G. et al. (1995) Cytokine 7, 237–241.

IL-5R

Interleukin 5 receptor

Subunits
CDw125 (α chain)
CDw131 (βc chain)

Molecular weights

Polypeptide	CDw125	45 557
	CDw131	95 707

Carbohydrate

N-linked sites	CDw125	6
	CDw131	3
O-linked	CDw125	unknown
	CDw131	unknown

Human gene location
CDw125: 3p26
CDw131: 22q12.2–q13.1

CDw125 CDw131

Domains
CDw125

Domains
CDw131

Tissue distribution

In human and mouse the IL-5R is expressed on eosinophils and basophils. Mouse IL-5R is also expressed on B cells [1,2].

Structure

The IL-5R is formed by the association of CDw125 and a common β chain (CDw131) that is also a component of the receptors for IL-3 and GM-CSF (see **IL-3R**) [1-3]. The extracellular region of CDw125 consists of an N-terminal region of about 100 amino acids with sequence similarities to the equivalent regions in CDw123 (IL-3R α chain) and CD116 (GM-CSFR α chain), followed by a cytokine receptor domain and a fibronectin type III domain that includes the WSXWS motif [1,2,4]. Both membrane bound and secreted forms of CDw125 exist, probably arising from alternative splicing [1,4]. The structure of CDw131 is described in the **IL-3R** entry. The molecular weights of CDw125 and CDw131, as determined by chemical crosslinking, are 55–60 kDa and 120–140 kDa, respectively [1,4].

Ligands and associated molecules

CDw125 binds IL-5 ($K_d = 1$ nM) and associates with CDw131, which does not bind IL-5, to generate a functional high-affinity receptor for IL-5 ($K_d = 50$–250 pM) [1,4].

Function

IL-5 promotes the growth and differentiation of eosinophil precursors and activates mature eosinophils[2]. Mouse IL-5 is also a B cell growth and differentiation factor[2,5,6]. The secreted form of CDw125 has antagonistic properties and is able to inhibit IL-5-induced eosinophil proliferation and differentiation[1].

Comments

In vivo administration of mAbs against the IL-5R inhibits eosinophilia in transgenic mice overexpressing IL-5[7].

Database accession numbers

	PIR	SWISSPROT	EMBL/GENBANK	REFERENCE
Human CDw125	A40267	Q01344	X61176-X61178, X62156	4
Mouse CDw125	S12357	P21183	D90205	8

The accession numbers and amino acid sequence of CDw131, which is common to the IL-3R, IL-5R and GM-CSFR, are given in the **IL-3R** entry.

Amino acid sequence of human CDw125

```
MIIVAHVLLI LLGATEILQA                                           -1
DLLPDEKISL LPPVNFTIKV TGLAQVLLQW KPNPDQEQRN VNLEYQVKIN          50
APKEDDYETR ITESKCVTIL HKGFSASVRT ILQNDHSLLA SSWASAELHA         100
PPGSPGTSIV NLTCTTNTTE DNYSRLRSYQ VSLHCTWLVG TDAPEDTQYF         150
LYYRYGSWTE ECQEYSKDTL GRNIACWFPR TFILSKGRDW LSVLVNGSSK         200
HSAIRPFDQL FALHAIDQIN PPLNVTAEIE GTRLSIQWEK PVSAFPIHCF         250
DYEVKIHNTR NGYLQIEKLM TNAFISIIDD LSKYDVQVRA AVSSMCREAG         300
LWSEWSQPIY VGNDEHKPLR EWFVIVIMAT ICFILLILSL ICKICHLWIK         350
LFPPIPAPKS NIKDLFVTTN YEKAGSSETE IEVICYIEKP GVETLEDSVF         400
```

References

1. Tavernier, J. et al. (1991) Cell 66, 1175–1184.
2. **Takatsu, K. et al. (1994) Adv. Immunol. 57, 145–190.**
3. Nicola, N.A. and Metcalf, D. (1991) Cell 67, 1–4.
4. Murata, Y. et al. (1992) J. Exp. Med. 175, 341–351.
5. Arai, K. et al. (1990) Annu. Rev. Biochem. 59, 783–836.
6. Callard, R.E. and Gearing, A.J.H. (1994) The Cytokine FactsBook. Academic Press, London.
7. Hitoshi, Y. et al. (1991) Int. Immunol. 3, 135–139.
8. Takaki, S. et al. (1990) EMBO J. 9, 4367–4374.

Subunits

CD126 (α chain)
CD130 (β chain; gp130)

Molecular weights

Polypeptide	CD126	49 869
	CD130	101 041

SDS-PAGE		
reduced	CD126	80 kDa
	CD130	130 kDa

Carbohydrate

N-linked sites	CD126	5
	CD130	10
O-linked	CD126	unknown
	CD130	unknown

Human gene location

CD126: 1q21
CD130: 5q11

CD130

CD126

CD126

Domains

CD130

Domains

Tissue distribution

The IL-6R is expressed at high levels on activated and EBV-transformed B cells, plasma cells and myelomas but it is also present at lower levels on most leucocytes, epithelial cells, fibroblasts, hepatocytes and neural cells [1].

Structure

The functional high-affinity receptor for human IL-6 is formed by the non-covalent association of two subunits, CD126 and CD130 [2]. CD126 contains a C2-set IgSF domain, followed by a cytokine receptor domain and a fibronectin type III domain, which includes the WSXWS motif conserved in many cytokine receptors [3–5]. The second chain, CD130, does not bind IL-6 in isolation [6] and consists of a C2-set IgSF domain, a cytokine receptor domain and four fibronectin type III domains, the first of which contains the WSXWS motif[2]. CD130 is structurally similar to the G-CSFR (CD114)[7].

Ligands and associated molecules

CD126 binds IL-6 with low affinity $(K_d = 1 \, \text{nM})$[3]. CD130 binding stabilizes the CD126/IL-6 complex resulting in the formation of a high-affinity receptor $(K_d = 10 \, \text{pM})$[2].

Function

IL-6 is a growth factor for myelomas, B cell hybridomas, activated and EBV-transformed B cells and T cell lines[1,8]. IL-6 also induces differentiation and proliferation of haematopoietic precursors, mediates the acute phase response of hepatocytes and affects differentiation of neural cell lines[1,8]. CD130 mediates signal transduction and is Tyr phosphorylated in cells stimulated with IL-6[2,9]. Mutational analyses indicate that a membrane-proximal cytoplasmic region is important for the signal transduction activity of CD130[9].

Comments

Several other cytokines, including IL-11, leukaemia inhibitory factor (LIF), ciliary neurotrophic factor (CNTF), oncostatin M and cardiotrophin 1 (CT-1) utilize CD130 as a common signal transducer component of their receptors[10].

Database accession numbers

	PIR	SWISSPROT	EMBL/GENBANK	REFERENCE
Human CD126	JU0080	P08887	X12830	3
Human CD130	A36337	P40189	M57230	2
Mouse CD126	JL0145	P22272	X51975	11
Mouse CD130		Q00560	M83336	13
Rat CD126	A37986	P22273	J05668	12
Rat CD130	A44257	P40190	M92340	14

Amino acid sequence of human CD126

```
MLAVGCALLA ALLAAPGAA                                            -1
LAPRRCPAQE VARGVLTSLP GDSVTLTCPG VEPEDNATVH WVLRKPAAGS          50
HPSRWAGMGR RLLLRSVQLH DSGNYSCYRA GRPAGTVHLL VDVPPEEPQL         100
SCFRKSPLSN VVCEWGPRST PSLTTKAVLL VRKFQNSPAE DFQEPCQYSQ         150
ESQKFSCQLA VPEGDSSFYI VSMCVASSVG SKFSKTQTFQ GCGILQPDPP         200
ANITVTAVAR NPRWLSVTWQ DPHSWNSSFY RLRFELRYRA ERSKTFTTWM         250
VKDLQHHCVI HDAWSGLRHV VQLRAQEEFG QGEWSEWSPE AMGTPWTESR         300
SPPAENEVST PMQALTTNKD DDNILFRDSA NATSLPVQDS SSVPLPTFLV         350
AGGSLAFGTL LCIAIVLRFK KTWKLRALKE GKTSMHPPYS LGQLVPERPR         400
PTPVLVPLIS PPVSPSSLGS DNTSSHNRPD ARDPRSPYDI SNTDYFFPR         449
```

Amino acid sequence of human CD130

```
MLTLQTWVVQ ALFIFLTTES TG                                  -1
ELLDPCGYIS PESPVVQLHS NFTAVCVLKE KCMDYFHVNA NYIVWKTNHF     50
TIPKEQYTII NRTASSVTFT DIASLNIQLT CNILTFGQLE QNVYGITIIS    100
GLPPEKPKNL SCIVNEGKKM RCEWDGGRET HLETNFTLKS EWATHKFADC    150
KAKRDTPTSC TVDYSTVYFV NIEVWVEAEN ALGKVTSDHI NFDPVYKVKP    200
NPPHNLSVIN SEELSSILKL TWTNPSIKSV IILKYNIQYR TKDASTWSQI    250
PPEDTASTRS SFTVQDLKPF TEYVFRIRCM KEDGKGYWSD WSEEASGITY    300
EDRPSKAPSF WYKIDPSHTQ GYRTVQLVWK TLPPFEANGK ILDYEVTLTR    350
WKSHLQNYTV NATKLTVNLT NDRYLATLTV RNLVGKSDAA VLTIPACDFQ    400
ATHPVMDLKA FPKDNMLWVE WTTPRESVKK YILEWCVLSD KAPCITDWQQ    450
EDGTVHRTYL RGNLAESKCY LITVTPVYAD GPGSPESIKA YLKQAPPSKG    500
PTVRTKKVGK NEAVLEWDQL PVDVQNGFIR NYTIFYRTII GNETAVNVDS    550
SHTEYTLSSL TSDTLYMVRM AAYTDEGGKD GPEFTFTTPK FAQGEIEAIV    600
VPVCLAFLLT TLLGVLFCFN KRDLIKKHIW PNVPDPSKSH IAQWSPHTPP    650
RHNFNSKDQM YSDGNFTDVS VVEIEANDKK PFPEDLKSLD LFKKEKINTE    700
GHSSGIGGSS CMSSSRPSIS SSDENESSQN TSSTVQYSTV VHSGYRHQVP    750
SVQVFSRSES TQPLLDSEER PEDLQLVDHV DGGDGILPRQ QYFKQNCSQH    800
AADAFGPGTE GQVERFETVG MEAATDEGMP KSYLPQTVRQ GGYMPQ        896
ESSPDISHFE RSKQVSSVNE EDFVRLKQQI SDHISQSCGS GQMKMFQEVS    850
```

References

1. **Van Snick, J. (1990) Annu. Rev. Immunol. 8, 253–278.**
2. Hibi, M. et al. (1990) Cell 63, 1149–1157.
3. Yamasaki, K. et al. (1988) Science 241, 825–828.
4. Bazan, J.F. (1990) Proc. Natl Acad. Sci. USA 87, 6934–6938.
5. Patthy, L. (1990) Cell 61, 13–14.
6. Taga, T. et al. (1989) Cell 58, 573–581.
7. Larsen, A. et al. (1990) J. Exp. Med. 172, 1559–1570.
8. Callard, R.E. and Gearing. A.J.H. (1994) The Cytokine FactsBook. Academic Press, London.
9. Murakami, M. et al. (1991) Proc. Natl Acad. Sci. USA 88, 11349–11353.
10. **Kishimoto, T. et al. (1994) Cell 76, 253–262.**
11. Sugita, T. et al. (1990) J. Exp. Med. 171, 2001–2009.
12. Baumann, M. et al. (1990) J. Biol. Chem. 265, 19853–19862.
13. Saito, M. et al. (1992) J. Immunol. 148, 4066–4071.
14. Wang, Y. et al. (1992) Genomics 14, 666–672.

Subunits
CD127 (α chain)
CD132 (γc chain)

Molecular weights

Polypeptide	CD127	49 483
	CD132	39 920

CD127   CD132

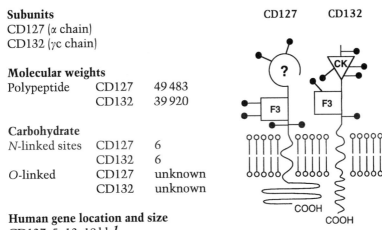

Carbohydrate

N-linked sites	CD127	6
	CD132	6
O-linked	CD127	unknown
	CD132	unknown

Human gene location and size
CD127: 5p13; 19 kb [1]
CD132: Xq13; 4.2 kb [2]

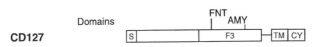

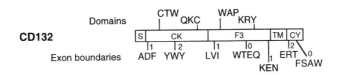

Tissue distribution

The IL-7R is expressed on bone marrow lymphoid precursors, pro-B cells, thymocytes, mature T cells and monocytes [1,3].

Structure

The extracellular domain of CD127 consists of an N-terminal region of about 100 amino acids with no clear sequence similarity to other proteins (see Chapter 3) followed by a fibronectin type III domain containing the WSXWS motif found in many cytokine receptors [3,4]. CD127 associates with CD132 (see **IL-2R**) to form a heterodimeric receptor complex at the cell surface [5]. A soluble form of human CD127 is produced by alternative splicing of the CD127 gene [1,3].

Ligands and associated molecules

Two classes of IL-7R with low- ($K_d = 5$–$10\,\text{nM}$) and high-affinity ($K_d = 100\,\text{pM}$) have been described [3]. The association of CD127 and CD132 augments both IL-7 binding and internalization [5].

Function

IL-7 stimulates the proliferation of pro-B and pre-B cells, thymocytes and mature T cells and induces the activation of monocytes [6-8]. IL-7R engagement stimulates Tyr phosphorylation and phosphatidylinositol turnover in B cell precursors and thymocytes [9,10].

Database accession numbers

	PIR	SWISSPROT	EMBL/GENBANK	REFERENCE
Human CD127	A34791–C34791	P16871	M29696	3
Mouse CD127	D34791	P16872	M29697	3

The accession numbers and amino acid sequence of CD132, which is common to the IL-2R, IL-4R, IL-7R, IL-9R and IL-15R, are given in the **IL-2R** entry.

Amino acid sequence of human CD127

```
MTILGTTFGM VFSLLQVVSG                                         -1
ESGYAQNGDL EDAELDDYSF SCYSQLEVNG SQHSLTCAFE DPDVNTTNLE        50
FEICGALVEV KCLNFRKLQE IYFIETKKFL LIGKSNICVK VGEKSLTCKK        100
IDLTTIVKPE APFDLSVIYR EGANDFVVTF NTSHLQKKYV KVLMHDVAYR        150
QEKDENKWTH VNLSSTKLTL LQRKLQPAAM YEIKVRSIPD HYFKGFWSEW        200
SPSYYFRTPE INNSSGEMDP ILLTISILSF FSVALLVILA CVLWKKRIKP        250
IVWPSLPDHK KTLEHLCKKP RKNLNVSFNP ESFLDCQIHR VDDIQARDEV        300
EGFLQDTFPQ QLEESEKQRL GGDVQSPNCP SEDVVVTPES FGRDSSLTCL        350
AGNVSACDAP ILSSSRSLDC RESGKNGPHV YQDLLLSLGT TNSTLPPPFS        400
LQSGILTLNP VAQGQPILTS LGSNQEEAYV TMSSFYQNQ                    439
```

References

1 Pleiman, C.M. et al. (1991) Mol. Cell. Biol. 11, 3052–3059.
2 Noguchi, M. et al. (1993) J. Biol. Chem. 268, 13601–13608.
3 **Goodwin, R.G. et al. (1990) Cell 60, 941–951.**
4 Patthy, L. (1990) Cell 61, 13–14.
5 **Noguchi, M. et al. (1993) Science 262, 1877–1880.**
6 Arai, K. et al. (1990) Annu. Rev. Biochem. 59, 783–836.
7 Callard, R.E. and Gearing, A.J.H. (1994) The Cytokine FactsBook. Academic Press, London.
8 Alderson, M.R. et al. (1991) J. Exp. Med. 173, 923–930.
9 Uckun, F.M. et al. (1991) Proc. Natl Acad. Sci. USA 88, 3589–3593.
10 Uckun, F.M. et al. (1991) Proc. Natl Acad. Sci. USA 88, 6323–6327.

Other names
CDw128: CXCR1

Molecular weights
Polypeptide   CDw128   39 806
               IL-8RB   40 760

Carbohydrate
N-linked sites   CDw128   4
                  IL-8RB   3
O-linked   CD128A   unknown
                  IL-8RB   unknown

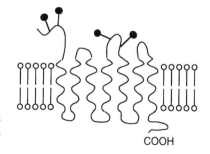

Human gene location and size
CDw128: 2q35
IL-8RB: 2q35; ~11 kb[1]

Tissue distribution

CDw128 and IL-8RB are expressed on neutrophils[2,3]. IL-8Rs are also expressed on basophils, eosinophils, a subset of T cells, monocytes, endothelial cells, keratinocytes and melanoma cells[4,5].

Structure

Both CDw128 and IL-8RB contain seven hydrophobic transmembrane domains and are members of the G protein-coupled receptor superfamily[2,3,6]. CDw128 and IL-8RB have 77% amino acid identity and contain potential Ser and Thr phosphorylation sites near the C-terminus[2,3].

Ligands and associated molecules

CDw128 binds IL-8 with high affinity ($K_d = 3.6$ nM)[2]. IL-8RB binds IL-8 with lower affinity and also functions as the receptor for three other IL-8-related CXC chemokines: melanoma growth-stimulating activity (MGSA/GRO), neutrophil-activating peptide 2 (NAP-2) and ENA-78[7,8].

Function

IL-8 induces chemotaxis of neutrophils, basophils and T lymphocytes. It activates neutrophils and basophils and increases neutrophil and monocyte adhesion to endothelial cells[4,5]. IL-8 binding to both CDw128 and IL-8RB induces a transient increase in intracellular calcium levels[2,3]. The activation of phospholipase D and the respiratory burst of neutrophils in response to

IL-8 can be blocked with an antibody specific for CDw128, but not with an anti-IL-8RB antibody [9].

Comments

The cDNA clone originally reported to encode the rabbit N-formyl peptide receptor is now identified as the rabbit homologue of CDw128 (79% identity) [10,11].

Database accession numbers

	PIR	SWISSPROT	EMBL/GENBANK	REFERENCE
Human CDw128	A39445	P25024	M68932	2
Human IL-8RB	A39446	P25025	M73969	3
Mouse IL-8RB	A53677	P35343	L13239	12
Rat IL-8RB	S42096	P35407	X77797	
Rabbit CDw128	A23669	P21109	M58021	10
Rabbit IL-8RB	A53752	P35344	L24445	13

Amino acid sequence of human CDw128

```
MSNITDPQMW DFDDLNFTGM PPADEDYSPC MLETETLNKY VVIIAYALVF    50
LLSLLGNSLV MLVILYSRVG RSVTDVYLLN LALADLLFAL TLPIWAASKV   100
NGWIFGTFLC KVVSLLKEVN FYSGILLLAC ISVDRYLAIV HATRTLTQKR   150
HLVKFVCLGC WGLSMNLSLP FFLFRQAYHP NNSSPVCYEV LGNDTAKWRM   200
VLRILPHTFG FIVPLFVMLF CYGFTLRTLF KAHMGQKHRA MRVIFAVVLI   250
FLLCWLPYNL VLLADTLMRT QVIQETCERR NNIGRALDAT EILGFLHSCL   300
NPIIYAFIGQ NFRHGFLKIL AMHGLVSKEF LARHRVTSYT SSSVNVSSNL   350
```

Amino acid sequence of human IL-8RB

```
MEDFNMESDS FEDFWKGEDL SNYSYSSTLP PFLLDAAPCE PESLEINKYF    50
VVIIYALVFL LSLLGNSLVM LVILYSRVGR SVTDVYLLNL ALADLLFALT   100
LPIWAASKVN GWIFGTFLCK VVSLLKEVNF YSGILLLACI SVDRYLAIVH   150
ATRTLTQKRY LVKFICLSIW GLSLLLALPV LLFRRTVYSS NVSPACYEDM   200
GNNTANWRML LRILPQSFGF IVPLLIMLFC YGFTLRTLFK AHMGQKHRAM   250
RVIFAVVLIF LLCWLPYNLV LLADTLMRTQ VIQETCERRN HIDRALDATE   300
ILGILHSCLN PLIYAFIGQK FRHGLLKILA IHGLISKDSL PKDSRPSFVG   350
SSSGHTSTTL                                              360
```

References
1 Sprenger, H. et al. (1994) J. Biol. Chem. 269, 11065–11072.
2 **Holmes, W.E. et al. (1991) Science 253, 1278–1280.**
3 **Murphy, P.M. and Tiffany, H.L. (1991) Science 253, 1280–1283.**
4 Oppenheim, J.J. et al. (1991) Annu. Rev. Immunol. 9, 617–648.
5 Callard, R.E. and Gearing, A.J.H. (1994) The Cytokine FactsBook. Academic Press, London.
6 Watson, S. and Arkinstall, S. (1994) The G–protein Linked Receptor FactsBook. Academic Press, London.
7 LaRosa, G.J. et al. (1992) J. Biol. Chem. 267, 25402–25406.
8 Walz, A. et al. (1991) J. Exp. Med. 174, 1355–1362.
9 Jones, S.A. et al. (1996) Proc. Natl Acad. Sci. USA 93, 6682–6686.

[10] Thomas, K.M. et al. (1990) J. Biol. Chem. 265, 20061–20064.
[11] Thomas, K.M. et al. (1991) J. Biol. Chem. 266, 14839–14841.
[12] Bozic, C.R. et al. (1994) J. Biol. Chem. 269, 29355–29358.
[13] Prado, G.N. et al. (1994) J. Biol. Chem. 269, 12391–12394.

IL-9R Interleukin 9 receptor

Subunits
CD129 (α chain)
CD132 (γc chain)

Molecular weights
Polypeptide	CD129	52 888
	CD132	39 920

Carbohydrate
N-linked sites	CD129	2
	CD132	6
O-linked	CD129	unknown
	CD132	unknown

Human gene location and size
CD129: Xq28, Yq12; ~17 kb [1]
CD132: Xq13; 4.2 kb [2]

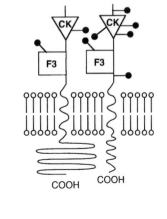

CD129   CD132

Domains: CHW SEC   WSI FIH

CD129 | S | CK | F3 | TM | CY |

Domains: CTW QKC   WAP KRY

CD132 | S | CK | F3 | TM | CY |
Exon boundaries: |1 |2 |1 |0 |2
ADF YWY   LVI   WTEQ   ERT 0
KEN   FSAW

Tissue distribution

The IL-9R is expressed on activated T cells, T cell lines, B cells, a mega-karyoblastic leukaemia cell line (Mo7E) and both erythroid and myeloid precursors [3–6].

Structure

The functional IL-9R consists of a complex formed through the association of CD129 and CD132 (see **IL-2R**) [7]. The extracellular region of CD129 consists of a cytokine receptor domain and a fibronectin type III domain that contains the WSXWS motif [3]. The cytoplasmic tail of CD129 (231 amino acids) contains a high percentage of Ser and Pro residues, including a stretch of nine successive Ser residues [3]. Crosslinking analysis identified mouse CD129 as a 64 kDa glycoprotein, which is reduced to 54 kDa following N-glycosidase F treatment [8]. A soluble form of mouse CD129 has been identified [3].

Ligands and associated molecules

The IL-9R binds IL-9 with a K_d of ~100 pM as demonstrated for the receptor on a mouse T cell clone [8]. The complex formed between CD129 and CD132 is essential for IL-9-dependent signal transduction [7].

Function

IL-9 promotes the growth of activated T cells and a megakaryoblastic leukaemia cell line (Mo7E), and supports the generation of erythroid and myeloid precursors [4-6]. IL-9 also potentiates the IL-4-induced production of IgG and IgE from B cells [9]. IL-9 stimulation of Mo7E cells induces Tyr phosphorylation of four unidentified proteins [10].

Database accession numbers

	PIR	SWISSPROT	EMBL/GENBANK	REFERENCE
Human CD129	B45268	Q01113	M84747	3
Mouse CD129	A45268	Q01114	M84746	3

The accession numbers and amino acid sequence of CD132, which is common to the IL-2R, IL-4R, IL-7R, IL-9R and IL-15R, are given in the **IL-2R** entry.

Amino acid sequence of human CD129

```
MGLGRCIWEG WTLESEALRR DMGTWLLACI CICTCVCLGV          -1
SVTGEGQGPR SRTFTCLTNN ILRIDCHWSA PELGQGSSPW LLFTSNQAPG  50
GTHKCILRGS ECTVVLPPEA VLVPSDNFTI TFHHCMSGRE QVSLVDPEYL  100
PRRHVKLDPP SDLQSNISSG HCILTWSISP ALEPMTTLLS YELAFKKQEE  150
AWEQAQHRDH IVGVTWLILE AFELDPGFIH EARLRVQMAT LEDDVVEEER  200
YTGQWSEWSQ PVCFQAPQRQ GPLIPPWGWP GNTLVAVSIF LLLTGPTYLL  250
FKLSPRVKRI FYQNVPSPAM FFQPLYSVHN GNFQTWMGAH RAGVLLSQDC  300
AGTPQGALEP CVQEATALLT CGPARPWKSV ALEEEQEGPG TRLPGNLSSE  350
DVLPAGCTEW RVQTLAYLPQ EDWAPTSLTR PAPPDSEGSR SSSSSSSSSN  400
NNNYCALGCY GGWHLSALPG NTQSSGPIPA LACGLSCDHQ GLETQQGVAW  450
VLAGHCQRPG LHEDLQGMLL PSVLSKARSW TF                     482
```

References

1. Kermouni, A. et al. (1995) Genomics 29, 371–382.
2. Noguchi, M. et al. (1993) J. Biol. Chem. 268, 13601–13608.
3. **Renauld, J-C. et al. (1992) Proc. Natl Acad. Sci. USA 89, 5690–5694.**
4. **Renauld, J-C. et al. (1993) Adv. Immunol. 54, 79–97.**
5. Donahue, R.E. et al. (1990) Blood 75, 2271–2275.
6. Holbrook, S.T. et al. (1991) Blood 77, 2129–2134.
7. Kimura, Y. et al. (1995) Int. Immunol. 7, 115–120.
8. Druez, C. et al. (1990) J. Immunol. 145, 2494–2499.
9. Dugas, B. et al. (1993) Eur. J. Immunol. 23, 1687–1692.
10. Miyazawa, K. et al. (1992) Blood 80, 1685–1692.

IL-10R
Interleukin 10 receptor

Molecular weight
Polypeptide   60 753

Carbohydrate
N-linked sites   6
O-linked   unknown

Human gene location
11

Domains

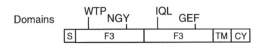

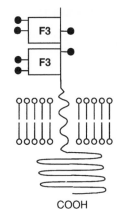

COOH

Tissue distribution

The IL-10R is expressed mainly by haematopoietic cells including T cells, B cells, NK cells, monocytes and macrophages[1,2].

Structure

The IL-10R belongs to the class II cytokine receptor family, which includes CD119 (IFNγR), CD118 (IFNα/βR), tissue factor (CD142) and viral CD119 homologues[2]. The IL-10R consists of two extracellular fibronectin type III domains, followed by a transmembrane region and a 318 amino acid cytoplasmic tail[2]. The WSXWS motif characteristic of Class I cytokine receptors is absent from both extracellular fibronectin type III domains. The human IL-10R has been identified as a 90–110 kDa protein by crosslinking experiments[2].

Ligands and associated molecules

The human IL-10R binds IL-10 with high affinity ($K_d = 200–250$ pM)[2].

Function

IL-10 inhibits cytokine synthesis by activated T cells, NK cells, monocytes and macrophages and blocks the accessory cell function of macrophages. IL-10 also co-stimulates human B cell proliferation and differentiation and synergizes with TGFβ to stimulate IgA production[1]. Mouse IL-10 also enhances the proliferation of thymocytes, T cells and mast cells, upregulates MHC Class II expression on B cells and sustains the viability of mouse B cells and mast cell lines *in vitro*[1,3].

Database accession numbers

	PIR	SWISSPROT	EMBL/GENBANK	REFERENCE
Human IL-10R			U00672	2
Mouse IL-10R			L12120	3

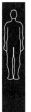

Amino acid sequence of human IL-10R

```
MLPCLVVLLA ALLSLRLGSD A                                           -1
HGTELPSPPS VWFEAEFFHH ILHWTPIPNQ SESTCYEVAL LRYGIESWNS            50
ISNCSQTLSY DLTAVTLDLY HSNGYRARVR AVDGSRHSNW TVTNTRFSVD           100
EVTLTVGSVN LEIHNGFILG KIQLPRPKMA PANDTYESIF SHFREYEIAI           150
RKVPGNFTFT HKKVKHENFS LLTSGEVGEF CVQVKPSVAS RSNKGMWSKE           200
ECISLTRQYF TVTNVIIFFA FVLLLSGALA YCLALQLYVR RRKKLPSVLL           250
FKKPSPFIFI SQRPSPETQD TIHPLDEEAF LKVSPELKNL DLHGSTDSGF           300
GSTKPSLQTE EPQFLLPDPH PQADRTLGNG EPPVLGDSCS SGSSNSTDSG           350
ICLQEPSLSP STGPTWEQQV GSNSRGQDDS GIDLVQNSEG RAGDTQGGSA           400
LGHHSPPEPE VPGEEDPAAV AFQGYLRQTR CAEEKATKTG CLEEESPLTD           450
GLGPKFGRCL VDEAGLHPPA LAKGYLKQDP LEMTLASSGA PTGQWNQPTE           500
EWSLLALSSC SDLGISDWSF AHDLAPLGCV AAPGGLLGSF NSDLVTLPLI           550
SSLQSSE                                                          557
```

References

[1] Moore, K.W. et al. (1993) Annu. Rev. Immunol. 11, 165–190.

[2] **Liu, Y. et al. (1994) J. Immunol. 152, 1821–1829.**

[3] Ho, A.S.Y. et al. (1993) Proc. Natl Acad. Sci. USA 90, 11267–11271.

Subunits
IL-11R α chain
CD130 (gp130)

Molecular weights

Polypeptide	α chain	43 131
	CD130	101 041

SDS-PAGE
reduced	CD130	130 kD

Carbohydrate

N-linked sites	α chain	2
	CD130	10
O-linked	α chain	unknown
	CD130	unknown

Human gene location
α chain: 9p13
CD130: 5q11

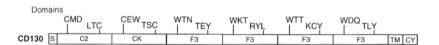

Tissue distribution

The IL-11R is expressed on multipotential haematopoietic progenitors, mega-karyocytes, B cells, macrophages, hepatocytes, adipocytes, muscle cells and osteoclasts [1,2].

Structure

The functional high-affinity receptor for human IL-11 is formed by the non-covalent association of two subunits, IL-11R α chain (sequence shown below) and CD130. The extracellular region of the IL-11R α chain consists of an N-terminal C2-set IgSF domain, followed by a cytokine receptor domain and a fibronectin type III domain, which includes the WSXWS motif, and is structurally related to CD126 (IL-6R α chain) and the α chain of the receptor for ciliary neurotrophic factor (CNTF). CD130, which does not bind IL-11 in isolation, consists of a C2-set IgSF domain, a cytokine receptor domain and four fibronectin type III domains, the first of which contains the WSXWS motif (see **IL-6R**). Alternative splicing of the IL-11R α chain gene results in a form of the molecule which lacks the entire cytoplasmic tail [2].

Ligands and associated molecules

The mouse IL-11R α chain has a relatively low affinity for IL-11 ($K_d = 10$ nM) and this interaction fails to transduce a biological signal. The generation of a high-affinity receptor for IL-11 ($K_d = 400$–800 pM) capable of signal transduction, requires co-expression of the IL-11R α chain and CD130[3].

Function

IL-11 is a growth factor for multipotential haematopoietic progenitors. IL-11 also stimulates erythropoiesis, enhances megakaryocyte and platelet formation, promotes osteoclastogenesis, functions as a macrophage maturation/activation factor and upregulates immunoglobulin secretion from activated B cells[1,2]. IL-11 also acts on various non-haematopoietic cell types, resulting in the inhibition of lipoprotein lipase activity in adipocytes, stimulation of acute phase protein synthesis by hepatocytes and the regulation of neuronal differentiation[1].

Database accession numbers

	PIR	SWISSPROT	EMBL/GENBANK	REFERENCE
Human IL-11Rα			Z38102	2
Mouse IL-11Rα	S51619		U14412	3

The accession numbers and amino acid sequence of CD130 (the β chain of the IL-11R), which is common to the IL-6R, LIFR, CNTFR, OSMR and CT-1R are given in the **IL-6R** entry.

Amino acid sequence of human IL-11R α chain

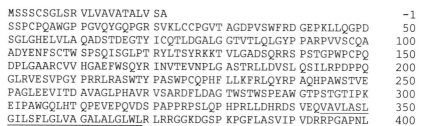

```
MSSSCSGLSR VLVAVATALV SA                             -1
SSPCPQAWGP PGVQYGQPGR SVKLCCPGVT AGDPVSWFRD GEPKLLQGPD   50
SGLGHELVLA QADSTDEGTY ICQTLDGALG GTVTLQLGYP PARPVVSCQA  100
ADYENFSCTW SPSQISGLPT RYLTSYRKKT VLGADSQRRS PSTGPWPCPQ  150
DPLGAARCVV HGAEFWSQYR INVTEVNPLG ASTRLLDVSL QSILRPDPPQ  200
GLRVESVPGY PRRLRASWTY PASWPCQPHF LLKFRLQYRP AQHPAWSTVE  250
PAGLEEVITD AVAGLPHAVR VSARDFLDAG TWSTWSPEAW GTPSTGTIPK  300
EIPAWGQLHT QPEVEPQVDS PAPPRPSLQP HPRLLDHRDS VEQVAVLASL  350
GILSFLGLVA GALALGLWLR LRRGGKDGSP KPGFLASVIP VDRRPGAPNL  400
```

References
[1] Du, X.X. and Williams, D.A. (1994) Blood 83, 2023–2030.
[2] **Chérel, M. et al. (1995) Blood 86, 2534–2540.**
[3] Hilton, D.J. et al. (1994) EMBO J. 13, 4765–4775.

IL-12R

Interleukin 12 receptor β chain

Molecular weight
Polypeptide   70 422

Carbohydrate
N-linked sites   6
O-linked   unknown

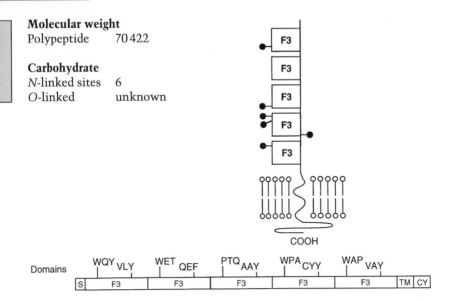

Tissue distribution

The IL-12R is expressed on activated CD4$^+$ and CD8$^+$ T cells, IL-2-activated CD56$^+$ NK cells and an IL-2-dependent CD4$^+$ T cell line (Kit225)[1,2].

Structure

The IL-12R is predicted to comprise a heterodimer formed between the designated IL-12R β subunit, cloned in both human and mouse, and an as yet unidentified second chain. The human IL-12R β chain consists of five extra-cellular fibronectin type III domains, followed by a transmembrane domain and a relatively short (91 amino acids) cytoplasmic tail and shows a high degree of amino acid sequence similarity to CD130 (gp130), G-CSFR (CD114) and LIFR α chain[3]. Crosslinking experiments using unlabelled human IL-12 and ^{125}I-labelled PHA-activated lymphoblasts have identified two proteins of approximately 110 kDa and 85 kDa which may associate to form a functional IL-12R[1].

Ligands and associated molecules

Three classes of IL-12 binding sites have been demonstrated on activated human T cells and the T cell line, Kit225; high-affinity ($K_d = 5$–20 pM), intermediate-affinity ($K_d = 50$–200 pM) and low-affinity ($K_d = 2$–6 nM)[3]. The IL-12R β chain (shown below) binds both human and mouse IL-12 with an apparent affinity of 2–5 nM[3].

Function

IL-12 has pleiotropic effects on NK cells and T cells, including the stimulation of cell proliferation, induction of IFNγ secretion, enhancement of cytolytic responses and promotion of a T_H1-type immune response[4].

Comments

COS-7 cells transfected with the IL-12R β chain cDNA express both monomers and disulfide-linked dimers, or oligomers, of the IL-12R β subunit on their surface[3]. Oligomerization of the IL-12R β subunit is independent of IL-12, while the dimers/oligomers but not the monomers bind IL-12 with low affinity ($K_d = 2$–5 nM).

Database accession numbers

	PIR	SWISSPROT	EMBL/GENBANK	REFERENCE
Human IL-12R β		P42701	U03187	[3]
Mouse IL-12R β			U23922	[5]

Amino acid sequence of human IL-12R β chain

```
MEPLVTWVVP LLFLFLLSRQ GAAC                                    -1
RTSECCFQDP PYPDADSGSA SGPRDLRCYR ISSDRYECSW QYEGPTAGVS        50
HFLRCCLSSG RCCYFAAGSA TRLQFSDQAG VSVLYTVTLW VESWARNQTE        100
KSPEVTLQLY NSVKYEPPLG DIKVSKLAGQ LRMEWETPDN QVGAEVQFRH        150
RTPSSPWKLG DCGPQDDDTE SCLCPLEMNV AQEFQLRRRQ LGSQGSSWSK        200
WSSPVCVPPE NPPQPQVRFS VEQLGQDGRR RLTLKEQPTQ LELPEGCQGL        250
APGTEVTYRL QLHMLSCPCK AKATRTLHLG KMPYLSGAAY NVAVISSNQF        300
GPGLNQTWHI PADTHTEPVA LNISVGTNGT TMYWPARAQS MTYCIEWQPV        350
GQDGGLATCS LTAPQDPDPA GMATYSWSRE SGAMGQEKCY YITIFASAHP        400
EKLTLWSTVL STYHFGGNAS AAGTPHHVSV KNHSLDSVSV DWAPSLLSTC        450
PGVLKEYVVR CRDEDSKQVS EHPVQPTETQ VTLSGLRAGV AYTVQVRADT        500
AWLRGVWSQP QRFSIEVQVS DWLIFFASLG SFLSILLVGV LGYLGLNRAA        550
RHLCPPLPTP CASSAIEFPG GKETWQWINP VDFQEEASLQ EALVVEMSWD        600
KGERTEPLEK TELPEGAPEL ALDTELSLED GDRCKAKM                     638
```

References

1 Chizzonite, R. et al. (1992) J. Immunol. 148, 3117–3124.
2 Desai, B.B. et al. (1992) J. Immunol. 148, 3125–3132.
3 **Chua, A.O. et al. (1994) J. Immunol. 153, 128–136.**
4 Trinchieri, G. (1994) Blood 84, 4008–4027.
5 Chua, A.O. et al. (1995) J. Immunol. 155, 4286–4294.

Note added in proof

A second component of the functional IL-12R, designated IL-12R β2 subunit, has been characterized through the isolation of human and mouse cDNA clones (Presky, D.H. et al. (1996) Proc. Natl Acad. Sci. USA 93, 14002–14007). These sequences are available using GENBANK accession numbers U64198 and U64199. The IL-12R β chain described in this entry has therefore been renamed IL-12R β1 chain.

Subunits
IL-13R α chain
CD124 (IL-4R α chain)

Molecular weights
| Polypeptide | IL-13R α chain | 41 457 |
| | CD124 | 87 067 |

Carbohydrate
N-linked sites	IL-13R α chain	4
	CD124	6
O-linked	IL-13R α chain	unknown
	CD124	unknown

Human gene location
CD124: 16p11.2–p12.1

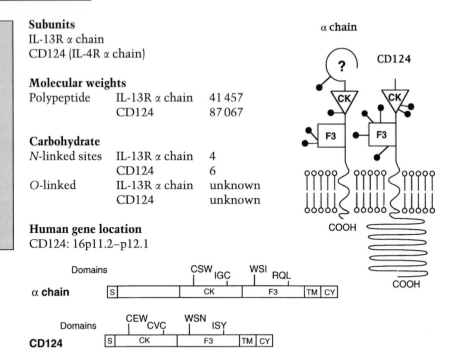

α chain

Tissue distribution

The IL-13R is expressed on B cells, monocytes, fibroblasts and endothelial cells [1,2].

Structure

The IL-13R α chain shows structural homology to CDw125 (IL-5R α chain), with 51% amino acid sequence similarity and 27% identity [2]. Similar to CDw125, the extracellular region of the IL-13R α chain consists of an N-terminal region of about 100 amino acids with sequence similarity to the equivalent portion of CDw123 (IL-3R α chain) and CD116 (GM-CSFR α chain), followed by a cytokine receptor domain and a fibronectin type III domain that includes the WSXWS motif [2].

Ligands and associated molecules

The human IL-13R α chain expressed in COS-7 cells binds human IL-13 with high affinity ($K_d = 220–280$ pM), whereas COS-7 cells transfected with the mouse IL-13R α chain cDNA bind mouse IL-13 with a low affinity ($K_d = 2–10$ nM) [2,3]. In both species, the IL-13R α chain also associates with CD124 to form a receptor capable of binding both IL-13 and IL-4 with high affinity and mediating signal transduction events [2–4]. This interaction may explain the apparent discrepancy in the ability of human, but not mouse, IL-13R α chain to bind IL-13 with high affinity, since untransfected COS-7 cells express low levels of CD124 which might associate with transfected human, but not mouse, IL-13R α chain to form a functional high-affinity binding site for IL-13. Crosslinking experiments have identified an IL-13 binding protein of approximately 60–70 kDa, which probably corresponds to the IL-13R α chain[2].

Function

IL-13 and IL-4 mediate similar biological functions except that, unlike IL-4, IL-13 does not regulate T cell functions[1,5].

Comments

The published human and mouse IL-13R α chain sequences share the same overall topology, but show only limited amino acid sequence identity[2,3]. It remains to be determined whether additional IL-13R subunits exist and whether, in fact, these molecules are true species homologues.

Database accession numbers

	PIR	SWISSPROT	EMBL/GENBANK	REFERENCE
Human IL-13R α			X95302	2

The accession numbers and amino acid sequence of CD124 are given in the **IL-4R** entry.

Amino acid sequence of human IL-13R α chain

```
MAFVCLAIGC LYTFLISTTF GCTSSS                                    -1
DTEIKVNPPQ DFEIVDPGYL GYLYLQWQPP LSLDHFKECT VEYELKYRNI          50
GSETWKTIIT KNLHYKDGFD LNKGIEAKIH TLLPWQCTNG SEVQSSWAET         100
TYWISPQGIP ETKVQDMDCV YYNWQYLLCS WKPGIGVLLD TNYNLFYWYE         150
GLDHALQCVD YIKADGQNIG CRFPYLEASD YKDFYICVNG SSENKPIRSS         200
YFTFQLQNIV KPLPPVYLTF TRESSCEIKL KWSIPLGPIP ARCFDYEIEI         250
REDDTTLVTA TVENETYTLK TTNETRQLCF VVRSKVNIYC SDDGIWSEWS         300
DKQCWEGEDL SKKTLLRFWL PFGFILILVI FVTGLLLRKP NTYPKMIPEF         350
FCDT                                                          354
```

References

1 Zurawski, G. and de Vries, J.E. (1994) Immunol. Today 15, 19–26.
2 **Caput, D. et al. (1996) J. Biol. Chem. 271, 16921–16926.**
3 Hilton, D.J. et al. (1996) Proc. Natl Acad. Sci. USA 93, 497–501.
4 **Lin, J-X. et al. (1995) Immunity 2, 331–339.**
5 Punnonen, J. et al. (1993) Proc. Natl Acad. Sci. USA 90, 3730–3734.

IL-14R | Interleukin 14 receptor, high molecular weight B cell growth factor receptor

Molecular weight
SDS-PAGE
  reduced   48–50 kDa
  unreduced   48 kDa and 90 kDa

Tissue distribution

The IL-14R is expressed at a low level on resting B cells, but at high levels on activated B cells and B cell leukaemias [1,2].

Structure

IL-14R cDNA clones have not yet been isolated. However the BA5 monoclonal antibody, believed to recognize the human IL-14R, immunoprecipitates a protein of approximately 90 kDa which may consist of two distinct subunits [1]. Crosslinking experiments using ^{125}I-labelled IL-14 also identified an IL-14-binding protein of approximately 90 kDa [1,2].

Ligands and associated molecules

The IL-14R on leukaemic B cells binds IL-14 with low affinity ($K_d = 20$ nM) [2]. Bb, the activation fragment of complement Factor B, competes with IL-14 for binding to the IL-14R [3,4].

Function

IL-14 induces proliferation of activated B cells and inhibits immunoglobulin secretion [5,6]. In B cells, levels of intracellular cAMP, diacylglycerol and calcium are increased following IL-14 binding to the IL-14R [4].

References
1 Ambrus, J.L. et al. (1988) J. Immunol. 141, 861–869.
2 Uckun, F.M. et al. (1989) J. Clin. Invest. 84, 1595–1608.
3 Peters, M.G. et al. (1988) J. Exp. Med. 168, 1225–1235.
4 Ambrus, J.L. et al. (1991) J. Biol. Chem. 266, 3702–3708.
5 Ambrus, J.L. et al. (1990) J. Immunol. 145, 3949–3955.
6 **Ambrus, J.L. et al. (1993) Proc. Natl Acad. Sci. USA 90, 6330–6334.**

Subunits

IL-15R α chain
CD122 (IL-2R β chain)
CD132 (γc chain)

Molecular weight

Polypeptide	α chain	24 997
	CD122	58 359
	CD132	39 920
SDS-PAGE reduced	CD122	70–75 kDa
	CD132	64 kDa

Carbohydrate

N-linked sites	α chain	1
	CD122	4
	CD132	6
O-linked	α chain	probable +
	CD122	unknown
	CD132	unknown

Human gene location and size

α chain: 10p14–p15
CD122: 22q11.2–q13; 24.3 kb [1]
CD132: Xq13; 4.2 kb [2]

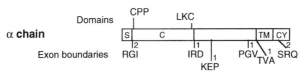

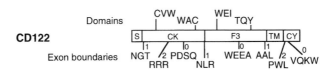

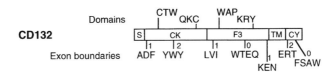

Tissue distribution

The IL-15R is expressed on activated T cells, T cell lines, NK cells and activated B cells [3-5].

Structure

The functional IL-15R is a heterotrimeric structure comprising the IL-15R α chain, CD122 (IL-2R β chain) and the common γ chain (CD132)[3-6]. The IL-15R α chain contains a single extracellular CCP domain, followed by a region rich in Ser and Thr residues, and has a 41 amino acid cytoplasmic tail that is dispensable for signal transduction[4]. The IL-15R α chain is structurally related to CD25 (IL-2R α chain). Three alternatively spliced forms of the human IL-15R α chain have been cloned[4].

Ligands and associated molecules

The IL-15R α chain binds IL-15 with high affinity (K_d = 10 pM)[4,5]. However, the interaction between the IL-15R α chain and CD122/CD132 is required to form a functional high-affinity IL-15R capable of mediating signal transduction[3-6]. High concentrations of IL-15 (450 ng/ml) can bind to, and signal through, a complex of CD122/CD132 in the absence of the IL-15R α chain[4].

Function

IL-15 shares biological activities with IL-2, such as the activation and proliferation of T cells, generation of cytotoxic T cells and lymphokine-activated killer (LAK) cells, and the proliferation of NK cells and B cells[3-5,7,8].

Comments

The IL-15R α chain and CD25 genes have a similar intron/exon organization and are closely linked in both human and mouse[4]. IL-15R α chain mRNA is expressed on a wide range of cell types, in contrast to CD25[4,5]. Since CD122 and CD132 are essential for IL-15 signalling in haematopoietic cell types and their expression patterns are more restricted than the IL-15R α chain, the possibility exists that the IL-15R α chain may associate with alternative signalling subunits in other cell types[4].

Database accession numbers

	PIR	SWISSPROT	EMBL/GENBANK	REFERENCE
Human IL-15Rα			U31628	4
Mouse IL-15Rα			U22339	5

The accession numbers and amino acid sequences of CD122 and CD132 are given in the **IL-2R** entry.

Amino acid sequence of human IL-15R α chain

```
MAPRRARGCR TLGLPALLLL LLLRPPATRG                       -1
ITCPPPMSVE HADIWVKSYS LYSRERYICN SGFKRKAGTS SLTECVLNKA  50
TNVAHWTTPS LKCIRDPALV HQRPAPPSTV TTAGVTPQPE SLSPSGKEPA  100
ASSPSSNNTA ATTAAIVPGS QLMPSKSPST GTTEISSHES SHGTPSQTTA  150
KNWELTASAS HQPPGVYPQG HSDTTVAIST STVLLCGLSA VSLLACYLKS  200
RQTPPLASVE MEAMEALPVT WGTSSRDEDL ENCSHHL               237
```

References
[1] Shibuya, H. et al. (1990) Nucleic Acids Res. 18, 3697–3703.
[2] Noguchi, M. et al. (1993) J. Biol. Chem. 268, 13601–13608.
[3] Grabstein, K.H. et al. (1994) Science 264, 965–968.
[4] **Anderson, D.M. et al. (1995) J. Biol. Chem. 270, 29862–29869.**
[5] **Giri, J.G. et al. (1995) EMBO J. 14, 3654–3663.**
[6] Giri, J.G. et al. (1994) EMBO J. 13, 2822–2830.
[7] Carson, W.E. et al. (1994) J. Exp. Med. 180, 1395–1403.
[8] Armitage, R.J. et al. (1995) J. Immunol. 154, 483–490.

IL-17R
Interleukin 17 receptor

Molecular weight
Polypeptide   94 416

SDS-PAGE
   reduced   120 kDa

Carbohydrate
N-linked sites   8
O-linked   unknown

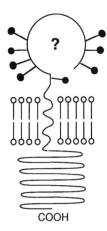

COOH

Tissue distribution

Mouse IL-17R mRNA is expressed by a wide range of haematopoietic and non-haematopoietic tissues and cell lines [1].

Structure

The mouse IL-17R is a type I transmembrane protein consisting of a 291 amino acid extracellular domain, a transmembrane domain and a very large (521 amino acids) cytoplasmic tail [1]. There are two acidic regions and a Ser-rich region in the cytoplasmic tail, similar to those found in CD122 (IL-2R β chain), CD124 (IL-4R α chain) and the G-CSFR (CD114) [1]. The IL-17R sequence is unrelated to previously identified cytokine receptors.

Ligands and associated molecules

The IL-17R binds to IL-17 and HVS13, a herpesvirus saimiri-encoded IL-17 homologue that shows 72% amino acid sequence identity to human IL-17 [1-3].

Function

IL-17 has been shown to induce secretion of IL-6 and IL-8 from fibroblasts, upregulate fibroblast expression of CD54 (ICAM-1), activate the transcription factor NF-κB and enhance the proliferative response of purified T cells to suboptimal concentrations of the mitogen PHA [1,3].

Comment

The mouse IL-17R gene maps to chromosome 6 [1].

Database accession numbers

	PIR	SWISSPROT	EMBL/GENBANK	REFERENCE
Mouse IL-17R			U31993	[1]

Amino acid sequence of mouse IL-17R

```
MAIRRCWPRV VPGPALGWLL LLLNVLAPGR A                           -1
SPRLLDFPAP VCAQEGLSCR VKNSTCLDDS WIHPKNLTPS SPKNIYINLS       50
VSSTQHGELV PVLHVEWTLQ TDASILYLEG AELSVLQLNT NERLCVKFQF      100
LSMLQHHRKR WRFSFSHFVV DPGQEYEVTV HHLPKPIPDG DPNHKSKIIF      150
VPDCEDSKMK MTTSCVSSGS LWDPNITVET LDTQHLRVDF TLWNESTPYQ      200
VLLESFSDSE NHSCFDVVKQ IFAPRQEEFH QRANVTFTLS KFHWCCHHHV      250
QVQPFFSSCL NDCLRHAVTV PCPVISNTTV PKPVADYIPL WVYGLITLIA      300
ILLVGSVIVL IICMTWRLSG ADQEKHGDDS KINGILPVAD LTPPPLRPRK      350
VWIVYSADHP LYVEVVLKFA QFLITACGTE VALDLLEEQV ISEVGVMTWV      400
SRQKQEMVES NSKIIILCSR GTQAKWKAIL GWAEPAVQLR CDHWKPAGDL      450
FTAAMNMILP DFKRPACFGT YVVCYFSGIC SERDVPDLFN ITSRYPLMDR      500
FEEVYFRIQD LEMFEPGRMH HVRELTGDNY LQSPSGRQLK EAVLRFQEWQ      550
TQCPDWFERE NLCLADGQDL PSLDEEVFED PLLPPGGGIV KQQPLVRELP      600
SDGCLVVDVC VSEEESRMAK LDPQLWPQRE LVAHTLQSMV LPAEQVPAAH      650
VVEPLHLPDG SGAAAQLPMT EDSEACPLLG VQRNSILCLP VDSDDLPLCS      700
TPMMSPDHLQ GDAREQLESL MLSVLQQSLS GQPLESWPRP EVVLEGCTPS      750
EEEQRQSVQS DQGYISRSSP QPPEWLTEEE ELELGEPVES LSPEELRSLR      800
KLQRQLFFWE LEKNPGWNSL EPRRPTPEEQ NPS                        833
```

References
[1] Yao, Z. et al. (1995) **Immunity 3, 811–821.**
[2] Albrecht, J-C. et al. (1992) J. Virol. 66, 5047–5058.
[3] Yao, Z. et al. (1995) J. Immunol. 155, 5483–5486.

Integrin β7 subunit

Molecular weights
Polypeptide   84 881

SDS-PAGE
  reduced   110 kDa
  unreduced   105 kDa

Carbohydrate
N-linked sites   8
O-linked sites   unknown

Human gene location and size
12q13.13, ~10 kb [1].

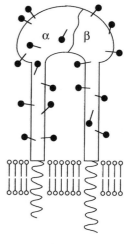

α4(CD49d)/β7

Tissue distribution

β7 combines with the α4 subunit (CD49d) to form the α4β7 integrin and with the αE subunit (CD103) to form the αEβ7 integrin (HML-1). Both antigens are expressed on mucosal lymphocytes [2]. Adult human lymphocytes have heterogeneous expression of α4β7, whereas expression on newborn lymphocytes is more homogeneous [3,4]. α4β7 is also expressed on NK cells and eosinophils [3]. αEβ7 is expressed on 95% of intraepithelial lymphocytes but only 1–2% of peripheral blood lymphocytes [2]. Its level of expression on lymphocytes can be upregulated by lymphocyte mitogens [5].

Structure

The β7 integrin subunit is most closely related to the β2 integrin subunit (CD18) including the cytoplasmic segment, in which two NPX(Y/F) motifs for potential tyrosine kinase binding are found. Most integrin β subunits have 56 conserved cysteine residues in their extracellular portion; the last two cysteines are missing from the β7 subunit [6,7]. The N-terminus has been determined by protein sequencing [2].

Ligands and associated molecules

Like the α4β1 integrin, α4β7 binds CD106 (VCAM-1) and the CS1 region of fibronectin [8,9]. In addition, α4β7 binds the mucosal addressin MAdCAM-1 [10,11]. αEβ7 binds E-cadherin on epithelial cells [12].

Function

The α4β7 integrin mediates the binding of lymphocytes to MAdCAM-1 on the high endothelial venules, thereby directing the homing of lymphocytes into

Peyer's patches and the intestinal lamina propria [10,11]. The interaction between αEβ7 and E-cadherin may be of importance in the homing and retention of αEβ7-expressing lymphocytes to the intestinal epithelium [12,13].

Database accession numbers

	PIR	SWISSPROT	EMBL/GENBANK	REFERENCE
Human	A40526	P26010	M62880	6
			M68892	7
Mouse	A46271	P26011	M68903	14
			M95632	15

Amino acid sequence of human β7 integrin subunit

```
MVALPMVLVL LLVLSRGES                                          -1
ELDAKIPSTG DATEWRNPHL SMLGSCQPAP SCQKCILSHP SCAWCKQLNF         50
TASGEAEARR CARREELLAR GCPLEELEEP RGQQEVLQDQ PLSQGARGEG        100
ATQLAPQRVR VTLRPGEPQQ LQVRFLRAEG YPVDLYYLMD LSYSMKDDLE        150
RVRQLGHALL VRLQEVTHSV RIGFGSFVDK TVLPFVSTVP SKLRHPCPTR        200
LERCQSPFSF HHVLSLTGDA QAFEREVGRQ SVSGNLDSPE GGFDAILQAA        250
LCQEQIGWRN VSRLLVFTSD DTFHTAGDGK LGGIFMPSDG HCHLDSNGLY        300
SRSTEFDYPS VGQVAQALSA ANIQPIFAVT SAALPVYQEL SKLIPKSAVG        350
ELSEDSSNVV QLIMDAYNSL SSTVTLEHSS LPPGVHISYE SQCEGPEKRE        400
GKAEDRGQCN HVRINQTVTF WVSLQATHCL PEPHLLRLRA LGFSEELIVE        450
LHTLCDCNCS DTQPQAPHCS DGQGHLQCGV CSCAPGRLGR LCECSVAELS        500
SPDLESGCRA PNGTGPLCSG KGHCQCGRCS CSGQSSGHLC ECDDASCERH        550
EGILCGGFGR CQCGVCHCHA NRTGRACECS GDMDSCISPE GGLCSGHGRC        600
KCNRCQCLDG YYGALCDQCP GCKTPCERHR DCAECGAFRT GPLATNCSTA        650
CAHTNVTLAL APILDDGWCK ERTLDNQLFF FLVEDDARGT VVLRVRPQEK        700
GADHTQAIVL GCVGGIVAVG LGLVLAYRLS VEIYDRREYS RFEKEQQQLN        750
WKQDSNPLYK SAITTTINPR FQEADSPTL                              779
```

References
1. Jiang, W.M. et al. (1992) Int. Immunol. 4, 1031–1040.
2. **Parker, C. M. et al. (1992) Proc. Natl Acad. Sci. USA 89, 1924–1928.**
3. **Erle, D.J. et al. (1994) J. Immunol. 153, 517–528.**
4. Andrew, D.P. et al. (1996) Eur. J. Immunol. 26, 897–905.
5. Schieferdecker, H.L. et al. (1990) J. Immunol. 144, 2541–2549.
6. Erle, D.J. et al. (1991) J. Biol. Chem. 266, 11009–11016.
7. Yuan, Q. et al. (1990) Int. Immunol. 2, 1097–1118; Corr. (1991) Int. Immunol. 3, 1373–1374.
8. Lobb, R.R. and Hemler, H.E. (1994) J. Clin. Invest. 94, 1722–1728.
9. Kilger, G. et al. (1995) J. Biol. Chem. 270, 5979–5984.
10. Berlin, C. et al. (1993) Cell 74, 185–195.
11. Rott, L.S. et al. (1996) J. Immunol. 156, 3727–3736.
12. **Cepek, K.L. et al. (1994) Nature 372, 190–193.**
13. Cepek, K.L. et al. (1993) J. Immunol. 150, 3459–3470.
14. Yuan, Q. et al. (1992) J. Biol. Chem. 267, 7352–7358.
15. Hu, M.C.T. (1992) Proc. Natl Acad. Sci. USA 89, 8254–8258.

Members (Modified from refs 1–4; sequences from refs 5–10)

(KIR molecules reactive with the mAbs EB6 and GL183 have been assigned the CD numbers CD158a and CD158b, respectively.)

cDNA clones	Other names[a]	IgSF domains	Cytoplasmic domain[b]	Putative ligands[c]	Reactive mAbs	Closely related cDNA clones
KIR-cl.42	NKAT1, p58.1	2	long	HLA-C group 1	EB6	KIR-cl.47.11[d]
KIR-cl.6	NKAT2, p58.2	2	long	HLA-C group 2	GL183	NKAT2a[d], NKAT2b[d], NKAT2b ΔIg2[e]
KIR-cl.43	p58.2	2	long	HLA-C group 2	GL183	NKAT6[d]
KIR-cl.49	NKAT5, p50.2	2	short	HLA-C group 2	GL183	NKAT5 ΔIg1/Ig2[e] NKAT5 ΔIg1[e] p183-ActI[d]
KIR-cl.39	NKAT8	2	short	?	5.133	
pEB6-ActI	p50.1	2	short	HLA-C group 1	EB6	
NKAT7		2	short	?		
NKAT9		2	short	?		
KIR-cl.11[f]	NKAT3, p70	3	long	HLA-Bw4	DX9, 5.133	NKAT3 ΔIg1[e]
KIR-cl.2[f]	NKB1, p70	3	long	HLA-Bw4	DX9, 5.133	NKB1B[e]
NKAT4		3	long	HLA-A3	5.133	KIR-cl.5[d], NKAT4a[d], NKAT4b[d]
NKAT10		3	short	?		

[a] Encode identical protein sequence.

[b] The additional peptide sequence in KIRs with long cytoplasmic domains contains two copies of the motif V/IXYXXL separated by 24 amino acids. These motifs are involved in recruiting the cytoplasmic tyrosine phosphatases SHP-1 and SHP-2.

[c] HLA-C group 1 (with Asn77 and Lys80) includes Cw2, Cw4, Cw5, and Cw6 alleles; group 2 (with Ser77, Asn80) includes Cw1, Cw3, Cw7, and Cw8 alleles.

[d] These clones encode proteins with ≤2 amino acid differences and might, therefore, represent allelic variants or cloning/sequencing errors, rather than transcripts from separate genes.

[e] These clones are identical except for deletions consistent with alternative splicing.

[f] KIR-cl.11 and KIR-cl.2 differ by only four amino acid substitutions.

Molecular weights

(KIRs can be grouped into four size groups according to number of IgSF domains and lengths of cytoplasmic domains (see Table). Examples are given from each group.)

Polypeptide
KIR-cl.42	36 253
KIR-cl.49	31 232
KIR-cl.11	46 906
NKAT10	40 573

SDS-PAGE (unreduced and reduced)
KIR-cl.42 (p58)	~58 kDa
KIR-cl.49 (p50)	~50 kDa
KIR-cl.11 (p70)	~70 kDa
NKAT10	unknown

Carbohydrate

N-linked sites	KIR-cl.42	4
	KIR-cl.11	4
O-linked	KIR-cl.42	none
	KIR-cl.11	none

Human gene location
19q13.4 [11]

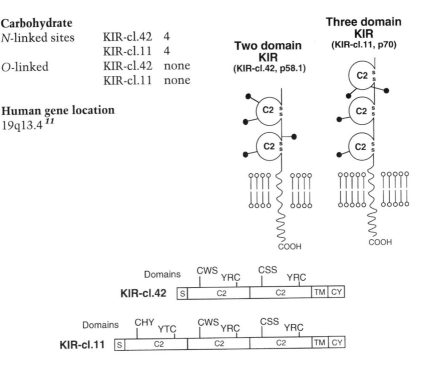

Two domain KIR
(KIR-cl.42, p58.1)

Three domain KIR
(KIR-cl.11, p70)

KIR-cl.42 Domains: CWS YRC CSS YRC — S | C2 | C2 | TM | CY

KIR-cl.11 Domains: CHY YTC CWS YRC CSS YRC — S | C2 | C2 | C2 | TM | CY

Tissue distribution

Individual KIRs are expressed on overlapping subsets of NK cells and T cells [1-3]. Expression of specific KIRs varies considerably between individuals. For example KIR-cl.2 (NKB1) expression on NK cells varies from 0 to >75% between individuals [12]. Interestingly, although the expression pattern appears to be genetically determined it is not correlated with MHC haplotype [12].

Structure

KIRs are a closely related multigene family of transmembrane glycoproteins having either two or three C2-set IgSF domains in the extracellular portion. The leader and extracellular portion of the two-domain KIRs show a high degree of similarity (>74%) with the leader and two membrane-proximal domains of the three-domain KIRs. KIRs either have a longer cytoplasmic domain (76–84 amino acids) containing two V/IXYXXL motifs or a truncated cytoplasmic domain (27–39 amino acids) lacking this motif. Molecules lacking the V/IXYXXL motifs have, within their transmembrane region, a charged residue in consensus sequence KXPXTI.

Ligands and associated molecules

Individual KIRs bind directly to specific MHC class I alleles [1-3]. KIRs have been identified which bind to HLA-A, -B, and -C [4] alleles. Binding specificity correlates with sequence similarity in the extracellular region of the KIRs, including the number of IgSF domains. Binding involves MHC Class I residues (77–83) in the C-terminal end of the α1-domain α helix, adjacent to the peptide binding groove, but does not require glycosylation of the adjacent N-glycan site [13]. Although KIRs do not recognize specific peptides, the nature of the peptide in the groove does affect binding [14]. KIRs with two IgSF domains contain a zinc-binding motif (HExxH) at their N-terminus and have been reported to bind zinc affinity columns and to require zinc for target recognition [15]. Most KIRs possess V/IXYXXL motifs in their cytoplasmic domain which, when phosphorylated, mediate association with and activation of the cytoplasmic tyrosine phosphatases SHP-1 and SHP-2 [16–18]. Ligation of KIRs leads to recruitment and activation of SHP-1, and catalytically-active SHP-1 is required for inhibition of NK cell killing [16–18].

Function

KIRs on NK cells and cytotoxic T lymphocytes are involved in recognition of MHC Class I molecules on target cells. Ligation of KIRs generally inhibits killing by NK or T cells, thereby protecting target cells which express autologous MHC class I molecules [1–3]. Since targets lacking suitable MHC Class I molecules are susceptible to killing, KIRs enable NK cells to recognize the 'absence of self' on cells. NK cells can express multiple, functionally independent KIRs [1–3]. The precise role of KIRs on T cells is not clear but the recent observation that KIRs are preferentially expressed on memory cells is consistent with a role in limiting and/or terminating activation through the T cell receptor [2]. Preliminary reports suggest that KIRs lacking the cytoplasmic I/VXXYXXL motif might transmit activation signals [1,3].

Database accession numbers for human KIR cDNA clones

cDNA	PIR	SWISSPROT	EMBL/GENBANK	REFERENCE
KIR-cl.42/NKAT1		P43626	U24076/L41267	5,6
KIR-cl.6/NKAT2		P43628	U24074/L41268	5,6
KIR-cl.43		P43627	U24075	5
KIR-cl.49/NKAT5		P43631	U24079/L41347	5,6
KIR-cl.39/NKAT8		P43632	U24077/L76671	5,10
p183-ActI			X89893	9
pEB6-ActI			X89892	9
NKAT7			L76670	10
NKAT9			L76672	10
KIR-cl.2/NKB1			U31416	7,8
KIR-cl.11/NKAT3		P43629	U30274/L41269	6,8
NKAT4		P43630	L41270	6
NKAT10			L76661	10

Amino acid sequence of KIR-cl.42 (NKAT1)

```
MSLLVVSMAC VGFFLLQGAW P                                          -1
HEGVHRKPSL LAHPGPLVKS EETVILQCWS DVMFEHFLLH REGMFNDTLR           50
LIGEHHDGVS KANFSISRMT QDLAGTYRCY GSVTHSPYQV SAPSDPLDIV          100
IIGLYEKPSL SAQPGPTVLA GENVTLSCSS RSSYDMYHLS REGEAHERRL          150
PAGPKVNGTF QADFPLGPAT HGGTYRCFGS FHDSPYEWSK SSDPLLVSVT          200
GNPSNSWPSP TEPSSKTGNP RHLHILIGTS VVIILFILLF FLLHRWCSNK          250
KNAAVMDQES AGNRTANSED SDEQDPQEVT YTQLNHCVFT QRKITRPSQR          300
PKTPPTDIIV YTELPNAESR SKVVSCP                                   327
```

Amino acid sequence of KIR-cl.11 (NKAT3)

```
MSLMVVSMAC VGLFLVQRAG P                                      -1
HMGGQDKPFL SAWPSAVVPR GGHVTLRCHY RHRFNNFMLY KEDRIHIPIF       50
HGRIFQESFN MSPVTTAHAG NYTCRGSHPH SPTGWSAPSN PVVIMVTGNH      100
RKPSLLAHPG PLVKSGERVI LQCWSDIMFE HFFLHKEGIS KDPSRLVGQI      150
HDGVSKANFS IGPMMLALAG TYRCYGSVTH TPYQLSAPSD PLDIVVTGPY      200
EKPSLSAQPG PKVQAGESVT LSCSSRSSYD MYHLSREGGA HERRLPAVRK      250
VNRTFQADFP LGPATHGGTY RCFGSFRHSP YEWSDPSDPL LVSVTGNPSS      300
SWPSPTEPSS KSGNPRHLHI LIGTSVVIIL FILLLFFLLH LWCSNKKNAA      350
VMDQEPAGNR TANSEDSDEQ DPEEVTYAQL DHCVFTQRKI TRPSQRPKTP      400
PTDTILYTEL PNAKPRSKVV SCP                                   423
```

Comparison of KIR-cl.42 (NKAT1) and KIR-cl.49 (NKAT5, p183-ActI) transmembrane and cytoplasmic domains

```
KIR-cl.42 ILIGTSVVII LFI-LLFFLL HRWCSNKKNA AVMDQESAGN RTANSEDSDE   30
KIR-cl.49 VLIGTSVVKI PFTILLFFLL HRWCSNKKNA AVMDQEPAGN RTVNSEDSDE   30

KIR-cl.42 QDPQEVTYTQ LNHCVFTQRK ITRPSQRPKT PPTDIIVYTE LPNAESRSKV   80
KIR-cl.49 QDHQEVSYA- ---------- ---------- ---------- ----------   39

KIR-cl.42 VSCP                                                    84
KIR-cl.49 ----
```

Note: **Bold**, I/VXYXXL motifs; double underlined, KXPXTI motif.

References

[1] Moretta, A. et al. (1996) Annu. Rev. Immunol. 14, 619–648.

[2] **Lanier, L.L. and Phillips, J.H. (1996) Immunol. Today 17, 86–91.**

[3] Colonna, M. (1996) Curr. Opin. Immunol. 8, 101–107.

[4] Döhring, C. et al. (1996) J. Immunol. 156, 3098–3101.

[5] Wagtmann, N. et al. (1995) Immunity 2, 439–449.

[6] Colonna, M. and Samaridis, J. (1995) Science 268, 405–408.

[7] D'Andrea, A. et al. (1995) J. Immunol. 155, 2306–2310.

[8] Wagtmann, N. et al. (1995) Immunity 3, 801–809.

[9] Biassoni, R. et al. (1996) J. Exp. Med. 183, 645–650.

[10] **Döhring, C. et al. (1996) Immunogenetics 44, 227–230.**

[11] Baker, E.A. et al. (1995) Chromosome Res. 3, 511–512.

[12] Gumperz, J.E. et al. (1996) J. Exp. Med. 183, 1817–1827.

[13] Gumperz, J.E. and Parham, P. (1995) Nature 378, 245–248.

[14] Peruzzi, M. et al. (1996) J. Exp. Med. 184, 1585–1590.

[15] Rajagopalan, S. et al. (1995) J. Immunol. 155, 4143–4146.

[16] Burshtyn, D.N. et al. (1996) Immunity 4, 77–85.

[17] Campbell, K.S. et al. (1996) J. Exp. Med. 184, 93–100.

[18] Fry, A.M. et al. (1996) J. Exp. Med. 184, 295–300.

Molecular weights
Polypeptide   137 731

SDS-PAGE
  reduced   200 kDa

Carbohydrate
N-linked sites   20
O-linked sites   unknown

Human gene location and size
Xq28; ~16 kb [1].

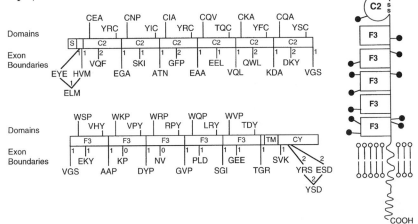

Tissue distribution

L1 is expressed on cell bodies of post-mitotic neurons and on axons of post-migratory neurons. It is also expressed on Schwann cells [2]. L1 is present on lymphoid and granulocyte precursor cells in the bone marrow, mature T cells in the thymus and both B and T cells in the spleen [3]. L1 is also expressed on peripheral blood monocytes, B lymphocytes, and CD4+ T lymphocytes, but not CD8+ T lymphocytes [4]. Although about 10–20% of the peripheral blood lymphocytes express both L1 and CD31, the majority express only one or the other [4].

Structure

The extracellular portion of L1 is organized into six Ig C2-like domains followed by five fibronectin type III domains [5]. Two peptide sequences, YEGHH and RSLE (both shown in bold in the sequence below), are coded for by exons 2 and 27 of the L1 gene and appear to be specifically spliced out in haematopoietic cells [4,6,7].

Ligands and associated molecules

L1 mediates homotypic adhesion [8]. L1 has been shown to bind the integrin CD51/CD61 ($\alpha V\beta 3$) [4,9]. L1 binding to the integrin CD49b/CD29 ($\alpha 5\beta 1$) has been demonstrated in the mouse but not in humans [9,10]. One possible explanation is that while there are two RGD motifs (RGDG and RGDS) in the sixth IgSF domain of mouse L1, only one of these (RGDG) is found in the human [4,5,11].

Function

L1 mediates homotypic adhesion between neural cells, which can be synergistically enhanced if L1 is associated with NCAM (CD56) on the membrane [8]. It also mediates neurite outgrowth on the ligand axonin-1 [12]. Activated B lymphocytes can undergo L1-dependent homotypic aggregation [13]. Since CD31 and L1 are expressed on different subsets of lymphocytes, it is proposed that CD51/CD61–L1 interaction may serve as an alternative to CD51/CD61–CD31 interaction for lymphocyte arrest and initiation of migration on endothelial cells [4]. Mutations in L1 are a feature of several X-linked neurological syndromes including hydrocephalus (HSAS), MASA syndrome, spastic paraparesis (SP1) and corpus collosum agenesis (ACC) [14].

Database accession numbers

	PIR	SWISSPROT	EMBL/GENBANK	REFERENCE
Human	A41060	P32004	X59847	5
Mouse	S05479	P11627	X12875	11

Amino acid sequence of human L1 antigen

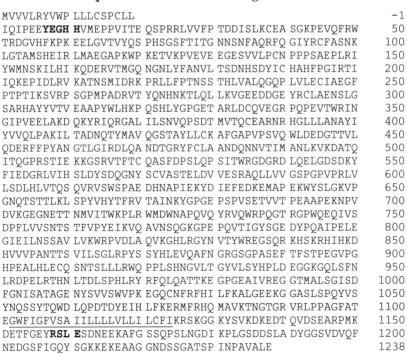

```
MVVVLRYVWP LLLCSPCLL                                              -1
IQIPEEYEGH HVMEPPVITE QSPRRLVVFP TDDISLKCEA SGKPEVQFRW            50
TRDGVHFKPK EELGVTVYQS PHSGSFTITG NNSNFAQRFQ GIYRCFASNK           100
LGTAMSHEIR LMAEGAPKWP KETVKPVEVE EGESVVLPCN PPPSAEPLRI           150
YWMNSKILHI KQDERVTMGQ NGNLYFANVL TSDNHSDYIC HAHFPGIRTI           200
IQKEPIDLRV KATNSMIDRK PRLLFPTNSS THLVALQGQP LVLECIAEGF           250
PTPTIKSVRP SGPMPADRVT YQNHNKTLQL LKVGEEDDGE YRCLAENSLG           300
SARHAYYVTV EAAPYWLHKP QSHLYGPGET ARLDCQVEGR PQPEVTWRIN           350
GIPVEELAKD QKYRIQRGAL ILSNVQPSDT MVTQCEARNR HGLLLANAYI           400
YVVQLPAKIL TADNQTYMAV QGSTAYLLCK AFGAPVPSVQ WLDEDGTTVL           450
QDERFFPYAN GTLGIRDLQA NDTGRYFCLA ANDQNNVTIM ANLKVKDATQ           500
ITQGPRSTIE KKGSRVTFTC QASFDPSLQP SITWRGDGRD LQELGDSDKY           550
FIEDGRLVIH SLDYSDQGNY SCVASTELDV VESRAQLLVV GSPGPVPRLV           600
LSDLHLVTQS QVRVSWSPAE DHNAPIEKYD IEFEDKEMAP EKWYSLGKVP           650
GNQTSTTLKL SPYVHYTFRV TAINKYGPGE PSPVSETVVT PEAAPEKNPV           700
DVKGEGNETT NMVITWKPLR WMDWNAPQVQ YRVQWRPQGT RGPWQEQIVS           750
DPFLVVSNTS TFVPYEIKVQ AVNSQGKGPE PQVTIGYSGE DYPQAIPELE           800
GIEILNSSAV LVKWRPVDLA QVKGHLRGYN VTYWREGSQR KHSKRHIHKD           850
HVVVPANTTS VILSGLRPYS SYHLEVQAFN GRGSGPASEF TFSTPEGVPG           900
HPEALHLECQ SNTSLLLRWQ PPLSHNGVLT GYVLSYHPLD EGGKGQLSFN           950
LRDPELRTHN LTDLSPHLRY RFQLQATTKE GPGEAIVREG GTMALSGISD          1000
FGNISATAGE NYSVVSWVPK EGQCNFRFHI LFKALGEEKG GASLSPQYVS          1050
YNQSSYTQWD LQPDTDYEIH LFKERMFRHQ MAVKTNGTGR VRLPPAGFAT          1100
EGWFIGFVSA IILLLLVLLI LCFIKRSKGG KYSVKDKEDT QVDSEARPMK          1150
DETFGEYRSL ESDNEEKAFG SSQPSLNGDI KPLGSDDSLA DYGGSVDVQF          1200
NEDGSFIGQY SGKKEKEAAG GNDSSGATSP INPAVALE                       1238
```

References

[1] Rosenthal, A. et al. (1994) EMBL/GenBank accession number Z29373.
[2] Schachner, M. (1990) Ciba Foundation Symp. 145, 156–172.
[3] Kowitz, A. et al. (1992) Eur. J. Immunol. 22, 1199–1205.
[4] **Ebeling, O. et al. (1996) Eur. J. Immunol. 26, 2508–2516.**
[5] Kobayashi, M. et al. (1991) Biochim. Biophys. Acta 1090, 238–240.
[6] Reid, R.A. and Hemperly, J.J. (1992) J. Mol. Neurosci. 3, 127–135.
[7] Jouet, M. et al. (1995) Mol. Brain Res. 30, 378–380
[8] Kadmon, G. et al. (1990) J. Cell Biol. 110, 193–208.
[9] Montgomery, A.M.P. et al. (1996) J. Cell Biol. 132, 475–485
[10] Ruppert, M. et al. (1995) J. Cell Biol. 131, 1881–1891.
[11] Moos, M. et al. (1988) Nature 3345, 701–703.
[12] Kuhn, T.B. et al. (1991) J. Cell Biol. 115, 1113–1126.
[13] Kowitz, A. et al. (1993) Clin. Exp. Metastasis 11, 419–429.
[14] **http://dnalab–www.uia.ac.be/dnalab/l1.html**

LAG-3

Lymphocyte activation gene 3

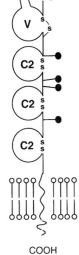

Molecular weights

Polypeptide   51 296

SDS-PAGE
   reduced   70 kDa
   unreduced   70 kDa

Carbohydrate
N-linked sites   4
O-linked   unknown

Human gene location and size
12p13.3; 6.6 kb [1]

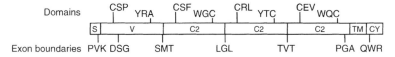

Domains

	CSP	YRA	CSF	WGC	CRL	YTC	CEV	WQC		
S	V		C2		C2		C2		TM	CY

Exon boundaries PVK DSG   SMT   LGL   TVT   PGA QWR

Tissue distribution

LAG-3 is expressed in activated T and NK cells, but not in activated B cells or monocytes [2]. Staining of sections identified scattered cells in germinal centres and T cell areas of lymphoid organs but not in non-lymphoid tissue [2]. On cultured IL-2-dependent T cells, expression of LAG-3 was 7-fold higher on CD8+ cells than CD4+ cells [2].

Structure

The cDNA encodes a transmembrane glycoprotein consisting of an IgSF V-set domain followed by three IgSF C2-set domains, a transmembrane sequence and a highly charged cytoplasmic domain. The first IgSF domain contains an extra loop of about 30 amino acids and an unusual disulfide bond is proposed between strands B and G (not F) in this domain [1]. Based on sequence similarities and intron/exon organization LAG-3 is likely to have shared an immediate ancestor in evolution with CD4. The CD4 and LAG-3 genes are closely linked (see page 141).

Ligands and associated molecules

LAG-3 binds MHC Class II in a cell rosetting assay [3]. Binding was inhibited by LAG-3 mAbs and by LAG-3-Ig [3,4]. A 45 kDa protein is co-precipitated with LAG-3 from activated T cells under reducing and non-reducing conditions [3].

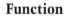

Function

A role for LAG-3 in downregulating an antigen-specific response is suggested by the effects of LAG-3 mAbs or LAG-3-Ig in prolonging an antigen-specific immune response by a MHC Class II-restricted CD4[+] T cell line[5]. However, LAG-3-deficient mice display normal MHC Class II-restricted responses[6]. Crossing LAG-3-deficient mice with CD4-deficient mice revealed that LAG-3 does not substitute for CD4[6].

Database accession numbers

	PIR	SWISSPROT	EMBL/GENBANK	REFERENCE
Human	S11246	P18627	X51985	1
Mouse			X98113	

Amino acid sequence of human LAG-3

```
MWEAQFLGLL FLQPLWVAPV KPLQPGAE                                  -1
VPVVWAQEGA PAQLPCSPTI PLQDLSLLRR AGVTWQHQPD SGPPAAAPGH          50
PLAPGPHPAA PSSWGPRPRR YTVLSVGPGG LRSGRLPLQP RVQLDERGRQ         100
RGDFSLWLRP ARRADAGEYR AAVHLRDRAL SCRLRLRLGQ ASMTASPPGS         150
LRASDWVILN CSFSRPDRPA SVHWFRNRGQ GRVPVRESPH HHLAESFLFL         200
PQVSPMDSGP WGCILTYRDG FNVSIMYNLT VLGLEPPTPL TVYAGAGSRV         250
GLPCRLPAGV GTRSFLTAKW TPPGGGPDLL VTGDNGDFTL RLEDVSQAQA         300
GTYTCHIHLQ EQQLNATVTL AIITVTPKSF GSPGSLGKLL CEVTPVSGQE         350
RFVWSSLDTP SQRSFSGPWL EAQEAQLLSQ PWQCQLYQGE RLLGAAVYFT         400
ELSSPGAQRS GRAPGALPAG HLLLFLTLGV LSLLLLVTGA FGFHLWRRQW         450
RPRRFSALEQ GIHPRRLRAR                                          470
```

References
1 Triebel, F. et al. (1990) J. Exp. Med. 171, 1393–1405.
2 Huard, B. et al. (1994) Immunogenetics 39, 213–217.
3 Baixeras, E. et al. (1992) J. Exp. Med. 176, 327–337.
4 **Huard, B. et al. (1995) Eur. J. Immunol. 25, 2718–2721.**
5 Huard, B. et al. (1994) Eur. J. Immunol. 24, 3216–3221.
6 Miyazaki, T. et al. (1996) Int. Immunol. 8, 725–729.

Low-density lipoprotein receptor

Molecular weights
Polypeptide   93 095

SDS-PAGE
   reduced   160 kDa

Carbohydrate
N-linked sites   5
O-linked   + abundant

Human gene location and size
19p13.2–p13.12; >45 kb[1]

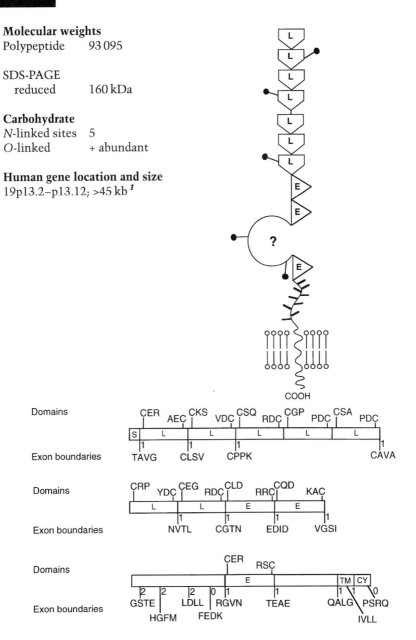

Domains		CER	AEC	CKS	VDC	CSQ	RDC	CGP	PDC	CSA	PDC
	S	L		L		L		L		L	
	1			1		1					1
Exon boundaries	TAVG		CLSV		CPPK						CAVA

Domains	CRP	YDC	CEG	RDC	CLD	RRC	CQD	KAC
	L		L		E		E	
	1		1		1		1	
Exon boundaries	NVTL		CGTN		EDID		VGSI	

Domains					CER	RSC			
				E				TM	CY
	2	2	2	0	1	1		1	1	0
Exon boundaries	GSTE		LDLL	RGVN	TEAE		QALG	PSRQ
		HGFM		FEDK				IVLL

Tissue distribution

The LDLR is found in most tissues with highest levels of expression on hepatocytes and in the adrenal cortex[2,3]. It is also present on lymphocytes, monocytes and macrophages[4]. The LDLR is regulated by cholesterol levels, such that cells incubated in cholesterol-free media upregulate LDLR expression and addition of LDL or cholesterol can lead to a decrease in receptor expression[4].

Structure

The mature LDLR protein is composed of several functional domains[5]. The N-terminal 288 amino acids of the protein contain seven Cys-rich repeats called LDLR domains. This region of the protein was shown to be important for the ligand binding function of the receptor by mutagenesis studies[6]. The structure of the first LDLR domain has been determined by NMR[7]. The next 350 amino acids show 33% homology to the EGF precursor and includes three EGF domains. The intron/exon boundaries for the EGF domains are preserved between the EGF precursor and the LDLR[8]. The first EGF domain participates in ligand binding, and it has also been shown that this entire region is important for the dissociation of ligand from receptor in an intracellular acidic compartment[9]. The membrane-proximal region contains sites for O-linked carbohydrate attachment[5]. The cytoplasmic domain contains a short motif, based around Tyr807, which serves to localize the receptor into coated pits and to mediate internalization[10]. This short motif is postulated to form a tight turn, similar to a sequence in the intracellular domain of the transferrin receptor (CD71)[11]. The N-terminal protein sequence has been determined for the purified bovine receptor, which is very similar to the human protein[5].

Ligands and associated molecules

The LDLR binds apoB-100- and apoE-containing lipoprotein particles. The receptor–ligand complex is internalized in coated pits, and the ligand dissociates from the receptor in acidic endosomes. The free LDLR is then recycled to the cell surface[2].

Function

The LDLR delivers cholesterol-containing lipoproteins to cells for use in membrane biogenesis, synthesis of bile acids and steroid hormone synthesis[2,3]. The ability of receptor levels to be increased on activated macrophages may contribute to foam cell formation and generation of atherosclerotic plaques[12]. Transgenic mice overexpressing human LDLR clear intravenously injected LDL 8–10 times more rapidly than normal mice, while their plasma concentrations of apoB-100 and apoE are reduced by greater than 90%[13].

Comments

Naturally occurring mutations which affect human LDLR expression, ligand binding, or internalization lead to familial hypercholesterolaemia which is characterized by high blood cholesterol levels and myocardial infarction (or atherosclerosis) early in life[2,3]. These are reviewed in OMIM entry 143890 (see Chapter 1 for methods to access OMIM).

Database accession numbers

	PIR	SWISSPROT	EMBL/GENBANK	REFERENCE
Human	A01383	P01130	L00336–L00352	1,5
Mouse	JN0461	P35951	Z19521	14
Rat	S03430	P35952	X13722	15

Amino acid sequence of human LDL receptor

```
MGPWGWKLRW TVALLLAAAG T                                              -1
AVGDRCERNE FQCQDGKCIS YKWVCDGSAE CQDGSDESQE TCLSVTCKSG              50
DFSCGGRVNR CIPQFWRCDG QVDCDNGSDE QGCPPKTCSQ DEFRCHDGKC             100
ISRQFVCDSD RDCLDGSDEA SCPVLTCGPA SFQCNSSTCI PQLWACDNDP             150
DCEDGSDEWP QRCRGLYVFQ GDSSPCSAFE FHCLSGECIH SSWRCDGGPD             200
CKDKSDEENC AVATCRPDEF QCSDGNCIHG SRQCDREYDC KDMSDEVGCV             250
NVTLCEGPNK FKCHSGECIT LDKVCNMARD CRDWSDEPIK ECGTNECLDN             300
NGGCSHVCND LKIGYECLCP DGFQLVAQRR CEDIDECQDP DTCSQLCVNL             350
EGGYKCQCEE GFQLDPHTKA CKAVGSIAYL FFTNRHEVRK MTLDRSEYTS             400
LIPNLRNVVA LDTEVASNRI YWSDLSQRMI CSTQLDRAHG VSSYDTVISR             450
DIQAPDGLAV DWIHSNIYWT DSVLGTVSVA DTKGVKRKTL FRENGSKPRA             500
IVVDPVHGFM YWTDWGTPAK IKKGGLNGVD IYSLVTENIQ WPNGITLDLL             550
SGRLYWVDSK LHSISSIDVN GGNRKTILED EKRLAHPFSL AVFEDKVFWT             600
DIINEAIFSA NRLTGSDVNL LAENLLSPED MVLFHNLTQP RGVNWCERTT             650
LSNGGCQYLC LPAPQINPHS PKFTCACPDG MLLARDMRSC LTEAEAAVAT             700
QETSTVRLKV SSTAVRTQHT TTRPVPDTSR LPGATPGLTT VEIVTMSHQA             750
LGDVAGRGNE KKPSSVRALS IVLPIVLLVF LCLGVFLLWK NWRLKNINSI             800
NFDNPVYQKT TEDEVHICHN QDGYSYPSRQ MVSLEDDVA                         839
```

References

1 Sudhof, T.C. et al. (1985) Science 228, 815–822.
2 **Brown, M.S. and Goldstein, J.L. (1986) Science 232, 34–47.**
3 Soutar, A.K. and Knight, B.L. (1990) Br. Med. Bull. 46, 891–916.
4 Cuthbert, J.A. et al. (1989) J. Biol. Chem. 264, 1298–1304.
5 Yamamoto, T. et al. (1984) Cell 39, 27–38.
6 Esser, V. et al. (1988) J. Biol Chem. 263, 13282–13290.
7 **Daly, N.L. et al. (1995) Proc. Natl Acad. Sci. USA 92, 6334–6338.**
8 Sudhof, T.C. et al. (1985) Science 228, 893–895.
9 Davis, C.G. et al. (1987) Nature 326, 760–765.
10 Davis, C.G. et al. (1987) J. Biol. Chem. 262, 4075–4082.
11 Collawn, J.F. et al. (1991) EMBO J. 10, 3247–3253.
12 Griffith, R.L. et al. (1988) J. Exp. Med. 168, 1041–1059.
13 Hoffman, S.L. et al. (1988) Science 239, 1277–1281.
14 Hoffer, M.J.V. et al. (1993) Biochem. Biophys. Res. Commun. 191, 880–886.
15 Lee, L.Y. et al. (1989) Nucleic Acids Res. 17, 1259–1260.

LPAP Lymphocyte phosphatase-associated phosphoprotein

Other names
CD45-AP (CD45-associated protein) (mouse)
LSM-1 (mouse)

Molecular weights
Polypeptide   21 196

SDS-PAGE
   reduced   29, 32 kDa (resting T cells)
              30, 31 kDa (activated T cells)

Carbohydrate
N-linked sites   nil
O-linked   nil

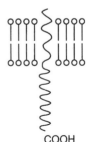

COOH

Tissue distribution

The expression of LPAP is restricted to resting and activated B and T lymphocytes and to lymphocyte cell lines[1].

Structure

The LPAP molecule has a short extracellular region, a transmembrane region and a large C-terminal cytoplasmic domain[1]. The first 50 amino acids of the cytoplasmic region share sequence similarity to WW domains, which have the potential to be involved in protein interaction[2]. LPAP is expressed in at least two different isoforms, LPAP29 and LPAP32, in resting T cells. These are replaced by LPAP30 and LPAP31 isoforms in activated T cells. The four isoforms appear to be generated by differential phosphorylation *in vivo*[1]. The discrepancy between the molecular weight of the polypeptide backbone and the apparent molecular weight determined by SDS-PAGE does not result from the attachment of phosphate groups as *in vitro* translated material has a similar M_r[1]. The N-terminus has been determined by protein sequencing[1].

Ligands and associated molecules

LPAP associates non-covalently with CD45. The LPAP–CD45 interaction is mediated by the transmembrane regions of the two molecules[2,3]. An extracellular ligand for LPAP has not been identified.

Function

LPAP was characterized as a CD45-associated molecule that was detected following *in vitro* kinase reactions of CD45 immunoprecipitates[1,4]. LPAP may function as an adapter molecule that links CD45 with other proteins, possibly through interactions with the putative WW domain. LPAP is unlikely to play a major role in linking CD45 to the protein tyrosine kinase Lck, because the LPAP–Lck interaction is weak[2].

Database accession numbers

	PIR	SWISSPROT	EMBL/GENBANK	REFERENCE
Human	A55412		X81422	1
Mouse	A49957		U03856	4

Amino acid sequence of human LPAP

```
MALPCTLGLG MLLALPGALG                                          -1
SGGSAEDSVG SSSVTVVLLL LLLLLLATGL ALAWRRLSRD SGGYYHPARL         50
GAALWGRTRR LLWASPPGRW LQARAELGST DNDLERQEDE QDTDYDHVAD        100
GGLQADPGEG EQQCGEASSP EQVPVRAEEA RDSDTEGDLV LGSPGPASAG        150
GSAEALLSDL HAFAGSAAWD DSARAAGGQG LHVTAL                       186
```

References
1. Schraven, B. et al. (1994) J. Biol. Chem. 269, 29102–29111.
2. **McFarland, E.D.C. and Thomas, M.L. (1995) J. Biol. Chem. 270, 28103–28107.**
3. Bruyns, E. et al. (1995) J. Biol. Chem. 270, 31372–31376.
4. Takeda, A. et al. (1994) J. Biol. Chem. 269, 2357–2360.

Molecular weights
Polypeptide   90 005

SDS-PAGE   100 kDa

Carbohydrate
N-linked sites   3
O-linked   unknown

Human gene location
15q13–21

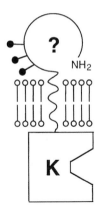

Tissue distribution

mRNA for human ltk has been found in haematopoietic cell lines, in a neuro-blastoma cell line and in placenta [1,2]. In the mouse, ltk message is specific to pre-B cell lines and is highest in adult but not embryonic brain [3]. Staining of mouse brain with polyclonal antiserum was specific for cerebral neurons [3]. Immunohistochemical staining with peptide mAbs of Hofbauer cells in human placenta has been reported but in general the level of expression of ltk is too low to detect with mAbs [2,4].

Structure

The extracellular domain does not show similarities with any known protein [2]. The cytoplasmic tyrosine kinase domain is closely related to that of c-ros [4]. Alternatively spliced ltk mRNAs predict the existence of receptors which are soluble or lack a cytoplasmic domain [2]. The predicted protein sequence of murine ltk begins at a CTG start codon and does not contain an identifiable signal sequence [3]. ltk cDNAs isolated which predicted a protein devoid of a large extracellular domain probably represent short or aberrant cDNA clones [2].

Ligands and associated molecules

In transfection studies in COS cells, ltk associated with PLC-γ, PI 3-kinase, GAP and raf-1 and the association was dependent on Met544 in a putative ATP binding site [4]. Analysis of a chimeric receptor revealed that in a ligand-dependent manner, the cytoplasmic domain of ltk associates with Shc through Tyr862 and Tyr485 which are both contained within an Shc binding motif [5].

Function

Ltk probably functions as a receptor for an unidentified growth factor. In an *in vitro* kinase assay in COS cells, ltk had kinase activity and was tyrosine phosphorylated [4]. A chimeric receptor containing the cytoplasmic domain of ltk was autophosphorylated in response to ligand [5].

Database accession numbers

	PIR	*SWISSPROT*	*EMBL/GENBANK*	*REFERENCE*
Human	S17452	P29376	D16105	2
Mouse	S00904	P08923	X07984	3

Amino acid sequence of human ltk

```
MGCWGQLLVW FGAAGA                                             -1
ILCSSPGSQE TFLRSSPLPL ASPSPQDPKV SAPPSILEPA SPLNSPGTEG        50
SWLFSTCGAS GRHGPTQTQC DGAYAGTSVV VTVGAAGQLR GVQLWRVPGP       100
GQYLISAYGA AGGKGAKNHL SRAHGVFVSA IFSLGLGESL YILVGQQGED       150
ACPGGSPESQ LVCLGESRAV EEHAAMDGSE GVPGSRRWAG GGGGGGGATY       200
VFRVRAGELE PLLVAAGGGG RAYLRPRDRG RTQASPEKLE NRSEAPGSGG       250
RGGAAGGGGG WTSRAPSPQA GRSLQEGAEG GQGCSEAWAT LGWAAAGGFG       300
GGGGACTAGG GGGGYRGGDA SETDNLWADG EDGVSFIHPS SELFLQPLAV       350
TENHGEVEIR RHLNCSHCPL RDCQWQAELQ LAECLCPEGM ELAVDNVTCM       400
DLHKPPGPLV LMVAVVATST LSLLMVCGVL ILVKQKKWQG LQEMRLPSPE       450
LELSKLRTSA IRTAPNPYYC QVGLGPAQSW PLPPGVTEVS PANVTLLRAL       500
GHGAFGEVYE GLVIGLPGDS SPLQVAIKTL PELCSPQDEL DFLMEALIIS       550
KFRHQNIVRC VGLSLRATPR LILLELMSGG DMKSFLRHSR PHLGQPSPLV       600
MRDLLQLAQD IAQGCHYLEE NHFIHRDIAA RNCLLSCAGP SRVAKIGDFG       650
MARDIYRASY YRRGDRALLP VKWMPPEAFL EGIFTSKTDS WSFGVLLWEI       700
FSLGYMPYPG RTNQEVLDFV VGGGRMDPPR GCPGPVYRIM TQCWQHEPEL       750
RPSFASILER LQYCTQDPDV LNSLLPMELG PTPEEEGTSG LGNRSLECLR       800
PPQPQELSPE KLKSWGGSPL GPWLSSGLKP LKSRGLQPQN LWNPTYRS        848
```

References
1. Krolewski, J.J. and Dalla-Favera, R. (1991) EMBO J. 10, 2911–2919.
2. Toyoshima, H. et al. (1993) Proc. Natl Acad. Sci. USA 90, 5404–5408.
3. Bernards, A. and de la Monte, S.M. (1990) EMBO J. 9, 2279–2287.
4. Kozutsumi, H. et al. (1994) Oncogene 9, 2991–2998.
5. **Ueno, H. et al. (1995) J. Biol. Chem. 270, 20135–20142.**

Molecular weights
Ly-6A.2   8649

SDS-PAGE
  reduced   14–18 kDa
  unreduced   10–14 kDa

Carbohydrate
N-linked sites   0
O-linked sites   unknown

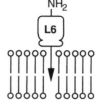

Mouse locus location and gene sizes
15 band E, ~3 kb (Ly-6A.2/E.1, Ly-6C.1); ~4 kb (Ly-6F.1, Ly-6G.1) [1–3].

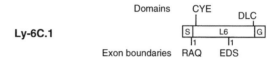

The Ly-6 genetic complex

The mouse Ly-6 locus spans approximately 630 kb and contains at least 18 genes [1,2]. Hybridization studies show that several of these genes are related to Ly-6. The Ly-6 lymphoid antigens were originally characterized with alloantisera, but subsequent cDNA cloning showed that they were the products of two genes, namely Ly-6A/E and Ly-6C [4,5]. Recently two further genes (Ly-6F and Ly-6G) have been identified in the region which are clearly related to Ly-6A/E and Ly-6C [3]. The mouse thymocyte B cell antigen (ThB) also has sequence homology (~25%) to the Ly-6A/E and Ly-6C molecules and its gene has been mapped to chromosome 15, raising the possibility that it too may lie within the Ly-6 complex [6]. The gene encoding the antigen Ly-6B has yet to be characterized. No human Ly-6 homologues have been identified to date.

Tissue distribution

The four mouse Ly-6 genes have different expression patterns, as do the alleles of the Ly-6A/E gene [3–5]. Ly-6A/E is expressed on haematopoietic stem cells [7]. The allele Ly-6A.2 is also present on 30% of CD4⁻/CD8⁻ thymocytes, 50–70% of peripheral lymphocytes, and on all activated B and T cells. In contrast, the allele Ly-6E.1 is expressed on only 10–15% of peripheral lymphocytes and on activated T and B cells. Ly-6C is expressed on bone marrow cells, monocytes, neutrophils and 50% of peripheral CD8⁺ T cells. Ly-6G.1 is expressed in the bone marrow. Transfection studies suggest that the Ly-6G.1 cDNA does not encode a protein that is recognized by anti-Ly-6B antibodies [5]. Ly-6F.1 mRNA is not detected in the bone marrow, spleen or thymus, but is detected in several non-lymphoid tissues including testes [3].

Structure

Ly-6A/E and Ly-6C are both GPI-anchored cell surface glycoproteins [4], as are the predicted proteins encoded by the Ly-6F.1 and Ly-6G.1 genes [3]. The Ly-6 gene products share ~50% amino acid sequence identity. The N-termini of Ly-6C.2 and Ly-6E.1 have been confirmed by protein sequencing [8,9]. The sites of attachment of the GPI anchors are not known, but they are predicted to be Asn76/79 based on known attachment sites of similar GPI-anchored proteins [4,10]. The Ly-6 antigens are similar to CD59 and presumably have a similar fold [10].

Function

The expression patterns of Ly-6A/E, Ly-6C and Ly-6G suggest a role in the development and maturation of lymphocytes [3]. Anti-Ly-6 antibodies can activate T cells but this generally requires secondary antibody cross-linking and phorbol esters, and is dependent on TCR/CD3 expression [11]. This activation requires the GPI anchor [12]. B cell activation can be induced by anti-Ly-6 antibodies in the presence of IL-4 and IFNγ [13]. Ly-6 expression is induced in a complex manner by interferons and TNF [5,14].

Database accession numbers

	PIR	SWISSPROT	EMBL/GENBANK	REFERENCE
Mouse A.2	A32506	P05533	M18184	[15]
	A31935		J03636	[16]
	A35921		M37707	[17]
Mouse E.1	A25708	P05533	X04653	[18]
Mouse C.1		P09568	M21734	[19]
Mouse C.2		P09568	M18466	[8]
Mouse F.1		P35460	X70922	[3]
Mouse G.1		P35461	X70920	[3]
Rat A			M30692	[20]
Rat B	A45835		M30689	[20]
Rat C	D45835		M30690	[20]

Amino acid sequence of mouse Ly-6 antigens

```
A.2 MDTSHTTKSC LLILLVALLC AERAQG                        -1
E.1 ---------- ---------- ------                        -1
C.1 --ST-A---- ---------- -G----                        -1
C.2 --ST-A---- ---------- -G----                        -1
F.1 --SC------ V-----V--- ------                        -1
G.1 --SC------ V-----V--- ------                        -1

A.2 LECYQCYGVP FETSCPSITC PYPDGVCVTQ EAAVIVDSQT RKVKNNLCLP 50
E.1 ---------- ---------- ---------- ------G--- ---------- 50
C.1 -Q--E----- I-----AV-- RAS--F-IA- NIEL-E---R --L-TRQ--S 50
C.2 -Q--E----- I-----AV-- RAS--F-IA- NIEL-E---R --L-TRQ--S 50
F.1 ----N-L--S LGIA-K---- ----A--IS- QVEL-----R -----K--F- 50
G.1 ----N-I--- P----NTT-- -FS--F--AL -IE-----HR S---S----- 50
```

```
A.2 ICPPNIESME ILGTKVNVKT SCCQEDLCN          79
E.1 ---------- ---------- ---------          79
C.1 F--AGV...P -RDPNIRER- ---S-----          76
C.2 F--AGV...P -KDPNIRER- ---S-----          76
F.1 F--A-L-N-- ----T---N- ---K-----          79
G.1 ---TTLDNT- -T-NA----- Y--K-----          79

A.2 VAVPNGGSTW TMAGVLLFSL SSVLLQTLL         +29
E.1 A--------- ---------- ---------         +29
C.1 A---TA---- ---------- ---V-----         +29
C.2 A---TA---- ---------- ---I-----         +29
F.1 APFST----- --TR---LN- G--F-----         +29
G.1 A---T---S- ---------- V------F-         +29
```

Dashes represent residues identical to that in the top sequence; dots represent a gap in alignment.

References

1   LeClair, K.P. et al. (1987) Proc. Natl Acad. Sci. USA 84, 1638–1643.
2   Kamiura, S. et al. (1992) Genomics 12, 89–105.
3   **Fleming, T.J. et al. (1993) J. Immunol. 150, 5379–5390.**
4   **Shevah, E.M. and Korty, P.E. (1989) Immunol. Today 10, 195–200.**
5   Rock, K.L. et al. (1989) Immunol. Rev. 111, 195–224.
6   Gumley, T.P. et al. (1992) J. Immunol. 149, 2516–2518.
7   van de Rijn, M. et al. (1989) Proc. Natl Acad. Sci. USA 86, 4634–4638.
8   Palfree, R.G. et al. (1988) J. Immunol. 140, 305–310.
9   Reiser, H. et al. (1987) Proc. Natl Acad. Sci. USA 84, 3370–3374.
10 Kieffer, B. et al. (1994) Biochemistry 33, 4471–4482.
11 Sussman, J.J. et al. (1988) J. Immunol. 140, 2520–2526.
12 Su, B. et al. (1991) J. Cell Biol. 112, 377–384.
13 Codias, E.K. and Malek, T.R. (1990) J. Immunol. 144, 2197–2204.
14 Malek, T.R. et al. (1989) J. Immunol. 142, 1929–1936.
15 Palfree, R.G. et al. (1987) Immunogenetics 26, 389–391.
16 Reiser, H. et al. (1988) Proc. Natl Acad. Sci. USA 85, 2255–2259.
17 Khan, K.D. et al. (1990) Mol. Cell. Biol. 10, 5150–5159.
18 LeClair, K.P. et al. (1986) EMBO J. 5, 3227–3234.
19 Bothwell, A.L.M. et al. (1988) J. Immunol. 140, 2815–2820.
20 Friedman, S. et al. (1990) Immunogenetics 31, 104–111.

Ly-9

Molecular weights
Polypeptide   67 278

SDS-PAGE
  reduced   90–120 kDa

Carbohydrate
N-linked sites   8
O-linked   unknown

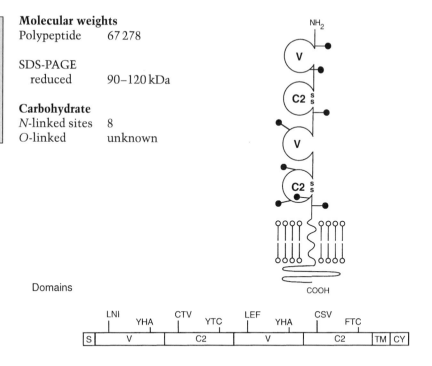

Domains

Tissue distribution

Expressed on mouse thymocytes and mature T and B cells[1].

Structure

Ly-9 is an IgSF domain-containing glycoprotein with structural features which place it within the CD2 family, which includes CD48, CD58, 2B4 and CD150[1,2]. Ly-9 differs from the other CD2 family members in having four rather than two IgSF domains. Domains 1 and 3 are very similar to each other, as are domains 2 and 4, suggesting that Ly-9 arose from a progenitor with one V and one C2 domain, such as CD48[1]. The Ly-9 locus lies within 1100 kb of the CD48 gene on mouse chromosome 1[3]. It is possible that Ly-9 and CD48 arose by gene duplication from a common ancestor with a second duplication step leading to the four domain structure of Ly-9. The gene for a putative human homologue of Ly-9 lies within 410 kb of the CD48 locus in human chromosome 1q22[3,4].

Function

Unknown.

Database accession numbers

	PIR	SWISSPROT	EMBL/GENBANK	REFERENCE
Mouse	A46500	Q01965	M84412	1
Human			L42621	4

Amino acid sequence of mouse Ly-9

```
MSQQQIFSPI LWIPLLFLIM GLGASG                            -1
KETPPTVISG MLGGSVTFSL NISKDAEIEH IIWNCPPKAL ALVFYKKDIT   50
ILDKGYNGRL KVSEDGYSLY MSNLTKSDSG SYHAQINQKN VILTTNKEFT  100
LHIYEKLQKP QIIVESVTPS DTDSCTFTLI CTVKGTKDSV QYSWTREDTH  150
LNTYDGSHTL RVSQSVCDPD LPYTCKAWNP VSQNSSQPVR IWQFCTGASR  200
RKTAAGKTVV GILGEPVTLP LEFRATRATK NVVWVLNTSV ISQERRGAAT  250
ADSRRKPKGS EERRVRTSDQ DQSLKISQLK MEDAGPYHAY VCSEASRDPS  300
VRHFTLLVYK RLEKPSVTKS PVHMMNGICE VVLTCSVDGG GNNVTYTWMP  350
LQNKAVMSQG KSHLNVSWES GEHLPNFTCT AHNPVSNSSS QFSSGTICSG  400
PERNKRFWLL LLLVLLLLML IGGYFILRKK KQCSSLATRY RQAEVPAEIP  450
EPPTGHGQFS VLSQRYEKLD MSAKTTRHQP TPTSDTSSES SATTEEDDEK  500
TRMHSTANSR NQLYDLVTHQ DIAHALAYEG QVEYEAITPY DKVDGSMDEE  550
DMAYIQVSLN VQGETPLPQK KEDSNTIYCS VQKPKKTAQT PQQDAESPES  600
PYL                                                    603
```

References
1. Sandrin, M.S. et al. (1992) J. Immunol. 149, 1636–1641.
2. Davis, S.J. and van der Merwe, P.A. (1996) Immunol. Today 17, 177–187.
3. Kingsmore, S.F. et al. (1995) Immunogenetics 42, 59–62.
4. Sandrin, M.S. et al. (1996) Immunogenetics 43, 13–19.

Ly-49 family

Members

Mouse	Ly-49A (A1, YE1/48)
	Ly-49B
	Ly-49C (5E6)
	Ly-49D
	Ly-49E
	Ly-49F
	Ly-49G (LGL-1)
	Ly-49H
Rat	rLy-49.9
	rLy-49.12
	rLy-49.29

Molecular weights (Ly-49A)

Polypeptide   30 648

SDS-PAGE
  reduced   44–50 kDa
  unreduced   85–95 kDa

Carbohydrate

N-linked sites   3
O-linked   unknown

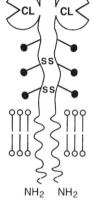

Gene location and size

Mouse: chromosome 6[1]; ~19 kb[2]
Rat: chromosome 4[3]

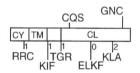

Domain

Exon boundaries

Ly-49 and the NK gene complex

The NK gene complex (NKC) is a chromosomal region containing several genes and multigene families which encode cell surface C-type lectins expressed on NK cells[4,5]. It was first identified in the mouse (chromosome 6)[4] and subsequently in humans (chromosome 12)[4] and the rat (chromosome 4)[3]. Ly-49, NKR-P1 and CD69 genes have been identified in the mouse NKC. NKR-P1, CD69, CD94 and NKG2 genes have been identified in the human NKC. Ly-49 and NKR-P1 genes have been identified in the rat NKC[3,5]. cDNA clones have been obtained corresponding to eight mouse and three rat Ly-49 genes, but no human Ly-49 homologues have been identified[3,4,6]. In the mouse multiple alleles have been identified for some genes (Ly-49A, Ly49C[7], and Ly-49G[8]) and mice heterozygous for Ly-49A and Ly-49C may undergo allelic exclusion at these loci[7]. Four probable splice varients of Ly-49G have been identified[9,10], one of which (Ly-49G2) corresponds to LGL-1[8].

Tissue distribution

Ly-49A is expressed at low levels on mouse thymocytes and T cells and at higher levels on 15–20% of NK cells. Ly-49C is expressed on a similar proportion (~26%) of NK cells, with ~5% of cells expressing both Ly-49A and C[10]. Ly-49G (LGL-1) is expressed on ~40% of NK cells with 8% expressing both Ly-49G and Ly49A[8]. Because of a lack of suitable reagents, the expression pattern of other mouse and rat Ly-49 molecules is not known.

Structure

Proteins within the rat and mouse Ly-49 gene families share 62–90%[3] and 48–91%[9] amino acid identity, respectively, and there is 46–81% identity between the rat and mouse Ly-49 families[3]. Sequence comparisons suggest that all members have a similar overall structure[9,10]. They are type II transmembrane proteins with no signal peptide and an extracellular C-type lectin domain. Ly-49A, Ly-49C and Ly-49G (LGL-1) have been shown to be expressed as disulfide-linked homodimers[6,8]. The cytoplasmic regions show some heterogeneity which may reflect different signalling functions. For example ITIM motifs ((I/V)XYXX(L/V)) are found in mouse Ly-49A, C, F, G1, and G4 and rat Ly-49.9[11] and putative G_i-binding motifs are found in mouse Ly-49A and D and rat Ly-49.9[3].

Ligands and associated molecules

Ly-49A has been shown to bind to the MHC Class I alleles $H-2D^d$ and $H-2D^{k}$[5] whereas Ly-49C interacts with the $H-2D^{b,d,k, and s}$ alleles[10,12]. Preliminary evidence suggests that Ly-49G (LGL-1) interacts with $H-2D^d$ and $H-2L^{d}$[8]. Ly-49A and Ly49C have both been shown to interact with carbohydrates, presumably through their C-type lectin domains, and there is suggestive evidence that their interaction with MHC Class I molecules involves carbohydrate determinants[13,14]. Peptides comprising the phosphorylated ITIM motif of Ly-49A bind to the cytoplasmic tyrosine phosphatases SHP-1 (PTP1C) and SHP-2 (PTP1D, SYP)[11], suggesting a mechanism for the inhibitory effect of this receptor.

Function

Several members of the Ly-49 family (Ly-49A, Ly-49C, and Ly-49G) have been implicated in the recognition by murine NK cells of MHC Class I molecules on target cells[6,8]. Of these the role of Ly-49A is the best documented[6]. In general, ligation of Ly-49 members by MHC Class I molecules inhibits NK cell function, consistent with the notion that Ly-49 molecules are involved in recognition of the 'missing self' on target cells[5]. No human Ly-49 homologues have been identified. Instead CD94/NKG-2 receptors and IgSF domain-containing killer inhibitory receptors (KIR) appear to have an equivalent function on human NK cells[5].

Database accession numbers

	PIR	SWISSPROT	EMBL/GENBANK	REFERENCE
Mouse LY-49A		P20937	M25775	15,16
Mouse LY-49B	I49058		U10304	17
Mouse LY-49C	I49059		U10305	9
Mouse LY-49D			U10090	9
Mouse LY-49E			U10091	9
Mouse LY-49F			U10092	9
Mouse LY-49G1			U10093	9
Mouse LY-49G2			U10094	9
Mouse LY-49G3			U10095	9
Mouse LY-49G4			U12890	10
Mouse LY-49H			U12889	10
Rat Ly-49.9			U56863	3
Rat Ly-49.12			U56822	3
Rat Ly-49.29			U56824	3

Amino acid sequence of mouse Ly-49A

```
MSEQEVTYSM VRFHKSAGLQ KQVRPEETKG PREAGYRRCS FHWKFIVIAL    50
GIFCFLLLVA VSVLAIKIFQ YDQQKKLQEF LNHHNNCSNM QSDINLKDEM   100
LKNKSMECDL LESLNRDQNR LYNKTKTVLD SLQHTGRGDK VYWFCYGMKC   150
YYFVMDRKTW SGCKQTCQSS SLSLLKIDDE DELKFLQLVV PSDSCWVGLS   200
YDNKKKDWAW IDNRPSKLAL NTRKYNIRDG GCMLLSKTRL DNGNCDQVFI   250
CICGKRLDKF PH                                           262
```

References

1 Yokoyama, W.M. et al. (1990) J. Immunol. 145, 2353–2358.
2 Kubo, S. et al. (1993) Gene 136, 329–331.
3 Dissen, E. et al. (1996) J. Exp. Med. 183, 2197–2207.
4 Yokoyama, W.M. and Seaman, W.E. (1993) Annu. Rev. Immunol. 11, 613–635.
5 Gumperz, J.E. and Parham, P. (1995) Nature 378, 245–248.
6 **Yokoyama, W.M. et al. (1995) Semin. Immunol. 7, 89–101.**
7 Held, W. et al. (1995) Nature 376, 355–358.
8 Mason, L.H. et al. (1995) J. Exp. Med. 182, 293–303.
9 Smith, H.R.C. et al. (1994) J. Immunol. 153, 1068–1079.
10 Brennan, J. et al. (1994) J. Exp. Med. 180, 2287–2295.
11 Olcese, L. et al. (1996) J. Immunol. 156, 4531–4534.
12 Colonna, M. (1996) Curr. Opin. Immunol. 8, 101–107.
13 Brennan, J. et al. (1995) J. Biol. Chem. 270, 9691–9694.
14 Daniels, B.F. et al. (1991) Immunity 1, 785–792.
15 Chan, P.Y. and Takei, F. (1989) J. Immunol. 142, 1727–1736.
16 Yokoyama, W.M. et al. (1989) J. Immunol. 143, 1379–1386.
17 Wong, S. et al. (1991) J. Immunol. 147, 1417–1423.

Mac-2-BP

Other names
Mac-2 binding protein
CyAP (cyclophilin C-associated protein)
L3 antigen
MAMA

Molecular weights
Polypeptide   63 277

SDS-PAGE
  reduced   97 kDa
  unreduced   97 kDa

Carbohydrate
N-linked sites   7
O-linked   unknown

Human gene location
17q25

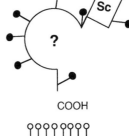

COOH

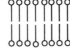

Domain

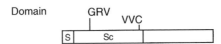

Tissue distribution

Human Mac-2-BP is present in extracellular fluids with a high concentration in breast milk and is secreted by cultured tumour cells [1,2]. Mouse Mac-2-BP is expressed on the surface of activated macrophages and mRNA is found in many organs but not brain [2]. Mouse Mac-2-BP mRNA is strongly increased in response to adherence and moderately to TNF and IFNγ [2].

Structure

Mac-2-BP contains an N-terminal scavenger receptor cysteine-rich domain [1-3]. Mac-2-BP is susceptible to cleavage and there is a dibasic cleavage site at residue 417 [1]. There is no obvious transmembrane sequence or a site for the attachment of a GPI anchor. The native molecular size of human Mac-2-BP is in the order of several million kDa [1].

Ligands and associated molecules

Mac-2 BP binds galectin 3 (formerly known as Mac-2) [1] and to cyclophilin C [4]. Binding of Mac-2-BP to galectin 3 is lactose dependent [1]. Binding of cyclophilin C to Mac-2-BP is inhibited by cyclosporin [4]. Mac-2-BP is reported to bind to CD14 in the presence of LPS [5].

Function

Unknown.

Database accession numbers

	PIR	SWISSPROT	EMBL/GENBANK	REFERENCE
Human			L13210	1
Mouse			L16894	4

Amino acid sequence of human Mac-2-BP

```
MTPPRLFWVW LLVAGTQG                                              -1
VNDGDMRLAD GGATNQGRVE IFYRGQWGTV CDNLWDLTDA SVVCRALGFE           50
NATQALGRAA FGQGSGPIML DEVQCTGTEA SLADCKSLGW LKSNCRHERD          100
AGVVCTNETR STHTLDLSRE LSEALGQIFD SQRGCDLSIS VNVQGEDALG          150
FCGHTVILTA NLEAQALWKE PGSNVTMSVD AECVPMVRDL LRYFYSRRID          200
ITLSSVKCFH KLASAYGARQ LQGYCASLFA ILLPQDPSFQ MPLDLYAYAV          250
ATGDALLEKL CLQFLAWNFE ALTQAEAWPS VPTDLLQLLL PRSDLAVPSE          300
LALLKAVDTW SWGERASHEE VEGLVEKIRF PMMLPEELFE LQFNLSLYWS          350
HEALFQKKTL QALEFHTVPF QLLARYKGLN LTEDTYKPRI YTSPTWSAFV          400
TDSSWSARKS QLVYQSRRGP LVKYSSDYFQ APSDYRYYPY QSFQTPQHPS          450
FLFQDKRVSW SLVYLPTIQS CWNYGFSCSS DELPVLGLTK SGGSDRTIAY          500
ENKALMLCEG LFVADVTDFE GWKAAIPSAL DTNSSKSTSS FPCPAGHFNG          550
FRTVIRPFYL TNSSGVD                                             567
```

References

1 Koths, K. et al. (1993) J. Biol. Chem. 268, 14245–14249.
2 **Chicheportiche, Y. and Vassalli, P. (1994) J. Biol. Chem. 269, 5512–5517.**
3 Resnick, D. et al. (1994) Trends Biochem. Sci. 19, 5–8.
4 Friedman, J. et al. (1993) Proc. Natl Acad. Sci. USA 90, 6815–6819.
5 Yu, B. and Wright, S.D. (1995) J. Inflammation 45, 115–125.

Macrophage lectin

Other names
Macrophage asialoglycoprotein binding protein (M-ASGP-BP) (rat)
Macrophage galactose/N-acetylgalactosamine-specific lectin (MMGL) (mouse)

Molecular weights
Polypeptide   32 937

SDS-PAGE
   reduced   34.5–36.5 kDa

Carbohydrate
N-linked sites   1
O-linked   unknown

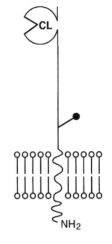

Domain

CY | TM | CL

CQL   DVC

Tissue distribution

This has not been established by immunohistological techniques, however RNA analysis suggests that in the mouse the molecule is expressed at low levels by resident peritoneal macrophages and is upregulated on thio-glycollate-elicited peritoneal macrophages[1]. Similarly, in the rat the antigen appears to be restricted to macrophages[2].

Structure

Human macrophage lectin (HML) is a type II transmembrane molecule containing a single extracellular C-type lectin domain[3]. It is the homologue of the rat macrophage asialoglycoprotein receptor (M-ASGP-BP), the mouse macrophage galactose/N-acetylgalactosamine-specific lectin (MMGL) and is closely related to other human C-type lectins (human hepatic lectin 1 (HHL-1); 56% identity and human hepatic lectin 2 (HHL-2); 45% identity). The C-type lectin domains of the lectins have the greatest similarity: 69% between HML and HHL-1, and 63% between HML and HHL-2[3]. The cytoplasmic domains of the lectins are more poorly conserved[3]. Additionally, the HML and HHL-1/HHL-2 proteins differ through the presence of a 24 amino acid insertion in the extracellular neck region of HML which is also found in the mouse and rat homologues[1,3,4]. In the rat the N-terminus of M-ASGP-BP has been confirmed by protein sequencing[5].

Ligands and associated molecules

HML is a lectin that binds galactose and N-acetylgalactosamine carbohydrate groups in a calcium-dependent manner[3]. A weaker interaction between HML and fucose is also observed.

Function

The presence of a YENF internalization motif in the cytoplasmic domain suggests that the lectin is likely to be involved in receptor-mediated endocytosis. Recombinant HML expressed in *E. coli* has been shown to strongly bind glycopeptides carrying three consecutive *N*-acetylgalactosamine-Ser/Thr residues known as Tn antigen, which is a human carcinoma-associated epitope, implicating a role in recognition by tumoricidal macrophages[3].

Database accession numbers

	PIR	*SWISSPROT*	*EMBL/GENBANK*	*REFERENCE*
Human			D50532	3
Mouse		P49300	S36676	1
Rat		P49301	J05495	4

Amino acid sequence of human macrophage lectin

```
MTRTYENFQY LENKVKVQGF KNGPLPLQSL LQRLRSGPCH LLLSLGLGLL      50
LLVIICVVGF QNSKFQRDLV TLRTDFSNFT SNTVAEIQAL TSQGSSLEET     100
IASLKAEVEG FKQERQAVHS EMLLRVQQLV QDLKKLTCQV ATLNNNGEEA     150
STEGTCCPVN WVEHQDSCYW FSHSGMSWAE AEKYCQLKNA HLVVINSREE     200
QNFVQKYLGS AYTWMGLSDP EGAWKWVDGT DYATGFQNWK PGQPDDWQGH     250
GLGGGEDCAH FHPDGRWNDD VCQRPYHWVC EAGLGQTSQE SH             292
```

References

1 Sato et al. (1992) J. Biochem. 111, 331–336.
2 Kawasaki, T. et al. (1986) Carbohydrate Res. 151, 197–206.
3 **Suzuki, N. et al. (1996) J. Immunol. 156, 128–135.**
4 Ii, M. et al. (1990) J. Biol. Chem. 265, 11295–11298.
5 Ii, M. et al. (1988) Biochem. Biophys. Res. Commun. 155, 720–725.

MAdCAM-1 | Mucosal addressin cell adhesion molecule 1

Molecular weights
Polypeptide   40 909

SDS-PAGE
  reduced   58–66 kDa
  unreduced   54–62 kDa

Carbohydrate
N-linked sites   2
O-linked   +

Mouse gene location
10c1–2; ~3.5 kb [1]

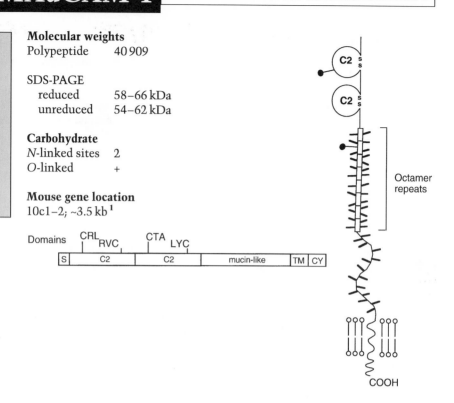

Domains

| S | C2 | C2 | mucin-like | TM | CY |

Tissue distribution

MAdCAM-1 is expressed at high levels on high endothelial venules of Peyer's patches and mesenteric lymph nodes and on flat-walled venules within the gut lamina propria [1–5]. It is also expressed on vascular endothelium in mammary glands, pancreas and the spleen marginal sinus. Expression is induced *in vitro* by TNFα and IL-1 and MAdCAM-1 has been detected on blood vessels within areas of chronic inflammation [3].

Structure

The N-terminal half of the extracellular region contains two C2-set IgSF domains. These domains are closely related to the two membrane-distal IgSF domains of CD106 (VCAM-1), which binds the integrins α4β1 (CD49d/CD29) and α4β7 [4,6]. MAdCAM-1 and CD106 are structurally related to three other integrin-binding molecules: CD50, CD54 and CD102. Features shared by these molecules include an atypical disulfide between the B–C and F–G loops and an (I/L)(D/E)(S/T)XL motif (LDTSL in MAdCAM-1) in the C–D loop [6]. The IgSF domains are followed by a mucin-like region rich in Ser, Thr, and Pro residues, which includes eight copies of the octameric repeat (P/S)PDTTS(Q/P)E [4]. The two IgSF domains, but not the mucin-like portions, are reasonably well-conserved between species [4].

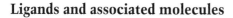

Ligands and associated molecules

MAdCAM-1 binds the integrin a4β7 through its IgSF portion [7,8]. It can also bind CD62L (L-selectin) through poorly characterized sialoglycoconjugates present in the mucin-like portion of a subpopulation of MAdCAM-1 molecules [9]. The α4β7 binding site incorporates the LDTSL motif in the C-D loop of domain 1, which also forms part of the binding site on other integrin-binding IgSF domains [6,8].

Function

Through its interaction with the lymphocyte adhesion molecules CD62L and α4β7, MAdCAM-1 contributes to the recirculation of naive lymphocytes to Peyer's patches and mesenteric lymph nodes, and the homing of a sub-population of activated or memory lymphocytes to the lamina propria of the gut mucosa [2,5]. MAdCAM-1 is involved in the initial tethering and rolling of lymphocytes on endothelial surfaces (through CD62L and α4β7 binding) as well as the subsequent activation-induced arrest of these cells (through α4β7 binding) prior to extravasation [5].

Database accession numbers

	PIR	SWISSPROT	EMBL/GENBANK	REFERENCE
Human			U43628	4
Mouse	S33601		L21203	10

Amino acid sequence of human MAdCAM

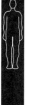

```
MDFGLALLLA GLLGLLLG                                          -1
QSLQVKPLQV EPPEPVVAVA LGASRQLTCR LACADRGASV QWRGLDTSLG       50
AVQSDTGRSV LTVRNASLSA AGTRVCVGSC GGRTFQHTVQ LLVYAFPDQL       100
TVSPAALVPG DPEVACTAHK VTPVDPNALS FSLLVGGQEL EGAQALGPEV       150
QEEEEEPQGD EDVLFRVTER WRLPPLGTPV PPALYCQATM RLPGLELSHR       200
QAIPVLHSPT SPEPPDTTSP EPPNTTSPES PDTTSPESPD TTSQEPPDTT       250
SQEPPDTTSQ EPPDTTSPEP PDKTSPEPAP QQGSTHTPRS PGSTRTRRPE       300
ISQAGPTQGE VIPTGSSKPA GDQLPAALWT SSAVLGLLLL ALPTYHLWKR       350
CRHLAEDDTH PPASLRLLPQ VSAWAGLRGT GQVGISPS                    388
```

References

1. Sampaio, S.O. et al. (1995) J. Immunol. 155, 2477–2486.
2. Picker, L.J. and Butcher, E.C. (1992) Annu. Rev. Immunol. 10, 561–591.
3. Sikorski, E.E. et al. (1993) J. Immunol. 151, 5239–5250.
4. **Shyjan, A.M. et al. (1996) J. Immunol. 156, 2851–2857.**
5. **Butcher, E.C. and Picker, L.J. (1996) Science 272, 60–66.**
6. Jones, E.Y. et al. (1995) Nature 373, 539–544.
7. Berlin, C. et al. (1993) Cell 74, 185–195.
8. Briskin, M.J. et al. (1996) J. Immunol. 156, 719–726.
9. Berg, E.L. et al. (1993) Nature 366, 695–698.
10. Briskin, M.J. et al. (1993) Nature 363, 461–464.

Mannose receptor

Molecular weights
Polypeptide   164 120

SDS-PAGE
  reduced   175–190 kDa

Carbohydrate
N-linked sites   8
O-linked   unknown

Human gene location and size
10p13; ~70 kb [1]

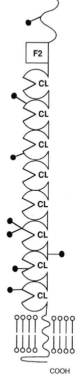

COOH

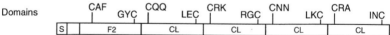

Domains

```
        CAF    CQQ      CRK      CNN      CRA
          | GYC |   LEC  |   RGC  |   LKC  |   INC
        |_|_____|_____|_____|_____|_____|
        |S|  F2  |   CL  |   CL  |   CL  |  CL  |
```

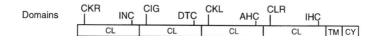

Domains

```
      CKR    CIG      CKL      CLR
        | INC |   DTC  |   AHC  |   IHC
      |_____|_____|_____|_____|__|__|
      |  CL  |   CL  |   CL  |   CL  |TM|CY|
```

Tissue distribution

The mannose receptor is expressed on mature tissue macrophages, hepatic sinusoidal cells and in the placenta [2–4]. Its expression on macrophages is upregulated in response to IL-4, IL-13 or anti-inflammatory steroids and down-regulated by IFNγ or IFNα [5–8].

Structure

The mannose receptor is a type I membrane glycoprotein. The N-terminus has a Cys-rich domain that shows sequence similarity to the B subunit of the plant protein ricin D, followed by a fibronectin type II domain, eight C-type lectin domains, transmembrane and cytoplasmic regions [2,3,9]. The overall

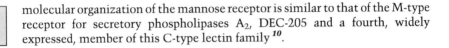

molecular organization of the mannose receptor is similar to that of the M-type receptor for secretory phospholipases A_2, DEC-205 and a fourth, widely expressed, member of this C-type lectin family [10].

Ligands and associated molecules

The mannose receptor binds oligomannose-containing carbohydrates. In addition, the Cys-rich domain of the mouse mannose receptor, fused to the Fc region of human IgG1, binds to macrophage populations in the splenic marginal zone (metallophilic macrophages) and the lymph node subcapsular sinus [11]. The ligand(s) for the Cys-rich domain is also expressed in germinal centres of the spleen and follicular areas of lymph nodes in immunized mice [11].

Function

The mannose receptor mediates phagocytosis by macrophages of micro-organisms with cell walls containing oligomannose carbohydrates. COS-1 cells transfected with full length mannose receptor cDNA bind and internalize *Candida albicans* yeast particles. Cells transfected with a cDNA mutated to delete the cytoplasmic region express the protein, but do not ingest particles [3].

Comment

The human mannose receptor gene is divided into 30 exons [1]. Due to the complex nature of the gene, with no simple correlation between the 26 exons that encode the eight lectin C-type domains, the positions of the intron/exon boundaries are not shown on the domain diagram.

Database accession numbers

	PIR	SWISSPROT	EMBL/GENBANK	REFERENCE
Human	A36563	P22897	J05550	2
Mouse	A48925		Z11974	12

Amino acid sequence of human mannose receptor

```
MRLPLLLVFA SVIPGAVL                                          -1
LLDTRQFLIY NEDHKRCVDA VSPSAVQTAA CNQDAESQKF RWVSESQIMS        50
VAFKLCLGVP SKTDWVAITL YACDSKSEFQ KWECKNDTLL GIKGEDLFFN       100
YGNRQEKNIM LYKGSGLWSR WKIYGTTDNL CSRGYEAMYT LLGNANGATC       150
AFPFKFENKW YADCTSAGRS DGWLWCGTTT DYDTDKLFGY CPLKFEGSES       200
LWNKDPLTSV SYQINSKSAL TWHQARKSCQ QQNAELLSIT EIHEQTYLTG       250
LTSSLTSGLW IGLNSLSFNS GWQWSDRSPF RYLNWLPGSP SAEPGKSCVS       300
LNPGKNAKWE NLECVQKLGY ICKKGNTTLN SFVIPSESDV PTHCPSQWWP       350
YAGHCYKIHR DEKKIQRDAL TTCRKEGGDL TSIHTIEELD FIISQLGYEP       400
NDELWIGLND IKIQMYFEWS DGTPVTFTKW LRGEPSHENN RQEDCVVMKG       450
KDGYWADRGC EWPLGYICKM KSRSQGPEIV EVEKGCRKGW KKHHFYCYMI       500
GHTLSTFAEA NQTCNNENAY LTTIEDRYEQ AFLTSFVGLR PEKYFWTGLS       550
DIQTKGTFQW TIEEEVRFTH WNSDMPGRKP GCVAMRTGIA GGLWDVLKCD       600
EKAKFVCKHW AEGVTHPPKP TTTPEPKCPE DWGASSRTSL CFKLYAKGKH       650
EKKTWFESRD FCRALGGDLA SINNKEEQQT IWRLITASGS YHKLFWLGLT       700
```

```
YGSPSEGFTW SDGSPVSYEN WAYGEPNNYQ NVEYCGELKG DPTMSWNDIN    750
CEHLNNWICQ IQKGQTPKPE PTPAPQDNPP VTEDGWVIYK DYQYYFSKEK    800
ETMDNARAFC KRNFGDLVSI QSESEKKFLW KYVNRNDAQS AYFIGLLISL    850
DKKFAWMDGS KVDYVSWATG EPNFANEDEN CVTMYSNSGF WNDINCGYPN    900
AFICQRHNSS INATTVMPTM PSVPSGCKEG WNFYSNKCFK IFGFMEEERK    950
NWQEARKACI GFGGNLVSIQ NEKEQAFLTY HMKDSTFSAW TGLNDVNSEH   1000
TFLWTDGRGV HYTNWGKGYP GGRRSSLSYE DADCVVIIGG ASNEAGKWMD   1050
DTCDSKRGYI CQTRSDPSLT NPPATIQTDG FVKYGKSSYS LMRQKFQWHE   1100
AETYCKLHNS LIASILDPYS NAFAWLQMET SNERVWIALN SNLTDNQYTW   1150
TDKWRVRYTN WAADEPKLKS ACVYLDLDGY WKTAHCNESF YFLCKRSDEI   1200
PATEPPQLPG RCPESDHTAW IPFHGHCYYI ESSYTRNWGQ ASLECLRMGS   1250
SLVSIESAAE SSFLSYRVEP LKSKTNFWIG LFRNVEGTWL WINNSPVSFV   1300
NWNTGDPSGE RNDCVALHAS SGFWSNIHCS SYKGYICKRP KIIDAKPTHE   1350
LLTTKADTRK MDPSKPSSNV AGVVIIVILL ILTGAGLAAY FFYKKRRVHL   1400
PQEGAFENTL YFNSQSSPGT SDMKDLVGNI EQNEHSVI               1438
```

References
1 Kim, S.J. et al. (1992) Genomics 14, 721–727.
2 Taylor, M.E. et al. (1990) J. Biol. Chem. 265, 12156–12162.
3 **Ezekowitz, R.A.B. et al. (1990) J. Exp. Med. 172, 1785–1794.**
4 Lennartz, M.R. et al. (1987) J. Biol. Chem. 262, 9942–9944.
5 Mokoena, T. and Gordon, S. (1985) J. Clin. Invest. 75, 624–631.
6 Shepherd, V.L. et al. (1985) J. Biol. Chem. 260, 160–164.
7 Stein, M. et al. (1992) J. Exp. Med. 176, 287–292.
8 Doyle, A.G. et al. (1994) Eur. J. Immunol. 24, 1441–1445.
9 Harris, N. (1994) Biochem. Biophys. Res. Commun. 198, 682–692.
10 Wu, K. et al. (1996) J. Biol. Chem. 271, 21323–21330.
11 Martínez-Pomares, L. et al. (1996) J. Exp. Med. 184, 1927–1937.
12 Harris, N. et al. (1992) Blood 80, 2363–2373.

MARCO

Molecular weights
Polypeptide   52 730

SDS-PAGE
  reduced   80 kDa
  unreduced   210 kDa

Carbohydrate
N-linked sites   2
O-linked   unknown

represents one third of
the collagen-like region

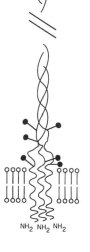

Domains

	GRA	VEC
CY	TM		Sc

Tissue distribution

MARCO is expressed by macrophages in the marginal zone of spleen and in the medullary cord of lymph nodes but not in liver or lung [1].

Structure

MARCO is a type II glycoprotein and is expressed as a disulfide-linked trimer at the cell surface [1]. MARCO has a 49 amino acid N-terminal cytoplasmic sequence, a 25 amino acid transmembrane sequence, a 75 amino acid putative spacer sequence containing two cysteine residues, followed by 270 amino acids predicted to be a collagen-like domain and at the C-terminus, a scavenger receptor cysteine-rich SF domain [1-3]. The predicted structure of MARCO is similar to scavenger receptor but differs in that MARCO has a longer collagenous domain where scavenger receptor has a coiled-coil region followed by a short collagen-like region [1-3]. The scavenger receptor domains of MARCO and scavenger receptor type I show 49% amino acid sequence identity and each contain six cysteines [1-3].

Ligands and associated molecules

COS cells expressing MARCO bind acetylated low-density lipoprotein and bacteria, specifically, *E. coli* and *S. aureus* [1,3].

Function

Unknown.

Database accession numbers

	PIR	SWISSPROT	EMBL/GENBANK	REFERENCE
Mouse	A55840		U18424	1

Amino acid sequence of mouse MARCO

```
MGSKELLKEE DFLGSTEDRA DFDQAMFPVM ETFEINDPVP KKRNGGTFCM    50
AVMAIHLILL TAGTALLLIQ VLNLQEQLQM LEMCCGNGSL AIEDKPFFSL   100
QWAPKTHLVP RAQGLQALQA QLSWVHTSQE QLRQQFNNLT QNPELFQIKG   150
ERGSPGPKGA PGAPGIPGLP GPAAEKGEKG AAGRDGTPGV QGPQGPPGSK   200
GEAGLQGLTG APGKQGATGA PGPRGEKGSK GDIGLTGPKG EHGTKGDKGD   250
LGLPGNKGDM GMKGDTGPMG SPGAQGGKGD AGKPGLPGLA GSPGVKGDQG   300
KPGVQGVPGP QGAPGLSGAK GEPGRTGLPG PAGPPGIAGN PGIAGVKGSK   350
GDTGIQGQKG TKGESGVPGL VGRKGDTGSP GLAGPKGEPG RVGQKGDPGM   400
KGSSGQQGQK GEKGQKGESF QRVRIMGGTN RGRAEVYYNN EWGTICDDDW   450
DNNDATVFCR MLGYSRGRAL SSYGGGSGNI WLDNVNCRGT ENSLWDCSKN   500
SWGNHNCVHN EDAGVECS                                     518
```

References
1 **Elomaa, O. et al. (1995) Cell 80, 603–609.**
2 Resnick, D. et al. (1994) Trends Biochem. Sci. 19, 5–8.
3 Pearson, A.M. (1996) Curr. Opin. Immunol. 8, 20–28.

Other names
Colony-stimulating factor (CSF)-1 receptor
c-fms proto-oncogene

Molecular weights
Polypeptide   105 619

SDS-PAGE
   reduced   150 kDa

Carbohydrate
N-linked sites   11
O-linked   unknown

Human gene location and size
5q33.2–q33.3; ~60 kb [1]

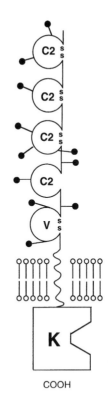

COOH

Domains

| | CVG | | CLL | | CSA | | LKV | | CAA | | | | |
	YRC		YQC		YSC		YSF		YEC				
S	C2		C2		C2		C2		V		TM	K	

Tissue distribution

CD115 is expressed on monocytes and their progenitors, macrophages, placental cells and choriocarcinoma cells [1].

Structure

CD115 is encoded by the c-fms proto-oncogene [2]. It belongs to subclass III within the family of growth factor receptors with tyrosine kinase activity, which also includes CD117 (c-kit) and the PDGF receptors type A and B (CD140a and CD140b) [1,3]. The extracellular domain of CD115 consists of five IgSF domains (four C2-set and one V-set). The cytoplasmic region contains a protein tyrosine kinase domain, interrupted by an insertion of about 70 amino acids [1–3]. This insertion is necessary for the association of

CD115 with phosphatidylinositol 3-kinase (PI 3-kinase)[4]. Lys593 (mature numbering) is predicted to be the site of ATP binding (*) and is preceded by the conserved GXGXXG motif[3] as shown below:

```
                    *
FGKTLGAGAFGKVVEATAFGLGKEDAVLKVAVKMLKSTAH
```

Ligands and associated molecules

The binding of M-CSF to CD115 ($K_d = 50$ pM) induces or stabilizes dimerization of the receptor[5]. This results in kinase activation and Tyr phosphorylation of CD115 itself and other cytoplasmic proteins, including PI 3-kinase[1,6]. CD115 is also associated with a G protein, stimulates the translocation of protein kinase C to the membrane, and induces phosphatidylcholine hydrolysis and gene expression (reviewed in ref. 6).

Function

M-CSF stimulates the survival, proliferation and differentiation of monocytes and macrophages and their bone marrow progenitors[1,7]. Human CD115 acquires transforming activity following mutation of Leu278 (equivalent to 301 in the precursor form) to Ser, and this oncogenic activity is increased by further substitutions near the C-terminus[1]. The loss of both alleles of CD115 has been demonstrated in patients with myelodysplastic syndrome[8].

Database accession numbers

	PIR	SWISSPROT	EMBL/GENBANK	REFERENCE
Human	A24533	P07333	X03663	2
Mouse	S01880	P09581	X06368	9

Amino acid sequence of human CD115

```
MGPGVLLLLL VATAWHGQGI PVI                                    -1
EPSVPELVVK PGATVTLRCV GNGSVEWDGP ASPHWTLYSD GSSSILSTNN       50
ATFQNTGTYR CTEPGDPLGG SAAIHLYVKD PARPWNVLAQ EVVVFEDQDA      100
LLPCLLTDPV LEAGVSLVRV RGRPLMRHTN YSFSPWHGFT IHRAKFIQSQ      150
DYQCSALMGG RKVMSISIRL KVQKVIPGPP ALTLVPAELV RIRGEAAQIV      200
CSASSVDVNF DVFLQHNNTK LAIPQQSDFH NNRYQKVLTL NLDQVDFQHA      250
GNYSCVASNV QGKHSTSMFF RVVESAYLNL SSEQNLIQEV TVGEGLNLKV      300
MVEAYPGLQG FNWTYLGPFS DHQPEPKLAN ATTKDTYRHT FTLSLPRLKP      350
SEAGRYSFLA RNPGGWRALT FELTLRYPPE VSVIWTFING SGTLLCAASG      400
YPQPNVTWLQ CSGHTDRCDE AQVLQVWDDP YPEVLSQEPF HKVTVQSLLT      450
VETLEHNQTY ECRAHNSVGS GSWAFIPISA GAHTHPPDEF LFTPVVVACM      500
SIMALLLLLL LLLLYKYKQK PKYQVRWKII ESYEGNSYTF IDPTQLPYNE      550
KWEFPRNNLQ FGKTLGAGAF GKVVEATAFG LGKEDAVLKV AVKMLKSTAH      600
ADEKEALMSE LKIMSHLGQH ENIVNLLGAC THGGPVLVIT EYCCYGDLLN      650
FLRRKAEAML GPSLSPGQDP EGGVDYKNIH LEKKYVRRDS GFSSQGVDTY      700
VEMRPVSTSS NDSFSEQDLD KEDGRPLELR DLLHFSSQVA QGMAFLASKN      750
CIHRDVAARN VLLTNGHVAK IGDFGLARDI MNDSNYIVKG NARLPVKWMA      800
PESIFDCVYT VQSDVWSYGI LLWEIFSLGL NPYPGILVNS KFYKLVKDGY      850
QMAQPAFAPK NIYSIMQACW ALEPTHRPTF QQICSFLQEQ AQEDRRERDY      900
TNLPSSSRSG GSGSSSSELE EESSSEHLTC CEQGDIAQPL LQPNNYQFC       949
```

References

[1] **Sherr, C.J. (1990) Blood 75, 1–12.**

[2] Coussens, L. et al. (1986) Nature 320, 277–280.

[3] **Ullrich, A. and Schlessinger, J. (1990) Cell 61, 203–212.**

[4] Ghosh Choudhury, G. et al. (1991) J. Biol. Chem. 266, 8068–8072.

[5] Li, W. and Stanley, E.R. (1991) EMBO J. 10, 277–288.

[6] Vairo, G. and Hamilton, J.A. (1991) Immunol. Today 12, 362–369.

[7] Nicola, N.A. (1989) Annu. Rev. Biochem. 58, 45–77.

[8] Boultwood, J. et al. (1991) Proc. Natl Acad. Sci. USA 88, 6176–6180.

[9] Rothwell, V.M. and Rohrschneider, L.R. (1987) Oncogene Res. 1, 311–324.

Other names
P170
Multidrug transporter

Molecular weights
Polypeptide   141 504

SDS-PAGE
    reduced   170 kDa

Carbohydrate
N-linked sites   3
O-linked   unknown

Human gene location and size
7q21.1; >100 kb [1]
The *MDR1* gene contains 28 introns, of which 26 interrupt the protein coding sequence (see ref. 1 for a detailed description of the gene structure).

Tissue distribution

The P-glycoprotein (P-gp) product of the *MDR1* gene is expressed in small intestine, colon, kidney, liver and adrenal, with very low levels of expression in most other tissues. Normal peripheral blood and bone marrow cells express very low amounts of P-gp, but it is expressed in practically all haematopoietic progenitor cells with the highest levels in pluripotent stem cells [1].

Structure

MDR1 belongs to the ABC superfamily of ATP-binding transport proteins that includes the product of the cystic fibrosis gene (*CFTR*), the *Plasmodium falciparum* multidrug resistance protein (pfMDR) and a large number of bacterial periplasmic transport proteins [2]. *MDR1* cDNA encodes a glycoprotein with 12 transmembrane domains. The protein consists of two halves which share a high degree of sequence similarity. The genomic organization of *MDR1* suggests that this gene arose by fusion of two related, but independently evolved genes, rather than by gene duplication [1]. Each half of the protein consists of a short hydrophilic N-terminal sequence, a long hydrophobic region containing six transmembrane segments, and a relatively hydrophilic region containing an ATP binding cassette of about 200 amino acids [3].

Function

P-gp has been shown to utilize ATP to pump hydrophobic drugs out of cells, thus decreasing their intracellular concentration and hence their toxicity [1]. The *MDR1* gene is amplified in multidrug-resistant cell lines [1]. However the actual physiological role of P-gp is not clear, although recent evidence suggests two possibilities that are not mutually exclusive. First, P-gp appears to be a flippase which translocates, or "flips", phospholipids from the inner leaflet of the lipid bilayer to the outer leaflet, or vice versa, to maintain the asymmetric distribution of different phospholipids in cell membranes[4]. The flippase model would explain how P-gp can export a wide range of drugs but not most normal cellular constituents: hydrophobic drug molecules could initially intercalate into the inner leaflet of the bilayer, then interact with P-gp and be "flipped" from the inner to the outer leaflet and subsequently into the aqueous phase[4]. Secondly, P-gp appears to regulate cell volume by modulating the activity of an endogeonous chloride channel, rather than being itself an ion channel[5].

Database accession numbers

	PIR	SWISSPROT	EMBL/GENBANK	REFERENCE
Human	A25059	P08183	M14758	6
Rat		P43245	M81855	7
Mouse	A33719	P06795	M14757	8

Amino acid sequence of human *MDR1* gene product

```
MDLEGDRNGG AKKKNFFKLN NKSEKDKKEK KPTVSVFSMF RYSNWLDKLY     50
MVVGTLAAII HGAGLPLMML VFGEMTDIFA NAGNLEDLMS NITNRSDIND    100
TGFFMNLEED MTRYAYYYSG IGAGVLVAAY IQVSFWCLAA GRQIHKIRKQ    150
FFHAIMRQEI GWFDVHDVGE LNTRLTDDVS KINEVIGDKI GMFFQSMATF    200
FTGFIVGFTR GWKLTLVILA ISPVLGLSAA VWAKILSSFT DKELLAYAKA    250
GAVAEEVLAA IRTVIAFGGQ KKELERYNKN LEEAKRIGIK KAITANISIG    300
AAFLLIYASY ALAFWYGTTL VLSGEYSIGQ VLTVFFSVLI GAFSVGQASP    350
SIEAFANARG AAYEIFKIID NKPSIDSYSK SGHKPDNIKG NLEFRNVHFS    400
YPSRKEVKIL KGLNLKVQSG QTVALVGNSG CGKSTTVQLM QRLYDPTEGM    450
VSVDGQDIRT INVRFLREII GVVSQEPVLF ATTIAENIRY GRENVTMDEI    500
EKAVKEANAY DFIMKLPHKF DTLVGERGAQ LSGGQKQRIA IARALVRNPK    550
ILLLDEATSA LDTESEAVVQ VALDKARKGR TTIVIAHRLS TVRNADVIAG    600
FDDGVIVEKG NHDELMKEKG IYFKLVTMQT AGNEVELENA ADESKSEIDA    650
LEMSSNDSRS SLIRKRSTRR SVRGSQAQDR KLSTKEALDE SIPPVSFWRI    700
MKLNLTEWPY FVVGVFCAII NGGLQPAFAI IFSKIIGVFT RIDDPETKRQ    750
NSNLFSLLFL ALGIISFITF FLQGFTFGKA GEILTKRLRY MVFRSMLRQD    800
VSWFDDPKNT TGALTTRLAN DAAQVKGAIG SRLAVITQNI ANLGTGIIIS    850
FIYGWQLTLL LLAIVPIIAI AGVVEMKMLS GQALKDKKEL EGAGKIATEA    900
IENFRTVVSL TQEQKFEHMY AQSLQVPYRN SLRKAHIFGI TFSFTQAMMY    950
FSYAGCFRFG AYLVAHKLMS FEDVLLVFSA VVFGAMAVGQ VSSFAPDYAK   1000
AKISAAHIIM IIEKTPLIDS YSTEGLMPNT LEGNVTFGEV VFNYPTRPDI   1050
PVLQGLSLEV KKGQTLALVG SSGCGKSTVV QLLERFYDPL AGKVLLDGKE   1100
IKRLNVQWLR AHLGIVSQEP ILFDCSIAEN IAYGDNSRVV SQEEIVRAAK   1150
EANIHAFIES LPNKYSTKVG DKGTQLSGGQ KQRIAIARAL VRQPHILLLD   1200
EATSALDTES EKVVQEALDK AREGRTCIVI AHRLSTIQNA DLIVVFQNGR   1250
VKEHGTHQQL LAQKGIYFSM VSVQAGTKRQ                         1280
```

References

1 Gottesman, M.M. and Pastan, I. (1993) Annu. Rev. Biochem. 62, 385–427.
2 **Higgins, C.F. (1995) Cell 82, 693–696.**
3 Kast, C. et al. (1996) J. Biol. Chem. 271, 9240–9248.
4 **van Helvoort, A. et al. (1996) Cell 87, 507–517.**
5 Valverde, M.A. et al. (1996) EMBO J. 15, 4460–4468.
6 Chen, C.J. et al. (1986) Cell 47, 381–389.
7 Silverman, J.A. et al. (1991) Gene 106, 229–236.
8 Gros, P. et al. (1986) Cell 47, 371–380.

Other names
HLA-A, -B and -C (human)
H-2K, -D, -L (mouse)
RT1A, RT1C (rat)

Molecular weights

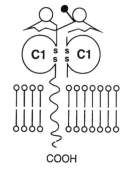

Polypeptide HLA-A2	α chain	38 412
	β_2-microglobulin	11 731
SDS-PAGE reduced	α chain	44 kDa
	β_2-microglobulin	12 kDa

Carbohydrate

N-linked sites	α chain	1
	β_2-microglobulin	nil
O-linked	α chain	nil
	β_2-microglobulin	nil

Human gene location
α chain: 6p21.3
β_2-microglobulin: 15q21–q22.2
The organization of genes within the human MHC complex is reviewed in ref. 1.

HLA-A2 α chain

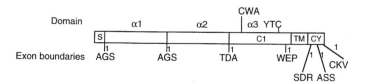

β_2-microglobulin

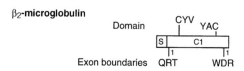

Tissue distribution

The "classical" MHC Class I molecules (HLA-A, -B and -C in man) are expressed on most nucleated cells but expression varies on different cell types. Interferons α, β and γ and tumour necrosis factor α increase the expression of MHC Class I molecules[2]. Expression can be low on virus-infected or tumour cells[3]. "Non-classical" MHC molecules generally have a broad distribution[4]. HLA-G is expressed only on cytotrophoblasts[4].

Structure

MHC Class I molecules consist of heterodimers of highly polymorphic α chains non-covalently associated with the invariant β_2-microglobulin subunit[5-7]. β_2-Microglobulin and the $\alpha3$ domain are Ig-related and of the C1-set. The $\alpha1$ and $\alpha2$ domains form a platform consisting of a single β pleated sheet topped by α helices[5-7]. A groove between the two α helices binds peptides[5-7]. The polymorphic amino acids of Class I molecules are concentrated along the peptide binding groove[5-7]. Endogenous proteins in the cell are degraded by proteasomes and resultant peptides transported by TAP proteins to be assembled in MHC Class I molecules before being expressed stably on the cell surface[2,8]. Peptides are usually nine amino acid residues long and anchored via residues, typically 2 and 9, in pockets on the peptide binding groove[5-7]. "Non-classical" MHC molecules have a similar structure to "classical" MHC molecules[4].

Ligands and associated molecules

Peptide antigen bound to MHC Class I antigens is recognized by the α/β TCR (on CD8$^+$ T cells) and γ/δ TCR heterodimers[9,10]. The affinity of the interaction between the TCR and the MHC/peptide complex is in the range 10^{-7}–10^{-4} M[11]. CD8 interacts with the non-polymorphic $\alpha3$ domain[12]. MHC Class I antigens bind the human and mouse NK receptors, CD158 IgSF molecules and Ly-49 C-type lectins respectively[3,13].

Function

The "classical" MHC Class I molecules present endogenously synthesized peptides to CD8$^+$ lymphocytes, which are usually cytotoxic T cells[2,14]. MHC Class I molecules expressed on thymic epithelial cells regulate the positive and negative selection of CD8$^+$ T cells during T cell maturation[14]. Expression of Class I molecules depends on the expression of β_2-micro-globulin and mice lacking a functional β_2-microglobulin gene do not express Class I molecules on the cell surface. These animals lack mature CD4$^-$CD8$^+$ T cells and have defective cell-mediated cytotoxicity[14]. Recognition of MHC Class I by NK receptors can protect from lysis by NK cells[3,14].

Comments

1 Allogeneic MHC molecules on transplanted organs can induce potent graft rejection[15].
2 Certain auto-immune diseases are linked to MHC Class I haplotype, e.g. ankylosing spondylitis is linked to HLA-B27[15].

Database accession numbers

	PIR	SWISSPROT	EMBL/GENBANK	REFERENCE
Human HLA-A2α	A02191	P01892	M32322	[16]
Human β_2-microglobulin	A02179	P01884	M17986	[17]
Rat β_2-microglobulin	A26842	P07151	Y00441	[18]
Mouse β_2-microglobulin	A02182	P01887	X01838	[19]

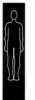

Amino acid sequence of human HLA-A2 α chain

```
MAVMAPRTLV LLLSGALALT QTWA                                   -1
GSHSMRYFFT SVSRPGRGEP RFIAVGYVDD TQFVRFDSDA ASQRMEPRAP       50
WIEQEGPEYW DGETRKVKAH SQTHRVDLGT LRGYYNQSEA GSHTVQRMYG      100
CDVGSDWRFL RGYHQYAYDG KDYIALKEDL RSWTAADMAA QTTKHKWEAA      150
HVAEQLRAYL EGTCVEWLRR YLENGKETLQ RTDAPKTHMT HHAVSDHEAT      200
LRCWALSFYP AEITLTWQRD GEDQTQDTEL VETRPAGDGT FQKWAAVVVP      250
SGQEQRYTCH VQHEGLPKPL TLRWEPSSQP TIPIVGIIAG LVLFGAVITG      300
AVVAAVMWRR KSSDRKGGSY SQAASSDSAQ GSDVSLTACK V              341
```

Amino acid sequence of human β_2-microglobulin

```
MSRSVALAVL ALLSLSGLEA                                        -1
IQRTPKIQVY SRHPAENGKS NFLNCYVSGF HPSDIEVDLL KNGERIEKVE       50
HSDLSFSKDW SFYLLYYTEF TPTEKDEYAC RVNHVTLSQP KIVKWDRDM        99
```

References

1   Trowsdale, J. (1995) Immunogenetics 41, 1–17.
2   **York, I.A. and Rock, K.L. (1996) Annu. Rev. Immunol. 14, 369–396.**
3   Gumperz, J.E. and Parham, P. (1995) Nature 378, 245–248.
4   Shawar, S. et al. (1994) Annu. Rev. Immunol. 12, 839–880.
5   **Stern L. and Wiley, D.C. (1994) Curr. Biol. 2, 245–251.**
6   Wilson, I.A. and Fremont, D.H. (1993) Semin. Immunol. 5, 75–80.
7   Young, A.C.M. et al. (1995) FASEB J. 9, 26–36.
8   Lehner, P.J. and Cresswell, P. (1996) Curr. Opin. Immunol. 8, 59–67.
9   Garcia, K.C. et al. (1996) Science 274, 209–219.
10 Garboczi, D.N. et al. (1996) Nature 384, 134–141.
11 Fremont, D.H. et al. (1996) Curr. Opin. Immunol. 8, 93–100.
12 Zamoyska, R. (1994) Immunity 1, 243–246.
13 Lanier, L.L. and Phillips, J.H. (1996) Immunol. Today 17, 86–91.
14 Raulet, D.H. (1994) Adv. Immunol. 55, 381–421.
15 Vyse, T.J. and Todd, J.A. (1996) Cell 85, 311–318.
16 Bjorkman, P.J. et al. (1987) Nature 329, 506–512.
17 Güsson, D. et al. (1987) J. Immunol. 139, 3133–3138.
18 Mauxion, F. and Kress, M. (1987) Nucleic Acids Res. 15, 7638.
19 Daniel, F. et al. (1983) EMBO J. 2, 1061–1065.

MHC Class II

Major histocompatibility complex Class II antigen

Other names
HLA-DP, -DQ and -DR (human)
I-A and I-E (mouse)
RT1B and RT1D (rat)

Molecular weights

SDS-PAGE
   reduced α chain   33–35 kDa
                 β chain   28–30 kDa

Carbohydrate
N-linked sites α chain   2
                    β chain   1
O-linked α chain   nil
                    β chain   nil

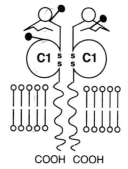

Human gene location
6p21.3
The organization of genes within the human MHC complex is reviewed in ref. 1.

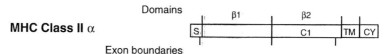

MHC Class II α

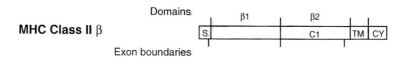

MHC Class II β

Tissue distribution

MHC Class II molecules are expressed on dendritic cells, B cells, monocytes, macrophages, myeloid and erythroid precursors and some epithelial cells. MHC Class II is expressed on activated T cells in human and rat[2]. Expression of MHC Class II is regulated by cytokines including interferon γ, which also induces expression on fibroblasts, epithelial and endothelial cells[2].

Structure

MHC Class II molecules are heterodimers of non-covalently associated α and β chains. Both chains are comprised of two IgSF domains and have transmembrane sequences and short cytoplasmic tails. Multiple alleles of α and β chains exist and they are highly polymorphic. Because of the extensive polymorphism of MHC Class II molecules, accession numbers and sequence data are not included in this entry. Crystal structure of the MHC Class II antigen HLA-DR1 is a similar structure to that of the MHC Class I antigen HLA-A2 (see page 566)[3]. The crystals contained dimers of the $\alpha\beta$ heterodimer. Polymorphic residues are positioned at the peptide antigen binding site[3,4]. Unlike MHC Class I, length is not critical for peptides bound to MHC Class II and they make several contacts along the length of the peptide binding groove[4]. MHC Class II molecules are first associated with CD74 (the invariant or Ii chain) in the endoplasmic reticulum. CD74 is degraded in the endosomal/lysosomal pathway leaving a CLIP (MHC Class II-associated Ii chain) peptide attached to the MHC Class II molecule. The CLIP peptide is dissociated by binding to Class II-related HLA-DM and replaced by peptides generated from exogenous proteins[5].

Ligands and associated molecules

Peptide antigen bound to MHC Class II bind to TCR on CD4[+] cells. The affinity of the interaction between the TCR and the MHC/peptide complex is in the range of $10^{-7}-10^{-4}$ M[6]. Superantigens as intact proteins bind to MHC Class II differently from peptides[6]. CD4 interacts directly with non-polymorphic residues on MHC Class II and both domain 1 and 2 of the β chain are implicated in binding[7,8].

Function

MHC Class II molecules present exogenously derived antigen to CD4[+] T lymphocyes, which are usually helper T cells[9]. MHC Class II molecules expressed on thymic stromal cells play a key role in the positive and negative selection of CD4[+] T cells during thymopoiesis and genetically engineered mice that do not express MHC Class II antigens lack CD4[+] T cells in the periphery[10]. Signalling can occur through MHC Class II[11].

Comments

Certain HLA Class II molecules are associated with auto-immune diseases such as coeliac disease, insulin-dependent diabetes mellitus, rheumatoid arthritis, myasthenia gravis, multiple sclerosis and pemphigus vulgaris[12].

References
1 Trowsdale, J. (1995) Immunogenetics 41, 1–17.
2 Seddon, B. and Mason, D. (1996) Int. Immunol. 8, 1185–1193.
3 Brown, J.H. et al. (1993) Nature 364, 33–39.
4 **Stern L. and Wiley, D.C. (1994) Structure 2, 245–251.**
5 **Cresswell, P. (1996) Cell 84, 505–507.**
6 Fremont, D.H. et al. (1996) Curr. Opin. Immunol. 8, 93–100.
7 Littman, D.R. (ed.) (1996) The CD4 Molecule. Curr. Top. Microbiol. Immunol. 205, 19–46.
8 Sakihama, T. et al. (1995) Immunol. Today, 16, 581–587.
9 Rudensky, A.Y. (1995) Semin. Immunol. 7, 399–409.
10 Cardell, S. et al. (1994) Adv. Immunol. 55, 423–440.
11 Scholl, P.R. and Geha, R.S. (1994) Immunol. Today 15, 418–422.
12 Vyse, T.J. and Todd, J.A. (1996) Cell, 85, 311–318.

MS2

Molecular weight
Polypeptide   88 465

SDS-PAGE
  reduced   89 kDa
  unreduced   75 kDa

Carbohydrate
N-linked sites 5
O-linked   unknown

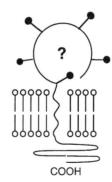

COOH

Tissue distribution

MS2 mRNA is expressed in macrophages and macrophage cell lines [1]. The level of expression of MS2 transcripts is upregulated following macrophage stimulation with LPS, phorbol ester or lymphokines.

Structure

MS2 is a type I membrane glycoprotein. The extracellular region contains a Cys-rich domain with no clear similarities to other Cys-rich domains. The cytoplasmic region contains a large number of Pro, Arg and Lys residues and encodes tandem repeats with homology to corresponding sequences in CD2 and CD122 (IL-2Rβ chain) [1]. Based on amino acid sequence similarity, the MS2 molecule is predicted to be a member of the zinc-dependent metalloprotease family.

Ligands and associated molecules

Unknown.

Function

The function of MS2 is unknown.

Database accession numbers

	PIR	SWISSPROT	EMBL/GENBANK	REFERENCE
Mouse	A60385	Q05910	X13335	1

Amino acid sequence of mouse MS2

```
MLGLWLLSVL WTPA                                              -1
VAPGPPLPHV KQYEVVWPRR LAASRSRRAL PSHWGQYPES LSYALGTSGH       50
VFTLHLRKNR DLLGSSYTET YSAANGSEVT EQLQEQDHCL YQGHVEGYEG      100
SAASISTCAG LRGFFRVGST VHLIEPLDAD EEGQHAMYQA KHLQQKAGTC      150
GVKDTNLNDL GPRALEIYRA QPRNWLIPRE TRYVELYVVA DSQEFQKLGS      200
REAVRQRVLE VVNHVDKLYQ ELSFRVVLVG LEIWNKDKFY ISRYANVTLE      250
NFLSWREQNL QGQHPHDNVQ LITGVDFIGS TVGLAKVSAL CSRHSGAVNQ      300
DHSKNSIGVA STMAHELGHN LGMSHDEDIP GCYCPEPREG GGCIMTESIG      350
SKFPRIFSRC SKIDLESFVT KPQTGCLTNV PDVNRFVGGP VCGNLFVEHG      400
```

```
EQCDCGTPQD CQNPCCNATT CQLVKGAECA SGTCCHECKV KPAGEVCRLS    450
KDKCDLEEFC DGRKPTCPED AFQQNGTPCP GGYCFDGSCP TLAQQCRDLW    500
GPGARVAADS CYTFSIPPGC NGRMYSGRIN RCGALYCEGG QKPLERSFCT    550
FSSNHGVCHA LGTGSNIDTF ELVLQGTKCE EGKVCMDGSC QDLRVYRSEN    600
CSAKCNNHGV CNHKRECHCH KGWAPPNCVQ RLADVSDEQA ASTSLPVSVV    650
VVLVILVAAM VIVAGIVIIR KAPRQIQRRS VAPKPISGLS NPLFYTRDSS    700
LPAKNRPPDP SETVSTNQPP RPIAKPKRPP PAPPGAVSSS PLPVPVYAPK    750
IPNQFRPDPP TKPLPELKPK QVKPTFAPPT PPVKPGTGGT VPGATQGAGG    800
PKVALKVPIQ KR                                            812
```

Reference
[1] Yoshida, S. et al. (1990) Int. Immunol. 2, 585–591.

NKG2 family

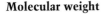

Molecular weight
Polypeptide (NKG2-A)
         26 270

SDS-PAGE
  unreduced   70 kDa (NKG2A/CD94 heterodimer)
  reduced   43 kDa (NKG2A plus 30 kDa CD94)

Carbohydrate
N-linked sites 3 (NKG2-A)
O-linked   none

Human gene location
12p12.3–p13.1 (all members) [1,2]

CD94 **NKG2**

NKG2A

Domain

CPE YHC

| CY | TM | CL |

Tissue distribution

NKG2 transcripts are expressed in NK cell lines and in some T cell clones and lines [3]. NKG2 proteins are expressed as disulfide-linked heterodimers with CD94 on the surface of NK cells and T cells [4]. Different NK cell clones may express one or more NKG2 glycoproteins.

Structure

NKG2 was originally identified as five closely related cDNAs (NKG2-A, NKG2-B, NKG2-C, NKG2-D and NKG2-E). NKG2-A and -B are alternatively spliced transcripts of the same gene [1,2]. NKG2 genes encode type II integral membrane proteins with an extracellular C-type lectin domains. Molecules of the NKG2 family are structurally related to several other molecules (Ly-49 family, NKR-P1 family, CD69 and CD94) encoded within the mouse and/or human NK gene complexes which contribute to NK cell function (see **Ly-49**) [5]. NKG2 proteins are disulfide-bonded to CD94 proteins and expressed as heterodimers on the surface of NK cells and some T cells [4]. Transfection studies suggest that NKG2 glycoproteins may also be expressed as disulfide-linked homodimers [6]. The cytoplasmic domain of NKG2A/B has two (I/V)XYXXL motifs but these are absent from other NKG2 molecules.

Ligands and associated molecules

CD94/NKG2 receptors have been implicated in the recognition of HLA-A, -B and -C [4,7], but there is currently no evidence for direct binding. A soluble form of NKG2-C binds to an unidentified ligand on K562 cells and binding correlated with their susceptibility to NK cell lysis [6]. NKG2A has been shown to associate with the cytoplasmic tyrosine phosphatase SHP-1, presumably through its cytoplasmic (I/V)XYXXL motifs [9].

Function

CD94/NKG2 receptors have been implicated in activation or inhibition of NK cell cytotoxicity and cytokine secretion [4,8]. Whereas NKG2A is inhibitory, NKG2C activates NK cells [9].

Database accession numbers

	PIR	SWISSPROT	EMBL/GENBANK	REFERENCE
NKG2A	PT0372	P26715	X54867	3
NKG2B	PT0373	P26716	X54868	3
NKG2C	PT0374	P26717	X54860	3
NKG2D	PT0374	P26718	X54870	3
NKG2E			L14542	

Amino acid sequence of human NKG2A

```
MDNQGVIYSD LNLPPNPKRQ QRKPKGNKSS ILATEQEITY AELNLQKASQ      50
DFQGNDKTYH CKDLPSAPEK LIVGILGIIC LILMASVVTI VVIPSTLIQR     100
HNNSSLNTRT QKARHCGHCP EEWITYSNSC YYIGKERRTW EESLLACTSK     150
NSSLLSIDNE EEMKFLSIIS PSSWIGVFRN SSHHPWVTMN GLAFKHEIKD     200
SDNAELNCAV LQVNRLKSAQ CGSSIIYHCK HKL                       233
```

Note: (I/V)XYXXL motifs in **bold**.

References

1. Yabe, T. et al. (1993) Immunogenetics 37, 455–460.
2. Plougastel, B. et al. (1996) Immunogenetics 44, 286–291.
3. Houchins, J.P. et al. (1991) J. Exp. Med. 173, 1017–1020.
4. **Lazetic, S. et al. (1996) J. Immunol. 157, 4741–4745.**
5. Gumperz, J.E. and Parham, P. (1995) Nature 378, 245–248.
6. Düchler, M. et al. (1995) Eur. J. Immunol. 25, 2923–2931.
7. Phillips, J.H. et al. (1996) Immunity 5, 163–172.
8. Pérez-Villar, J.J. et al. (1995) J. Immunol. 154, 5779–5788.
9. Houchins, J.P., L.L. Lanier, E.C. Niemi, J.H. Phillips, and J.C. Ryan, submitted.

Molecular weights
Polypeptide   27 928

SDS-PAGE
    reduced   47 kD (rat thymocytes)
              41 kD (rat brain)

Carbohydrate
N-linked sites   6
O-linked   nil

Human gene location and size
3q12–q13; 8 kb [1]
It is probable that a further 5′ exon exists in the human gene.

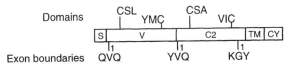

Tissue distribution

The OX2 antigen was originally named MRC OX2 after the first antibody. Human OX2 mRNA is expressed in normal brain and in B cell lines, but not in normal liver, T cell lines, a myeloma line or a monocyte cell line [1]. In the rat, OX2 is expressed in thymocytes, B cells, follicular dendritic cells, vascular endothelium, trophoblasts, neurons and some smooth muscle as assessed by mAb binding (reviewed in ref. 2). OX2 is also expressed on activated T cells (Seddon, B., unpublished).

Structure

The extracellular region consists of two IgSF domains, followed by a hydrophobic transmembrane domain and a cytoplasmic domain [2]. The carbohydrate composition of rat thymus and brain OX2 has been determined [3].

Ligands and associated molecules

Recombinant soluble OX2 antigen binds to an unidentified ligand on rodent peritoneal macrophages (Preston, S., Brown, M.H. and Barclay, A.N., unpublished).

Function

Unknown.

Database accession numbers

	PIR	SWISSPROT	EMBL/GENBANK	REFERENCE
Human	A47639	P41217	M17229	1
Rat	A02114	P04218	X01785	4

Amino acid sequence of human OX2

```
VIRMPFSHLS TYSLVWVMAA VVLCTA                              -1
QVQVVTQDER EQLYTTASLK CSLQNAQEAL IVTWQKKKAV SPENMVTFSE     50
NHGVVIQPAY KDKINITQLG LQNSTITFWN ITLEDEGCYM CLFNTFGFGK    100
ISGTACLTVY VQPIVSLHYK FSEDHLNITC SATARPAPMV FWKVPRSGIE    150
NSTVTLSHPN GTTSVTSILH IKDPKNQVGK EVICQVLHLG TVTDFKQTVN    200
KGYWFSVPLL LSMFSLVILL VLISILLYWK RHRNQDRGEL SQGVQKMT      248
```

References
[1] **McCaughan, G.W. et al. (1987) Immunogenetics 25, 329–335.**
[2] McCaughan, G.W. et al. (1987) Immunogenetics 25, 133–135.
[3] Barclay, A.N. and Ward, H.A. (1982) Eur. J. Biochem. 129, 447–458.
[4] Clark, M.J. et al. (1985) EMBO J. 4, 113–118.

OX40L CD134L

Molecular weights
Polypeptide   21 051

SDS-PAGE
  reduced   32–34 kDa

Carbohydrate
N-linked sites   4
O-linked   unknown

Human gene location
1q25 [1]

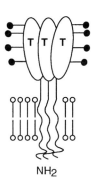

NH2

Domains

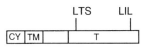

LTS   LIL

Tissue distribution

OX40L is expressed on activated T and B lymphocytes [1-3]. It is also expressed on HTLV-1 transformed and activated B lymphoblastoid and monocytic cell lines [2,4] and vascular endothelial cells [5]. Messenger RNA for mouse OX40L is widespread [1].

Structure

OX40L is a member of the TNF superfamily [2,6]. Like other members of this superfamily, it is a type II membrane protein expressed as a trimer with the similarity to TNF being in the C-terminal extracellular region [1,2,4].

Ligand and associated molecules

OX40 ligand binds to CD134 and there is no evidence for another ligand [7]. The affinity of monomeric CD134 for OX40L is 190 nM and of trimeric OX40L for CD134 on the surface of activated T cells is 0.2 nM [8]. Three CD134 receptors bind one OX40L molecule [8].

Function

Crosslinking OX40L on activated B cells stimulates proliferation and Ig production [3]. Similarly, blocking the OX40L–CD134 interaction reduced IgG production, suggesting a role in differentiation into plasma cells [9]. OX40L mAbs block binding of activated T cells to endothelial cell lines [5]. OX40L binding to CD134 on T cells co-stimulates proliferation [1,2].

Database accession numbers

	PIR	SWISSPROT	EMBL/GENBANK	REFERENCE
Human	A39680	P23510	X79929	2
Mouse		P43488	U12763	3

Amino acid sequence of human OX40L

```
MERVQPLEEN VGNAARPRFE RNKLLLVASV IQGLGLLLCF TYICLHFSAL    50
QVSHRYPRIQ SIKVQFTEYK KEKGFILTSQ KEDEIMKVQN NSVIINCDGF   100
YLISLKGYFS QEVNISLHYQ KDEEPLFQLK KVRSVNSLMV ASLTYKDKVY   150
LNVTTDNTSL DDFHVNGGEL ILIHQNPGEF CVL                     183
```

References

1. Baum, P.R. et al. (1994) EMBO J. 13, 3992–4001.
2. Gruss, H.-J. and Dower, S.K. (1995) Blood 85, 3378–3404.
3. **Stuber, E. et al. (1995) Immunity 2, 507–521.**
4. Godfrey, W.R. et al. (1994) J. Exp. Med. 180, 757–762.
5. Imura, A. et al. (1996) J. Exp. Med. 183, 2185–2195.
6. Armitage, R.J. (1994) Curr. Opin. Immunol. 6, 407–413.
7. Al-Shamkhani, A. et al. (1996) Eur. J. Immunol. 26, 1695–1699.
8. Al-Shamkhani, A. et al. (1997) J. Biol. Chem. 272, 5275–5282.
9. Stuber, E. and Strober, W. (1996) J. Exp. Med. 183, 979–989.

PC-1   EC 3.1.4.1, EC 3.6.1.9

Molecular weights
Polypeptide   99 930

SDS-PAGE
reduced   115–120 kDa
unreduced   220 kDa

Carbohydrates
N-linked sites   9
O-linked sites   unknown

Human gene location
6q22–q23

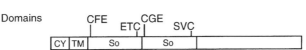

Domains

CFE   CGE
ETC   SVC

| CY | TM | So | So | |

Tissue distribution

PC-1 is expressed on plasma cells [1]. It is also expressed in non-lymphoid tissues including epithelial cells in testis, salivary gland, kidney, brain capillaries and bone chondrocytes [1].

Structure

PC-1 is a disulfide linked homodimeric type II membrane protein [2-4]. The membrane-proximal region contains two somatomedin-B like domains, followed by a catalytic domain characteristic of 5′ nucleotidases. Two consensus sequences of EF-hand like divalent cation binding motifs are found between residues 265–294 and 739–767 [5].

Function

PC-1 is an ecto-enzyme with alkaline phosphodiesterase I (EC 3.1.4.1) and nucleotide pyrophosphatase (EC 3.6.1.9) activities [6,7]. PC-1 was also found to have autophosphorylation activity [8], and autophosphorylation inactivates its other two enzymatic activities [9]. It has been suggested that auto-phosphorylation at low ATP concentration is a regulatory mechanism which prevents depletion of nucleotides when they are scarce [9].

Database accession numbers

	PIR	SWISSPROT	EMBL/GENBANK	REFERENCE
Human	A39216	P22413	M57736	3
			D12485	4
Mouse	A27410	P06802	J02700	10

Amino acid sequence of human PC-1

```
MDVGEEPLEK AARARTAKDP NTYKVLSLVL SVCVLTTILG CIFGLKPSCA      50
KEVKSCKGRC FERTFGNCRC DAACVELGNC CLDYQETCIE PEHIWTCNKF     100
RCGEKRLTRS LCACSDDCKD KGDCCINYSS VCQGEKSWVE EPCESINEPQ     150
CPAGFETPPT LLFSLDGFRA EYLHTWGGLL PVISKLKKCG TYTKNMRPVY     200
PTKTFPNHYS IVTGLYPESH GIIDNKMYDP KMNASFSLKS KEKFNPEWYK     250
GEPIWVTAKY QGLKSGTFFW PGSDVEINGI FPDIYKMYNG SVPFEERILA     300
VLQWLQLPKD ERPHFYTLYL EEPDSSGHSY GPVSSEVIKA LQRVDGMVGM     350
LMDGLKELNL HRCLNLILIS DHGMEQGSCK KYIYLNKYLG DVKNIKVIYG     400
PAARLRPSDV PDKYYSFNYE GIARNLSCRE PNQHFKPYLK HFLPKRLHFA     450
KSDRIEPLTF YLDPQWQLAL NPSERKYCGS GFHGSDNVFS NMQALFVGYG     500
PGFKHGIEAD TFENIEVYNL MCDLLNLTPA PNNGTHGSLN HLLKNPVYTP     550
KHPKEVHPLV QCPFTRNPRD NLGCSCNPSI LPIEDFQTQF NLTVAEEKII     600
KHETLPYGRP RVLQKENTIC LLSQHQFMSG YSQDILMPLW TSYTVDRNDS     650
FSTEDFSNCL YQDFRIPLSP VHKCSFYKNN TKVSYGFLSP PQLNKNSSGI     700
YSEALLTTNI VPMYQSFQVI WRYFHDTLLR KYAEERNGVN VVSGPVFDFD     750
YDGRCDSLEN LRQKRRVIRN QEILIPTHFF IVLTSCKDTS QTPLHCENLD     800
TLAFILPHRT DNSESCVHGK HDSSWVEELL MLHRARITDV EHITGLSFYQ     850
QRKEPVSDIL KLKTHLPTFS QED                                 873
```

References
1. Harahap, A.R. and Goding, J.W. (1988) J. Immunol. 141, 2317–2320.
2. Goding, J.W. and Shen, F.W. (1982) J. Immunol. 129, 2636–2640.
3. Buckley, M.F. et al. (1990) J. Biol. Chem. 265, 17506–17511.
4. Funakoshi, I. et al. (1992) Arch. Biochem. Biophys. 295, 180–187.
5. Belli, S.I. et al. (1994) Biochem. J. 304, 75–80.
6. Rebbe, N. et al. (1991) Proc. Natl Acad. Sci. USA 88, 5192–5196.
7. **Belli, S.I. and Goding, J.W. (1994) Eur. J. Biochem. 226, 433–443.**
8. Belli, S.I. et al. (1995) Eur. J. Biochem. 228, 669–676.
9. **Stefan, C. et al. (1996) Eur. J. Biochem. 241, 338–342.**
10. van Driel, I.R. and Goding, J.W. (1987) J. Biol. Chem. 262, 4882–4887.

PD-1

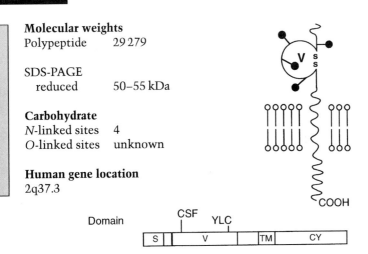

Molecular weights
Polypeptide   29 279

SDS-PAGE
 reduced   50–55 kDa

Carbohydrate
N-linked sites   4
O-linked sites   unknown

Human gene location
2q37.3

Domain

Tissue distribution

Mouse PD-1 was isolated by subtractive hybridization from the T cell line 2B4.11 and the haematopoietic progenitor cell line LyD9 under conditions designed to detect genes expressed following the induction of programed cell death (PCD). Analysis of mRNA indicates that the expression of PD-1 is associated with cells undergoing classical apoptosis, but not with cells undergoing non-apoptotic PCD [1]. PD-1 is expressed on 3–5% of normal thymocytes but on ~35% of CD4⁻/CD8⁻ cells. PD-1-expressing thymocytes can be divided into two distinct populations [2]: the high-level PD-1-expressing thymocytes are of the $\gamma\delta$ TCR lineage; PD-1 is also expressed at the transition phase between CD4⁻/CD8⁻ to CD4⁺/CD8⁺ stage on thymocytes of the $\alpha\beta$ TCR lineage. Expression of PD-1 on thymocytes, as well as T cells in the spleen and lymph nodes, can be stimulated *in vivo* with anti-CD3 antibodies [2,3]. PD-1 expression is not readily detected in the brain, heart, lung, spleen or kidney [1].

Structure

PD-1 is a type I membrane protein with one IgSF domain in the extracellular region. The cytoplasmic segment contains two ITAM motifs [1,2].

Function

From mRNA analysis it appears that PD-1 expression is strongly associated with the apoptotic programmed cell death [1,3]. It has been suggested that PD-1 may play a role in clonal selection of lymphocytes [4].

Database accession numbers

	PIR	*SWISSPROT*	*EMBL/GENBANK*	*REFERENCE*
Human			L27440	4
Mouse	S28029	Q02242	X67914	1

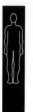

Amino acid sequence of human PD-1

```
MQIPQAPWPV VWAVLQLGWR                                          -1
PGWFLDSPDR PWNPPTFSPA LLVVTEGDNA TFTCSFSNTS ESFVLNWYRM        50
SPSNQTDKLA AFPEDRSQPG QDCRFRVTQL PNGRDFHMSV VRARRNDSGT       100
YLCGAISLAP KAQIKESLRA ELRVTERRAE VPTAHPSPSP RSAGQFQTLV       150
VGVVGGLLGS LVLLVWVLAV ICSRAARGTI GARRTGQPLK EDPSAVPVFS       200
VDYGELDFQW REKTPEPPVP CVPEQTEYAT IVFPSGMGTS SPARRGSADG       250
PRSAQPLRPE DGHCSWPL                                          268
```

References
[1] **Ishida, Y. et al. (1992) EMBO J. 11, 3887–3895.**
[2] Nishimura, H. et al. (1996) Int. Immunol. 8, 773–780.
[3] Agata, Y. et al. (1996) Int. Immunol. 8, 765–772.
[4] Shinohara, T. et al. (1994) Genomics 23, 704–706.

RT6

Molecular weights
SDS-PAGE
reduced	RT6.1	24, 27, 30–35 kDa
	RT6.2	25, 28 kDa
unreduced	RT6.1	21, 23, 27–32 kDa
	RT6.2	21, 24 kDa

Carbohydrate
N-linked sites	RT6.1	1
	RT6.2	0
O-linked	RT6.1	unknown
	RT6.2	nil

Human gene location
11q13

RT6.1

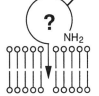

Tissue distribution

RT6 is a specific marker for peripheral T lymphocytes. In the rat, RT6 is expressed on the majority of mature peripheral T cells, but not on thymocytes or any other haematopoietic cells. Recent thymic emigrants are RT6[−]/Thy-1[+] and these mature to RT6[+]/Thy-1[−] cells[1]. Intestinal intra-epithelial T cells express RT6 at particularly high levels[2]. At the mRNA level, the expression of mouse Rt-6 is similar to that in the rat[3]. The human RT6 gene is transcriptionally inactive[4].

Structure

RT6.1 and RT6.2 are the products of separate alleles of the rat RT6 locus[1]. Both are GPI-anchored and a proportion of RT6.1 is N-glycosylated. The cDNA sequences of RT6.1 and RT6.2 differ at 18 positions leading to 12 amino acid substitutions and the presence of a glycosylation site in the translated sequence of RT6.1[1,5]. In the mouse, two closely linked genes encode different RT6 proteins, Rt6-1 and Rt6-2, both of which are polymorphic[3,6]. Remarkably, the single copy gene for human RT6 is a pseudogene as a result of three premature in-frame stop codons[4]. RT6 shows sequence homology to a family of bacterial toxins that function as mono-ADP-ribosyltransferases[7].

Ligands and associated molecules

RT6 co-immunoprecipitates with the Src family tyrosine kinases Fyn and Lck in rat T cells[8].

Function

RT6 has NAD-metabolizing activity and can undergo auto-ADP-ribosylation on arginine residues. RT6 may also ADP-ribosylate other target proteins at the cell surface thereby modulating their function (reviewed in ref. 7). This may help to explain the susceptibility to autoimmune disease of some experimental animals which have deficient RT6 expression [7]. Incubation of mouse cytotoxic T cells with NAD suppresses their ability to lyse target cells, an effect mediated through a GPI-anchored ADP-ribosyltransferase. This has prompted speculation that the transferase is RT6, suggesting a possible link between low RT6 expression and enhanced T cell autoreactivity [7].

Database accession numbers

	PIR	SWISSPROT	EMBL/GENBANK	REFERENCE
Human			X65050	4
Rat RT6.1	S08464	P17982	X52082	5
Rat RT6.2	A34866	P20974		1
Mouse Rt6–1	S12738	P17981	X52991	9

Amino acid sequences of the allelic forms of rat RT6

```
RT6.1 MPSNICKFFL TWWLIQQVTG                                        -1
RT6.2 ---------- ----------                                        -1

RT6.1 LTGPLMLDTA PNAFDDQYEG CVNKMEEKAP LLLKEDFNKS EKLKVAWEEA       50
RT6.2 ---------- ---------- --------- ----Q----MN A---------       50

RT6.1 KKRWNNIKPS MSYPKGFNDF HGTALVAYTG SIGVDFNRAV REFKENPGQF      100
RT6.2 ---------- R--------- --------- ---A------- ----------      100

RT6.1 HYKAFHYYLT RALQLLSNGD CHSVYRGTKT RFHYTGAGSV RFGQFTSSSL      150
RT6.2 ---------- ---------- ---------- ---------- ----------      150

RT6.1 SKTVAQSPEF FSDDGTLFII KTCLGVYIKE FSFYPDQEEV LIPGYEVYQK      200
RT6.2 --K----Q-- ---H------ ---------- ---R------ ----------      200

RT6.1 VRTQGYNEIF LDSPKRKKSN YNCLYSS                               227
RT6.2 ---C------ ---------- -------                               227

RT6.1 AGTRESCVSL FLVVLTSLLV QLLCLAEP                              +28
RT6.2 --A------- -----P---- --------                              +28
```

Residues different between RT6.1 and RT6.2 are shown with identical residues indicated by dashes.

References
1 Koch, F. et al. (1990) Proc. Natl Acad. Sci. USA 87, 964–967.
2 Fangmann, J. et al. (1991) Eur. J. Immunol. 21, 753–760.
3 Prochazka, M. et al. (1991) Immunogenetics 33, 152–156.
4 Haag, F. et al. (1994) J. Mol. Biol. 243, 537–546.
5 Haag, F. et al. (1990) Nucleic Acids Res. 18, 1047.
6 Koch-Nolte, F. et al. (1995) Immunogenetics 41, 152–155.
7 **Koch-Nolte, F. et al. (1996) Immunol. Today 17, 402–405.**
8 Rigby, M.R. et al. (1996) Diabetes 45, 1419–1426.
9 Koch, F. et al. (1990) Nucleic Acids Res. 18, 3636.

Sca-2

Stem cell antigen 2, thymic shared antigen 1 (TSA-1)

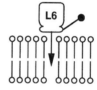

Molecular weights
Polypeptide   8828

Carbohydrate
N-linked sites   1
O-linked   unknown

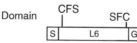

Domain

Tissue distribution

Sca-2 is expressed on intrathymic lymphoid precursors, immature thymocytes, B220[+] bone marrow cells and mature B cells, but is absent from mature thymocytes and peripheral T cells [1,2].

Structure

Sca-2 is a small Cys-rich GPI-linked protein containing a single Ly-6 domain [3].

Ligands and associated molecules

Unknown.

Function

Fetal thymic organ cultures repopulated with very early pre-T cells (CD44⁻CD25⁻TCRαβ⁻CD4⁻CD8⁻) and treated with MTS 35 (anti-TSA-1/ Sca-2 mAb) show a skewed development towards TCRαβ⁺CD4⁻CD8⁺ cells, and a decreased number of TCRαβ⁺CD4⁺CD8⁻ cells [4]. This suggests a role for Sca-2 in the positive selection of thymocytes or lineage commitment towards the CD4⁺ or CD8⁺ pathways.

Comments

The deduced amino acid sequences of Sca-2 and TSA-1 are identical, except at position −7 within the N-terminal leader sequence where a Gly residue has been reported for Sca-2 and an Arg residue has been reported for TSA-1 [3,4]. The mouse *Tsa-1 (Sca-2)* locus is linked to *Ly6* on chromosome 15 [4].

Database accession numbers

	PIR	SWISSPROT	EMBL/GENBANK	REFERENCE
Mouse	I48910		U04268	3
Chicken			L34554	

Amino acid sequence of mouse Sca-2

```
MSATSNMRVF LPVLLAALLG MEQVHS                            -1
LMCFSCTDQK NNINCLWPVS CQEKDHYCIT LSAAAGFGNV NLGYTLNKGC   50
SPICPSENVN LNLGVASVNS YCCQSSFCNF SA                      82
AGLGLRASIP LLGLGLLLSL LALLQLSP                          +28
```

References
[1] Wu, L. et al. (1991) J. Exp. Med. 174, 1617–1627.
[2] Spangrude, G.J. et al. (1988) J. Immunol. 141, 3697–3707.
[3] **Classon, B.J. and Coverdale, L. (1994) Proc. Natl Acad. Sci. USA 91, 5296–5300.**
[4] MacNeil, I. et al. (1993) J. Immunol. 151, 6913–6923.

Scavenger RI and II

SR-A1 and SR-AII

Molecular weights

Polypeptide	type I	49 762
	type II	39 583

SDS-PAGE
reduced	77 kDa
unreduced	220 kDa

Carbohydrate

N-linked sites	7
O-linked	unknown

SCAVENGER RECEPTOR I   SCAVENGER RECEPTOR II

collagen like

alpha
helical
coiled
coil

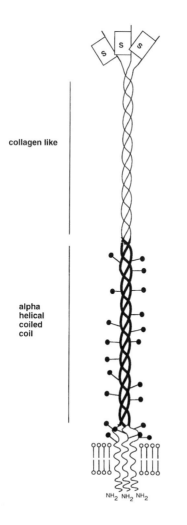
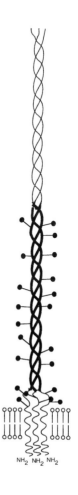

Human gene location
8 [1]

Scavenger Receptor I

Domains

| | | | | | GRV | VTC |

```
        ┌──┬──┬──────────────┬──┬─────────┐
        │CY│TM│              │  │   Sc    │
        └──┴──┴──────────────┴──┴─────────┘
```

Tissue distribution

The major sites of scavenger receptors I and II expression are tissue macrophages [1-3]. Inflammatory stimuli upregulate expression [1]. Scavenger receptor has been identified in atherosclerotic lesions of human tissues [1,2].

Structure

Both receptors are type II glycoproteins and are present as trimers at the cell surface [1]. It is not known if naturally occurring receptors are homotrimers or heterotrimers of type I and II proteins. The bovine sequence was determined first and is 70% identical to the human sequence [1,4]. The mature type I receptor has a 50 amino acid N-terminal cytoplasmic sequence, a 26 amino acid transmembrane sequence, a 75 amino acid sequence with no homology to other proteins, a 121 amino acid sequence predicted to have an α helical coiled-coil structure, a 69 amino acid collagen-like domain, and a C-terminal scavenger receptor cysteine-rich domain. The type II receptor is identical to the type I receptor to the end of the collagen-like sequence, but the C-terminal scavenger receptor domain is replaced by a 17 amino acid segment [5]. The two scavenger receptors are generated by alternative mRNA splicing [1]. The type I receptor has an overall structure similar to MARCO, both having a C-terminal domain scavenger receptor cysteine-rich domain [2,4]. Scavenger receptor has a shorter collagenous region than MARCO [2].

Ligands and associated molecules

Scavenger receptors I and II bind modified low-density lipoproteins [1,2]. Both receptors have a similar broad specificity for polyanionic ligands including cell surface components of gram-positive and gram-negative bacteria [1,2]. There is evidence from mutagenesis studies for their ligand binding properties being located in the collagenous region [1]. Scavenger receptors I and II bind β-amyloid fibrils [6].

Function

Roles in clearance of microbes and damaged or apoptotic cells and in recirculation are postulated [1,3].

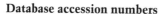

Database accession numbers

	PIR	SWISSPROT	EMBL/GENBANK	REFERENCE
Human type I	A38415	P21757	D90187	7
Human type II	B38415	P21759	D90188	7
Mouse type I	A38860	P30204	M36817, M59445	8
Mouse type II		P30204	M36818, M59446	8

Amino acid sequence of human scavenger receptor I

```
MEQWDHFHNQ QEDTDSCSES VKFDARSMTA LLPPNPKNSP SLQEKLKSFK    50
AALIALYLLV FAVLIPLIGI VAAQLLKWET KNCSVSSTNA NDITQSLTGK   100
GNDSEEEMRF QEVFMEHMSN MEKRIQHILD MEANLMDTEH FQNFSMTTDQ   150
 RFNDILLQLS TLFSSVQGHG NAIDEISKSL ISLNTTLLDL QLNIENLNGK   200
IQENTFKQQE EISKLEERVY NVSAEIMAMK EEQVHLEQEI KGEVKVLNNI   250
TNDLRLKDWE HSQTLRNITL IQGPPGPPGE KGDRGPTGES GPRGFPGPIG   300
PPGLKGDRGA IGFPGSRGLP GYAGRPGNSG PKGQKGEKGS GNTLTPFTKV   350
RLVGGSGPHE GRVEILHSGQ WGTICDDRWE VRVGQVVCRS LGYPGVQAVH   400
KAAHFGQGTG PIWLNEVFCF GRESSIEECK IRQWGTRACS HSEDAGVTCT   450
L                                                        451
```

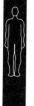

Amino acid sequence of human scavenger receptor II

```
MEQWDHFHNQ QEDTDSCSES VKFDARSMTA LLPPNPKNSP SLQEKLKSFK    50
AALIALYLLV FAVLIPLIGI VAAQLLKWET KNCSVSSTNA NDITQSLTGK   100
GNDSEEEMRF QEVFMEHMSN MEKRIQHILD MEANLMDTEH FQNFSMTTDQ   150
RFNDILLQLS TLFSSVQGHG NAIDEISKSL ISLNTTLLDL QLNIENLNGK   200
IQENTFKQQE EISKLEERVY NVSAEIMAMK EEQVHLEQEI KGEVKVLNNI   250
TNDLRLKDWE HSQTLRNITL IQGPPGPPGE KGDRGPTGES GPRGFPGPIG   300
PPGLKGDRGA IGFPGSRGLP GYAGRPGNSG PKGQKGEKGS GNTLRPVQLT   350
DHIRAGPS                                                 358
```

References

1 Kreiger, M. and Herz, J. (1994) Annu. Rev. Biochem. 63, 601–637.
2 **Pearson, A.M. (1996) Curr. Opin. Immunol. 8, 20–28.**
3 Hughes, D.A. et al. (1995) Eur. J. Immunol. 25, 466–473.
4 Resnick et al. (1994) Trends Biochem. Sci. 19, 5–8.
5 Ashkenas, J. et al. (1993) J. Lipid Res. 983–1000.
6 Khoury, J. El (1996) Nature 382, 716–719.
7 Matsumoto, A. et al. (1990) Proc. Natl Acad. Sci. USA 87, 9133–9137.
8 Freeman, M. et al. (1990) Proc. Natl Acad. Sci. USA 87, 8810–8814.

Sialoadhesin — Sheep erythrocyte receptor

Molecular weights
Polypeptide   181 065

SDS-PAGE
    unreduced   175 kDa
    reduced   185 kDa

Carbohydrate
N-linked sites   15
O-linked   nil

Human gene location
20p13 [1]

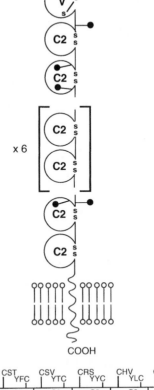

COOH

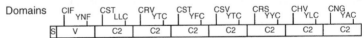

Domains								
CIF YNF	CST LLC	CRV YTC	CST YFC	CSV YTC	CRS YYC	CHV YLC	CNG YAC
S	V	C2	C2	C2	C2	C2	C2	C2

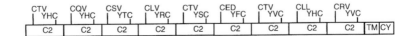

CTV YHC	CQV YHC	CSV YTC	CLV YRC	CTV YSC	CED YFC	CTV YVC	CLL YHC	CRV YVC		
C2	C2	C2	C2	C2	C2	C2	C2	C2	TM	CY

Tissue distribution

Sialoadhesin is expressed on subsets of macrophages in both bone marrow and secondary lymphoid organs [2,3].

Structure

Sialoadhesin is the eponymous member of a structurally related group of IgSF domain-containing sialic acid binding proteins called the sialoadhesin family, which includes CD22, CD33 and myelin-associated glycoprotein (MAG) [4]. Members of this family share ~35% identity between their 2–4 membrane-distal IgSF domains. Like other members of the sialoadhesin family, sialoadhesin is predicted to have an unusual disulfide bond between β strands B and E in domain 1 and a disulfide bond between domains 1 and 2 [4]. Full-length sialoadhesin has 17 IgSF domains in the extracellular region [3].

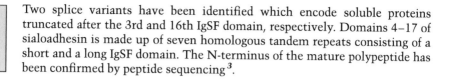

Two splice variants have been identified which encode soluble proteins truncated after the 3rd and 16th IgSF domain, respectively. Domains 4–17 of sialoadhesin is made up of seven homologous tandem repeats consisting of a short and a long IgSF domain. The N-terminus of the mature polypeptide has been confirmed by peptide sequencing[3].

Ligands and associated molecules

Sialoadhesin binds to sialoglycoconjugates NeuAcα2 → 3Galβ1 → 3(4)GlcNAc and NeuAcα2 → 3Galβ1 → 3GalNAc which are present on glycoproteins and glycolipids. The sialic acid binding site has been localized to the GFCC'C'' β sheet of the membrane-distal IgSF domain and includes a conserved arginine (residue 97)[5].

Function

Cell-adhesion studies suggest that sialoadhesin can mediate preferential recognition by macrophages of cells of the granulocytic lineage[6]. The biological role of such interactions are unknown but trophic and/or phagocytic functions have been suggested[6]. Sialoadhesin can also mediate adhesion to lymphocytes in spleen section overlay assays[7].

Database accession numbers

	PIR	SWISSPROT	EMBL/GENBANK	REFERENCE
Mouse	S50065		Z36293	3

Amino acid sequence of mouse sialoadhesin

```
MCVLFSLLLL ASVFSLGQT                                          -1
TWGVSSPKNV QGLSGSCLLI PCIFSYPADV PVSNGITAIW YYDYSGKRQV         50
VIHSGDPKLV DKRFRGRAEL MGNMDHKVCN LLLKDLKPED SGTYNFRFEI        100
SDSNRWLDVK GTTVTVTTDP SPPTITIPEE LREGMERNFN CSTPYLCLQE        150
KQVSLQWRGQ DPTHSVTSSF QSLEPTGSYH QTTLHMALSW QDHGRTLLCQ        200
FSLGAHSSRK EVYLQVPHAP KGVEILLSSS GRNILPGDPV TLTCRVNSSY        250
PAVSAVQWAR DGVNLGVTGH VLRLFSAAWN DSGAYTCQAT NDMGSLVSSP        300
LSLHVFMAEV KMNPAGPVLE NETVTLLCST PKEAPQELRY SWYKNHILLE        350
DAHASTLHLP AVTRADTGFY FCEVQNAQGS ERSSPLSVVV RYPPLTPDLT        400
TFLETQAGLV GILHCSVVSE PLATVVLSHG GLTLASNSGE NDFNPRFRIS        450
SAPNSLRLEI RDLQPADSGE YTCLAVNSLG NSTSSLDFYA NVARLLINPS        500
AEVVEGQAVT LSCRSGLSPA PDTRFSWYLN GALLLEGSSS SLLLPAASST        550
DAGSYYCRTQ AGPNTSGPSL PTVLTVFYPP RKPTFTARLD LDTSGVGDGR        600
RGILLCHVDS DPPAQLRLLH KGHVVATSLP SRCGSCSQRT KVSRTSNSLH        650
VEIQKPVLED EGVYLCEASN TLGNSSAAAS FNAKATVLVI TPSNTLREGT        700
EANLTCNGNQ EVAVSPANFS WFRNGVLWTQ GSLETVRLQL LARTDAAVYA        750
CRLLTEDGAQ LSAPVVLSVL YAPDPPKLSA LLDVGQGHMA VFICTVDSYP        800
LAHLSLFRGD HLLATNLEPQ RPSHGRIQAK ATANSLQLEV RELGLVDSGN        850
YHCEATNILG SANSSLFFQV RGAWVRFTIT ELREGQAVVL SCQVPTGVSE        900
GTSYSWYQDG RPLQESTSST LRIAAISLRQ AGAYHCQAQA PDTAIASLAA        950
PVSLHVSYTP RHVTLSALLS TDPERLGHLV CSVQSDPPAQ LQLFHRNRLV       1000
ASTLQGADEL AGSNPRLHVT VLPNELRLQI HFPELEDDGT YTCEASNTLG       1050
QASAAADFDA QAVRVTVWPN ATVQEGQQVN LTCLVWSTHQ DSLSYTWYKG       1100
GQQLLGARSI TLPSVKVLDA TSYRCGVGLP GHAPHLSRPV TLDVLHAPRN       1150
```

```
LRLTYLLETQ GRQLALVLCT VDSRPPAQLT LSHGDQLVAS STEASVPNTL    1200
RLELQDPRPS NEGLYSCSAH SPLGKANTSL ELLLEGVRVK MNPSGSVPEG    1250
EPVTVTCEDP AALSSALYAW FHNGHWLQEG PASSLQFLVT TRAHAGAYFC    1300
QVHDTQGTRS SRPASLQILY APRDAVLSSF RDSRTRLMVV IQCTVDSEPP    1350
AEMVLSHNGK VLAASHERHS SASGIGHIQV ARNALRLQVQ DVTLGDGNTY    1400
VCTAQHTLGS ISTTQRLLTE TDIRVTAEPG LDWPEGTALN LSCLLPGGSG    1450
PTGNSSFTWF WNRHRLHSAP VPTLSFTPVV RAQAGLYHCR ADLPTGATTS    1500
APVMLRVLYP PKTPTLIVFV EPQGGHQGIL DCRVDSEPLA ILTLHRGSQL    1550
VASNQLHDAP TKPHIRVTAP PNALRVDIEE LGPSNQGEYV CTASNTLGSA    1600
SASAYFGTRA LHQLQLFQRL LWVLGFLAGF LCLLLGLVAY HTWRKKSSTK    1650
LNEDENSAEM ATKKNTIQEE VVAAL                              1675
```

References

[1] Mucklow, S. et al. (1995) Genomics 28, 344–346.

[2] Crocker, P.R. et al. (1991) EMBO J. 10, 1661–1669.

[3] Crocker, P.R. et al. (1994) EMBO J. 13, 4490–4503.

[4] **Crocker, P.R. et al. (1996) Biochem. Soc. Trans. 24, 150–156.**

[5] Vinson, M. et al. (1996) J. Biol. Chem. 271, 9267–9272.

[6] Crocker, P.R. et al. (1995) J. Clin. Invest. 95, 635–643.

[7] van den Berg, T.K. et al. (1992) J. Exp. Med. 176, 647–655.

Thrombopoietin receptor

Other names
Mpl (myeloproliferative leukemia)

Molecular weights
Polypeptide   68 555

SDS-PAGE
   reduced   82–84 kDa

Carbohydrate
N-linked   4
O-linked   unknown

Human gene location and size
1p34; 17 kb [1]

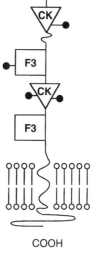

COOH

| Domains | | CFW | | WEE | | CQW | | WQH | | | |
		YVC		NSY		SRC		SRY			
S	CK		F3		CK		F3			TM	CY
	1	2	1	0	1	2	1	0	1	2	0

Exon boundaries   QDV   VGL   AVA   AVR   TAW   SPPK
                  PRE   REAS   DRY   WKVL   YRR

Tissue distribution

Thrombopoietin receptor is restricted to the megakaryocyte lineage and is expressed on megakaryocytes, platelets and weakly on CD34+ primitive stem cells [2].

Structure

Thrombopoietin receptor was originally defined as the cellular counterpart of the myeloproliferative leukemia virus oncogene [3,4]. Thrombopoietin receptor belongs to the cytokine receptor superfamily [5].

Ligands and associated molecules

Thrombopoietin was revealed as a ligand by virtue of its stimulatory activity on a cell line expressing thrombopoietin receptor [6].

Function

Thrombopoietin binding to its receptor stimulates growth and differentiation of megakaryocytes progenitors [6]. Mice lacking thrombopoietin receptor are deficient in megakaryocytes and their precursors [6]. Mutations of thrombopoietin receptor such as the introduction of cysteines into the predicted dimer interface result in an activated, ligand-independent phenotype with functional consequences similar to those observed in the myeloproliferative disease induced by mplv in mice [7]. Binding of thrombopoietin to thrombopoietin receptor activates the JAK–STAT signal transduction pathway [8].

Database accession numbers

	PIR	SWISSPROT	EMBL/GENBANK	REFERENCE
Human	A45266	P40238	M90102	3
Mouse	S35317	G08351	Z22649	4

Amino acid sequence of human thrombopoietin receptor

```
MPSWALFMVT SCLLLAPQNL AQVSS                                   -1
QDVSLLASDS EPLKCFSRTF EDLTCFWDEE EAAPSGTYQL LYAYPREKPR        50
ACPLSSQSMP HFGTRYVCQF PDQEEVRLFF PLHLWVKNVF LNQTRTQRVL       100
FVDSVGLPAP PSIIKAMGGS QPGELQISWE EPAPEISDFL RYELRYGPRD       150
PKNSTGPTVI QLIATETCCP ALQRPHSASA LDQSPCAQPT MPWQDGPKQT       200
SPSREASALT AEGGSCLISG LQPGNSYWLQ LRSEPDGISL GGSWGSWSLP       250
VTVDLPGDAV ALGLQCFTLD LKNVTCQWQQ QDHASSQGFF YHSRARCCPR       300
DRYPIWENCE EEEKTNPGLQ TPQFSRCHFK SRNDSIIHIL VEVTTAPGTV       350
HSYLGSPFWI HQAVRLPTPN LHWREISSGH LELEWQHPSS WAAQETCYQL       400
RYTGEGHQDW KVLEPPLGAR GGTLELRPRS RYRLQLRARL NGPTYQGPWS       450
SWSDPTRVET ATETAWISLV TALHLVLGLS AVLGLLLLRW QFPAHYRRLR       500
HALWPSLPDL HRVLGQYLRD TAALSPPKAT VSDTCEEVEP SLLEILPKSS       550
ERTPLPLCSS QAQMDYRRLQ PSCLGTMPLS VCPPMAESGS CCTTHIANHS       600
YLPLSYWQQP                                                   610
```

References
1 Mignotte, V. et al. (1994) Genomics 20, 5–12.
2 Debili, N. et al. (1995) Blood 85, 391–401.
3 Vigon, I. et al. (1992) Proc. Natl Acad. Sci. 89, 5640–5644.
4 Skoda, R.C. et al. (1993) EMBO J. 12, 2645–2653.
5 Sprang, S.R. and Bazan, J.F. (1993) Curr. Opin. Struct. Biol. 3, 815–827.
6 **Alexander, W.S. et al. (1996) Blood 87, 2162–2170.**
7 Alexander, W.S. et al. (1995) EMBO J. 14, 5569–5578.
8 Pallard, C. et al. (1995) EMBO J. 14, 2847–2856.

WC1 WC1 (cattle) antigen

Molecular weights
Polypeptide   154 197

SDS-PAGE
  reduced   220 kDa
  unreduced   220 kDa

Carbohydrate
N-linked sites   17
O-linked sites   unknown

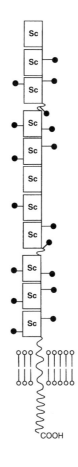

Domains

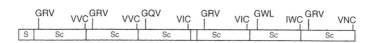

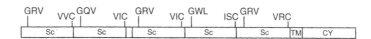

Tissue distribution

The WC1 antigens are expressed exclusively on CD4⁻/CD8⁻ γδ T lymphocytes (>90% of circulating γδ T cells) in cattle[1], sheep (the T19 antigen)[2], and pig[3]. WC1⁺ cells are found in the thymus, lymph nodes, spleen, in the dermis of the skin and the lamina propria of the gastrointestinal tract[1]. The T19 antigen in the sheep has a similar distribution[2]. Multiple WC1 genes (estimated to be in the order of 10 genes within a region of ~1 Mb) are found in cattle[4] which encode heterogenous WC1 antigens with overlapping epitopes. Using mAb specific for each of three WC antigens (WC1.1, WC1.2 and WC1.3) it was found that the WC1.1 and WC1.2 antigens are expressed on non-overlapping subsets of peripheral blood $\gamma\delta$ T cells, whereas the WC1.3[+] subset is contained within the WC1.1[+] subset [4]. The number of T19 genes in sheep is estimated to be between 50 and 100 [5]. WC1 genomic sequences have been identified in human and mouse but, in contrast to ruminants, there appear to be only one or two copies of the gene [4].

Structure

WC1.1 is a type I membrane protein [6]. The extracellular region consists of 11 SRCR domains. Domains 2–6 and domains 7–11 appear to be coded for by a higher order repeating element with a gap between the second and third domains (i.e. between repeats 3 and 4, and between repeats 8 and 9 of WC1.1). A similar type of repeating element is found in CD163 [7]. The two other WC1 cDNA clones that have been isolated (WC1.2 and WC1.3) are highly homologous (~85% identity) to WC1.1 [4].

Function

The function of WC1 is not known. It has been speculated that they may be the CD4/CD8 homologue of $\gamma\delta$ T cells [2,4]. Alternatively, they could be involved in the control of $\gamma\delta$ T cell homing to various tissues [4].

Database accession numbers

	PIR	SWISSPROT	EMBL/GENBANK	REFERENCE
Cattle (WC1.1)	A46496	P30205	X63723	6

Amino acid sequence of cattle WC1.1 antigen

```
MALGRHLSLR GLCVLLLGTM VGG                                -1
QALELRLKDG VHRCEGRVEV KHQGEWGTVD GYRWTLKDAS VVCRQLGCGA    50
AIGFPGGAYF GPGLGPIWLL YTSCEGTEST VSDCEHSNIK DYRNDGYNHG   100
RDAGVVCSGF VRLAGGDGPC SGRVEVHSGE AWIPVSDGNF TLATAQIICA   150
ELGCGKAVSV LGHELFRESS AQVWAEEFRC EGEEPELWVC PRVPCPGGTC   200
HHSGSAQVVC SAYSEVRLMT NGSSQCEGQV EMNISGQWRA LCASHWSLAN   250
ANVICRQLGC GVAISTPGGP HLVEEGDQIL TARFHCSGAE SFLWSCPVTA   300
LGGPDCSHGN TASVICSGNQ IQVLPQCNDS VSQPTGSAAS EDSAPYCSDS   350
RQLRLVDGGG PCAGRVEILD QGSWGTICDD GWDLDDARVV CRQLGCGEAL   400
NATGSAHFGA GSGPIWLDNL NCTGKESHVW RCPSRGWGQH NCRHKQDAGV   450
ICSEFLALRM VSEDQQCAGW LEVFYNGTWG SVCRNPMEDI TVSTICRQLG   500
CGDSGTLNSS VALREGFRPQ WVDRIQCRKT DTSLWQCPSD PWNYNSCSPK   550
EEAYIWCADS RQIRLVDGGG RCSGRVEILD QGSWGTICDD RWDLDDARVV   600
CKQLGCGEAL DATVSSFFGT GSGPIWLDEV NCRGEESQVW RCPSWGWRQH   650
NCNHQEDAGV ICSGFVRLAG GDGPCSGRVE VHSGEAWTPV SDGNFTLPTA   700
QVICAELGCG KAVSVLGHMP FRESDGQVWA EEFRCDGGEP ELWSCPRVPC   750
PGGTCLHSGA AQVVCSVYTE VQLMKNGTSQ CEGQVEMKIS GRWRALCASH   800
WSLANANVVC RQLGCGVAIS TPRGPHLVEG GDQISTAQFH CSGAESFLWS   850
CPVTALGGPD CSHGNTASVI CSGNHTQVLP QCNDFLSQPA GSAASEESSP   900
YCSDSRQLRL VDGGGPCGGR VEILDQGSWG TICDDDWDLD DARVVCRQLG   950
CGEALNATGS AHFGAGSGPI WLDDLNCTGK ESHVWRCPSR GWGRHDCRHK  1000
```

```
EDAGVICSEF LALRMVSEDQ QCAGWLEVFY NGTWGSVCRS PMEDITVSVI    1050
CRQLGCGDSG SLNTSVGLRE GSRPRWVDLI QCRKMDTSLW QCPSGPWKYS    1100
SCSPKEEAYI SCEGRRPKSC PTAAACTDRE KLRLRGGDSE CSGRVEVWHN    1150
GSWGTVCDDS WSLAEAEVVC QQLGCGQALE AVRSAAFGPG NGSIWLDEVQ    1200
CGGRESSLWD CVAEPWGQSD CKHEEDAGVR CSGVRTTLPT TTAGTRTTSN    1250
SLPGIFSLPG VLCLILGSLL FLVLVILVTQ LLRWRAERRA LSSYEDALAE    1300
AVYEELDYLL TQKEGLGSPD QMTDVPDENY DDAEEVPVPG TPSPSQGNEE    1350
EVPPEKEDGV RSSQTGSFLN FSREAANPGE GEESFWLLQG KKGDAGYDDV    1400
ELSALGTSPV TFS                                           1413
```

References

[1] Clevers, H.C. et al. (1990) Eur. J. Immunol. 20, 809–817.

[2] Mackay, C.R. et al. (1989) Eur. J. Immunol. 19, 1477–1483.

[3] Carr, M.M. et al. (1994) Immunology 81, 36–40.

[4] **Wijngaard, P.L.J. et al. (1994) J. Immunol. 152, 3476–3482.**

[5] Walker, I. D. et al. (1994) Immunology 83, 517–523.

[6] Wijngaard, P.L.J. et al. (1992) J. Immunol. 149, 3273–3277.

[7] Law, S.K.A. (1993) Eur. J. Immunol. 23. 2320–2325.

Index